a History of
SURGICAL PAEDIATRICS

Editors

ROBERT CARACHI
University of Glasgow, UK

DAN G. YOUNG
University of Glasgow, UK

CENK BUYUKUNAL
University of Istanbul, Turkey

a History of SURGICAL PAEDIATRICS

World Scientific

NEW JERSEY • LONDON • SINGAPORE • BEIJING • SHANGHAI • HONG KONG • TAIPEI • CHENNAI

Published by

World Scientific Publishing Co. Pte. Ltd.
5 Toh Tuck Link, Singapore 596224
USA office: 27 Warren Street, Suite 401-402, Hackensack, NJ 07601
UK office: 57 Shelton Street, Covent Garden, London WC2H 9HE

British Library Cataloguing-in-Publication Data
A catalogue record for this book is available from the British Library.

A HISTORY OF SURGICAL PAEDIATRICS

ISBN-13 978-981-277-226-8
ISBN-10 981-277-226-X

Typeset by Stallion Press
Email: enquiries@stallionpress.com

Printed by Fulsland Offset Printing (S) Pte Ltd, Singapore

FOREWORD

One aim of the International History Club at its inception nearly 25 years ago was to document the history and development of paediatric surgery. It has taken this length of time to realise this dream of publishing a book on the topic and as editors we are proud to have achieved this. It would of course not have been possible to write without the enormous contributions made by our international colleagues in this specialty which has grown so prodigiously in a relatively short period of time. The time is right for such a book to document accurately facts about the pioneers in paediatric surgery by many who can recall the earlier pioneers who have sadly passed away. We are indeed fortunate in having Dan as one of our editors who has such a worldwide network of friends all of whom, even if they wanted to, felt unable to refuse our gentle request to contribute to such a book. Despite some delays, almost all have contributed substantial material and we are grateful to them for the many hours of work amassing their material.

After some discussion between the three editors, we reached an agreement with World Scientific Publishing Co. Pte. Ltd. who agreed to publish "*A History of Surgical Paediatrics*". This was a great undertaking unlike other previously published textbooks, scientific material or papers. The plan was to create a history from as many parts of the world as possible rather than limit to certain local areas where individual contributions have been published in past years. Last summer we contacted friends and colleagues around the world asking for their support and for contributions in this venture. The specialty is rather exceptional in the enlarged "family" approach which has made strong bonds between paediatric surgeons internationally. Their common bond is in seeking to improve the health and welfare of the infants and children and not one controlled by the financial return which may be achieved.

"Paediatric Surgery" or "Surgical Paediatrics" are in fact synonymous terms and we had considerable discussion on which term we would use for the title. We settled on the latter as we are in practice paediatricians who look after the many infants and children with surgical disorders. In many places in the 19th century and well into the 20th century, the medical paediatricians preferred to have a surgeon "on call" for when they considered it appropriate to ask for surgical assistance. Where surgical beds and service were provided, it has been seen and recorded more than a century ago that more patients were referred to surgeons than to the medical paediatric clinics in these hospitals — a fact alluded to in at least two of the chapters, The specialty has developed from general surgeons who have had an interest in children's care and have developed expertise in the handling and management of the infants and children.

The book gives an indication of the development of the historical group in the specialty by the initiator, Jan Molenaar. Contributions for the second section on the development of the specialty in a wide range of countries, and to our pleasure, almost all of those asked have contributed interesting accounts of how the specialty has evolved in the vastly different social systems around the world. Following is a list of individuals whose names have been selected by asking a large number of our international colleagues to give us a list of individuals whom they felt had made major contributions to the development of the specialty. From the replies we have selected the most frequently quoted individuals in Section 3 and either referred to them there or indicated where they had received considerable mention in Section 2. The range of names received sometimes had a local dominance and from others the list given was very much reflected on the international standing. We felt it reasonable to limit the list to the 32 names although a great many others were mentioned. The one exception was the addition of Wilms.

We record our gratitude for the overwhelming support from all the contributors. The initial request was for an account of up to 3000 words for the countries or about 300 words on the individuals, but there is a wide variety in the responses. Limits have not been enforced, no doubt reflecting on the authors' respect of the request balanced against their view of the importance of recording of the innumerable facts they could have included. The exercise did help people get 'in touch' with colleagues' who were in retirement and reminisce about earlier days in the specialty and of colleagues, contributions and idiosyncrasies. Age has been no barrier; at least one 94-year old has recalled details that had not been documented previously.

Brief accounts of Associations and details of the current journals are followed by a selected group of contributions. They include two historical papers, a review of fetal surgery, a view on the minimally invasive surgery and one on modern imaging for our patients.

One of the Editors would like to acknowledge Professor V. G. Griffiths, whose interest in the history of surgery served as a beacon in those formative years at medical school.

Without the organisation and control of Kay Byrne of the Department of Surgical Paediatrics in Glasgow the finalised articles from so many different parts could not have been achieved. We wish to record our thanks to her for all her painstaking and careful work and in her contacts with the contributors, publishers and ourselves.

We hope you enjoy reading it as much as we enjoyed researching it.

Robert Carachi
Dan G. Young
Cenk Buyukunal

CONTENTS

---

* Indicates biography is within their country text.

SECTION D

CONTRIBUTORS

Al-Ejeilat, HJ, P.O Box 830280, Amman — 11183, Jordan.

Amjad, B. Royal Hospital for Sick Children, Yorkhill, Glasgow G3 8SJ, Scotland, UK.

Aronson, DC. Pediatric Surgical Center of Amsterdam, Emma Children's Hospital AMC, Academic Medical Center, P.O. Box 22700, 1100 DE Amsterdam, The Netherlands.

Audry, G, Hospital D'Enfants Armand Trousseau, Service De Chirurgie Viscerale Infantile, 26 Avenue Du Docteur Arnold Netter, 75571, Paris, Cedex 12, Paris, France.

Baglaj, M. M. Currie — Skolowskiej 50, 50–369 Wroclaw, Poland.

Beasley, SW. Christchurch Hospital, Private Bag 4710, Christchurch, New Zealand.

Bisset, WH. Deceased.

Boix-Ochoa, J. — see Grosfeld.

Boston, V. 69a Thornyhill Road, Killinchy, Co. Down, N. Ireland BT23 6SG.

Bradnam, M. Royal Hospital for Sick Children, Yorkhill, Glasgow, Scotland, UK.

Büyükünal, SNC. Cerrahpaşa Medical Faculty, University of Istanbul, Istanbul, Turkey.

Campbell, J. Department of Pediatric Surgery, 745 SW Gaines Road, CDW-7 Portland, Oregon 97239-2901, USA.

Carachi, R. University of Glasgow, Royal Hospital for Sick Children, Yorkhill, Glasgow G3 8SJ, Scotland, UK.

Coran, AG. C.S. Mott Children's Hospital, F3970 Pediatric Surgery, 1500 E. Medical Center Drive, Ann Arbor, MI 48109-0245, USA.

Coupris, L. Medical Faculty of Angers University, Teaching Hospital, Angers, France.

Cozzi, F. University of Rome, Policlinico Umberto I, University of Rome “La Sapienza”, Italy.

Czernik, J. M. M. Currie — Skolowskiej 50, 50–369 Wroclaw, Poland.

Daum, R. Heidelberg, Germany.

Deshmukh, SS. University in Bombay, Mumbai, India.

Ein, A. Canadian Association of Paediatric Surgeons, Canada.

Ein, S. University of Toronto, Division of General Surgery, Hospital for Sick Children, Toronto, Ontario, Canada, M5G 1X8.

Elhalaby, EA. Faculty of Medicine, Tanta University, Egypt, 5 Elhayaa St, Tanta, 31111, Egypt.

Frediani, S. Policlinico Umberto I, University of Rome “La Sapienza”, Italy.

Fitzgerald, R. Royal College of Surgeons of Ireland, St. Stephen’s Green, Dublin, 2, Ireland.

Fonkalsrud, EW. University of California, Los Angeles School of Medicine, 428 24th St., Santa Monica, California 90402, USA.

Gdanietz, K. Kinderchirurgische Klinik im Klinikum Berlin Buch, Germany private: Gudvangerstr. 21, 10439 Berlin, Germany.

Gentil Martins, A. Hospital de D. Estefânia Lisboa, Instituto Português de Oncologia Francisco Gentil Lisboa, Faculdade de Ciências Médicas da Universidade Nova de Lisboa, Portugal.

Genton, N. — see Lutz.

Grosfeld, JL. MD. Riley Children’s Hospital, 702 Barnhill Drive-Suite 2500, Indianapolis, IN 46202 USA.

Guiney, EJ. Royal College of Surgeons of Ireland, St. Stephen’s Green, Dublin, 2, Ireland.

Hadidi, A. Mannheim-Heidelberg University, Germany Max-Planck Str. 2, 63500-Seligenstadt, Germany.

Hagoort, K. Erasmus University Hospital, Sophia Children’s Hospital, Rotterdam, The Netherlands.

Hajivassiliou, CA. Royal Hospital for Sick Children, Yorkhill, Glasgow G3 8SJ, Scotland, UK.

Harrison, MR. Fetal Treatment Center, University of California, San Francisco, 513 Parnassus Avenue, HSW-1601, San Francisco, CA 94143-0570, USA.

Hashish, AA. Faculty of Medicine, Tanta University, Egypt, Borg Elmehata, Midan elmehata, Tanta, 31111, Egypt.

Holschneider, A. University of Cologne, Germany former Surgeon in Chief, Kinderkrankenhaus Amsterdamerstrasse, Cologne, Germany.

Hutson, J. Royal Children's Hospital, Flemington Road, Parkville VIC 3052, Australia.

Irwin, G. Royal Hospital for Sick Children, Yorkhill, Glasgow, Scotland, UK.

Jacobsen, AS. Department of Pediatric Surgery, K.K. Women's & Children's Hospital, Singapore.

Jaouni, WK. Al Wasl Maternity & Paediatric Hospital, Dubai, United Arab Emirates.

Kapila, L. 56 Main Street, Willoughby on the Wold, Leicestershire LE12 6SZ, UK.

Kaneko, M.

Keramidas, D. Mitera Women's and Children's Hospital, 6, Erythrou Stavrou Str, 15123 Maroussi, Greece.

Li, L. Department of Pediatric Surgery, The Capital Institution of Pediatrics, Beijing, China.

Liem, NT. Department of Surgery, National Institute of Pediatrics, Hanoi, Vietnam.

Lutz, N. Department of Paediatric Surgery, Centre Hospitalier Universitaire Vaudois, Lausanne, Switzerland.

Martin-Fiedler, P. Gyn. Gemeinschaftspraxis, Kellerstr, 38–40 Pfaffenhofen, 85276 Germany.

Maksoud, JG. University of São Paulo Medical School, Av. São Guálter, 400 CEP 05455-000, Brazil.

Mares, AJ. Ben Gurion University of the Negev, Be'er-Sheva, Israel.

Marques-Gubern, A. — see Tovar.

Menardi, G. Deceased.

Millar, AJW. Red Cross War Memorial Children's Hospital and University of Cape Town, South Africa.

Miyano, T. Junteno University, School of Medicine, 2-1-1, Hongo, Bunkyo-ku, Tokyo 113 8421, Japan.

Molenaar, JC. Erasmus University Rotterdam, The Netherlands.

Mustafawi, AR. Al Wasl Hospital, Dubai, United Arab Emirates.

Najmaldin, A. Level 08 — Gledhow Wing, St James's University Hospital, Leeds LS9 7TF, UK.

Nakagawara, A.

Nazir, Z. The Aga Khan University, POB 3500, Stadium Road, Karachi, Pakistan.

Nielsen, OH. Dronningens Tværgade 46, 3.-6, 1302 København K, Denmark.

Nissan, S. Hadassah University Mount Scopus Hospital, 6 Haela, Street Moza Illit, Jerusalem 90820, Israel.

O'Neill, J. Vanderbilt Children's Hospital, Suite 4150; 2200 Childrens Way; Nashville, TN 37232; USA.

Olsen, L. University Childrens Hospital, S-751 85, Uppsala, Sweden.

Päivi, S. Children's Hospital, Helsinki University Hospital, P.O. Box 281 00029 Helsinki, Finland.

Pinter, A. Pécs University /Faculty of Medicine, H-7623 József A. str. 7., Péc, Hungary.

Puri, P. Children's Research Centre, Our Lady's Children's Hospital, Crumlin, Dublin 12, Ireland.

Rasheed, K. Addenbrook's Hospital, Cambridge CB2 0QQ, UK.

Ribbink-Goslinga, AMC, Erasmus University Hospital, Sophia Children's Hospital, Rotterdam, The Netherlands.

Rode, H. Red Cross War Memorial Children's Hospital and University of Cape Town, South Africa.

Rokitansky, A. Langobardenstrasse 122, A-1220 Vienna.

Sari, N. Department of History of Medicine and Ethics, Cerrahpaşa Medical Faculty, University of Istanbul, Istanbul, Turkey.

Slim, M. New York Medical College, Munger Pavilion, Room 323, Valhalla, NY 10595, USA.

Smith, ED. 3/42 Severn St. Balwyn North, Victoria 3104, Australia.

Suita, S. 501, 1-7-9 Kusagae, Chuo-ku, Fukuokashi, 810-0045, Japan.

Tam, PKH, The University of Hong Kong, Hong Kong Medical Centre, Queen Mary Hosptial, Pokfulam Road, Hong Kong.

Tovar, JA. Hospital Universitario La Paz, P. Castellana 261, 28046, Madrid.

Udassin, R. Hadassah University Hospital, Jerusalem.

Ure, BM. Medizinische Hochschule, Hannover, Carl-Neuberg-Straße 1, 30625 Hannover, Germany.

Young, DG. Royal Hospital for Sick Children, Yorkhill, Glasgow G3 8SJ, Scotland, UK.

Zachariou, Z. University of Berne, Inselspital, Freiburgstr. 8, 3010 Berne, Switzerland.

Zhang, J-Z. China Department of Pediatric Surgery, Beijing Children's Hospital, Beijing, China.

Section A

THE INTERNATIONAL HISTORY CLUB

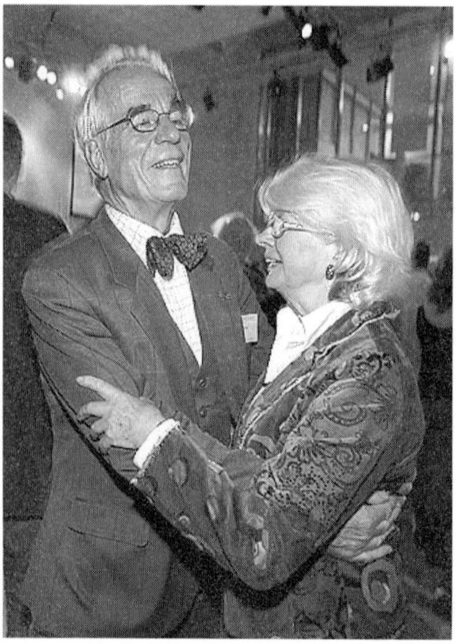

Jan C. Molenaar and his wife

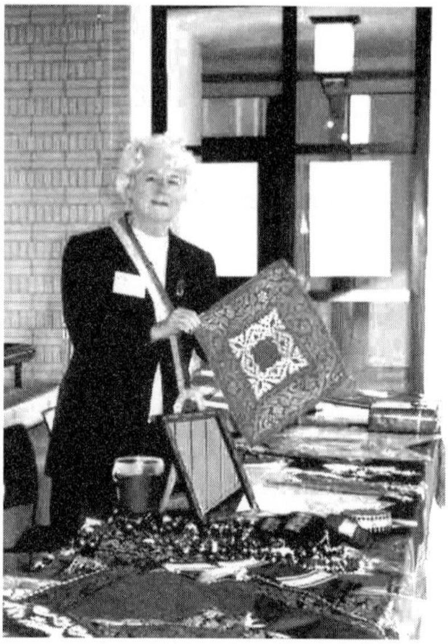

Alice M. C. Ribbink–Goslinga

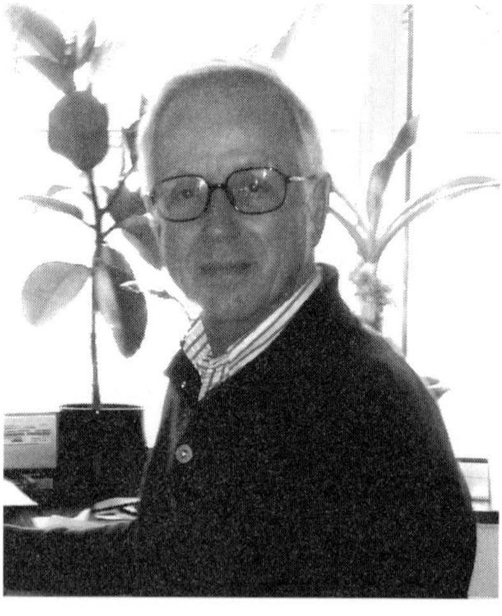

Ko Hagoort

THE BIRTH OF THE INTERNATIONAL SOCIETY FOR THE HISTORY OF PAEDIATRIC SURGERY: A NARRATIVE ACCOUNT

Jan C. Molenaar
Alice M. C. Ribbink–Goslinga
Ko Hagoort

In his Newsletter of April 1983, the Honorary Secretary and Treasurer of the British Association of Paediatric Surgeons, Sēan Corkery announced the upcoming 1983 London Meeting of BAPS. In his unparalleled style of writing he concluded his letter as follows:

"Jan Molenaar has had another rush of blood to the brain. This time he feels the need to see if there are enough interested members of the Association to form a "History Club". He would like all interested members to meet at lunchtime either on Thursday or Friday at the London Meeting, if you are interested please write to me so that we can know what size of room to book. At the moment we have reserved a telephone booth but if that is too spacious we can get something smaller! Appropriate signs will be posted at the Meeting — so watch out for them".

The response to this encouraging announcement was a rewarding one: 45 members of BAPS coming from 26 different countries attended. On Friday, July 22, 1983, the International Paediatric

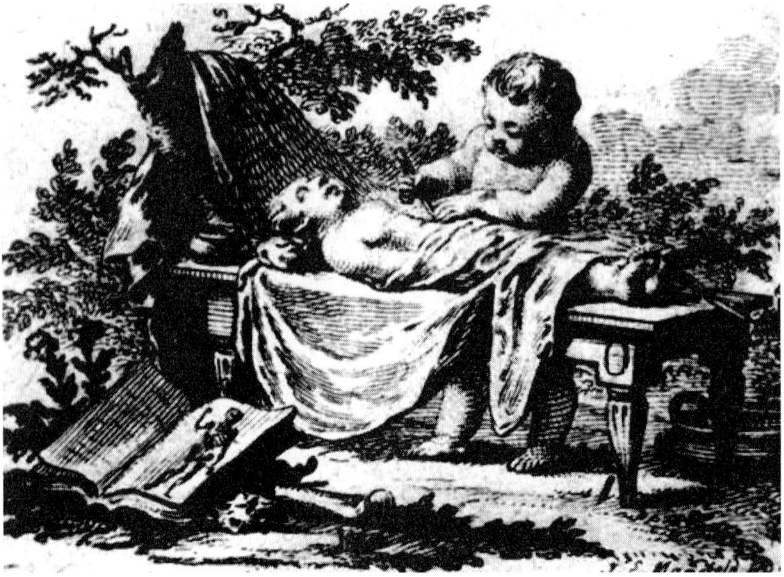

Fig. 1. Figure taken from book "*Primae Linea Anatomes*" (Vienna, 1775) by J. J. Plenck and made by the artist Johann Ernst Mansfeld.

Surgical History Club came into being. Membership was opened to everybody with an interest in the history of paediatric surgery and willing to contribute to the furtherance of this field. The aims of the club were defined as follows:

- to record for posterity how paediatric surgery came into being;
- to create a centralized bibliography concerning the development of paediatric surgery;
- to stimulate the writing of articles and the presentation of papers dealing with every single aspect of paediatric surgical history; and
- to accomplish our final aim: the publication of a comprehensive book on the history of paediatric surgery.

During a second probing session at lunchtime on Friday, July 27, 1984 at the next BAPS meeting in Liverpool, it was decided that our first scientific session would be held in conjunction with the upcoming 1986 BAPS meeting in Birmingham.

However earlier, in 1985 at the close of the Annual International Congress of the BAPS in Vienna, the hosts of BAPS, Dr Peter Wurnig and Mrs Wurnig, invited the President of BAPS and members of the History Club to attend a guided tour through the venerable Mautner Markhof Childrens's Hospital, founded in 1875. At that BAPS meeting it was decided, at the request of the History Club, that the History Club's biennial scientific meetings would be held on the Tuesday afternoon prior to the official start of the BAPS meeting on Wednesday. At the time, the membership totalled 115, with the largest contingent from the USA, followed by the UK and the remainder were spread out all over the world.

The Birmingham meeting in 1986 appeared to be a remarkable success. Subsequently, the membership rose to a total of 122 members spread over some 30 countries. Mr Peter Jones from Melbourne, who was in the audience, made the following account:

> "One of the most enjoyable and memorable events held in conjunction with the BAPS Meeting in Birmingham in 1986 was the meeting of the International Society for the History of Paediatric Surgery (ISHPS) on the day before the Scientific Programme began. Under the Chairmanship of Professor Jan Molenaar, the meeting was attended by some 50 paediatric surgeons form various countries, all of whom had a particular interest in the historical, cultural and social aspects of the specialty of paediatric surgery. The programme was as varied as its audience, and covered such subjects as the depiction of children in European paintings and various other works of art, and a most interesting account of the life, family and work of Ram(m)stedt, and his lasting contribution, serendipitously devised, to the treatment of pyloric stenosis".

The programme of this first meeting was as follows:

1) Why Paediatric Surgical History? J. C. Molenaar
2) The Contribution of Surgeons to Child Care through the Centuries. Mrs A. M. C. Ribbink–Goslinga
3) Dr Conrad Ramstedt, Paediatric Surgical Pioneer. G. Borgwardt

4) Children, Diseases and Doctors in Historical Pictures. P. J. Kuijjer
5) Paediatric Surgery in Birmingham and environs. P. Gornall

Mr Peter Jones continues: "Although it is perhaps invidious to select from among the excellent presentations, and the careful preparations demonstrated by every one of the speakers, Dr Görtz Borgwardt's tenacious search for Ramstedt's birthplace and the discovery of many of his relics, will be of particular interest and should, if feasible, be published in one of the paediatric surgical journals. Those who were unable to attend the meeting of the ISHPS will be delighted to know that Dr Borgwardt obtained a superb copy of the bust of Ramstedt sculpted by his obviously very talented daughter Tessa. The copy of the bust was later presented to the BAPS by Dr Borgwardt, to become one of the Society's permanent memorabilia.

There can be no doubt that the ISPH should go from strength to strength, and win a place as an adjunct to all BAPS meetings. It is very fitting that we should be better informed of those who have contributed to the ethos, the ethics, the philosophy and the expertise of our specialty. All of us are in a very real sense pygmies, advancing on the shoulders of surgical giants of the past. The more we know of their lives, times and innovations, the better we are able to appreciate their contributions, and the foundations of the specialty of paediatric surgery."

As an interesting note, Dr Borgwardt had serious difficulties in obtaining permission to leave his country, the DDR, and could do so only by special invitation of the History Club. Also in 1986, two interesting publications appeared:

- Vol. 20 of "*Progress in Pediatric Surgery*" was entirely devoted to "*Historical Aspects of Pediatric Surgery*" (Springer Verlag, Berlin, Heidelberg, 1986).
- "*Child Care through the Centuries*". Papers given at the Tenth Congress of the British Society for the History of Medicine, Swansea, April 1984, including a paper of one of our members,

John D. Atwell from Southampton, UK, who lectured on "*The History of Paediatric Surgery*" (STS Publishing, Cardiff).

In 1988 the BAPS was meeting at an unusual date; the end of September. On the afternoon of Tuesday, 20 September 1988, the ISHPS had its second meeting under the watchful eye of Pallas Athene at the Astir Palace Hotel in Athens. One of the highlights of this meeting was the lecture by Professor Mark Ravitch from Pittsburgh on the anatomist Fredericus Ruysch of Amsterdam (1638–1731). Earlier that year the logo of our society was coined into a beautiful bronze medal, financed by the Foundation University Fund Rotterdam. At the close of the BAPS meeting, this medal was presented for the first time by the President of BAPS to Drs Çenk Büyükünal and N. Sari from Istanbul, Turkey for their prize-winning presentation: *Sabuncuoglu Şerafedding (XVth Century), an outstanding personality in the Turkish history of paediatric surgery.*

The History Club has proceeded from then on with scientific meetings every two years prior to and in conjunction with the international meetings of BAPS, in close collaboration with Miss Dorothy Grant, staff secretary of BAPS, who has always been of great help from the very beginning.

A very special meeting was held in Istanbul on Tuesday morning July 22, 1997, in the historical setting of the Topkapi Palace. It was here that chairmanship of the History Club changed hands. As the History Club newsletter of June 1997 puts it: "This newsletter, we're afraid, is the last one to be sent from the Sophia Children's Hospital in Rotterdam. As already alluded to earlier, Jan C. Molenaar has now retired from his office, and wishes to hand over the chairmanship of our society as well. Excellent candidates, in his view, would be Prof. Cenk Büyükünal from Istanbul, and Mr Robert Carachi from Glasgow."

In conclusion, a new tradition within the BAPS organization has been established. Not all the aims formulated at the start of the International Society for the History of Paediatric Surgery were accomplished, but the final aim, the publication of a comprehensive book on the history of paediatric surgery, has now been instigated.

Section B

THE DEVELOPMENT OF SURGICAL PAEDIATRICS IN COUNTRIES

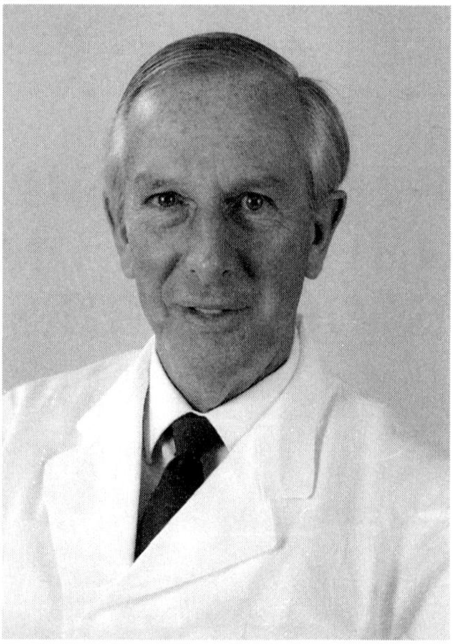

E. Durham Smith

AUSTRALIA

E. Durham Smith

It is one of the strange ironies of surgical history that one of the great contributors to the development of paediatric surgery, certainly in Britain, its colonies and in Europe, was an Australian who never practiced surgery for a single day in Australia. **Denis Browne*** graduated from Sydney University in 1915, immediately left to serve in the Australian Army overseas, and did not return to Australia for 50 years, by which time he had retired. His entire career was in Britain, but his Australian origins are of interest in determining the character and personality that had a dominating influence on the early development of the specialty.[1]

Prior to World War II (WWII)

Prior to World War II, Browne was not the only contributor to paediatric surgery in Australia, although at least to the end of World War I, children's surgery was mostly performed by practitioners who remained in family practice or in adult general surgery. Their contributions need to be seen in the context of the history of Australia.

European settlement began in Australia in 1788, when the first fleet of British ships established a penal colony in Port Jackson, Sydney, on the east coast. Indigenous Australian Aborigines, however, had occupied the land for at least 40,000 years. From their intimate knowledge of and respect for the land and its resources they had many empirical remedies from seeds and plants, but little is known of any of their surgical procedures. Of the many tribal groups some did employ a "sub-incision" in males as an initiation rite — virtually producing a hypospadias penis — perhaps to serve a contraceptive purpose, but there is no record of female genital interference. After European settlement, paediatric care was very limited in the 19th century. Surgeons attached to the military garrisons cared for the children of the soldiers, but no public facilities were available until children's hospitals were established, the first in Melbourne in 1870, and later in other cities. Surgical staff was appointed to these hospitals on a part-time and honorary basis, and always combined with adult practice as it was not considered financially viable to practice exclusively in paediatrics or paediatric surgery. Nevertheless there were some outstanding individuals in all Australian States from the end of the 19th century and not a few landmark contributions. In the State of Queensland, John Lockhart Gibson was an Honorary Medical Officer to the Hospital for Sick Children, Brisbane from 1884–1921, mainly as an ENT surgeon, and together with A. J. Turner identified the syndrome due to lead poisoning from the ingestion of particles of lead paint on domestic surfaces. Dr Lillian Cooper was the first woman to be registered as a surgeon in Australia, and was appointed to the hospital in 1894. Perhaps the most dominant personality in paediatric surgery in Queensland before WW2, and extending into the post-war period was **K. Fraser** (later **Sir Kenneth**), serving the hospital from 1923 for 34 years. He was a brilliant scholar, won University "Blues" in cricket, football and athletics, and became a national champion hurdler and sprinter. He had wide surgical experience but with a particular interest in cleft palate, in which he wrote a monograph in 1939, beautifully illustrated with his own sketches, although his technique was later criticised; in hypospadias, he developed a repair utilising a scrotal flap.[2] He was a powerful voice in medical circles, with a personality to match, serving on the Senate of the Queensland University, and was a principal influence in the formation of the University Department of Paediatrics. He was the founder of the St. John Ambulance Brigade in Queensland (1948) and Foundation Member of the Australian Paediatric Association, of which he was President from 1958 to 1959.

In New South Wales, the same pattern of holding other positions in surgery or general practice continued by surgeons appointed to the Sydney Hospital for Sick Children (later to become the Royal Alexandra Hospital for Children). Robert Wade was associated with the hospital from 1897 and Honorary Surgeon from 1912 to 1932. He specialised in orthopaedic surgery and became President of the Royal Australasian College of Surgeons (RACS) 1935 to 1937. He was the first surgeon to be associated with paediatric surgery to hold this position. The seminal surgical contribution of the hospital, however, was in the management of intussusception. **C. P. B. Clubbe** (later **Sir Charles**) had written a monograph on the diagnosis and treatment of intussusception,[3] and reported the first successful resection of an intussusception in a child in 1897, but it was the work of P. L. Hipsley in the next two decades that established the value of hydrostatic reduction of the mass. Although Hirschsprung of Copenhagen had described the technique in 1876, it was Hipsley who published a successful series of saline reductions in 1926,[4] which confirmed the value of non-operative management under the right conditions.

In the State of South Australia, another President of the Royal Australasian College of Surgeons, Henry S. Newland (later Sir Henry), President of the College (1929–1935) was a Consultant at the Children's Hospital from 1903 to 1928. **Douglas Mackay**, another staff surgeon appointed pre-war, continued a family practice combined with paediatric surgery. He was a co-author of an important paper with Robert Fowler and John Barnett of Melbourne on the aetiology and treatment of congenital hydrocele.[5]

In the State of Victoria, the Children's Hospital (later Royal, in 1953) commenced in 1870. Until 1902 little distinction was made between physicians and surgeons in appointments to the honorary staff, with one notable exception. **Robert Hamilton Russell** (1860–1933) (Fig. 1), born in England, had been house surgeon to Joseph Lister. He migrated to Australia in 1890. After a brief period in general practice he was appointed to the hospital in 1892 and served as an Honorary until 1902 when the (adult) Alfred Hospital persuaded him to join their staff. Nevertheless, after retirement

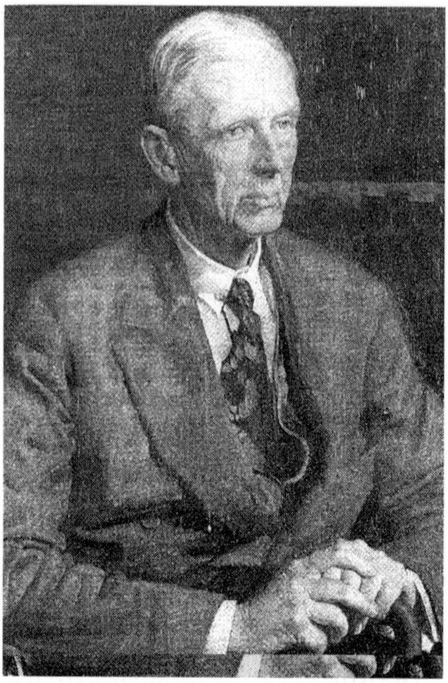

Fig. 1. Portrait of R. Hamilton Russell.

from the Alfred Hospital, his love of children drew him back and he returned to the active staff of the RCH in 1920 for 5 more years. Sadly, he was killed in a motor car accident in 1933. He was also a gifted pianist and his specific contributions to paediatric surgery covered a wide spectrum, but he was best known for his insistence that almost all, if not all, inguinal hernias in infancy and childhood were due to the persistence of a patent *processus vaginalis*, and that surgery only required the removal of the sac. It was a revolutionary concept in 1899 when he published it[6] and it was against the prevailing wisdom of the day, which was using procedures which carried a significant mortality and morbidity. His second contribution was in hypospadias. In 1900 Russell described a 'stole' operation, a pedicle tube of penile and preputial skin,[7] and in 1915, after excising a urethral stricture (not in hypospadias), he found that if the urethral ends or part of their circumference were joined together as a flat strip of mucosa and buried, the urethra re-formed.[8] Denis Browne always attributed his "buried strip" idea to Hamilton **Russell**, although

Duplay had actually described the concept in 1800. Russell is also well known for his method of simple 3-point traction for femoral fractures without a Thomas splint or plaster. He advocated prolonged rest and conservative support in a Thomas splint for tubercular hip and spine disease, against the destructive effects of surgical excision current at the time. He wrote about intussusception in 1902, stressing the "gentleness and care" of the gut in operative reduction; and in cleft palate repair he stressed that the operation should concentrate on the principles by which speech is produced and assured.

Charles C. Ryan, who was on the staff of RCH from 1882 to 1914, was one of the first surgeons to operate successfully on intussusception in 1899, just after Clubbe's success in 1897. Perhaps the best "all-rounder" was **Henry Douglas Stephens**, father of F. Douglas Stephens (see infra), who served the hospital for 50 years. In 1904 he entered private practice, largely as a paediatrician in association with a senior paediatrician, Hobill Cole, whose daughter he married. He acquired both MD and MS very quickly. At this time he also became the Honorary Pathologist to the RCH in 1914, stimulating his interest in congenital anomalies. By this time he had also acquired a good reputation as a skillful operative surgeon in a wide range of surgical conditions; he was confirmed as a Consultant Surgeon from 1909 to 1939, although even then, he was recalled to carry the burden due to WW2 due to the absence of younger surgeons in the Services. He held prestigious appointments in the hospital and in the profession generally. He was not only an experienced surgeon, but had an eager enthusiasm, an avidity for knowledge, and a flexibility of mind which together undoubtedly was the greatest inspiration to his son, Douglas. John Colquhoun (1930–1960) and E. E. Price (1936–1962) in orthopaedics, John G. Whitaker (1934–1955) and W. R. Forster (1944–1948) in general surgery, also served through the war years and beyond.

During the 1920's and 1930's in Australia, it was not easy to establish a surgical practice, and a number of surgeons who later became very successful and prominent surgeons had accepted appointments in Children's Hospitals only until they secured an appointment in an adult Teaching Hospital. The "pure" Paediatric Surgeon, committed entirely to the surgery of children, did not emerge until after WW2.

Ample records exist as to the spectrum of surgical conditions encountered. Prior to 1900, the list was dominated by infection, particularly tubercular glands, bone and joints, syphilis, abscesses, osteomyelitis and septicaemia. Injuries and burns were frequent, calculi, spinal deformity, congenital dislocation of the hip, Perthé's disease, talipes, poliomyelitis, cleft lip and palate, hypospadias, hernias, and intussusception. From 1900 onwards, these conditions continued and we hear more about pyloric stenosis (the first operation for this condition at the Melbourne RCH was in 1903, treated by a gastro-enterostomy, as the Ramstedt procedure was not developed until 1912), appendicitis, neck lesions, anal lesions, Wilms' tumour and tonsillectomy. Very little changed until the advent of better anaesthesia, understanding of fluid and electrolytes balance and the development of antibiotics, all of which were occurred during and after WW2.

During and After WWII

During the war years, older surgeons carried the load in children's hospitals. Despite the difficulties, two events are worth recording. In 1941, Norman Gregg (later Sir Norman), an ophthalmologist in Sydney, discovered the link between maternal rubella and the congenital anomalies of cataract, deafness, mental retardation and cardiac defects.[9] In March 1944, a patient, AG, was admitted to the Melbourne Children's Hospital, dying of osteomyelitis and septicaemia. The Superintendent, Dr Elizabeth Turner, obtained some penicillin from the Royal Melbourne Hospital, then occupied by the American Army, and empiric doses were injected. AG recovered completely, without any complications. The penicillin era had arrived, and with the subsequent development of other antibiotics, to revolutionise medicine and surgery.

The first generation 1945–1975. Post-war, surgeons returned from the Services and were appointed to their Children's Hospital posts.

Many had been Residents pre-war, and a few had already achieved a surgical appointment before enlisting, but not all saw a future in paediatric surgery. The change to a commitment to 'pure' paediatric surgery varied across the country. A confluence of far-seeing decisions and a significant personality determined that Melbourne became the earliest starter in the field, which set the pattern for other areas. Under the Presidency of Lady Ella Latham (1933–1954), the wife of a future Chief Justice of Australia, she had a vision that the hospital had to change from one "for the sick poor" to a centre for research, training and high standards. The Honorary system did not suit these objectives. At the same time, 1952, an equally remarkable Medical Director, Dr Vernon Collins, urged the appointment of full-time Directors of Departments, both in Research and in specialties like Neurosurgery and Plastic Surgery, and he instituted a system of sessional payment for visiting consultants and assistants. Immediately there was financial support for young surgeons to commit to paediatric surgery, and the numbers "took off".

The significant personality mentioned above was **Russell Norfolk Howard** (Fig. 2). After distinguishing himself with honours in all subjects at medical graduation from Melbourne University in 1928,

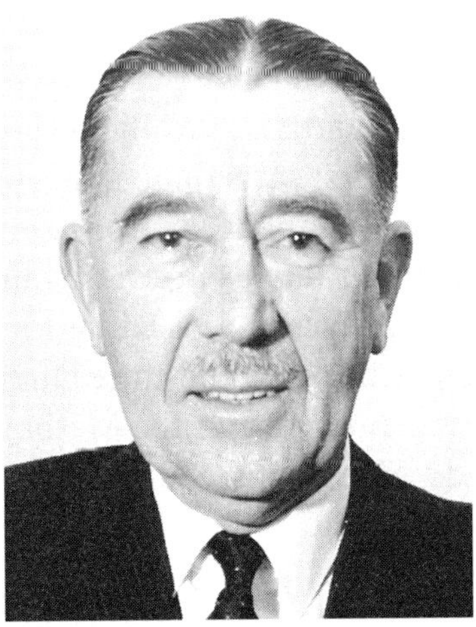

Fig. 2. Russell Howard.

he spent four years at the Children's Hospital as Resident, Registrar and Medical Superintendent, and a further residency at the Royal Women's Hospital. Surgical experience followed at St. James Hospital, Balham, in London and he completed degrees of MD, MRCOG, FRCS and FRACS. He served in the Australian Army in the Middle East and Southwest Pacific as a Lt. Col. in charge of a Surgical Division. Prior to the war, he had already been appointed as an Honorary Surgeon at both the Children's Hospital and at the Alfred Hospital, a senior Teaching Hospital of the University. After the war, he returned to both hospitals and quickly gained an enviable reputation as a dexterous and able operative surgeon, and a superb teacher. After seven years in both the disciplines of paediatric and adult surgery, a defining decision was made. He accepted an appointment as Chief General Paediatric Surgeon at the Children's Hospital in 1952 and gave up adult surgery. Here was a man who had the universal respect of his colleagues in adult surgery, and yet he chose paediatric surgery.

The significance was that it immediately gave paediatric surgery legitimacy, status and respect, unlike in most other areas of the country, and indeed the world. It was consolidated by the efforts of Howard in his role on the Council of the Royal Australasian College of Surgeons to establish a Fellowship in Paediatric Surgery in 1962. Howard's own surgical contributions were not only in organising a strong surgical department, which he did with an iron will and a fearless defense of standards, and specifically in thoracic surgery and in malignancies. He was the first surgeon in the southern hemisphere to have a successful result in oesophageal atresia in 1949. He performed the first ligation of a patent ductus arteriosus in 1946. He also realized that specialist anaesthesia was essential for the advance of surgery and secured the position of a full-time Director of Anaesthesia.

Russell Howard was not alone at the Melbourne Children's; one of the decisions made by the hospital in 1952 was to appoint two other staff surgeons to the hospital — Murray Clarke and Douglas Stephens. **A. Murray Clarke** had been a Resident before the war, served with distinction in the war, and returned on staff in 1946 until retirement in 1974. His contribution was to establish a Burns Unit in

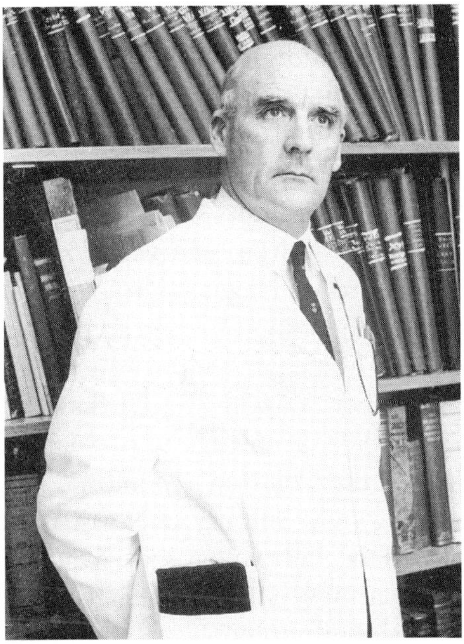

Fig. 3. Douglas Stephens.

1955, one of the first in the world. He, with Howard and Stephens, led one of the three general surgical units of the hospital.

Frank Douglas Stephens (Fig. 3) is one of the greatest contributors to the development of paediatric surgery. Stephens was an innovator, always breaking new ground and opening up new directions by original research. He is the master of patho-embryology. His studies of foetal material, his meticulous dissections and histological sections, literally by the thousands over a lifetime of research, have revolutionised the understanding and treatment of ano-rectal anomalies, and of many genito-urinary abnormalities. He was Director of Surgical Research from 1958 to 1975, but prior to this he had already been heavily engaged in research since his return from war service in 1946.

Douglas was born in Melbourne and graduated from Melbourne University in 1936. After Residencies at the Royal Melbourne Hospital and the Children's Hospital, he served in a Forward

Operating Team and Field Ambulance of the 6th Division of the Australian Army in the Middle East and in the Pacific, from 1940 to 1946. He was awarded a DSO (Distinguished Service Order) in 1942 for conspicuous gallantry under fire, an honour to which he never referred. On return to the hospital in 1946, he was then awarded a Nuffield Traveling Research Fellowship which took him to London to the Hospital for Sick Children for 3 years. Here, he worked with Denis Browne, T. Twistington Higgins (Urologist) and Martin Bodian (Pathologist) and the beginning of a research career. On his return from England in 1950, he began building a team of young research workers, including Robert Fowler and Durham Smith, and led his team for 25 years. In 1975, at the age of 61 years his unique talents were 'head-hunted' by the Children's Memorial Hospital in Chicago as Professor of Urology and Surgery of North West University. His research encompassed the embryology and pathological development of anomalies of the urinary tract, especially ureteric reflux, dysplasias, duplications and ureterocoeles; of the genital tract, including vaginal and cloacal anomalies; and of the vast range of ano-rectal anomalies in which his dissections defined the exact anatomy of each type, and especially the controlling sphincters in relation to each type. His landmark papers in the latter subject were published in 1953.[10–12] He destroyed the concept that a dilated urinary tract meant an obstruction somewhere, but rather can equally result from a motility dysfunction in a tube or from congenital dysplasia, thus saving thousands of children from serious unnecessary invasive procedures current at the time. His originality lay in the marriage of accurate clinical and operative observations with meticulous dissection of foetal material or of operative specimens, leading to postulates of development. He has prodigious energy and enthusiasm and as the time of writing 2007, Douglas is still writing papers at the age of 94 years, on the concept of how pressure on the developing foetus in utero can displace structures and result in abnormalities. His books and publications are now classics, especially on "*Ano-rectal Anomalies*," and "*Congenital Anomalies of Urinary and Genital Tracts*".[13] Space precludes discussion of his private life, but suffice to say he is no recluse. He has a happy family life and loves a party. An excellent

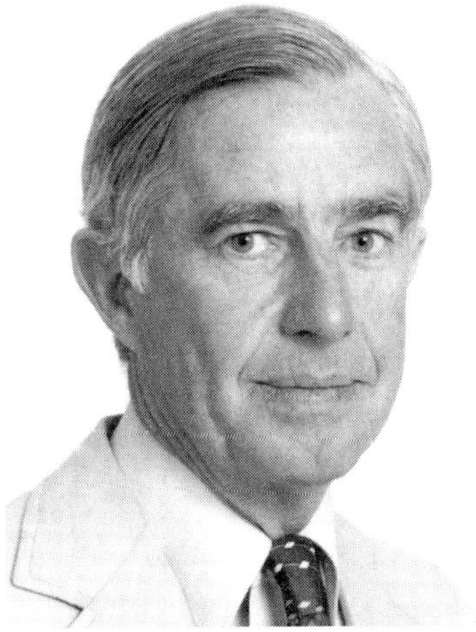

Fig. 4. Geoffrey Wyllie.

water-colour artist, a fly-fisherman, a modest golfer and tennis player, he remains enthusiastic and active well into his nineties.

In Adelaide, South Australia, **Geoffrey Wylie** (Fig. 4) was the outstanding surgeon, and was the first surgeon in South Australia to confine himself to paediatric surgery. He is remembered for advocating the conservative approach for ruptured spleens. He was supported later by Brian Douglas, Joseph Savage and Bruce Davey.

In Perth, Western Australia, the pattern of general surgeons with part-time commitment to children continued until **Alasdair Mackellar** (Fig. 5) was appointed to the Princess Margaret Hospital for Children in 1960. He had migrated from Scotland, first to New Zealand, then to Melbourne for further training, until he was invited to the Perth appointment. He established a Paediatric Surgical Department, an Intensive Care Unit, a burns unit, and development of neonatal studies and data collection systems. He was a leading advocate for injury prevention in children, and instrumental in setting up the Child Accident Prevention Foundation of Australasia. He died in 2007, thus defeating his determination to have a further visit to Europe and attend the BAPS Seniors meeting in Edinburgh as he died early in the year. Ian Penn, Gordon Baron–Hay and the

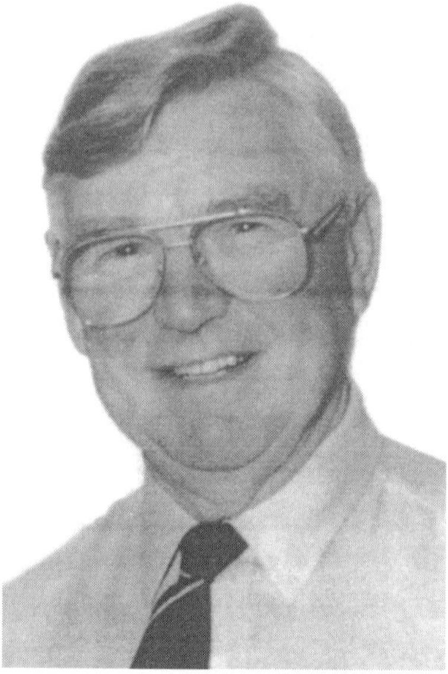

Fig. 5. Alisdair MacKellar.

late Philip King all worked with him in Perth but are now replaced by a new generation.

In Brisbane, Queensland, Des McGuckin was the first full-time paediatric surgeon in 1962, not productive of papers but a superb operator whose results excelled; J. **Fred Leditschke** (Fig. 6) trained in Adelaide and Toronto and accepted the first professorial appointment in the University Department in 1967. He has made impressive contributions to academic surgery and in burn management. Peter Grant, Tony Milne and Stuart Pegg, as general surgeons at the Brisbane Royal Children's Hospital, the latter especially in burns treatment, and Leonard Marriott, served at the Mater Children's Hospital from 1962 to 1985.

In Sydney, New South Wales, with the retirement of those surgeons who had served children's surgery well — T. Y. Nelson, J. Steingrad, E. Goulston and E. Stuckey — the next generation became committed to surgical paediatrics exclusively, except in some of the specialties, who retained appointments in adult hospitals.

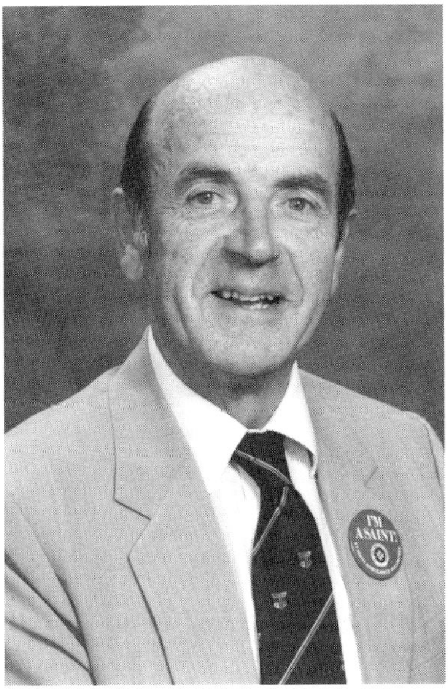

Fig. 6. Fred Leditschke.

David Dey, who had spent time at GOS in London, developed the Plastic Surgery Unit at Royal Alexandra Hospital for Children (RAH), followed later by Don Llewellyn. Denis Arnold in Urology also had dual appointments, until Bruce Filmer became a full-time paediatric urologist. Robert Jones developed Neurosurgery, Bruce Benjamin developed great expertise in Otolaryngology, and Patrick Gratton–Smith in advanced Paediatric Radiology, as did Douglas Rye in Pathology. John Gibson continued in general surgery, and **Arch Middleton** was a consultant at RAH from 1964, after previous experience in general practice and adult surgery. **Douglas Cohen** (Fig. 7), an early leader of the new direction of paediatric surgery in NSW, graduated in medicine in 1942 from Sydney University. After residency at the Royal Prince Alfred Hospital, at the end of 1943 he enlisted in the Australian Army and served in the Southwest Pacific until de-mobilisation in 1946. He then entered General practice and completed surgical training (MS and FRACS). He remained in General practice until 1953, simultaneously beginning an appointment as an

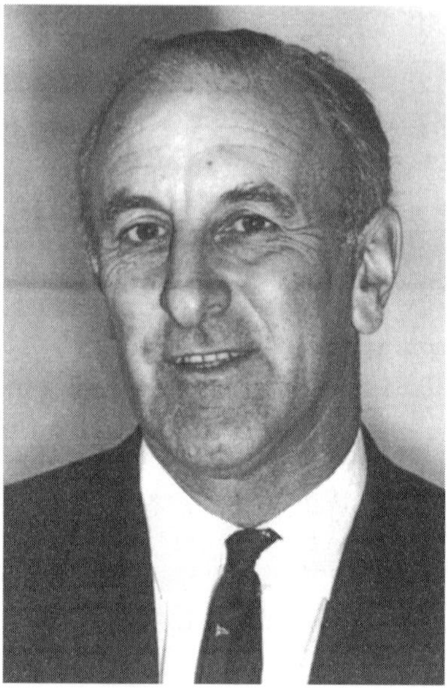

Fig. 7. Douglas Cohen.

assistant paediatric surgeon at RAH in 1951. He had further training at the Hospital for Sick Children, London (1954–1955) with David Waterston in general, cardiac and thoracic surgery. He returned to general adult surgery and surgical paediatrics, but from 1959, he was based exclusively in paediatrics in T. Y. Nelson's Unit at RAH, in both general and cardiac surgery. Together with Victor Hercus and an engineer, Vivian Ebsary, they developed the first heart-lung machine in Sydney in 1959, a machine which was commonly used in other parts of Australia and New Zealand. He remained as Head of Cardiac Surgery until Tim Cartmill was appointed and Douglas became Head of the Department of Surgery at the hospital in 1971. He was a pioneer in the early development of cardiac surgery in eastern Australia, and published papers on oesophageal surgery, tracheopexy, portal hypertension and solid tumours. **A. C. Bowring** (Fig. 8) was another major influence in the Sydney scene. He graduated in 1948 and after residencies in general surgery and at RAH, and a period in England, he was committed to full-time paediatric

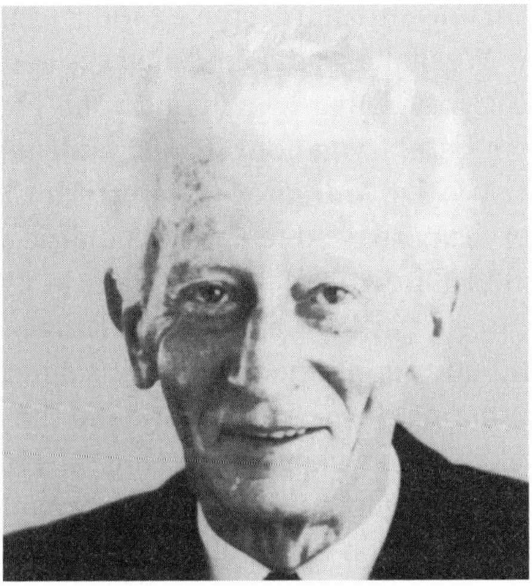

Fig. 8. A. C. (Toby) Bowring.

surgery as the first in New South Wales in 1956. After staff appointments at RAH, he became the first Head of Unit and Associate Professor of Paediatric Surgery at Prince of Wales Hospital, as a second children's hospital for Sydney under the auspices of the University of NSW. He had a special interest in child abuse. Ian Kerr later joined the unit.

Jim Cartledge established a unit in Hobart, Tasmania and rural surgical centres developed a little later, James Wright and Ian Reid in Newcastle, followed by Rodney Laing in Wollongong and Errol Simpson in Canberra.

Meanwhile in Victoria, under the stimulus of Howard and Stephens, paediatric surgery flourished in all fields. Departments were established in all the paediatric specialties between 1945 and 1954, and significant contributions were made by Reginald S. Hooper and later by Geoffrey Klug, in Neurosurgery; Alan Wakefield and George Gunter, and later by John Barnett, Tony Holmes, Bruce Levant, Bruce Johnson and Keith Mutimer in Plastic Surgery; Eric Price, John Colquhoun, **Peter Williams** and **Malcolm Menelaus** in Orthopaedic Surgery (Williams as a significant leader of paediatric orthopaedics in Australia and Menelaus wrote an authoritative book on orthopaedic management of spina bifida), later with Robert Dickens; George Westlake and Peter Clarke, and later by **Roger Mee** in Cardiac Surgery; Clive Pyman and John Floyd, and later by Warner Mooney in Oto-laryngology; **Roger Hall** and Alan Parker in Paediatric Dentristry; **Dr Margaret (Gretta) McClelland**, who had been leading a very experienced team of paediatric anesthetists since 1947 was appointed Director of Anaesthesia in 1956, followed by **John Stocks** as Director in 1970 and **Kestor Brown** in 1974.

Three General units continued, and it was agreed that all would remain 'general', sharing the neonatal work and the common lesions, but each would take on a special interest (Fig. 9). Howard's unit concentrated on thoracic surgery, oesophagus and diaphragm with Nate Myers, Max Kent and Helen Noblett, until the latter was appointed as Consultant at Bristol, UK; Murray's unit managed burns and the special requirements of liver and biliary surgery with Peter Jones and John Solomon; Stephens's unit concentrated on urology and ano-rectal work with Robert Fowler and Durham Smith. **Nate Myers** (Fig. 10) became a world authority on oesophageal atresia;[14] **Helen Noblett** did studies on meconium ileus management by Gastrografin enema,[15] and designed a biopsy instrument for rectal biopsies in

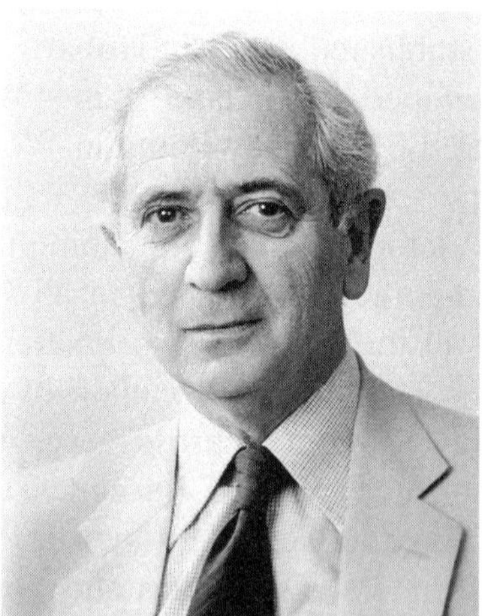

Fig. 9. Nate Myers.

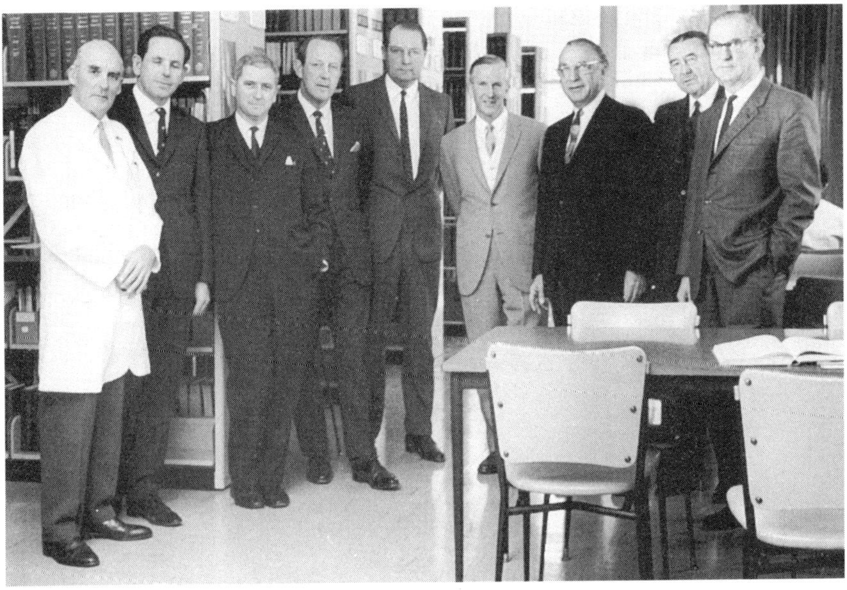

Fig. 10. Surgical staff at the Royal Children's Hospital, Melbourne (1968): Douglas Stephens, Max Kent, Nate Myers, Peter Jones, L. E. G. Sloane (Medical Director), Durham Smith, Mark Ravitch (Visitor), Russell Howard and Murray Clarke.

Hirschsprung's Disease; **Peter Jones** (Fig. 11) wrote a monograph on torticollis, and edited a widely used textbook for students "*Clinical Paediatric Surgery*"[16] and co-authored a book on tumours in children;[17] **John Solomon** continued to be a leader in the management of burns; **Robert Fowler** had a penetrating mind for research, initially in transplantation, and contributed to the ano-rectal work; **Durham Smith** was initially assistant to Hooper as a neurosurgeon, and wrote a monograph on spina bifida in 1959,[18] but under Stephens as both mentor and co-author, was associated with studies on ano-rectal lesions, hypospadias and general urology.

In Victoria, South Australia, Western Australia and Tasmania, paediatric urology remained within the orbit of general paediatric surgeons — indeed it remains to this day as a discipline within the curriculum requirements for the Paediatric Fellowship, rather than in adult urology — although specific paediatric urology units were established in New South Wales and Queensland.

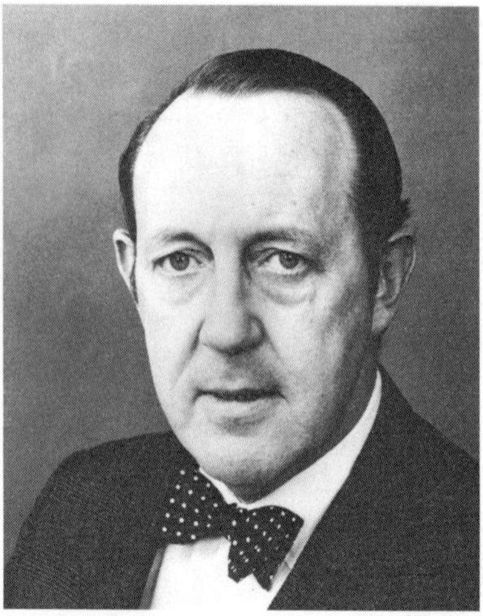

Fig. 11. Peter Jones.

In Melbourne, a second University was established in 1956 (Monash) and this included a new Medical School. A Department of Paediatric Surgery was developed under **Robert MacMahon**, and under his tutelage a strong clinical and research service was established.

In the 30 years since the end of WW2, paediatric surgery had moved from the periphery of adult practice to a specialty in its own right. Everywhere new procedures had been developed for conditions that previously were untouchable, in almost every organ of the body, and almost all the major surgical lesions encountered in children now had established techniques of diagnosis and treatment.

Perhaps the most outstanding development in the early post-war period was the advent of safe neonatal surgery. This was only made possible by the concurrent development of specifically paediatric anaesthesia, better understanding of neonatal physiology, the developments of incubators to control humidity and temperature, detailed understanding of fluid and electrolyte metabolism, and the developments of surgical techniques to deal with most of the lesions.

Spina bifida and myelomeningocele patients had largely been unmanageable prior to 1960 but changed dramatically when several disciplines combined their efforts. A Spina Bifida Clinic was set up in Melbourne in 1961, coordinating the disciplines of neurosurgery (Reginald Hooper), with careful back closure under antibiotic cover, and the recently developed ventricular shunts for hydrocephalus; orthopaedic surgery (Peter Williams, Malcolm Menelaus), with tendon transfers; urinary management (Durham Smith), with urinary diversion, external collection devices, intermittent catheterization, antispasm drugs, and later, implantable artificial sphincters and bladder augmentation; and a psychiatrist and social worker, and the whole program of rehabilitation and education under a Co-ordinator (G. Keys Smith). Major protocols were developed in the selection of patients for maximum effort and those whose quality of survival was judged to be untenable.

The survival of patients with oesophageal atresia and diaphragmatic hernia increased dramatically in all centres, with a particularly large experience under Russell Howard, with Nate Myers, Max Kent, Alex Auldist and Helen Noblett, whose work became internationally recognised. The ongoing interest in oesophageal atresia led to one of the first major studies of the long-term outcomes of survivors, and the text "*Oesophageal Atresia*" edited by three of the surgeons.[20] Tumour surgery was expanded by the development of newer and safer chemotherapeutic agents, and the establishment of Combined Clinics to maximize the contributions of surgeons, oncologists, and radiotherapists. The 5-year survival of Wilms tumour increased to over 90%, and significantly improved in neuroblastoma.

The exact anatomy of the ano-rectal sphincters was defined, both by dissections and radiographic means, under Douglas Stephens, Robert Fowler, Durham Smith, Ruth Magnus, and Justin Kelly, and a complete classification of the myriad anatomical types was developed as a guide to treatment in an International Conference, chaired by Douglas Stephens and Durham Smith in 1970 and repeated, with modifications, in the Wingspread Conference of 1984. Techniques of hypospadias repair were multiplying and the great era of cardiac surgery for a whole range of congenital anomalies began under Tim Cartmill in Sydney, Morgan Windsor in Brisbane, Darcy Sutherland in Adelaide and Roger Mee in Melbourne. In urology, the indications for surgery or conservative management of ureteric reflux were defined, and techniques for ureteric implantation, partial nephrectomy for dysplasia, ureteroceles and duplex ureters, bladder augmentation and implantation of artificial sphincters, and the endoscopic resection of urethral valves were developed. Murray Clarke, John Solomon, Julian Keogh, Fred Leditschke and Stuart Pegg improved burns management. Experience with endoscopy was just being developed under the introduction of fiber optic lighting and flexible endoscopes. Endoscopic intervention was largely confined to urology, the oesophagus and upper GI tract, colonoscopy, and ENT; the latter greatly contributed by **Bruce Benjamin** in Sydney.[19]

It was an exciting time for the surgeons of this era. Australian surgeons were productive in all these areas, and even as similar progress was taking place in the UK, USA and Europe, the standards achieved locally established the Antipodes as a location that provides good training opportunities for young surgeons from all over the world. The traffic in training opportunities was in both directions. For example, since the founding of the British Association of Paediatric Surgeons in 1953, over the next 30 years no fewer than 15 consultants in the UK had part of their training in Australian and New Zealand paediatric centres, and at the same time, at least 20 Australian and New Zealanders had similar training in the UK. Since 1983, the pattern of traffic in both directions for training has continued and extended, now between Australia, New Zealand, UK, USA, Canada, Africa and Asia.

The second generation 1975–2000. As could be expected, in the 1970's some of the first generation of Paediatric Surgeons began to retire. But major advances in anaesthesia, surgery and diagnosis were made and this called for a new breed of surgeons to embrace the new techniques. A second generation of surgeons became the seniors up to the turn of the century. They were the leaders of another great wave of progress, who adapted readily to the new modalities. The changes were as profound as in the golden era of the 30 years after WW2. Without identifying individuals with any particular advance, except in a few instances, the new breed in general paediatric surgery (with some overlap of the third generation to come) included, in Melbourne, **Keith Stokes, Alex Auldist, Alan Woodward, John Hutson, Justin Kelly, Spencer Beasley, Hock Tan, Russell Taylor, Neil McMullin, Robert Yardley, Chris Kimber, Robert Stunden, Patrick Dewan**; in Sydney, **Martin Glasson, Ralph Cohen, Genevieve Cummins, John Harvey, Hugh Martin, John Pitkin, Edward Shi, Albert Shun**; in Newcastle, **John Cassey, Patricia Davidson**; in Brisbane, **Tat-Hin Ong, Rosslyn Walker, Mervyn Lander, Peter Borzi, Athol Mackay, Roy Kimble**; in Adelaide, **John Freeman, Hock Tan** (in endoscopy), **Andrew Ford, Hiliary Boucart, Anthony Sparnon**; in Perth, **Ian Gollow, Philip King, Colin Kikiros, Andrew Barker**; in Canberra, **Errol Simpson, George Malecky**; and in Tasmania, **Ed Fenton**.

Major developments from 1975 were occurring all over the world, and were adopted by the above surgeons, each adding their own finesse.

Much had been achieved in Neonatal and Premature Baby Care by the first generation of surgeons, but a new leap now took place under a new discipline of intensive care specialists. In many units, Intensive Care became a separate department from Anesthesia, requiring special knowledge of the physiology and disturbed pathology of sick infants, supported by the exponential growth in electronic monitoring of almost every parameter of body functions. There is no doubt that the increased survival and quality of survival of neonatal infants can largely be attributed to the Intensive Care facilities, as indeed also in other conditions, heart surgery, and severe trauma.

Endoscopic Minimal Invasive Surgery has revolutionised the operative approach to an increasing number of paediatric lesions — in renal surgery for stone, pyeloplasty, partial and total nephrectomy, and drainage; in inguinal hernia, testicular exploration, appendicitis, pyloric stenosis, ano-rectal reconstruction, and bowel resection; in thoracic exploration; in hiatus hernia. The indications and effectiveness are still being assessed and expanded. Almost every organ can be visualised endoscopically, and the development of minute flexible endoscopes, better lenses and fiber optic lighting, minute cameras and electronic computerisation of images continues to expand. The new breed of surgeons have had to come to terms with the optics, electronics, and the different form of manual dexterity in manipulating the endoscope and surgical instruments through operative ports while looking at a television monitor. In Australia, **Hock Tan** and **Peter Borzi** were two of the leaders in this field, being quite innovative in its application to infants and young children.

A similar revolution has occurred in diagnostic imaging techniques to assess structure and function in many lesions, by cat scans, MRI, ultrasound, echocardiography, biliary and pancreatic intubation, angiography in various forms, perfusion of radio-opaque dyes, thallium and other nuclear scans.

Renal transplantation has been established for many years but paediatric surgeons are increasingly involved in liver transplants for biliary atresia and tumour surgery, and transplants of pancreas, lung, and bowel. It has become a specialty area, along with Microsurgery. The operating microscope made possible the exploration and treatment of fine structures in ophthalmology, and the anastomosis of minute vessels and nerves in plastic surgery and neurosurgery. Laser surgery has been refined for lesions in ophthalmology, skin lesions and urology.

The maxillofacial reconstruction of grossly deforming lesions of the face, jaws and skull has been made possible by computer planning, steriotactic imaging and cooperation between neurosurgeons, plastic surgeons, head and neck surgeons, maxillofacial surgeons and ophthalmologists.

With improved antenatal diagnosis by imaging techniques, foetal surgery intervention is a growing field in urinary obstruction, diaphragmatic hernia and other bowel anomalies.

Almost all the major centres for paediatric surgery in Australia have active surgical research programs. In general they are underfunded, but some time in research projects is encouraged in all surgical trainees. Genetics is strong in Melbourne (Murdoch Research Institute), e.g. cystic fibrosis research, as well as research in testicular development and intestinal neuronal dysplasia (**Professor John Hutson**); and in Sydney (**Professor Daniel Cass**), in Hirschsprung

Disease. The possibilities in tumour research, neuroblastomas, angiogenesis, short bowel syndrome and others continue to expand.

The third generation 2000–present. Currently there are about 70 paediatric surgeons in Australia and New Zealand in active full-time practice of the specialty (and 30 in retirement). If we exclude those surgeons listed in the second generation above, some of whom are still practicising, there are additionally 36 surgeons who have entered the field in the last 10–15 years. It is too soon to make an assessment of the individual contributions of these surgeons, and too many to list. No longer do we look for new operations for standard conditions, but endless variations are constantly being tried. An exception might be the new technique of repair of bladder extrophy, developed by Justin Kelly, which is revolutionising the outcome (in continence) in a previously notoriously disappointing lesion The extension of the electronic world in monitoring, in digital imaging and analysis, and into robotic surgery continues to grow; endoscopic instruments are getting smaller and smaller extending the range of intervention; genetic knowledge leading to better counseling and prevention, the definition of syndromes, and the possibilities of genetic manipulation through stem cell research — all will usher in yet another landmark advance.

Royal Australasian College of Surgeons. No survey of Australasian surgery would be complete without reference to the role the College has played in the development of paediatric surgery. Paediatric surgeons have played a disproportionate part in College affairs compared to their numbers. Mention has been made above that two early Presidents, Sir Henry Newland (1929–1935), and Sir Robert Wade (1935–1937), had paediatric appointments in children's hospitals for many years, although neither were primarily paediatric surgeons. Russell Howard was a Senior Vice-President and was largely responsible for the College to initiate a Paediatric Fellowship in 1962, equivalent in status to the Fellowships in other disciplines, decades ahead of any other surgical College. As a result, during the 1960's there were more paediatric surgeons in Melbourne than in London; in fact, there were more in Australia than in the United Kingdom! Douglas Stephens was Treasurer of the College Council in 1965. Durham Smith, who had been an Examiner and Chairman of the Court of Examiners, was elected President in 1987–1989 as the first full-time paediatric surgeon, and was instrumental in proposing mechanisms to define the complicated relationship between the Specialist Surgical Societies with the College, so that the Societies continued to have autonomy but work with the College in the setting of standards, the award of Fellowship, and recognizing the College as the legal authority to represent surgery with the State Authorities. It has kept the profession together, united with the broader concerns of the profession as a whole.

Acknowledgements

The author acknowledges with thanks the help received from a number of colleagues in assembling this data, and in particular Toby (A. C.) Bowring, Rick Cohen and the family of Douglas Cohen, Fred Leditschke, Rosslyn Walker, John Pearn and Gordon Baron-Hay.

References

1. Smith ED. Denis Browne: Maverick or master surgeon. *Aust NZ J Surg* 2000;70:770–777.
2. Fraser K. Hypospadias: A Queensland review of 31 major hypospadias repairs using a uniform technique. *Br J Surg* 1964;51:167–177.
3. Clubbe CPB. *The Diagnosis and Treatment of Intussusception.* Young J Pentland, Edinburgh, 1907.
4. Hipsley PL. Intussusception and its treatment by hydrostatic pressure: Based on an analysis of 100 consecutive cases so treated. *Med J Aust* 1926;2:201.
5. McKay DG, Fowler R Jr, Barnett JS. The pathogenesis and treatment of primary hydrocoeles in infancy and childhood. *Aust NZ J Surg* 1958;28:1.
6. Russell RH. The etiology and treatment of inguinal hernia in the young. *Lancet* 1988;2:1353.

7. Russell RH. Operation for severe hypospadias. *Br J Surg* 1900;Iii:1432.
8. Russell RH. The treatment of urethral stricture by excision. *Br J Surg* 1915;2:375.
9. Gregg N McA. Congenital cataract following German measles in the mother. Trans. Ophthalmol Soc Aust 1941;3:35–46.
10. Stephens FD. Congenital imperforate rectum, recto-urethral and recto-vaginal fistulae. *Aust NZ J Surg* 1953;22:161.
11. Stephens FD. Malformations of the anus. *Aust NZ J Surg* 1953;23:9.
12. Stephens FD. Imperforate rectum: A new surgical technique. *Med J Aust* 1953;1:202.
13. Stephens FD. *Congenital Malformations of the Rectum, Anus and Genito-Urinary Tract*. E & S Livingston, Inc. Edinburgh and London, 1963.
    Stephens FD, Smith ED. *AnoRectal Malformations in Children*. Year Book Medical Publishers, Inc, Chicago, 1971.
    Stephens FD, Smith ED. *AnoRectal Malformations in Children: Update 1988*. March of Dimes Birth Defects Foundation. Original Article Series, Vol. 24, No. 4. Alan R Liss, New York, 1988.
    Stephens FD, Smith ED, Hutson JM. *Congenital Anomalies of the Kidney, Urinary and Genital Tracts*, 2nd ed. Martin Dunitz Ltd, London, 2002.
14. Myers NA Oesphageal atresia: the epitome of modern surgery. *Ann R Coll Surg Eng* 1974;54:277.
15. Noblett Helen. Treatment of uncomplicated meconium ileus by Gastrographin enema: a preliminary report. *J Pediat Surg* 1969;4:190.
16. Jones PG, Woodward AA (eds.). *Clinical Paediatric Surgery: Diagnosis and Management*, 3rd ed., Blackwell Scientific Publications, Carlton, Victoria, 1986.
17. Jones PG, Campbell PE (eds.). *Tumours in Infancy and Childhood*. Blackwell Scientific Publications, Oxford, UK, 1976.
18. Smith ED. *Spina Bifida and the Total Care of Myelomeningocoele*. Charles C Thomas, Illinois, USA, 1965.
19. Beasley SW, Myers NA, Auldist AW. *Oesophageal Atresia*. Chapman and Hall Medical, London, UK, 1991.
20. Benjamin BNP. *Atlas of Paediatric Endoscopy: Upper Respiratory Tract and Oesophagus*. Oxford University Press, Oxford UK, 1981.

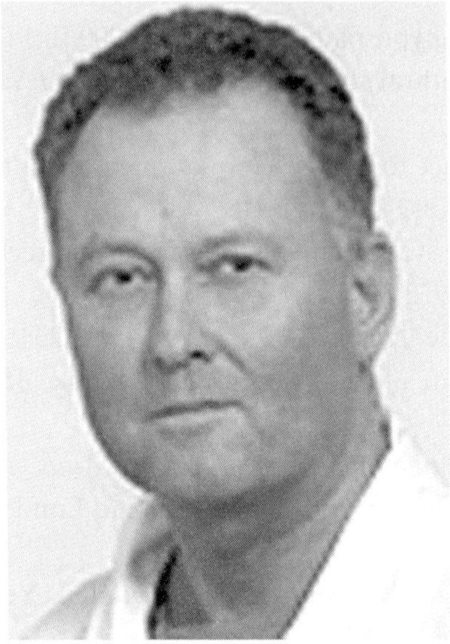

Alexander M. Rokitansky

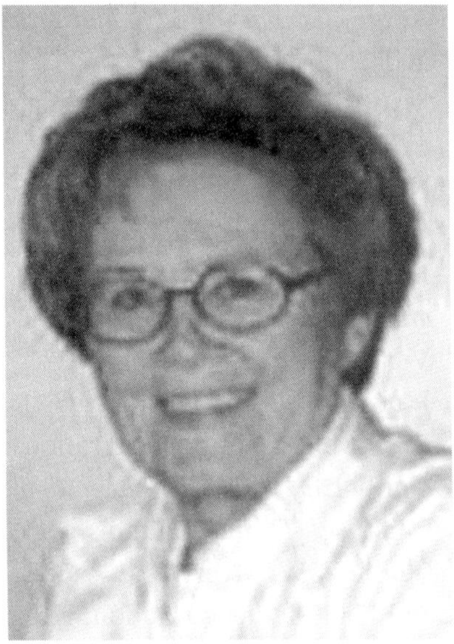

Gesine Menardi

AUSTRIA

Alexander M. Rokitansky
Gesine Menardi (1936–2007)

Specialised medical care of the child in Austria has made great advancements in the last 200 years. The roots are to be found in Vienna: at the end of the 18th century, two institutions focused on the treatment of children were founded simultaneously. The so-called *Wiener Allgemeines Krankenhaus* (Vienna General Hospital) founded under Kaiser Josef II (the son of Empress Maria Theresia) in 1784 and the ***Vienna Findelhaus*** (Vienna Foundling Hospital) were opened at the same time. During this time, infanticide and infant mortality were major topics of interest and were discussed within the scope of enlightened absolutism. At the Foundling Hospital illegitimate newborns and infants could be handed over, if desired even anonymously. An important reason for establishing this facility was to reduce the rate of child mortality, also in the interest of population policy. From the patient population at the Foundling Hospital **Alois Bednar** reported, on March 7, 1851, about a case of anal atresia. He perforated a "fluctuating lump" on the floor of the pelvis with a trocar and drained meconium. The Viennese paediatrician Alois Bednar (1816–1888) was the director of the Vienna Foundling Home. In the 126 years of its existence from 1784 to 1910, approximately 750,000 children were admitted at the Vienna Foundling Hospital. In 1787 the physician **Johann Josef Mastalier** (1757–1793) founded a private **Out-patient Service for Poor Children** at Wollzeile in Vienna. This institution provided counselling for mothers and also conducted house calls to treat children. The out-patient service was the precursor of the first

Public Children's Hospital in Vienna under **Anton Leopold Göllis** (1764–1827). Started in 1881, the Institute developed significantly under the management of the Slovak paediatrician **Max Kassowitz** (1842–1913). Special treatment rooms for surgery, orthopaedics, laryngology and ophthalmology were set up from 1882 to 1913. Besides, an operating room and a lecture hall were created. Sigmund Freud headed the Department of Neurology at this Institute.

In 1837, after paediatric hospitals had been founded in 1802 in Paris and 1830 at the Charité in Berlin, the first paediatric hospital in Austria was founded in the Viennese suburb of Schottenfeld by a philanthropist and erstwhile military doctor **Ludwig Wilhelm Mauthner** (1806–1858) at his own expense. This facility was shifted to Kinderspitalgasse 6 and was the forerunner of what is known today as ***St. Anna Kinderspital*, St. Anna Children's Hospital**. Mauthner was a member of the Vienna Medical Faculty, a surgeon, and a kind of "people's doctor". He was concerned with improving medical care for acutely ill children of poor parents. He also was interested in scientific research on paediatric diseases. His chief aim was to connect socially committed basic care with medical research and this remained a major determining factor for the development of the hospital. Mauthner's paediatric hospital became famous in scientific circles and many physicians came to the hospital to be trained. Mauthner struggled to obtain permission to teach at his hospital. In 1844 he was granted permission to hold clinical lectures. In 1850 the University Paediatric Clinic of Vienna was founded and established in the premises of *St. Anna Kinderspital*. In 1851 he received the first Associate Professorship for Paediatrics at the University of Vienna. This university facility was located at *St. Anna Kinderspital* until 1911.

After Mauthner's demise in 1858, a separate department of surgery was opened and **Friedrich Franz Salzer** (1827–1890) was appointed as the unpaid head of the institution. Under the subsequent director **Hermann Widerhofer** (1832–1901) and finally after the nomination of the surgeon **Josef Weinlechner**, surgery at *St. Anna Kinderspital* experienced a significant upsurge. Josef Weinlechner (1829–1906), a pioneer of paediatric surgery, was born in humble circumstances in a town named Altheim in Upper Austria. After a period of great privation Josef Weinlechner achieved his doctorate in 1854. He then completed his specialisation training at the University Clinic of Surgery in Vienna under **Franz Schuh**. Schuh belonged to the close circle of the council of professors at the Second Medical School under the rector **Carl Rokitansky**.

In 1864 Josef Weinlechner was asked to serve at *St. Anna Kinderspital*. Weinlechner's appointment marked a major upswing in paediatric surgery at *St. Anna Kinderspital*. During this time he also applied for an assistant professorship in surgery with special emphasis on paediatric surgery. This application was dated July 1, 1865: a milestone in the history of paediatric surgery because it was extremely unusual at the time to apply for a professor's degree in paediatric surgery. He submitted his thesis on the cleft lip and was awarded a professorship on October 10, 1865. Deformities and oncological operations were his favourite subjects from the very beginning. From 1866 onwards, the annual reports of *St. Anna Kinderspital* included detailed statistics about surgical work. Interestingly, the most frequently performed paediatric operations today, which are appendectomy, hernia surgery and hydrocele operations, do not feature in these statistics. Weinlechner treated hernias with a truss; hydroceles were punctured and then instilled with iodine. An important chapter in paediatric surgery at the time were life-saving tracheotomies for diphtheria; Weinlechner improved upon the technique.

Appendicitis belonged to the realm of internal medicine at the time. Only in 1886 was it discovered that the cause of the frequently fatal inflammation of the peritoneum was an inflammation of the appendix. In 1894 the American surgeon McBurney reported that the "internal-medicine problem" could be resolved by performing a small incision in the right lower abdomen and removing the vermiform appendix. For several years surgeons discussed whether it would be better to drain the abscess only. Even in 1907 appendectomy was one of the main topics of the German Congress of Surgeons.

When *St. Anna Kinderspital* was founded in Vienna, the so-called **Paediatric Hospital Associations** were founded under the patronage of aristocratic ladies and distinguished townswomen in Graz and Salzburg. In 1842, for instance, the **Paediatric Hospital Association** was founded in Graz under the special patronage of **Mrs. Anna Freiin von Brandhofen**, wife of Archduke Johann. The year 1843 marked the inauguration of a provisional paediatric hospital with eight beds in two hospital wards in Klosterwiesgasse. In 1846 this facility was shifted into a new single-storey building at Villefortgasse in Graz. In 1899 the Paediatric Clinic of Salzburg was opened, supported by the Archduchess Valerie. The paediatrician-in-charge, Hans Fiala (1858–1924), was appointed head of the institution and established paediatric surgery here. He completed a part of his training under Widerhofer and Weinlechner at *St. Anna Kinderspital* in Vienna and tried his best to introduce the Viennese standards of paediatric medicine in Salzburg. Thus, he created a separate department for ill children in need of surgery and a separate operating room.

After a two-year construction period, the new ***Anna Kinderspital*** (**Anna Paediatric Hospital**), named after **Countess Anna von Meran,** was inaugurated in Graz in 1877. In addition to the medical and surgical-oculistic departments, a department for children with infectious diseases was accommodated here. At the time **Benjamin Ipavic** was in charge of the Department of Paediatric Surgery. In 1899 the hospital was significantly developed by **Theodor Escherich** (1857–1911). A lecture hall and an isolation tract were built. **Hans Spitzy** (1872–1956) became head of the Surgical-Orthopaedic Department in 1905. He was succeeded by **Philipp Erlacher** in 1913. In 1906, more than 686 operations were performed here; anaesthesia was administered in 252 cases.

Until the beginning of the 20th century, paediatricians frequently performed surgery in children. For instance, the famous physician in Graz **Theodor Escherich** used the paraffin plug to treat umbilical hernia in children; the paraffin plug had been proposed by **Robert Gersuny** (1844–1927) for the treatment of rectal episodes. In 1903, in the monthly journal of paediatrics Escherich finally reported about more than 30 cases in which he used this method in children aged 1 to 14 months. Even from **Klagenfurt** we know that the chief paediatric physician **Gernot Brandesky** personally operated on children at the paediatric hospital until the Department of Paediatric Surgery was founded in 1974.

In 1875 the ***Kronprinz–Rudolf Kinderspital*** **(Crown Prince Rudolf Paediatric Hospital)** was inaugurated in Vienna and a Department of Paediatric Surgery was established here in 1903. It was headed by **Hans Salzer** (1871–1944), the second pioneer of paediatric surgery in Austria. Hans Salzer served as an assistant at the Second University Clinic of Surgery in Vienna under the chairmanship of **Carl Gussenbauer** (1842–1903). He had to leave the clinic in 1902 because of his marriage. At the time assistants working at a clinic were not permitted to marry. He moved to ***Kronprinz–Rudolf Kinderspital*** and also occupied the position of chief physician at the Vienna Polyclinic for some time. *Kronprinz–Rudolf Kinderspital* was re-named *Mauthner Markhofsches Kinderspital.* In 1924 Hans Salzer was appointed Director of *Mauthner Markhof'sches Kinderspital.* At this time he surrendered his chief physician position at the Polyclinic.

The Austrian Society of Paediatric and Adolescent Surgery, which arose from the study group of paediatric surgery in 1971, has been honouring Hans Salzer by awarding the **Hans Salzer prize** every year from 1976 onwards. Salzer's major merits included the establishment of a Department of Paediatric Surgery and also trend-setting work on highly relevant problems in paediatric surgery at the time. He focused his attention on three major fields. The first was the treatment of pneumococcal peritonitis in the young girl, the second was the treatment of congenital inguinal hernia and, thirdly, he became very famous through his publications on early bouginage of caustic alkali burns. At this time pneumococcal peritonitis in the young girl was a disease with a mean lethality of 50%. As the symptoms were similar to those of acute appendicitis, the children were commonly operated on. The combination of surgical trauma and pneumococcal peritonitis led to a lethality rate of nearly 100%. He was able to show that a limited conservative therapy later complemented by the administration of a pneumococcus serum helps to achieve a significantly better prognosis for the child affected by this condition. While treating inguinal hernia, he realised that all inguinal hernias in newborns, infants and young children are congenital; his treatment consisted of high ablation of the hernia sac and/or the vaginal process without any plastic coverage in the region of the inguinal canal. Hans Salzer was succeeded by **Rudolf Jonas**, the youngest brother of mayor and the Austrian president Franz Jonas, followed by **Peter Wurnig** who earned great merit in intensive medicine for children as well as neonatal surgery and was responsible for establishing Vienna as the venue of the 32nd BAPS Congress at the Hofburg in 1985. Finally, he was succeeded by **Ernst Horcher**, a student of **Fritz Helmer**.

Apart from the Department of Paediatric Surgery at Mauthner Markhofsches Kinderspital, surgical diseases in the child were also given attention at the University Clinic in Vienna. At the First Clinic of Surgery **Leopold Schönbauer** (1888–1963) was in charge of this sub-speciality. He was succeeded by **Huber**. At the Second University Department of Surgery **Fritz Demmer** (1884–1967), **Wolfgang Denk** (1882–1970) and finally **Georg Salzer** (1903–1995) son of Hans Salzer, frequently devoted their attention to treatment methods in paediatric surgery. As early as in 1921 **Fritz Demmer** reported on a successfully operated ileal atresia. The child, referred from the obstetric clinic to the Second University Clinic of Surgery on the first day after its birth, had a simultaneous small omphalocele (hernia in the cord). When exposing the umbilical hernia it was found that an additional ileal atresia with a microcolon was present. Demmer resected the markedly dilated distal end of the ileum and restored continuity by performing a side-to-side anastomosis between the ileum and the ascending colon. The child could be discharged from the hospital in healthy condition. This was the third published case of a successfully operated small bowel atresia in the global literature.

In 1930 **Leopold Schönbauer** presented to the Society of Surgeons in Vienna a successfully operated left-sided hernia of the diaphragm in a 3-month-old infant which he corrected in accordance with surgical principles valid even today. Besides his work as a consultant surgeon at the so-called ***Kinderklinik Glanzing*** (**Paediatric Clinic of Glanzing**), which had been founded with resources of the "*Jubiliäumsfonds für Kinder*" (Jubilee Fund for Children) in 1915, Leopold Schönbauer also had sufficient opportunity to operate on cases of hypertrophic pyloric stenosis and he published his experience in this field in 1931.

A remarkable study from this period reports his experience in treating intestinal obstruction due to invagination, which was presented by **Fritz Starlinger** from **Anton Eiselsberg's Clinic** in 1931 and drew attention, at this early point in time, to the option of hydrostatic repositioning of the invagination. In 1935 **Wolfgang Denk** presented his successful treatment of uni- and bilateral testicular retention (cryptorchidism) at the Society of Physicians, using extracts from male gonads. The above mentioned legendary Paediatric Clinic of Glanzing had no surgery facilities of its own. Until 1994 its numerous paediatric-surgery patients were treated at the University Clinic of Surgery in the General Hospital of Vienna by the consultant surgeons **Paul Huber**, **Georg Salzer**, **Fritz Helmer** and, after 1990, **Alexander Rokitansky**. From 1994 onward, paediatric surgery for the Paediatric Clinic of Glanzing was performed at ***Donauspital*** in Vienna. A centre of paediatric chest surgery and paediatric urology was developed here under Rokitansky.

The Paediatric Hospital Association in Graz was dissolved in 1939 and the surgical-orthopaedic department was shifted to ***Sanatorium Theresia***, which was located in close proximity. **Wilhelm Schäfer** became the successor of **Philipp Erlacher**. A resolution was passed and the construction of a new University Clinic of Paediatric Surgery in Graz was started in 1973. In 1974 **Hugo Sauer,** who came from the University of Innsbruck, took over the Clinic of Paediatric Surgery. Under Sauer's management, paediatric surgery in Graz received a major new impetus, particularly because its usual work was flanked by intensive attention to traumatology and the founding of an Austrian Committee of Accident Prevent in Children (1983). In addition to the regular spectrum of paediatric and adolescent surgery, accident prevention was pursued by his successor **Michael Höllwarth** at the Clinic in Graz.

The Department of Paediatric Surgery was founded in 1956 at the **Paediatric Clinic in Linz. Hermann Hartl** was in charge of this department from 1956 to 1987. In the 1950's, the first two corrections of oesophageal atresia in Austria were performed by **Hartl** in Linz and **Georg Salzer** in Vienna. From 1987 to 2002 **Michael Engels** was in charge of the large Department of Paediatric Surgery in Linz. He was the initiator and a major driving force behind the so-called **(*Kinderchirurgisches Donausymposium*) Danube Symposium on Paediatric Surgery**. In 1992 he performed laparoscopic surgical techniques in newborns, infants and children. In 2002 he was succeeded by **Wolfgang Pumberger**, a student of Peter Wurnig and Ernst Horcher, who then became the head of the Department of Paediatric Surgery at the Regional Paediatric Clinic of Linz.

After the Second World War an out-patient surgery department was set up at ***Gottfried v. Preyersches Kinderspital*** **(Gottfried von Preyer Paediatric Hospital).** This was followed by a Department of Paediatric Surgery under **Rudolf Rauhs**, established in 1961. His successor was Rehbein's student **Leopold Preier** who set up an interdisciplinary intensive care unit and modernised the operating rooms.

Peter Wurnig (1923–2005), appointed chief physician at the **(*Mauthner Markhofsches Kinderspital*) Mauthner Markhof Paediatric Hospital** in 1963, gave a new impetus to this institution. He developed surgery in the newborn and surgery for deformities, and also set up an intensive care unit. Peter Wurnig was able to establish Vienna as the venue of the **32nd BAPS Congress** in 1985. Wurnig's successor in 1989 was **Ernst Horcher**, a student of Fritz Helmer. Horcher switched to the newly built and largest Department of Paediatric Surgery in Vienna at *Donauspital* in 1992, which is headed by **Alexander Rokitansky** since 1994. Rokitansky is also a student of **Fritz Helmer**. Under Rokitansky Donauspital eventually took charge of paediatric surgery for *Mauthner–Markhof Kinderspital*. In 2003 he also took charge of surgery for *Preyersches Kinderspital*. At the large hospitals of Vienna, Rokitansky established paediatric surgery out-patient departments according to the so-called "model for out-patient care in paediatric surgery". These units provided care and also served as outposts of *Donauspital*'s paediatric surgery. In 1994 **Ernst Horcher** took over the **University Clinic of Paediatric Surgery** at the General Hospital of Vienna, which had been planned by Fritz Helmer and later by Alexander Rokitansky. He consolidated his cooperative work with *St. Anna Kinderspital* and devoted special attention to tumour surgery.

A **Department of Paediatric Surgery** was founded at the Regional Hospital of **Salzburg** in 1964. **Hans Henkel** was head of the department from 1964 to 1989. A new building for paediatric surgery was set up in 1989, and subsequently managed by **Irene Oesch** and **Thomas Böhmers**. Hugo Sauer's student **Günter Schimpl** from Graz took over the management in 2006.

In 1966 the University Clinic of Surgery in Innsbruck under **Hans Huber** received its own Department of Paediatric Surgery. **Hugo Sauer** headed this department from 1968 to 1976. He completed his training in paediatric surgery under Hartl in Linz and Rehbein in Bremen. **Gesine Menardi** (1936–2007) served as his assistant. After completing a period of training at Alder Hey Children's Hospital in Liverpool, she became head of the Department of Paediatric Surgery at the University Clinic of Surgery in Innsbruck in 1976. In 2001 **Josef Hager**, who had been her colleague for several years, became head of the department.

The **Study Group for Paediatric Surgery** was constituted in 1966. The **Austrian Society of Paediatric Surgery** emerged from this group in 1971 (Van Swieten Convention). The Presidents of the Society were Hermann Hartl from 1966 to 1971, Hugo Sauer from 1972 to 1976, Peter Wurnig from 1977 to 1978, Hans Henkel from 1979 to 1982, Gernot Brandesky from 1983 to 1986, Gesine Menardi from 1987 to 1990, Leopold Preier from 1991 to 1992, Michael Höllwarth from 1993 to 1996, Michael Engels from 1997 to 2000, Alexander Rokitansky from 2001 to 2004 and Josef Hager from 2005 onwards.

Since 1975 paediatric surgery is an **additional speciality in general surgery** with the additive subsidiary specialities of paediatrics, urology and traumatology. Thanks to Leopold Preier's diligent efforts, a separate **speciality of paediatric surgery** was created in 1994. In 2007 the regulation for physicians' training was amended and the speciality was renamed **paediatric and adolescent surgery**. The new name took the age spectrum of the patients into account.

A **special Department of Paediatric Surgery** under **Fritz Helmer**, a student of Wolfgang Denk, was set up at the Second Department of Surgery in Vienna. After a period of study in the USA, Helmer introduced hydrocephalus shunt surgery in Vienna and brought his comprehensive knowledge from Boston on the subject of paediatric heart surgery to Austria. A **Chairman's Post in Paediatric Surgery** was created under Helmer in 1984 and **Alexander Rokitansky** was assigned the new assistant's position in paediatric surgery. Rokitansky became Helmer's co-worker in paediatric surgery and remained in this position for several years. In 1994 **Ernst Horcher** was appointed head of the Department of Paediatric Surgery and head of the University Department of Paediatric Surgery in Vienna.

In 1974 the existing facility of paediatric medicine at the Regional Hospital in **Klagenfurt** was divided into an internal and a surgical department. It was headed for several years by **Gernot Brandesky**. Brandesky expanded the department and covered the entire spectrum of paediatric surgery including traumatology and urology. After him, the department was managed by the German paediatric surgeon **Peter Illing** and subsequently taken over by **Günter Fasching**, a student of Hugo Sauer. Fasching has been in charge of this department for some years now. In the last few years he has transformed paediatric and adolescent surgery in Klagenfurt into a centre of international renown.

In 1982 paediatric surgery in Graz was assigned the status of a University Clinic under **Hugo Sauer**. As the clinic developed, the premises in the Mozartgasse/Heinrichstrasse were sold. The ground-breaking ceremony for the new building in the premises of the University Clinics of Graz was held in 1989. In 1993 the new building of the University Clinic of Paediatric Surgery under Sauer in Graz was inaugurated. In 1989 **Michael Höllwarth** took over the management of the Clinic, which is currently the largest university clinic of paediatric surgery in Austria. In 1991 Höllwarth together with **Peter Schier** founded a **Children's Protection Group** and also set a milestone here in child care, as Sauer had done by introducing **accident prevention** for children.

Including the large Department of Paediatric Surgery at *Donauspital* in Vienna, inaugurated in 1992 and equipped with the most modern facilities, we currently have 4 paediatric surgery chair positions in Austria (Vienna, Graz, Innsbruck, Salzburg), a university-associated Teaching Department of Paediatric Surgery at *Donauspital* in Vienna, and two Departments of Paediatric Surgery in Linz and Klagenfurt.

Acknowledgement

I am indebted to Dr Elisabeth Peter–Bonelli and my staff member Karin Entrich for their assistance and review of the data material.

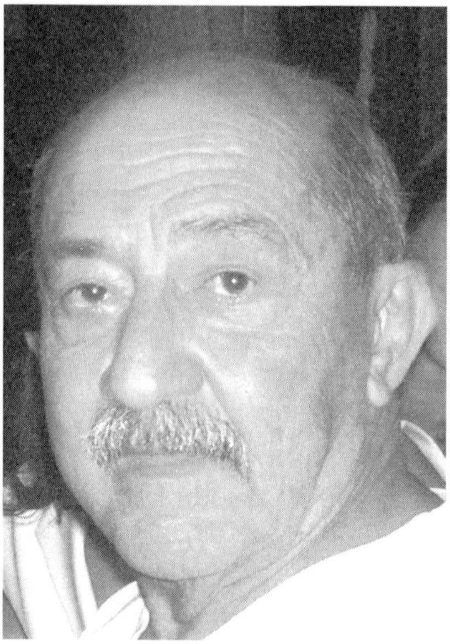

João Gilberto Maksoud

BRAZIL

João Gilberto Maksoud

The first notice on the exercise of the pediatric surgery in Brazil was at the end of the decade of the 1940s. At that time, the unique physician dedicated to the surgery of children was Dr Auro S. Amorim, working at the nursery of a popular maternity ward. He was responsible for the neo-natal surgery of the Maternity Leonor M. Barros (1947). Due to the fact that he was the first to work in such an unknown specialty, very little is known about his actual activities and accomplishments. However, in that year, the Service of Pediatric Surgery was founded in the Pediatric Department at the Matarazzo General Hospital, a private hospital, by Dr Virgílio Carvalho Pinto, working with Dr Vilhena de Moraes and Dr José Pinus, group of doctors that remained together for many years. At the end of the 1940's, Dr Fábio Dória do Amaral went to Seattle to spend some months with Dr Alexander Bill, one of the first generation of Dr Ladd's disciples. He was immediately followed by Dr Virgílio Alves de Carvalho Pinto, with a Rockefeller Foundation Fellowship, who spent some months with Dr Robert Gross at the Children's Hospital in Boston at the Harvard Medical School and Dr Octávio Freitas Vaz from Rio de Janeiro in Chicago, following the worldwide enthusiasm for the new rising specialty.

In the following years, Dr Carvalho Pinto became one of the most important and enthusiastic advocates of pediatric surgery in Brazil, promoting several courses to surgeons and pediatricians in order to define the field of actuation pediatric surgery. His first and significant accomplishment was his effort to include the pediatric surgery as a regular discipline in the regular Graduation Course in the Medical Schools all over Brazil. The effort and enthusiasm of all these pioneers led to the creation of the first official and regular discipline of pediatric surgery in a medical school in 1955, at the School Of Medicine of Sorocaba (Catholic University of São Paulo), where Dr Carvalho Pinto was the first full Professor of Pediatric Surgery in Brazil. In the next year, the discipline of pediatric surgery at the Paulista School of Medicine was created (presently UNIFESP-Federal University Medical School at the State of São Paulo), leaded by Dr José Pinus (Fig. 1). Over the next few years, many University Schools of Medicine following this worldwide trend set up their own disciplines of pediatric surgery.

In the University of São Paulo, the most prestigious school of medicine in Brazil, Dr Carvalho Pinto was the first full Professor at the University of São Paulo until he retired in 1983. In the middle of 1960's, Dr Primo Curti edited the first textbook on pediatric surgery. The textbook was disseminated in many cities of Brazil, with the creation of independent specialized services, such as with Dr Carvalheira in northeast of the country (Recife), Dr Ubirajara Motta in south (Porto Alegre), Dr Beltrão and Dr Faria in middle west (Curitiba) and Dr Duarte Lana (Belo Horizonte).

Before these years of consolidation of pediatric surgery in Brazil, in 1956, there was a case the first successful survival of a

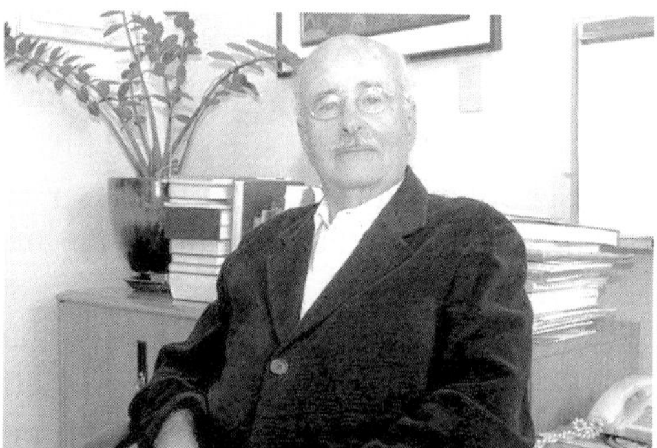

Fig. 1. Jose Pinus.

newborn with esophageal atresia through a primary anastomosis. This achievement was obtained by the team of surgeons working together, which composed of Dr Carvalho Pinto, Dr Pinus and Dr Vilhena. In 1964, the Brazilian Society of Pediatric Surgery (CIPE) was founded, two years after the foundation of the Argentinean Society of Pediatric Surgery, the first such society in South America. Two years later, in 1966, the Pan-American Association of Pediatric Surgery was founded by Dr J. Lozoya Solis from Mexico.

The first main office of Brazilian Society (CIPE) was located in the 5th floor of the University of São Paulo Medical School, and it remained there until the acquisition of the new independent head-office, under Dr Pinus's CIPE presidency. In 1967, the First Program of Residence in Pediatric Surgery was constituted in Brazil by the Service of Pediatric Surgery of the Department of Surgery, under the leadership of Dr João Gilberto Maksoud who succeeded Dr Carvalho Pinto as a full Professor of Pediatric Surgery in the University of São Paulo Medical School. In 1974, the Vth Brazilian Congress of Pediatric Surgery, the IVth Pan-American and the IIIrd World Symposium of Pediatric Surgery was held in São Paulo, with 1285 participants from 38 countries, an impressive number of participants at that time. The most important event of this Symposium was the foundation of the World Federation of Pediatric Surgery (WOFAPS), and Dr Pinus from Brazil elected as vice president. In 1994 the CIPESUR was founded; a Society of the Pediatric Surgery Associations from countries of the Lower South America — Argentina, Brazil Chile and Paraguay.

In 1975, the first Laboratory of Investigation in Pediatric Surgery in Brazil was created by Dr Maksoud. At this Research Laboratory, many technical advances were developed and it was the basis as well for the implantation of the Program of Liver Transplantation at the São Paulo University Medical School. The first Liver Transplantation at the Service of Pediatric Surgery was accomplished in September of 1989, by a team of pediatric surgeons lead by Dr Maksoud. Up to June 2007 around 350 liver transplants, including all technical varieties — whole liver, reduced, split-liver and liver-related liver transplants — have been accomplished. Experimental research was also carried out in this investigative laboratory, achieving many medical successes.

In 2000, was released the first complete textbook of "*Pediatric Surgery*", edited by Dr João Gilberto Maksoud (Cirurgia Pediátrica, ed. Revinter, 2000-Rio de Janeiro), through collaboration of many pediatric surgeons from all South America and USA.

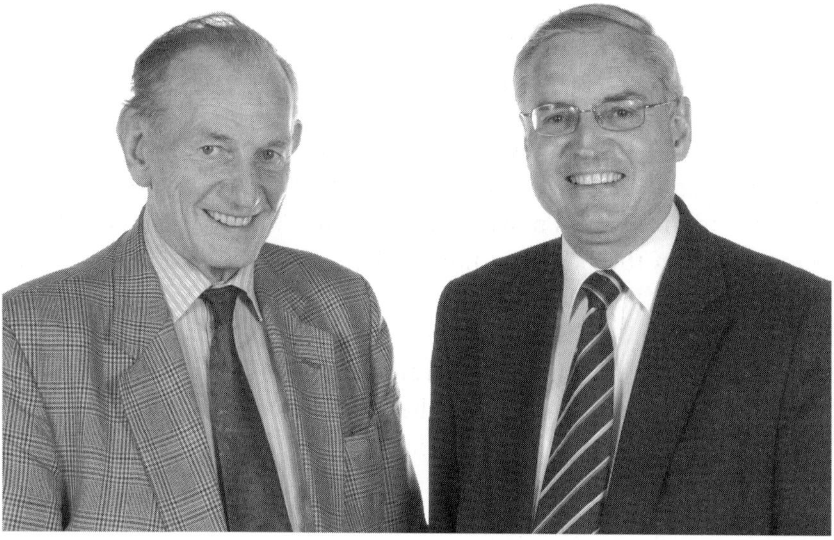

Dan G. Young and Robert Carachi

BRITAIN

Dan G. Young
Robert Carachi

"Let not worship of the past nor confusion of the present prevent us from preparing wisely for the future"[1]

The title "paediatrics"[2] was not used until the 19th century when it gradually came into use to designate the study of diseases and disorders of children. Even midway through the 20th century the term did not appear in the Shorter Oxford Dictionary. Although it is widely accepted, but the spelling changes to pediatrics in some countries. An additional complication was the distinction that some of our medical colleagues made and prefer the term "child health" as this indicates a wider remit than the ground covered by diseases in infants and children. Surgeons have not been concerned with this nomenclature dispute but have their own schizoid problem whether to call their specialty "paediatric surgery" or "surgical paediatrics".

From Charitable Institutions to Children's Hospitals

Paediatrics is a relatively new term but the study of children's diseases has been undertaken for centuries. In the 18th century effective therapeutic agents were limited and relatively little attention was paid to the problems of children. Society seems to have accepted that about half of the population would die before reaching the end of their first decade but the scourge of death in the young age group in Britain did stir the conscience of some individuals. Coram,[3] a retired sea captain, made a major impact in London in the 18th century.

After an extended battle lasting more than a decade he succeeded in establishing in London the Foundling Hospital or Home for Infants and Children who were in need of care. This was "London's most fashionable charity" for a time after it opened in 1739 but over the years it became less popular and among the accusations made against it was the concern that it may encourage illegitimate births. In consequence by the mid century it ran into financial difficulties and had to seek money from the Government. The condition on which the grant was given was that all who attended had to be accepted and this resulted in overcrowding and deterioration in the service. In the next four years with the "open to all policy" there were 14,934 babies received but only 4545 survived. The institution reverted to its previous charitable status without the strictures applied by the politicians. The Coram Foundation still retains its site in Guildford Street where adults cannot enter the fields unless they are accompanying a child or children.

Later in the 18th century George Armstrong[4] followed his brother, both to study medicine in Edinburgh and then move to London. At that time Scots, and in particular Edinburgh students, were not made welcome in London where approval was required by the College of Physicians before a practice can be set up in the city. William Armstrong was obstructed, as were many Edinburgh graduates, but George boldly proceeded to ignore the regulations imposed by the College of Physicians and set up a dispensary in Holborn — about a kilometre from the Coram Foundling Hospital — for the treatment of poor children. He is described as the instigator of a scientific approach to diseases in children and his meticulous notes formed the basis of Underwood's books. Apparently a very good doctor but a poor business man, he ultimately ran out of funds. He was desirous of establishing a hospital in-patient facility but this goal was not achieved for another three-quarters of a century.

After Armstrong's clinic closed, there was a significant change occurring in Europe. At the beginning of the 19th century, hospitals for children were opened in many of the major cities (Table 1). Britain lagged behind on this development. In 1849 the British and Foreign Medico-Chirurgical Review stated "*We need an Hôpital des*

Table 1. Children's hospitals built in the first half of the 19th century in Europe.

Children's Hospitals, Europe: 1800–1850	
1802	Paris
1834	St Petersburg
1837	Vienna
1839	Pest
1842	Moscow
1842	Prague
1843	Turin
1843	Berlin
1844	Berlin
1844	Graz
1845	Copenhagen
1845	Turin
1846	Munich

Enfans Malades in the metropolis, near the schools of medicine; we need men of admitted ability, professional, scientific, and literary, able to stand side by side with the officers of hospitals for adults, prosecuting the study of a special pathology and treatment in its wards, and hence able and willing to impart the results of their experience to the rising generation ...."[5]

In Britain, children's hospitals did develop rapidly in the second half of the century (Table 2). The **Hospital for Sick Children** in **Great Ormond Street**[6] was the first, and unlike so many of the other hospitals that were established then, it has continued without interruption and is known worldwide. The hospital was close to the site of the Coram Foundling Institution, being on the other side of Guildford Street. In its early days after being established by the intense work of Drs George West and the influential Henry Bence–Jones it progressed well, but in less than a decade, it ran into serious financial difficulties. However at the hospital's annual dinner Charles Dickens attended and made an extremely successful appeal which helped to sustain the hospital and remove the serious financial threat. A second much later benefactor,

Table 2. Children's Hospitals built in the second half of the 19th century in England and Scotland. (From E. M. R. Lomax, Small and Special: The Development of Hospitals for Children in Victorian Britain, Welcome Institute, London, 1996.)

Hospital for Sick Children	London	1852
Leeds Hospital for Women and Children	Leeds	1853
Jenny Lind Infirmary for Sick Children	Norwich	1853
Manchester Children's Hospital	Manchester	1856
Royal Edinburgh Hospital for Sick Children	Edinburgh	1859
Liverpool Infirmary for Children	Liverpool	1859
Royal Hospital for Women and Children, Waterloo Bridge Rd	London	1860
Birmingham and Midlands Children's Hospital	Birmingham	1861
Newcastle on Tyne Hospital for Sick Children	Newcastle	1861
Manchester Clinical Hospital for Women	Manchester	1865
Bristol Royal Hospital for Children and Women	Bristol	1866
Victoria Hospital for Children, Chelsea	London	1866
Alexandra Hospital for Children with Hip Disease	London	1867
Belgrave Hospital for Children	London	1867
North Eastern Hospital for Children	London	1867
Brighton Royal Alexandra Hospital for Sick Children	Brighton	1868
East London Hospital for Women and Children	London	1868
Birkenhead and Wirral Children's Hospital	Liverpool	1869
Evelina Hospital for Sick Children	London	1869
Nottingham Hospital for Children	Nottingham	1869
Victoria Hospital for Sick Children	Hull	1872
Royal Alexandra Children's Hospital and Convalescent Home	Rhyl	1872
Seven Oaks Hospital for Children with Hip Disease	Kent	1872
Sheffield Hospital for Sick Children	Sheffield	1876
Royal Aberdeen Hospital for Sick Children	Aberdeen	1877
Derbyshire Hospital for Sick Children	Derby	1877
Royal Hospital for Sick Children	Glasgow	1882
Bradford Children's Hospital	Bradford	1883
Paddington Green Children's Hospital	London	1883
Gateshead Children's Hospital	Gateshead	1887
St Mary's Hospital for Children	Plaistow	1894

Sir J. M. Barrie, in 1929 gave the royalties and the copyright income from the play and novel versions of Peter Pan to the hospital. This continues to aid the resources necessary to run the institution[6] to the present day.

Dr West opposed any surgical appointment to the hospital in London at the time of the opening but the Board insisted that a surgeon be appointed as well as physicians. The second surgeon — **Mr Athol Johnston** — to hold the post presented three long articles in the "*British Medical Journal*" in 1861,[7] which present a fascinating list of the paediatric surgical diseases of the time. His successor — Mr Holmes — published a 37-chapter book on the "*Surgical Treatment of the Diseases of Infancy and Childhood*".[8] The considerable resemblance and also the divergence from the 20th and 21st century surgical paediatrics are interesting.

An interesting fact of the developments of the surgery of infants and children was the divergence of opinion within the profession. It is difficult to understand the logic behind rationalising that the medical diseases of infants and children are sufficiently different from adult pathology and that paediatricians are required for this special management of the "medical" aspects but for children with the surgical diseases could be looked after by general surgeons in an adult environment. The dominance and belief in many centres of the expertise required for the child with "medical" problems compared to the one with "surgical" problems was often dominated by the relatively new doctors then becoming known as paediatricians.

The Hospital for Sick Children's Board in Glasgow did appoint an equal number of surgeons and physicians for the opening of the Hospital.[9] In Edinburgh surgeons were peripheral, although one was appointed for consultation when required. Those requiring surgery were transferred to the adult hospital (the Royal Infirmary). It was not until 1887, 27 years after the hospital opened, that it was agreed to institute a surgical ward for a trial period of 3 years. The operating theatre was created by a modification of the sewing room. In contrast, in Glasgow the Board appointed the same number of surgeons as physicians at the outset and had a surgical ward and an operating theatre active from opening in 1883.[10] Within two decades of opening there were more attendances to the surgical department than to the medical side and this balance has continued throughout the century since then.

The major stimuli to the development of paediatric surgery in the 19th century were from developments outwith the paediatric field. There were in the mid-19th century developments of anaesthesia (ether and chloroform) and shortly after that the introduction of the antiseptic approach to surgery. Pasteur's development of the understanding of bacteria and Lister's development of the antiseptic principle as practised in the Royal Infirmary in Glasgow had significant effects as well as the development of anaesthesia in the mid century. The society at that time became conscious of the huge infant mortality and the very high mortality in childhood. The plethora of children's hospitals opened in the second half of the 19th century was an indication of how the social conscience in Britain had been stirred. It was also the time when there was appreciation of the value of inoculation against smallpox which had been a regular killer, especially of the young patients. Another feature of these decades was the appointment and recognition of medical officers of health and their contribution to the health of the communities.

There was a problem in the paediatric field — most physicians and surgeons had to make a livelihood from their medical skills and the great part of the care required in paediatrics was for the poorer section of the community. The families needed all their earnings for housing, clothing and feeding their young family and did not have money for doctor's fees. These factors contributed to the delay in the paediatric specialty developing and why there were virtually no doctors working full-time with children until the 20th century.

The aims set out in 1859 for the hospital, which became the Royal Edinburgh Hospital for Sick Children (REHSC), were that it was for sick children to be given treatment and advice, to teach, to raise funds to fulfil its objectives and to establish a medical committee. Similar aims were set out by many of the new institutions. In some institutions teaching, including parenthood, was given significantly more emphasis as the years passed. Specialisation in paediatrics developed towards the end of the 19th and into the 20th century.

Twentieth Century

The intervention of the First World War was a stimulus to aid the progression of women in the medical profession. With the number of female graduates increasing there was gradually an increase in the number of females advancing in paediatric surgery. Individuals like Gertrude Hertzfeld were appointed as an assistant surgeon to Sir John Fraser in 1919 and continued on the staff to her retirement in 1946. Another notable example was Isabella Forshall, who built up the paediatric surgical unit in Liverpool. Peter Rickham, in delivering the Forshall lecture in 1981, used "Women in Paediatric Surgery" as his topic and discussed some aspects of the changing face of medicine. The change in the sex ratio is marked as at the beginning of this 21st century, where 70% of our undergraduates in the Medical faculty are female. Paediatric surgery has the highest proportion of female consultants of any branch of surgery in Britain at the present time.

It is interesting to note how many of the distinguished surgeons had a particular interest in paediatric surgery. The standing of these surgeons can be judged by the fact that each ultimately received a Knighthood in recognition of their outstanding contributions to society. In London the Scot, **Sir Arbuthnot Lane**, made significant progress in the surgical field in the earlier part of the century in London. In Glasgow three of the early consultants appointed at the Children's Hospital became **Sir William Macewen**, **Sir Hector Clare Cameron** and **Sir Kennedy Dalziel,** while in Edinburgh **Sir Harold Styles** and **Sir James Fraser** were the surgical "chiefs" in the Children's Hospital for many years. All of these surgeons were general surgeons with an interest in what has evolved as paediatric surgery.

The first hospital to demand full-time commitment to paediatric work by consultant staff was the Glasgow Children's Hospital just prior to the First World War.[11] They had just completed building a new hospital by 1914. The Directors ruled that "Visiting Physicians and Visiting Surgeons must visit their wards every day and must not hold a regular visiting appointment in any other hospital".[8]

This ruling did not apply to the dispensary surgeons as every developing surgeon attempted to hold these children's hospital posts for a time. Such appointments were very important on their C.V. Most of the "chiefs" of the general surgical units in the West of Scotland had served an apprenticeship in these posts, but contrary to the statement made by Peter Rickham in Japan about the short tenure by Scottish surgeons at the children's hospitals, that only applied to the Dispensary staff and those appointed as visiting surgeons or "chiefs" had a very long period of tenure of their positions.

Teaching has been a significant aspect of the function of children's hospitals. In the 1880s at the St Mungo College — later incorporated into the University of Glasgow — courses of lectures were given on "Surgical Diseases of Children" (Table 3), apparently with more consistency than the parallel course in "Medical Diseases of Children". Undergraduate teaching was incorporated into the northern hospitals very soon after their opening. One of the original aims of the children's hospitals was teaching. One aspect was to teach what would currently be called parenthood and the other was to teach and train nurses and doctors in paediatric pathology, treatment and care.

Academia and Paediatric Surgery

It was not until 1919 that the University of Glasgow in collaboration with the Board of the Royal Hospital for Sick Children established a Lectureship in the Medical Diseases of Infancy and Childhood and one on Surgery and Orthopaedics in relation to Infancy and Childhood. These posts were endowed appointments by Gow and Barclay respectively.[12] They were paid appointments but the remuneration from them was very low and private practice was necessary to supplement income until the NHS salaried structure was introduced in 1948. Since 1919 a University surgical appointee has been maintained, now a Professor and the Barclay lecturer.

In 1957 the Nuffield Chair in Paediatric surgery was established when Denis Browne retired from NHS practice at the Hospital for Sick Children, London. This significant development of an academic

Table 3. Surgical paediatric lectures to students given in the latter part of the 19th century in Glasgow.

Lecturer — James A Adams, M.D., F.F.P.S.G.,
Assistant Surgeon to the Royal Infirmary.

The Course will be delivered during the Summer Session at 11.30 a.m., on Tuesday and Thursdays, and will include a consideration of the following subjects:

1. The management of infants and children during illness.
2. Diathesis — Haemorrhagic; Tuberculosis; Struma; Rachitis, & c.
3. Syphilis.
4. Fractures.
5. Dislocations.
6. Affections of the Joints.
7. Diseases of Periosteum and Bone.
8. Glandular Disease — Cervical; Axillary; Femoral; Hodgkin's Disease.
9. Congenital Malformations — Hare Lip; Cleft Palate; Spina bifida and encephalocele; Talipes; Wry neck; Imperforate anus and rectum; malformations of foot and hand.
10. Tumours — Innocent; Malignant; Congenital.
11. Diphtheria — Laringitis; Croup; Tracheotomy and its alternatives.
12. Burns — Scalds; subsequent deformities.
13. Diseases of the spinal column — Caries; angular and lateral curvature.
14. Empyaema — Hydrothorax.
15. Paralysis — Psuedo-Hypertrophic, Tetany; Spastic Paralysis; Neuroninesis, & c.
16. Genito — Urinary Affections.-Extroversion of the bladder; Hypospadias; Phimosis; Paraphimosis; Masturbation; Hermaphroditism; Calculus; Lithotomy; Lithotrity; Incontinence of urine.
17. Hernia.
18. Abdominal diseases — Peritonitis; Obstruction; Tabes; Tumours; rectum and anus.
19. Organs of special sense.
20. Aural disease — Its influence upon intracranial abscess.
21. Foreign bodies in Eye, Ear, Nose, & c.

---

department was headed by Andrew Wilkinson — a committed "Scot" who never forgave the fact that he was born in England! Departments have been much slower to develop on the surgical side than in the medical. The lack of departments has also been part of the vicious circle that with the limited number of trainee academics there has been delay in advancing the specialty.

All of the undergraduate medical schools have paediatric departments but some of the delay in development of surgical departments has been due to some surgeons who felt strongly that paediatric surgery should be a postgraduate exercise, whereas in other universities paediatric surgery has been an essential part of the final examination for medical graduation. In general surgeons involved in research have retained connections to the larger university departments to obtain adequate funding rather than to concentrate fully on the paediatric field because better facilities exist.

Training of Paediatric Surgeons

Postgraduate training was in the main part of the 20th century largely done by the apprenticeship approach. By the last quarter of the century, substantial changes were evolving and an increasing amount of attention was focussed on training and of tuition of the younger surgeons. The Specialist Advisory Committees were established by agreement between the separate surgical colleges in the British Isles and these supervised the centres approved for training in the initial eight branches of surgery agreed at that time. Paediatric Surgery was one of these accepted specialist groups. Assessment by the older examination systems was gradually reviewed and in the 1980's the intercollegiate fellowship examinations were agreed as an "exit" assessment of the individuals toward the end of their official training. The first intercollegiate examination in paediatric surgery was held in 1989 so that now there is in effect an entrance hurdle — the FRCS exam, now revised to the MRCS — and an exit examination (FRCS) towards the end of their official surgical training.

Political input into the scene has become a significant factor in the last two decades. With the European Economic Community extending its areas of interest and activity, this has significant effects on training schedules. The substantial changes in the organisation of the medical training in the current decade have been attempted at a rate beyond which the system could cope and this has led to a current situation of difficulty for the young graduates to have much control over their progress in the specialties and to the political removal of the more ancient supervisory roles the Colleges have over the competence of individuals practising in specialties. Change has to continue to achieve a balance for the society's care. The move currently is for a means of establishing competence in many facets of activity that are necessary for the surgical competence. Proof of the value of this significant change is awaited.

Clubs and Associations

The development in 1948 of the Scottish Surgical Paediatric Club (SSPC), later to change to the Scottish Surgical Paediatric Society (SSPS), is documented in the Supplement to the *Journal of Paediatric Surgery* by Willie Bisset (1930–2008) and Robert Carachi.[13] The subsequent development (1953) of the British Association of Paediatric Surgeons (BAPS) is documented by the outstanding paediatric urologist — Sir David Innes Williams — who was in Great Ormond Street staff at the time and gives an accurate overview of the development.[14] He notes that the SSPC had a meeting in London in 1951 and that it was from that the concept of a Society developed. Twistington Higgins hosted a meeting in London at which he ensured that the Scots were included and the concept grew as reported until the first meeting was held in 1953. Denis Browne was the first President as the previous senior surgeon Twistington Higgins (TTH) had retired in 1952. TTH was described as "the gentlest of men whose every characteristic was the antithesis of his colleague" and was the first Honorary member of the SSPC. The first official meeting forming BAPS was held in November 1953. The first executive committee appointed with Denis Browne as Chairman. The inaugural meeting in 1954 was held in London and to which a number of overseas surgeons were invited. The international aspect of the association grew rapidly as the second meeting in Glasgow had 12 surgeons from overseas, but by 1962, 120 overseas surgeons attended the annual congress.

References

1. Johnston DG, quoting Abraham Lincoln. *J Pediatr Surg* 1980; 21:1019–1031.
2. Pearn J, *Arch Dis Child*: personal communication.
3. Franklin AW. In Poynter FNL (ed.), *The Evolution of Hospitals in Britain*. Pitman Publishing Co., London 1964, pp. 103–122.
4. Dunn PM. George Armstrong MD (1719–1789) and his dispensary for the infant poor. *Arch Dis Child* 2002;87:f228.
5. *British and Foreign Medico-Chirurgical Review*. 1849, p. 409.
6. Baldwin N. About Great Ormond Street Hospital (GOS), The history of GOSH; The whole story. http://www.ich.ucl.uk/ablut_gosh/history/story/index.html
7. Johnston A. Surgery of childhood. *Brit Med J* 1861;1:1–4, 41–47, 61–63.
8. Holmes T. *Surgical Treatment of the Diseases of Infancy and Childhood*. Longmans, Green, Reader and Dyer, London, 1868.
9. Young DG. *J Roy Col Surg Edin*. 1999;44:211–215.
10. Hospital for Sick Children, Glasgow Archives. *Minute Book* 1:134.
11. Royal Hospital for Sick Children, Glasgow Archives. *Minute Book* 5:360.
12. Royal Hospital for Sick Children, Glasgow, 36th Annual Report for the year ending 31st December 1918, p. 14.
13. Bisset WH, Carachi R. British Association of Paediatric Surgeons 50th Anniversary. *J Pediatr Surg* 2003;7(1):2–5.
14. Williams Sir DI. British Association of Paediatric Surgeons 50th Anniversary. *J Pediatr Surg* 2003;7(1):6–9.

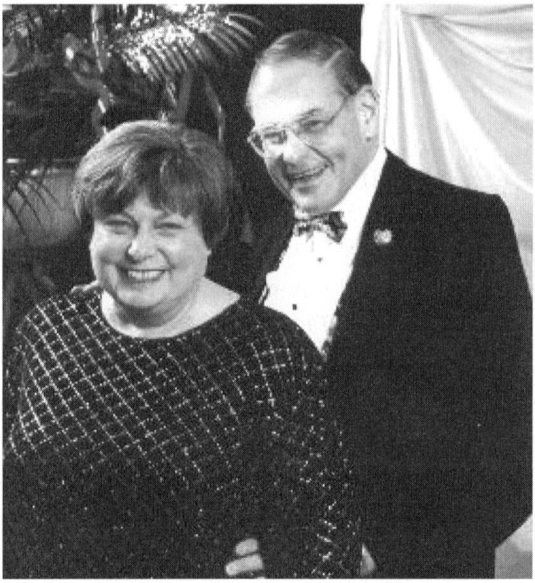

Arlene Ein and Sigmund H. Ein

CANADA

Sigmund H. Ein
Arlene Ein

Introduction

This chapter is dedicated to those men and women in Canada whose love of Pediatric (Paediatric) Surgery and its patients has made this specialty what it is today. We feel that once Pediatric Surgery was established in a certain area, our historical job was finished; our focus was on the history of its beginning.

For the most part today (December 2008), a Pediatric Surgeon is a General Surgeon who is trained, experienced and comfortable operating upon various organ systems in the infant's and child's body. However, the individual surgical disciplines have become subspecialized and many Pediatric Surgeons have obtained extra training in some surgical specialty.[1] Therefore, for the purpose of this historical review, the major focus has been on Pediatric Surgery, as practiced by Pediatric General Surgeons, focusing their expertise, generally-speaking, on the head and neck, chest and abdomen (including genitourinary and reproductive systems). Exceptions to this generalization can and do occur, according to the "when in Rome rule," and are so described herein, if and when the situation is appropriate.

At the time of writing this chapter, Canada is a large country (3.8 million square miles, nine million square kilometers)[2] with a small population (33 million).[3] It consists of ten provinces and three territories[2] with 60% of the population in Ontario and Québec, and almost 85% in Ontario, Québec, British Columbia and Alberta[3] concentrated in the areas close to the United States border. The three territories of Yukon Territory, Northwest Territories and Nunavut account for over a third of Canada's area, but have a smaller combined population than the smallest province, Prince Edward Island.[3] In Canada, there are presently >340,000 births per year, 14 births per 1000 population, and 28% of the population is < 19 years old.[4,5] From these births, there are almost 700 babies born with a congenital anomaly every year.[5] There are presently 50 Pediatric Surgeons practicing in Canada, with a ratio of 1/600,000 population.[6]

There were really two eras in the historical development of Canadian Pediatric Surgery:

(1) The first era started about 1900 in the big cities (Toronto, Montreal), where a few Adult General Surgeons did whatever Pediatric Surgery they could until the trained Pediatric Surgeons came along. Some Adult General Surgeons did it because they had to; others did it because they liked to. Regardless of the reason, they were the Real Pioneers, because they unofficially developed the specialty, but were never formally trained for it. As such, they were usually amalgamated into the new children's hospitals, if and when they came along in their area. The first of 16 present children's hospitals in Canada was the Hospital for Sick Children (HSC) in Toronto, Ontario, which opened in 1875.[7]
(2) The second era was in the 1950s and 1960s when the first "real" Pediatric Surgeons received their formal training and started practicing in each of the larger cities, like Vancouver, Regina, Calgary, Edmonton, Winnipeg, London, Toronto, Kingston, Ottawa, Montreal, Québec City, Halifax and St John's. Things became even more specialized and consolidated after the Canadian Association of Paediatric Surgeons (CAPS) formed in 1967.

Newfoundland and Labrador

St John's. The earliest surgery performed on children consisted mostly of tonsillectomies, adenoidectomies and hernias. The first major attempt to treat anomalies was done by Dr Nigel Rusted in 1950. He went to Toronto (Hospital for Sick Children, HSC) and spent some time with Dr Arthur LeMesurier (Chief of Surgery at HSC, 1944–1950) and learned the LeMesurier procedure for the repair of cleft lip and palate.[8]

In the late 1950s trained General Surgeons from various programs in Canada and the United States returned to Newfoundland and began performing more procedures on children with varying degrees of success.[8]

Prior to 1966, most of the Pediatric Surgery was done at **St John's General Hospital** initially by Drs Baird, Brownrigg, Cater, Horan, Neary and Rusted.[9] In 1959, Dr Richard Kennedy (trained in Montreal, Montreal Children's Hospital — MCH) started his Pediatric Surgical practice (the first to do so in Newfoundland) with admitting privileges at three hospitals. He became involved with the group promoting a separate children's hospital. When The **Janeway Children's Hospital** opened, he was appointed Chief of Surgery in December 1965, with the task of developing a surgical department.[8,9]

Nova Scotia

Nova Scotia has the only children's hospital in the three Maritime Provinces (Nova Scotia, New Brunswick, Prince Edward Island) established in Halifax in 1909.[9]

Halifax. Major abdominal and thoracic surgical procedures on Pediatric patients were first performed in the old children's hospital in the 1940s by a few Adult General Surgeons, especially Dr Merritt. In the late 1950s Dr Paul Nonamaker succeeded Dr Merritt and was the first to successfully treat esophageal atresia and congenital diaphragmatic hernia in Halifax.[9]

Dr Alexander Gillis (a Nova Scotian) joined the staff in 1961; he was the first Nova Scotian Pediatric Surgeon, and was trained at the Children's Memorial Hospital in Chicago by Drs Willis J. Potts, Orvar Swenson, and Paul Hollinger (Pediatric Otolaryngology).[9] He carried on with all aspects of Pediatric General Surgery, including endoscopy.

The new **Izaak Walton Killam Hospital** for children was opened in 1970 adjacent to the old Halifax Children's Hospital. Dr Gillis became the first Chief of Surgery.[9] In 1988, Dr Gillis established the sixth Canadian Pediatric Surgery Training Program, training one Chief Resident (Fellow) every two years.[10]

Prince Edward Island and New Brunswick

It is assumed that whatever Pediatric Surgical problems did arise in the past were either sent to the nearest children's hospital (St John's, Halifax, Québec City, Montreal), or handled locally by an Adult General Surgeon with an interest, but no formal training, in Pediatric Surgery.

Québec

Québec has two of the 16 children's hospitals in Canada, both in Montreal.[7] Pediatric Surgery is practiced at this point in time (October 2007) in three cities: Québec City, Montreal and Sherbrooke.

Québec City. The development of Pediatric Surgery in Québec City started in the late 1960s and early 1970s, due to the efforts of Drs Jacques Turcot (President of The Royal College of Physicians and Surgeons of Canada, and a Founding Member of the Canadian Association of Paediatric Surgeons), Wilfred Caron (Chief of the Department of Surgery at Laval University), and Louis Levasseur. In 1972, Dr Raymond Cloutier (trained in Montreal (St Justine) and Australia) joined Dr Levasseur and Pediatric Surgery was established.[11]

Most of the pediatric surgery continues to be practiced in the **Centre Mère Infant**, which is part of the **Centre Hospitalier Universitaire de Quebec** (CHUQ).[11]

Montreal. In Montreal, a bilingual city, Pediatric Surgery was always practiced in two locations, one primarily treating English-speaking

(Anglophone) and the other French-speaking (Francophone) patients.

The **Montreal Children's Hospital (MCH)** was founded in 1903, and has always been the children's hospital which treated a majority of English-speaking patients. Although, Dr Alexander Forbes, an Orthopedic Surgeon, played a key role at the MCH from 1904 to 1929, Dr Dudley Ross, who led the Department of Surgery from 1937–1954, was largely responsible for establishing the first modern children's surgical unit in The Province of Québec. In 1938, Canada's first operation to repair a congenital heart defect was performed at The MCH, and in 1948, Dr Ross reported the first successful repair of an esophageal atresia in Canada.[12,13]

Following Dr Ross, Dr David Murphy Sr. served as Chief of Pediatric Surgery from 1953 to 1974, and he started the fifth Pediatric Surgery Training Program in North America and the first in Canada; it graduates one trainee every year.[10] The MCH moved to its current location across from the old Montreal Forum (former home of The Montreal Canadiens hockey team), in 1956 and had 210 beds with more than 60 surgical beds.[13]

During his 20 years as Chief of Surgery, Dr David Murphy had on his staff his first trainee, Dr Harvey Beardmore, along with Drs Herb Owen and Gordon Karn. Dr Beardmore later went on to establish an international reputation both as a Pediatric Surgeon and as a spokesperson for this new specialty. In 1967 he was one of The Founding Members of the Canadian Association of Pediatric Surgeons and was its first President. He also became the Training Program Director in 1974 and he was influential in 1975 in convincing the previously (1950s and 1960s) reticent American Board of Surgery to grant a new Certificate of Special Competence in Pediatric Surgery to all qualified applicants.[12,13] He was truly a Pioneer in Canadian Pediatric Surgery.

Pediatrics did not exist as a specialty in Montreal in the early 1900s. Initially, **St Justine Hospital** was staffed by ten to 12 General Practitioners, who also formed the hospital's first Medical Board and then concentrated their practice on children's diseases, becoming self-taught Pediatric specialists.[10]

Dr Pierre-Paul Collin (trained in St Louis) came to the hospital in 1954 bringing Pediatric (especially Thoracic) Surgical experience. Prior to that, very little major Pediatric Surgery had been attempted in any of the French-speaking Montreal hospitals. Dr Paul Maurice Ricard at Notre-Dame Hospital had successfully repaired an esophageal atresia patient with a subcutaneous skin tube replacement.[9] The present hospital was opened in 1957 with 900 beds, after its frame stood incomplete for many years on Côte St Catherine Road. This site was purposely chosen to be located in close proximity to The University of Montreal and its Faculty of Medicine.[10]

Dr Collin became Chief of General Surgery in 1964 and in the same year the first Pediatric Surgery Training Program in Canada started, training a new Resident (Fellow) every year.[10] Soon after Dr Collin arrived in the mid-1950s (and ten years before the Training Program at St Justine became official), Dr Lucille Teasdale was the first Pediatric Surgery trainee at St Justine (and probably the first female Pediatric Surgeon in Canada); she soon moved to Uganda, where she opened a hospital.[14] A number of Canada's Chiefs of Pediatric Surgery, especially in Montreal, including Drs Frank Guttman, Hervé Blanchard, Salam Yazbeck and Jean-Martin Laberge were trained by Dr Collin.[10] In 1966, he became The Director of Surgery at St Justine.

Dr Jacques Duchrame (trained in Columbus) was recruited in 1960 and was the first fully trained Pediatric General Surgeon at St Justine, and succeeded Dr Collin as Director of the Department of Surgery. In 1980, Dr Hervé Blanchard (trained in Montréal, St Justine) followed Dr Collin as Program Director and also started the Liver Transplant Program. In 1986, Dr Jean Desjardins (trained in Toronto) became Chief of the Division of General Surgery and Program Director.[15]

The **University of Sherbrooke Medical School** was founded in the mid-1960s and at that time, in Sherbrooke, Adult General Surgeons did all of the Pediatric Surgery on older children, referring all of the neonatal and infant surgery as well as the complicated and oncology cases to Montreal.[15]

Pediatric Surgery was started there in 1971 when Dr Raymond Cloutier (trained in Montreal, at St Justine and Australia) arrived to start a Pediatric Surgery practice in a University Hospital setting, but in 1972 he moved to Québec City.[15] In 1999, Dr Sandeep K. Mayer, Jr. (trained in Montreal at St Justine), moved from Hamilton to Sherbrooke to become the second Pediatric Surgeon in the city (albeit 16 years apart).

Ontario

As of December 2008, Pediatric Surgery is practiced in Ottawa, Kingston, Toronto, Hamilton and London.

Ottawa. Dr Stanley Mercer (trained in Toronto) was the first Pediatric Surgeon in Ottawa and arrived in 1956. At that time, he found that the Ottawa General Hospital was the main teaching hospital of the University of Ottawa and was mostly French-speaking, while the Ottawa Civic Hospital, also a teaching institution, was affiliated with Queen's University in Kingston, Ontario. Shortly after Dr Mercer's arrival, both hospitals became formally affiliated with The Medical School at the University of Ottawa. At that time, there were children's wards at both hospitals and well-established Pediatric services, but no surgeons restricted their practices only to Pediatric Surgery. At the Civic Hospital, where Dr Mercer had his first appointment, Dr Kenneth Smith did a small volume of Pediatric Surgery. He offered strong support for Dr Mercer's efforts to gain specialty recognition for Pediatric Surgery in Ottawa.[9]

The **Children's Hospital of Eastern Ontario (CHEO)** in Ottawa is one of only two free-standing children's hospitals in Canada and the last one (1974) to be built;[7] it was a 278-bed facility in which all major specialties within Pediatric Surgery are fully available. Dr Mercer was the first Chief of The Department of Surgery, and the Division of General Surgery, as well as being Professor of Surgery at the University of Ottawa and firmly established Pediatric Surgery in Ottawa. A Pediatric Surgery Training Program was established in

1987 (the fifth in Canada) by Dr Mercer, and graduates one trainee every other year.[10]

KINGSTON. As with many cities throughout Canada, until the last few decades, most Pediatric Surgery was done by a handful of Adult General Surgeons with an interest, but no formal training, in Pediatric Surgery. Such was also the case in **Kingston**, 250 kilometers east of Toronto. Drs Jack Kerr and Giovanni Paloschi both did Pediatric Surgery as well as Adult General Surgery during the 1950s and 1960s. The **Kingston Children's Hospital** (not free-standing) was opened in 1953. In 1994, Dr Dan Poenaru (trained in Montreal at St Justine) was the first fully trained Pediatric Surgeon to locate in Kingston.[17]

Toronto. In Toronto, beside the Hospital for Sick Children (HSC), Pediatric Surgery has been practiced in three other large general hospitals: St Joseph's Health Center, North York General, and Toronto East General.

The **Hospital for Sick Children (HSC)** in Toronto was established in 1875 by Mrs. Elizabeth McMaster (whose husband founded McMaster University in Hamilton) and a group of visionary and dedicated women friends, and was the first children's hospital in Canada as well as in the British Empire, outside the United Kingdom.[18]

Many of the children who were admitted up to 1914, World War I, (WWI) required treatment for the complications of infections diseases, particularly tuberculosis. The latter often presented with spinal deformities and/or hip or knee joint disease. Some operations were undertaken, but it remains unclear in those early days just who were the operating surgeons. In 1913, Dr Clarence Starr (an Orthopedic Surgeon) became the first Surgeon-in-Chief. He and his Associate Chief of Surgery (Dr William Edward Gallie) completely reorganized the surgical staff, and chose what they considered to be promising young men for staff appointments. Starr remained as Chief of Surgery until 1921 (when he became Professor of Surgery at the University of Toronto). He was succeeded by Dr Gallie.[1]

Dr Donald E. Robertson succeeded Dr Gallie as Chief of Surgery in 1929 and carried the HSC Surgery Department through both the Great Depression and World War II (WWII). Regrettably, Dr Robertson died in February 1944. He is also remembered for a right upper quadrant subcostal muscle-splitting (Robertson) incision lateral to the right rectus muscle for the treatment of pyloric stenosis in marasmic (malnourished) infants. Of necessity, Dr Arthur B. LeMesurier became Chief of Surgery from 1944 to 1950. He was a Plastic and Orthopedic Surgeon, well-known for his cleft lip and spinal scoliosis operations.[1]

The sixth and present hospital was a new building (holding 800 beds) at 555 University Avenue; it was first occupied in February 1951. Dr Robert M. (Tim) Wansbrough was the fifth Chief of Surgery (1951–1956), and he performed the first emergency operation in this new hospital at noon[18] on the day of the move, for a baby with pyloric stenosis, using the Robertson incision. Dr Wansbrough was also responsible for the non-operative (conservative) management of the damaged spleen.[19]

It was not until Dr A. W. Farmer became the sixth Chief of Surgery at HSC in 1956 that the Division of General Surgery was created. Prior to that, the Pediatric Surgeons, without any formal training (Mustard, Wansbrough, Wilkinson, Walker, to name a few), did most Pediatric Surgical cases with very little specialization. When Dr Farmer returned to HSC after WWII, he was certified as a Plastic, Orthopedic and General Surgeon. He also brought his organizational experience that he had acquired as Medical Director at a Veterans' Hospital and he applied the concept of military stratification to create six Divisions (which remain today) within the Department of Surgery.[1]

In 1967, Dr Clinton Stephens succeeded Dr Stuart Thomson as Chief of General Surgery and during his ten years as Chief, he initiated the third Canadian Pediatric Surgery Training Program in 1967, with one of the authors (SHE) being the first trainee in the HSC two-year program.[10] He along with the help of his 2 close colleagues, Dr Jones Simpson (trained in Toronto and England) and Barry Shandling (trained in South Africa, England and Toronto) established Pediatric General Surgery at HSC, as we know it today.

Dr James Fallis (trained in Toronto) was initially on the Surgical Staff at The Hospital for Sick Children (HSC), Toronto from 1962 to 1968. In 1968, he became the Senior Pediatric Surgeon of The Imperial Order of the Daughters of the Empire (I.O.D.E.) at the new **North York General Hospital (NYGH)** when it opened that year; it was an independent children's wing of a new ultra-modern general hospital in Northern Toronto.[9] In 1980, Dr Noelle Grace (trained in Montreal) moved from the Montreal Children's Hospital to continue Pediatric Surgery at the NYGH. She[19] was the first formally trained female Pediatric Surgeon in Canada as well as the first female member of CAPS.[20]

When Dr Michael Allen finished his Pediatric Surgery training in Toronto, he started his long and successful practice of Pediatric Surgery at the **Toronto East General Hospital** in 1966, which continued until he retired in the mid-1990s.

In the western part of Toronto, at **St Joseph's Health Care Center**, two Adult General Surgeons, Drs John McIntyre and Michael Baida, did a fair amount of Pediatric General Surgery from the 1950s and 1960s until their retirement in the 1980s. Dr David Lindsay carries on in a similar vein since 1999.

Hamilton. Before Dr Gordon Cameron arrived, whatever Pediatric Surgery there was in Hamilton was done, suffice it to say, by Adult General Surgeons with pre- and post-operative care assisted by Pediatricians in the area.[7] Dr Cameron finished his Pediatric Surgical training Toronto in 1957, having been the first Chief Surgical Resident for both Chief of Surgery, Dr A. W. Farmer and Chief of The Division of General Surgery, Dr Stuart Thomson. After a 6 month stay at Great Ormand Street Hospital, London he then returned to Hamilton in 1958, where he became the very first Pediatric Surgeon in that city. In a few years, Pediatric Surgery was well established in Hamilton.[21]

By the end of the 1960s and early 1970s, McMaster Medical School was started and Drs Barry Sachs (trained in Pittsburgh) and George Lau (trained in Toronto) joined Dr Cameron in his busy practice which was divided between St Joseph's Hospital and the new University Hospital.[22]

As of October 2008, the Pediatric Surgery group at **McMaster Children's Hospital** headed by Dr Peter Fitzgerald became the 8th Canadian Pediatric Surgery Training Program.[23]

London. In May 1919, the construction of a children's hospital in London, Ontario was first proposed as a monument to those who participated in WWI from 1914 to 1918, and opened in 1923.[24,25]

By 1945, Dr Angus D. McLachlin had been made Professor and Head of the Department of Surgery, at the University of Western Ontario Medical School and also Chief of Surgery at the Victoria Hospital. He was the first surgeon in London to do some Pediatric Surgery, including esophageal atresia repairs.[24] Dr Donald Marshall (Trained in Toronto) was the first trained Pediatric Surgeon in London, arriving in 1957 and worked at both St Joseph's Hospital[22] and The Children's Hospital. In September 1975, a separate Division of Pediatric Surgery was initiated and supported by the Departments of Surgery, Pediatrics, and The Senate of the University of Western Ontario. This was one of the first universities in Canada to recognize Pediatric Surgery as an autonomous Division within the Department of Surgery.[25]

In 1995, The Children's Hospital of Western Ontario at the Victoria Hospital and the University Hospital merged into the London Health Sciences Centre (LHSC) although the Children's Hospital continues to have an autonomous Board of Directors.

Manitoba

Winnipeg. There were 2 hospitals in Winnipeg that were involved with the development of pediatric surgery: the Children's Hospital of Winnipeg and St Boniface General Hospital.[26]

The development of surgery at **The Children's Hospital of Winnipeg** may arbitrarily be divided into three phases. Phase 1 covers the first decade (1909–1919) and includes the first group of staff surgeons who were, for the most part, General Practitioners

(GP) in private practice, with some extra training and experience in surgery.[27]

The Children's Hospital of Winnipeg first opened its doors on February 6, 1909, in an old house on Beaconsfield Street in Winnipeg. The first three General Surgeons (who[24] did the Pediatric Surgical operations at that time) were Drs D. S. MacKay, William Kenny and Neil J. MacLean.

The second phase of surgical care lasted from the end of WWI (1919) until 1953. This period was featured by more effective organization of the Surgical Staff who were assigned responsibilities in their special field of interest. Dr J. D. McEachern (who joined the Staff in 1920), acted as Chief of Surgery from 1926–1940. Drs Stewart McInnes and Donald McIntyre were GPs with extra surgical training and experience; Dr McInnes specialized in the treatment of fractures and acute surgical emergencies (appendicitis, burns and bowel obstructions), and Dr McIntyre specialized in abdominal surgery. There continued to be regular additions to the Surgical Staff by mostly Manitoba graduates, who took special surgical training overseas. Among these were Dr Cecil Clark (a General Surgeon with a special interest in abdominal surgery in children), Dr Norman Merkeley (also a General Surgeon, with expertise in Plastic Surgery, especially the repair of cleft lips and palates), and Dr Gordon Fahrni (a General Surgeon trained at The Mayo Clinic and at the Hospital for Sick Children in Toronto).[27]

The third phase of development of Pediatric Surgery centered around a very young Dr Colin Ferguson. He was both a Winnipegger and a Manitoba graduated who joined the Surgical Staff of the Children's Hospital of Winnipeg in 1951 (after training in Montreal and Philadelphia), but was given two years leave of absence to complete his Pediatric Surgical training with Dr Robert Gross at the Children's Hospital in Boston. On January 1, 1954, he was also appointed as the Surgeon-in-Chief of the Children's Hospital of Winnipeg[28] and established a neonatal surgical unit and one for the correction of congenital heart disease.[9,29] He reorganized the surgical residency training at all of the teaching hospitals, to bring these programs entirely under university control, and established an experimental animal surgical laboratory at the Medical College.[29] It was obvious, he had great surgical expertise, teaching skills and a remarkable ability to attract excellent young people to take up this career.[30] In 1956, the Children's Hospital of Winnipeg moved from its Aberdeen Street location to be near the Medical School of the University of Manitoba and the Winnipeg General Hospital.[28]

St Boniface General Hospital has been a longstanding institution in Winnipeg, serving a large section of the Anglophone and Francophone population. Early on, as in most general hospitals, Pediatric Surgery was carried out by many Adult General Surgeons, however, in the 1970s, 1980s and 1990s, Drs Tom Goodhand and Nathan Wiseman were primarily involved in the Pediatric Surgery.[26]

The new era of Pediatric Surgery was underway. The main focus of Pediatric Surgery has always centered around the equivalent of the Children's Hospital of Winnipeg, now the Health Science Centre.[26]

Saskatchewan

Pediatric Surgery has been practiced (to a greater or lesser degree) in three Saskatchewan cities since the late 1940s: Moose Jaw, Regina and Saskatoon.[31,32] Following WWII, there was a continued comradery amongst those doctors who served in The Canadian Armed Forces. This led to the establishment of The Western Surgical Society, which was a multi-disciplinary society of all surgeons in the three Prairie Provinces. On a rotation basis, each province would host a Spring Meeting and it was expected that each member of the hosting province would present a paper. Pediatric Surgical subjects took a fairly prominent place each year.[33]

Dr Fred Morris was trained in Toronto and in 1964 he returned to **Moose Jaw** to do Adult General Surgery and some Pediatric Surgery.[33]

In **Regina**, in the 1940s, a number of practicing adult general and thoracic surgeons, like Drs Clayton Grosfie and Dr Frank

Schroeder, developed increasing skills in dealing with congenital problems (congenital bowel obstructions, cleft lips and palates, esophageal atresia, missing arteriosis ligation and Swenson pull-through procedures).[9,33]

In 1960–1961, Dr Murray Fraser spent six months learning Pediatric Surgery with Dr William Clatworthy in Columbus. About the same time (1962), Dr Angus Juckes was trained in Toronto and then headed back out West and landed in Regina temporarily, but stayed for the long term. He was joined by Dr Fraser, and both initially practiced Adult and Pediatric General Surgery.[31]

In 1978, Dr Juckes took the position of Director of Continuing Medical Education for southern Saskatchewan and by then was practicing Pediatric Surgery full-time together with Dr Fraser, who stopped doing Adult General Surgery in 1993.[31]

Saskatoon. Pediatric Surgery in Saskatoon (the surgical center for northern Saskatchewan) was largely non-existent as a specialty until after WWII in the late 1940s. Even then, what little there was, was done was by Adult General Surgeons. Dr Robert W. Cram (from Swift Current, Saskatchewan) was the first Pediatric Surgeon in Saskatoon (if not in Saskatchewan), arriving in 1952; he was trained in Toronto and Detroit. He confined his Pediatric Surgical practice to the City Hospital, where he served as Chief of Surgery and also became Clinical Professor Surgery at the University of Saskatchewan in Saskatoon, a position he maintained until he retired in 1982.[32] It was not until 1992 that Dr Grant Miller (trained in Vancouver) came to Saskatoon from Chicago as a full-time Pediatric Surgeon with the **University of Saskatoon**.[34]

Alberta

The only cities in Alberta where any Pediatric Surgery of note was (and is) practiced are Calgary and Edmonton.

Calgary. It was in Calgary in 1922 that the Red Cross developed the first children's hospital (Red Cross Children's Hospital) in Alberta in a rented house, where care was provided for 35 children with Orthopedic problems. Because no operating room (OR) facilities were included in this new small hospital, whatever operative treatment was necessary took place at the Calgary General Hospital.[9]

In 1952, a completely modern hospital on Richmond Road was constructed with 128 beds and two fully-equipped ORs. Dr Gordon Townsend, an Orthopedic Surgeon, was the driving force in the development of a separate children's hospital, at a time when the emphasis was on the care of disabled children. Since Orthopedic problems constituted the main initial workload, the hospitals' name was changed to the Alberta Crippled Children's Hospital in 1957, but in 1960, because an increasing variety of Pediatric cases were being admitted, it became known as the **Alberta Children's Hospital.**[9,35]

Dr Geoffrey Seagram arrived in Calgary in August 1972, after completing his training in Toronto. He was the first trained Pediatric Surgeon in Calgary.[35,36] Initially, as in other similar pioneering situations, his position was not readily supported by the General Surgeons, who had traditionally accepted responsibility for treating Pediatric Surgical problems.[36] In 2002, the Alberta Children's Hospital became the seventh Canadian Pediatric Surgical Training Program, training a resident every two years.[37]

Edmonton. Dr Sam Kling arrived in Edmonton in 1951 and was the first Pediatric Surgeon in Edmonton (as well as in Alberta, by more than 20 years). He was trained in Toronto and was the Chief Resident in General Surgery at the Hospital for Sick Children (HSC) in Toronto in 1950 under Dr Arthur B. LeMesurier, then Chief of Surgery at HSC. He had a keen interest in medical education and research, which he pursued at the University of Alberta as Professor of Surgery and Associate Dean of the Faculty of Medicine. He was also a Founding Member of CAPS in 1967. Since then, Pediatric Surgery has continued with Dr James Fischer (trained in Seattle) and Gordon Lees (trained in Seattle and the U.K.). In the mid to late 1990s, all Pediatric Surgery was consolidated at the **University of Alberta Hospital/Stollery Children's Hospital**. This tertiary and quaternary referral center was one of the first to have Pediatric Transplant, and congenital Cardiac Surgery programs for Western Canada. It is safe to say that, apart from the occasional appendicitis, virtually all Pediatric Surgical cases less than 17 years of age from Northwestern and Central Canada are referred to this and other Western Canadian Pediatric Surgical Centers.[38]

British Columbia

In this Province, Pediatric Surgery is presently practiced by fully trained Pediatric Surgeons only in Vancouver and Victoria.

Vancouver. Until the mid 1950s, the surgery of children had principally been carried out by Adult Surgeons in various specialties. Drs S. Elliott Harrison, George Saxton, William Trapp, and Ross Robertson all did occasional Pediatric Surgical cases at the **Vancouver General Hospital**, and Dr Robert Gourlay did the same at St Paul's Hospital, also in Vancouver. Dr J. Russell Neilson (General Surgeon) also saw an increasing number of children in his practice and was especially interested in cleft lip and palate surgery. He is considered to be the first surgeon in Vancouver to specialize, in Pediatric Surgery, as it was then known.[39] Dr Phil Ashmore (trained in Toronto) returned to Vancouver in 1957 and was the first to restrict his surgical practice to infants and children, apart from Dr Neilson, who had done no chest surgery. Following Dr Ashmore, two other surgeons with special training in Pediatric Surgery also commenced their practices in Vancouver: Dr Murray Kliman (trained in London at the Hospital for Sick Children at Great Ormond Street) and Dr Russ Marshall (trained in Toronto). They formed the core group of what became the first Department (Division) of Pediatric Surgery in Vancouver.[39] In 1967, Dr Graham Fraser (trained in London, the Hospital for Sick Children at Great Ormond Street) joined the above three Pediatric Surgeons. Pediatric Surgery was also now recognized as a Division of the Department of Surgery, at the University of British Columbia (UBC) Medical School.[39]

The new **British Columbia Children's Hospital** opened in 1982, and four years later it became the fourth (of eight, as of December 2008) Canadian Pediatric Surgery Training Program, with Dr Fraser as its first Director. One Pediatric Surgical trainee is graduated from this training program every other year.[10]

Victoria. Review of the earliest operating room records of The **Royal Jubilee Hospital** in Victoria around 1910 reveals that the surgeons of that day operated on some Pediatric patients with cleft lips, palates and neck masses. It was not until the late 1940s that the first surgeon (Dr H. S. Ford) with Pediatric Surgical exposure in his training (at the Hospital for Sick Children, Toronto) arrived in Victoria and performed major Pediatric Surgical procedures. In 1968 he was joined by Dr James C. Donald, who had just completed his training in Seattle, as the first Chief Resident at the Children's Hospital under Dr Alexander Bill. Dr Donald was the first fully trained and certified Pediatric Surgeon on Vancouver Island.[40]

At this time (late 1960s), most of the Pediatric Surgery was done at the **Royal Jubilee Hospital**, where the first Pediatric and Neonatal Intensive Care Units (PICU, NICU) were opened. By the 1970s, most of the major Pediatric Surgical procedures (except Cardiac) were now done in Victoria.[40]

Yukon Territory, Northwest Territory, Nunavut

Whatever Pediatric Surgical problems that do arise are either sent to the nearest children's hospital in Western Canada, or attended to locally by an Adult General Surgeon with an interest, but no formal training, in Pediatric Surgery.

References

1. Humphreys RP. *The History of the Department of Surgery at The Hospital for Sick Children.* Hospital for Sick Children, Toronto, 2007.
2. Land and fresh water area, by province and territory. *Statistics Canada,* 2005.

3. Population estimates. *Statistics Canada*, 1 January 2008.
4. Age groups and sex for population of Canada. *Statistics Canada*, 2006.
5. *Toronto Sun*. September 2007.
6. O'Neill JA Jr, Gautam S, Geiger JD, *et al.* A longitudinal analysis of the pediatric surgeon workforce. *Ann Surg* 2000;232:442–453
7. Stang AS, Joshi A. The evolution of freestanding children's hospitals in Canada. *Paediatr Child Health* 2000;11:501–506.
8. Kennedy R. *Personal communication*, 2008.
9. Delarue NC. *Thoracic Surgery in Canada*. Decker, Toronto, 1989.
10. Glick PL, Azizkhan RG. *A Genealagy of American Pediatric Surgery: From Ladd Until Now*, 1st ed. Quality Medical, St Louis, 1997.
11. Cloutier R. Personal communication, 2008.
12. Randolph J, Young DG. A brief history of pediatric surgery. In: Grosfeld JL, O'Neill JA Jr, Coran AG, Fonkalsrud EW (eds.) *Pediatric Surgery*. Mosby Elsevier, Philadelphia, 2006, p. 3–10.
13. Scriver JB. *The Montreal Children's Hospital. Years of Growth*. McGill-Queen's University Press, Montreal, 1979.
14. Bass J. Personal communication, 2008
15. Desjardins, J. Personal communication, 2008
16. Ouimet A. Personal communication, 2008.
17. Jones S. Personal communication, 2008.
18. Swyer PR. Babies. *The Fight for Intact Survival of The Hospital for Sick Children, Toronto, Canada, 1875–2000: A Personal View*. Hospital for Sick Children, Toronto, 2004.
19. Douglas GJ, Simpson JS. The conservative management of splenic-trauma. *J Pediatr Surg* 1971;6:565-570.
20. Grace N. Personal communication, 2008.
21 . Cameron G. Personal communication, 2008.
22. Sachs B. Personal communication, 2008.
23. Fitzgerald P. Personal communication, 2008.
24. Girvan D. Personal communication, 2008.
25. Marshall D. Letter, 1954.
26. Wiseman, N. Personal communication, 2008.
27. Medovy H. *A Vision Fulfilled. The Story of The Children's Hospital of Winnipeg 1909–1973*. Pegius Publishers, Winnipeg, 1979.
28. Ferguson CC. *Letter to Dr Barry Shandling*, 17 July 1980.

29. Ferguson CC. *One Hundred Years of Surgery 1883-1983: Professors of Surgery, The University of Manitoba*. Pegius Publishers, Winnipeg, 1983.
30. Goodhand T. Personal communication, 2008.
31. Juckes A. Personal communication, 2008.
32. Cram RW. *Letter to Dr Barry Shandling*, 27 June 1980.
33. Fraser M. Personal communication, 2008.
34. Miller G. Personal communication, 2008.
35. Wong A. Personal communication, 2008.
36. Seagram GC. Personal communication, 2008.
37. Sigalet D. Personal communication, 2008.
38. Lees GM. Personal communication, 2008.
39. Ashmore PG, Fraser G. Personal communication, 2008.
40. Hayashi A. Personal communication, 2008.

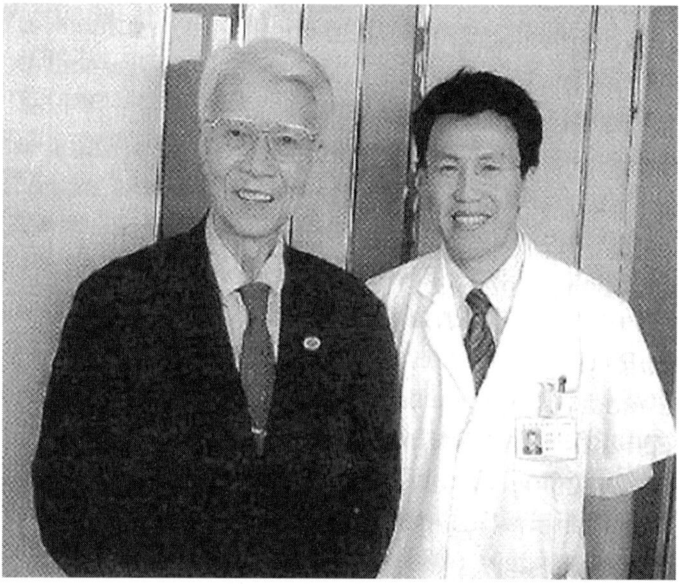

Jin-Zhe Zhang and Long Li

CHINA

Long Li
Jin-Zhe Zhang

A Brief History of China Society of Pediatric Surgeons

The term "pediatric surgery" appeared in China only after the founding of People's Republic of China (PRC) in 1949. There are historical records of cleft lip repair and the treatment of anorectal malformation in the 16th century, and occasional reports of surgical reduction of intussusception and incarcerated inguinal hernia in the modern Chinese medical literatures in the early 20th century. In July 1950, the First National Congress of Health-work and Medicine was held in Beijing. It was decided then to improve the maternal and child health care. This was the beginning of the history of pediatric surgery in China.

Before 1950, in the vast land of China, there were only two small pediatric clinics, located in Beijing and Shanghai respectively. China was a country 40 times the area of Britain with a population more than 20 times that of Britain. The government began to build children's hospitals, at least one in every province. It was under these circumstances, that the first and biggest hospital, the Beijing Children's Hospital was born in 1952. It was formally inaugurated on June 1, 1955. Dr Jin-Zhe Zhang (Fig. 1) moved from Peking University to take up the appointment as the Pediatric Surgeon-in-Chief. Much change has occurred in the succeeding years and the gradual evolution of pediatric services has been interrupted with national turmoil.

The great demand for pediatric service requires training of larger number of doctors in a short period of time. Special "Schools

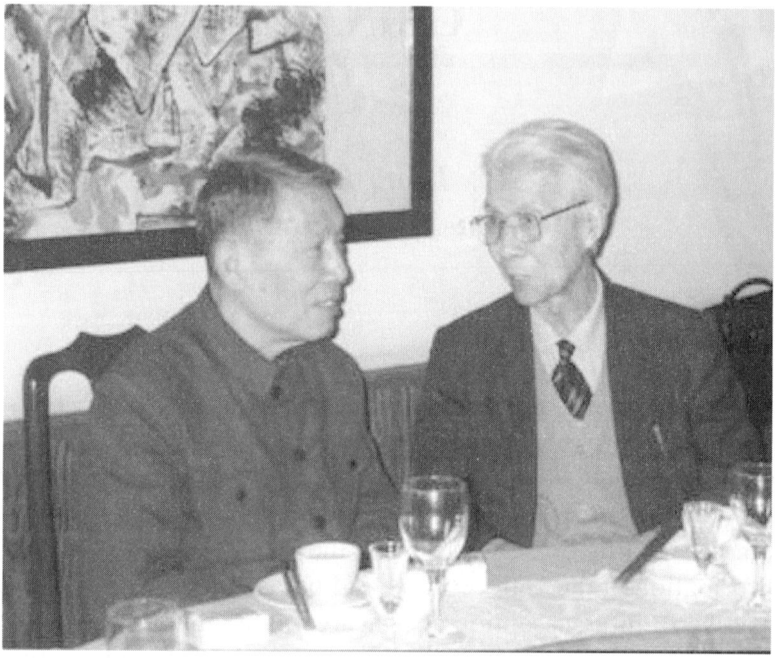

Fig. 1. Prof Jin-Zhe Zhang (right) and Prof Er-Chang Tong.

of Pediatrics" were established in several medical colleges. Pediatric surgery was one of the main courses in these pediatric teaching centers. In August 1950, Dr Jin-Zhe Zhang was appointed to establish the first pediatric surgical section with special clinic and surgical ward in the Department of Pediatrics of Peking University Hospital. Almost at the same time, Dr A Q Ma (Fig. 2) and Dr Y X She (Fig. 3) in Shanghai and, shortly after, Dr E C Tong in Wuhan and some others also established pediatric surgical specialties either in surgical departments or in pediatric departments of various medical colleges. In 1957, the Ministry of Health created a number of pediatric surgical training centers in Beijing and Shanghai to train general surgeons to perform pediatric surgery. Most of the earlier trainees became the first generation of leading pediatric surgeons, mainly in the new children's hospitals or the big medical centers in the provincial capital cities all over China.

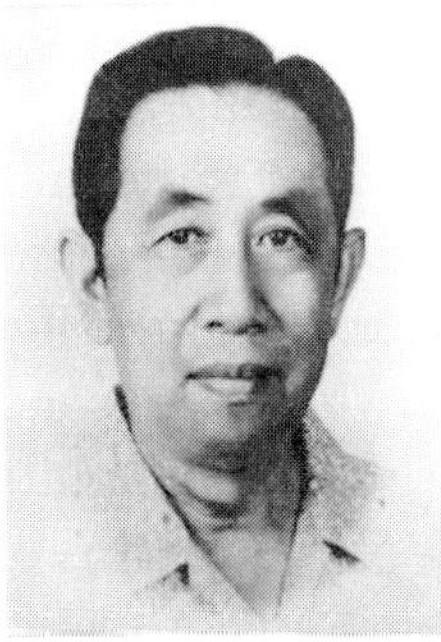

Fig. 2. Dr An-Quan MA.

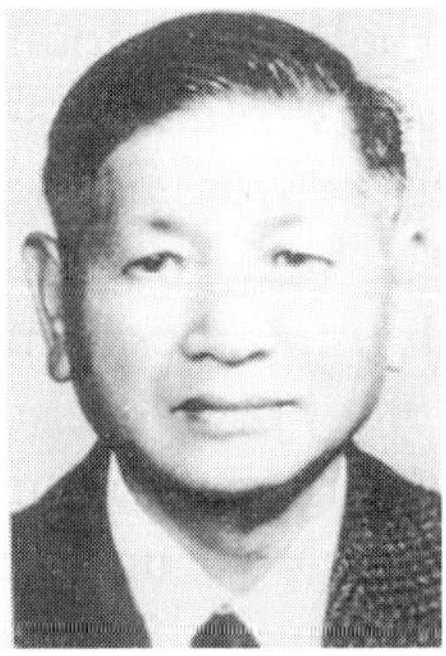

Fig. 3. Prof Yan-Xiong She.

At the 6th Congress of Pediatrics in Beijing, June 1964, some 20 delegates of pediatric surgeons from different parts of China had their first gathering. Those young pediatric surgeons identified two objectives: the first was to organize a pediatric surgical section in the Society of Pediatrics of Chinese Medical Association, and the second, to establish a journal of pediatric surgery. The second task was commissioned to Dr E C Tong who edited the "*Pediatric Surgical Journal*" affiliated to "*Wuhan Medical Journal*", which was published bimonthly in Wuhan. However the first suggestion was delayed by more than a decade as a consequence of the Cultural Revolution. It was not until June 1980, that the First Congress of Pediatric Surgeons of China was held in Harbin, a provincial capital city in North-east China. There an official Pediatric Surgical Section was organized and Drs J Z Zhang and Y X She were elected the President and Deputy President respectively. At the same time, the official "*Chinese Journal of Pediatric Surgery*" was started as a bimonthly publication under the editorship of Dr E C Tong. In 2002 in Changsha of Hunan Province, a second journal, the "*Journal of Clinical Pediatric Surgery*" began bimonthly publication. The name China Society of Pediatric Surgeons was officially adopted after the Third Congress of Pediatric Surgeons was held in Suzhou in 1987.

Through the second half of the 20th century, the education and training of pediatric surgeons in China changed rapidly. The first generation pediatric surgeons were practically self-trained general surgeons who graduated before the founding of PR China. From 1958, the special "Schools of Pediatrics" were progressively opened in ten big medical colleges. More than 1000 students graduated annually since 1963. Half of them were assigned to the newly built children's hospitals, and from these emerged the doctors who became the new generation of pediatric surgeons. They were called pediatric surgeons and although a six-month course of pediatric surgery was included in the five-year undergraduate medical curriculum of school of pediatrics, the training was still inadequate. After graduation, they underwent a five-year resident training including one-year chief resident training which was great experience. In Beijing Children's Hospital which had 750 beds, at least 1000 emergencies and critical cases a year were managed by the chief resident. With this experience, she or he will be able to handle the majority of urgent pediatric surgical problems, and to be qualified as a pediatric surgeon. Those who had no chance to be a chief resident were also trained for 4–5 years with adequate practical knowledge and to finally join a sub-specialty of pediatric surgery. Further training was to be received there.

Postgraduate schools for medicine once opened in early 1960's but were soon closed down by 1965. Since 1978, the regular high schools as well as medical colleges were re-opened after the ten-year disaster (the Cultural Revolution). Regular postgraduate medical schools re-opened and began to train young medical doctors for research Master or Doctor Degrees. Thereafter, papers on molecular medicine and genetics began to appear in Chinese medical journals. Entering the 21st century, the shortage of pediatricians and pediatric surgeons seemed to have been eased. In order to broaden the basic knowledge for medical students, the special "Schools of Pediatrics" were closed in all medical colleges. The next generation of pediatric surgeons will be selected from the well-trained general surgeons, who will then undergo further pediatric surgical training.

Evolution of Technology in Pediatric Surgery of China

The original knowledge of pediatric surgery in China came from the scientific thought and experience of Gross. In early 1950s, at the time that PR China was isolated from the modern world, Dr J Z Zhang began his pediatric surgical work based on two text books, namely "*Abdominal Surgery of Infancy and Childhood*" by Ladd and Gross (USA, 1941) and "*Childhood Surgery*" by Telnovsky (USSR, 1949). He developed his skill based on his own clinical experience and self-learning. The four pioneers of pediatric surgery in China: Ma, She, Tong and Zhang, graduated from different Medical Schools in Shanghai. Ma graduated from St. John's, speaking English; She from Zhendan, speaking French; Tong from Tongji, speaking German, and Zhang from Shanghai Medical College, a Chinese school. In Northeast Chinese cities, like Shenyang, our colleagues speak Japanese. The original information came from all parts of the world, but I would like to emphasize that the main technology was from Gross.

In the early years after the founding of PR China, people's living and sanitary conditions were very poor. People were devoted to their jobs and that left very little time for proper child care. Surgical emergencies were the most common challenge in pediatric surgery. These included accidental trauma, scalds, pyogenic infections and acute abdomen. They differ from spectrum seen in the Western countries, especially the surgical complications of ascariasis, such as intestinal obstruction, appendiceal perforation with ascaris peritonitis, and biliary ascariasis. In the 1960's, following the rapid improvement of the economical conditions, the above-mentioned diseases were largely reduced. People began to pay more attention to congenital anomalies. A great number of children with inguinal hernias needed operative repair. As there were not enough surgical beds for those requiring admission, day-surgery was developed. All those minor surgical conditions, like small superficial tumors, redundant prepuce, hydrocele, undescended testis, and simple cleft lip, which require little post-operative care, were operated in out-patient department with satisfactory results. This approach was welcomed by the mothers.

The 1980's saw the recovery of the national economy. The "opening policy" began to pay dividends. In the following years, prominent pediatric surgeons from developed countries visited China. They included Drs Kieswetter, S. L. Gans, C. E. Koop, H. W. Hendren, J. L. Grosfeld *et al.* from USA, and Drs J. Lister, D. G. Young, D. Lloyd, L. Kapila and L. Spitz from UK, etc. They brought with them the modern technology to China. At the same time, Chinese pediatric surgeons began to visit Western countries and Japan. These exchanges brought the gap of knowledge into our awareness and galvanized the Chinese pediatric surgeons to close the gap. Meanwhile, the living condition of people improved markedly. The epidemiology of pediatric surgical diseases also changed. The one-child policy of family planning improved the child-care immensely. Accidental injuries and infections due to poor care plummeted. Among the common acute abdominal emergencies, ascariasis was under control and was rarely seen among urban populations. Intussusception was managed mostly by rectal insufflation even in county hospitals. Acute appendicitis and incarcerated hernia were well managed by community hospitals. With the improvement of pediatric surgery and control of tuberculosis, intestinal obstruction due to adhesion was also reduced dramatically. Good results from the common surgical emergencies management were achieved in large centres. These include 10,000 cases of acute appendicitis in 20 years without mortality, 100 consecutive cases of strangulated intestinal obstruction with no death, 90% successful rate of reimplantation of severed finger and successful treatment of

90% burns in small children. In tertiary hospitals, elective surgery became a new priority. Sub-specialties of pediatric surgery were developed in most centers including pediatric orthopedics, pediatric urology, thoracic and cardiovascular surgery, neurosurgery, tumor surgery and plastic surgery. Ano-rectal surgery and biliary surgery were also separated from general pediatric surgery and neonatal surgery. Papers published in 1990s showed that most treatment results have become comparable to those achieved in the developed world. For instance, the survival rate of esophageal atresia and intestinal atresia in full-term newborns was about 90% and satisfactory results were achieved in 90% of ano-rectal anomaly, Hirschsprung's disease and choledochal cyst operations. The two- or five-year survival rate for the solid tumors, e.g. Wilms' tumor, rhabdomyosarcoma, hepatoblastoma and neuroblastoma, approximated 60–80%. Developmental dislocation of the hip, scoliosis, and leg lengthening in orthopedics, hypospadias repair and urinary dynamic disorders in urology, complex cardiovascular anomalies in infants, etc, all achieved similarly high standards with our modification of the conventional procedures.

Entering the 21st century, as the new generation of pediatric surgeons matured, new aspects of molecular medicine and genetics are studied in all pediatric surgical centers. Living-related liver transplantation began to be popular in big pediatric surgical centers since it means further advancement of surgery. Because of financial limitations in mainland China, we lag behind Hong Kong and Taiwan in adoption of new equipment. Another trendy entity, pediatric laparoscopic surgery, has caught on in China. In the last couple of years, thousands of appendectomies and hernia repairs and hundreds of hepatoenterostomies for choledochal cyst were reported. More than 50 types of surgical procedures were successfully performed with endoscopic technique in children of various ages. China is a huge developing country and that means that there are irregularities between regions in modernization. The gaps in some instances can be quite large.

In 1997, J Z Zhang was elected an academician to the China Academy of Engineering. Honors and recognition have enhanced the specialty as the scientific level of pediatric surgery in China is now accepted by Chinese scientists. In 2000 in Sorrento, Jin-Zhe Zhang was awarded by British Association of Paediatric Surgeons (BAPS) the Denis Browne Gold Medal. This indicates that the Chinese pediatric surgical community has joined the world pediatric surgical family.

Unique Approaches of Pediatric Surgical Work in China

The aim of China Society of Pediatric Surgeons was announced in Suzhou, 1997: "To set the standards and to popularize them to all surgeons." This is similar to that of British Association of Pediatric Surgeons, "The aim of pediatric surgery is to set a standard not to seek a monopoly." which is carved on the back of the Denis Browne Gold Medal. China is a big country with a huge population and poor transportation facilities. Three thousand full-time pediatric surgeons who are concentrated in city hospitals would not be able to solve the large pediatric surgical workload. In many instances, in practice, children with surgical emergencies have to be handled by the local general surgeons. Therefore we pediatric surgeons have to make the procedures simple and safe and the techniques easy to master by the adult surgeons. For example, in the early years, before the "opening policy", pediatric anaesthesia was the main problem in the community hospitals. Back then, they were unable to obtain appropriate endotracheal tubes for children. Thanks to the development of sedation and immobilization in a special frame, various kinds of operation could be done under local anesthesia. With the use of epidural anesthesia for abdominal operation, laparotomy in the neonatal group could also be performed smoothly, avoiding hypopnea secondary to general anaesthesia. Primary one-stage pull-through procedure without colostomy for Hirschsprung's disease and high anorectal malformation have simplified the home care greatly. Colostomy was avoided with the development of the "ring clamp" which crushes the spurs in Duhamel operation. Incision of the "adventitia rectalis" allows rectal mobilization in high anorectal malformation. Air enema, or insufflation treatment, for intussusception is widely practiced in the country with 90% reduction rate in early cases. The recently introduced fluid-enema under sonography monitoring obviates the risk of radiation, however, it is not as popular as air enema due to the unavailability of sonograph machine in some hospitals.

The one-child policy has generated a new challenge for the pediatric surgeons. Three couples (father and mother, maternal grandparents and paternal grandparents) are involved in the decision of the treatment. Every family hopes for their "only child" to be perfect. Any imperfection, no matter how minor, should be corrected as early as possible. On the other hand, people may show different philosophy to those severe anomalies, which need multi-staged operations with certain residual morbidity. They prefer to have another child rather than exhausting all means of treatment for the sick child. To meet the new expectation of the family and the society has become a great challenge to the Chinese pediatric surgeons.

Involvement of Chinese traditional medicine is unique in Chinese pediatric surgical practice. It is based on an entirely different paradigm of disease treatment, emphasizing instead on self-healing of human body; in a way, it is very much similar to the philosophy of homeopathy. The most well-known example is "acupuncture anesthesia." Rhythmic acupuncture stimulation at certain meridian points relieves pain by interfering with the sensation pathway of certain area. The senior author of this article underwent partial gastrectomy with acupuncture anesthesia, fully awake. The operation was completed smoothly. But frankly speaking, we don't advise the readers to try it at home. It is not uncommon among children that stomatitis and other cold-like symptoms may develop after major operations. Chinese herb tonic relieves the symptoms promptly, while antibiotics may do more harm than good.

A popular treatment of infantile anal fistula with seton stitch was modified from an old Chinese traditional treatment. A rubber band attached to a malleable probe was threaded through the anal fistula and tied. The rubber band cut through the overlying skin and sphincter muscle gradually and laid the tract fully open. The incision of the fistula and, the granulation take place simultaneously. The rubber band is coated with fine herb powder to relieve pain and promote healing. Once the tract is cut through and the rubber band drops by itself, the wound heals on following day. This 5-minute procedure under local anesthesia without any risk of bleeding or incontinence has the advantage over the conventional fistulectomy in small infants.

For fracture of femur in small kids, we put the child in a Bryant traction frame in combination with Chinese traditional small wooden splints to hold the thigh in alignment. Under traction, these splints can be removed and replaced every day for bath and cleansing. Several small splints all around the thigh will prevent the backward angulation and rotation of the fragments but allow free movement of the lower extremities in all directions under the traction frame. This constitutes the "fixation and active motion" treatment of fractures in Chinese traditional medicine. It minimizes the atrophy of both muscle and bone secondary to disuse.

Chinese traditional medicine is a great treasure trove to be explored. It has a great potential and we Chinese pediatric surgeons are delighted to share it with the rest of the world.

Outstanding Individuals Contributing to the Development of Surgical Pediatrics in China

Jin-Zhe Zhang (1920–present), sponsored by Ministry of Health, started the first surgical pediatric section in the department of pediatrics of Peking University Medical College in 1950, and built the multiclinic surgical department of Beijing Children's Hospital in 1955. He conducted the national training center for pediatric surgeons from 1957 onwards. He devoted himself to the organization of China Society of Pediatric Surgeons, being the first president in 1987–1991, and the honorary president thereafter.

An-Quan Ma (1911–1977) having been a surgical observer in Philadelphia Children's Hospital before the founding of new China, began to do some surgery in Shanghai Children's Hospital by 1950. He was the Chief Editor of the official "*Text Book of Pediatric Surgery*" for Chinese medical students. It was a pity that he died before the open policy of China.

Ya-Xiong She (1917–1995) established pediatric surgery in Shanghai 2nd Medical College in 1953. Devoting himself to medical education, he was the chief editor of the national textbook of pediatric surgery since its 2nd edition — that was established "*Air Enema Reduction*" of intussusception, rapidly popularized all over China.

Er-Chang Tong (1921–present) founded the pediatric surgery in Tongji Hospital of Wuhan and in 1964, established the "*Chinese Journal of Pediatric Surgery*", thence devoted his whole life to medical publication and remained being the Chief Editor of the *Chinese Journal of Pediatric Surgery* until his sick leave in 1995.

The above four people are the pioneers of the beginning generation.

Shao-Chuan Pan (1926–present) the co-worker of J. Z. Zhang, had many achievements in the orthopedic surgery of children, particularly in the deformities of spine. He combined the procedures of Ilizarov and Chinese traditional short splint in bony fixation with better results, particularly in the baby care, than the traditional plaster cast and bed-ridden traction.

Wen-Xiang Ding a co-worker of Y. X. She, made the self-designed heart-lung machine for small infant before the era of China where opened to the West. Most of the pediatric cardiac surgeons in children's hospitals of China were trained under his supervision.

Zhen-Gang Zhan was the chief anesthesiologist of Beijing Children's Hospital until his death in 1995. He developed epidural anesthesia under light central depression in neonates, which provided an excellent relaxation but avoided the post-operative prolonged intubation and respirator assistance in neonates or prematures.

Guang-Da Wang of Shenyang Medical University of China established saline enema reduction of intussusception under ultrasonic observation, avoiding the over exposure of X-rays.

The following have done prominent works in pediatric surgery and are famous in China:

Cheng-Ru Huang of Beijing Children's Hospital, the pioneer in pediatric urology; Zheng Li of Shenyang China Medical University, the authority on anorectal anomalies; Guo Wang of Wuhan Tongji Medical University and an expert of Hirschsprung's Disease; and Zhen-Dong Li of Hebei Medical University, known specially in the subject of choledochal cyst.

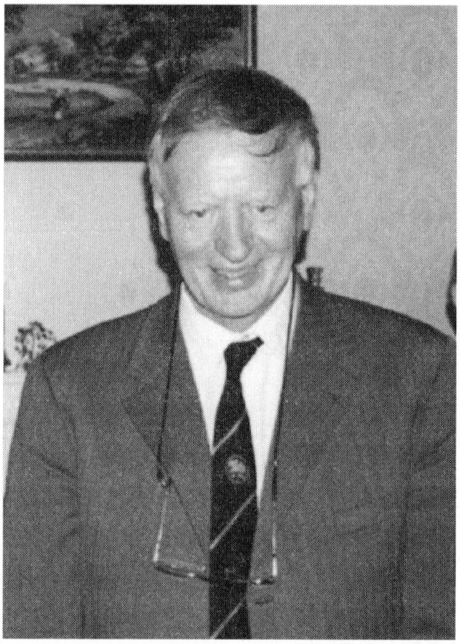

Ole H. Nielsen

DENMARK

Ole H. Nielsen

Before 1945

Paediatric surgery as we know it now, with congenital anomalies as the dominating theme, did not begin its development until after 1945, when the war-inspired invention of endotracheal intubation had made anaesthesia and surgery in children much safer. In the earlier centuries the pattern of surgery in children was different, consisting mostly of bone diseases and ENT surgery. There was little abdominal surgery, mostly bladder stones, but gradually also appendicitis and intussusception began to be treated.

The conditions in Scandinavia were quite similar to those in the western world as a whole. To begin with, surgery in children and adults was performed by the same surgeons, and in the same surroundings. Children's hospitals began to appear in the big cities in the 19th century, beginning in Paris 1802, and subsequently in the rest of Europe, including Scandinavia. In Copenhagen the first children's hospital opened in 1850. It moved to a new hospital under the name of Queen Louise's Children's Hospital in 1879 with Harald Hirschsprung as chief. In Stockholm, the Crown Princess Lovisa's Children's Hospital opened in 1854, and in Gothenburg, a children's hospital opened in 1859. In Norway no children's hospital was erected, but a paediatric department was opened in the University Hospital of Oslo, Rikshospitalet, in 1893.

The surgery in children moved gradually into these hospitals, but stayed in the adult departments in places without a children's hospital. The details about the development of paediatric surgery in Norway, Sweden and Finland are described in other chapters.

From Denmark the early contributions to international paediatric surgery have been rather sparse, but there are some significant events.

Harald Hirschsprung (1830–1916)

The Scandinavian doctor who has made the greatest contribution to the paediatric surgical profession during this period is probably the paediatrician Harald Hirschsprung (Fig. 1). He was the eldest son of an immigrant German tobacco manufacturer who came to Copenhagen in 1811. In opposition to his father's wish that he should be educated in the tobacco profession and take over the family business, he began a study of medicine at Copenhagen University in 1848. A severe epidemic of cholera occurred in 1853, while he was still in his studies, and he was involved in the fight of the epidemic, distributing medicine, finding the newly infected and admitting them

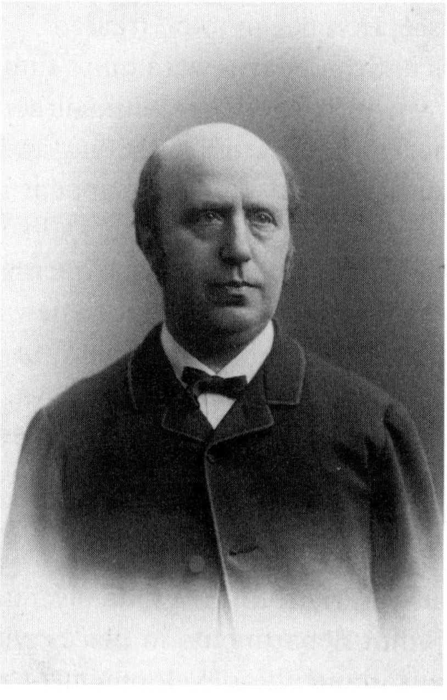

Fig. 1. Portrait photo of Harald Hirschsprung, about 1905.

to hospital treatment. He graduated in 1855. He worked in medical departments in Copenhagen hospitals and had a short spell as a general practitioner before he started working at the Copenhagen Children's Hospital in 1870. Here he taught paediatrics to the medical students and was appointed as professor in 1877. He was very fond of music and had been a member of the University Choir. His two daughters were skilled musicians and he was frequently hosting soirées with participation of the Copenhagen cultural elite.[1]

He was very interested in anatomical anomalies and rare diseases, and in his teaching of medical students he only reluctantly talked about more usual diseases. He was a frequent visitor in the operation theatre, and his research and publications were very relevant to surgery. His slightly selective teaching did not signify clinical arrogance. He was a very diligent clinician himself and taught his assistants to be thorough and comprehensive in their diagnostic work. He was fond of his patients and used to chat and play with them on ward rounds. His uncompromising care for the children was demonstrated during the building of the Queen Louise's Childrens' Hospital. Queen Louise wanted the wall spaces above doors to be decorated with biblical quotations for the edification of the children. Hirschsprung firmly refused this, and the Queen had to accept wall decorations with pictures of animals and flowers.

His doctoral thesis was written in 1860–1861. The title was "The congenital occlusion of the oesophagus and contributions to the knowledge about the congenital occlusion of the small intestine." He had met these anomalies during his short stay at the obstetric institution in 1859.[2] He reported 14 cases of oesophageal atresia, seven Danish cases, of which he had seen four and seven cases collected from the international literature. Concerning oesophageal atresia he concluded: "About the prognosis and treatment there is nothing to add. The disease is of such nature that it carries the seeds of a swift and inevitable death." However, he noted that surgical cure might be possible in the future.

In the section about intestinal atresia he reported 25 cases: 20 were from the literature, but he had autopsied three cases himself and a colleague had autopsied two. On this basis he proposed three types:

A: the congenital stricture of the small intestine;
B: the valvular occlusion; and
C: the total occlusion;

There were no survivors in the material, but it is mentioned that an attempt at treatment by enterostomy is possible.

After the thesis he published nothing for a long time, but following his appointment at the Children's Hospital he began collecting cases again. He published papers about hydronephrosis, hydrocephalus, pleural empyema, congenital occlusion of the biliary tract, congenital inguinal hernia, intubation of the larynx, and about the use of catheters in small children. But he made major contributions to paediatric surgery in three other areas: intussusception, Hirschsprung's disease, and congenital pyloric stenosis.

Intussusception. A very high mortality was connected to this disease at the time, because diagnosis was late and because recognition and treatment of fluid and electrolyte balance disturbance was lacking. In fact reduction by rectal fluid or indeed air instillation was known at the time but rarely utilised. Hirschsprung's merit in this connection was his demonstration that chloroform anaesthesia allowed palpation and easier reduction of the lump, and also an ascertainment of the result. (At the time X-rays had not yet been introduced.) He published reports of his results several times; the first seven cases were in 1875, and by 1905 he had accumulated 107.[3] The mortality was still considerable, about 40%, but that was lower than that of surgical treatment, which was then 100%. In spite of this he was unable to persuade the surgeons to switch to hydrostatic reduction.

Hirschsprung's disease. His paper about the disease which bears his name was read at the paediatric congress in Berlin, 1886. He had seen two cases, one in 1880, one in 1885. His observations of symptoms, clinical findings and pathological anatomy were described very lucidly, and in fact the description can not be much improved today. The title of his paper was: "Constipation in newborns caused by dilation and hypertrophy of the colon".[4] He published four additional papers about the disease, the last one in 1904, when he reported ten cases. He did not know the aetiology and pathogenesis of the condition. The definitive recognition of aganglionosis did not occur until the late 1940's (and the Swedish-born paediatric surgeon Orvar Swenson played a significant role in the development of successful treatment of this disease).

Congenital pyloric stenosis. Hirschsprung's name might as well have been connected to this disease as to aganglionosis of the colon. At a meeting in Wiesbaden, 1887, he read a paper entitled "2 cases of congenital pyloric stenosis observed in infants".[5] Such cases had been reported before, just like cases of Hirschsprung's disease, but in both instances Hirschsprung's precise description of the clinical picture opened the eyes of the medical world to the conditions, and since then an abundance of research and publications has occurred.

At a Scandinavian surgical congress in Copenhagen, 1901, Hirschsprung read a paper about the disease, describing the typical clinical picture with gastric peristalsis and palpable tumour. He also mentioned his persuasion that the future treatment would be surgical, but the time apparently was not ripe (Fig. 2). The first operation was done by Fredet in 1907.

The first survivor in duodenal atresia. There is one other interesting early Danish event: The first successful operation of duodenal atresia ever reported was done in Copenhagen on November 30, 1914. The surgeon was N. P. Ernst who was chief surgeon at St Elisabeth's Hospital. The patient was a boy, born at an uneventful delivery with a birth weight of 4300 g. He began explosive, bile-stained vomiting on the fourth day of life. He had late passage of meconium and very little urine output. Dr. Ernst first saw the boy on day 7. He made a diagnosis of intestinal atresia or stenosis and proposed surgery. The parents wanted the opinion of the paediatric professor, who suggested continued medical treatment for some days.

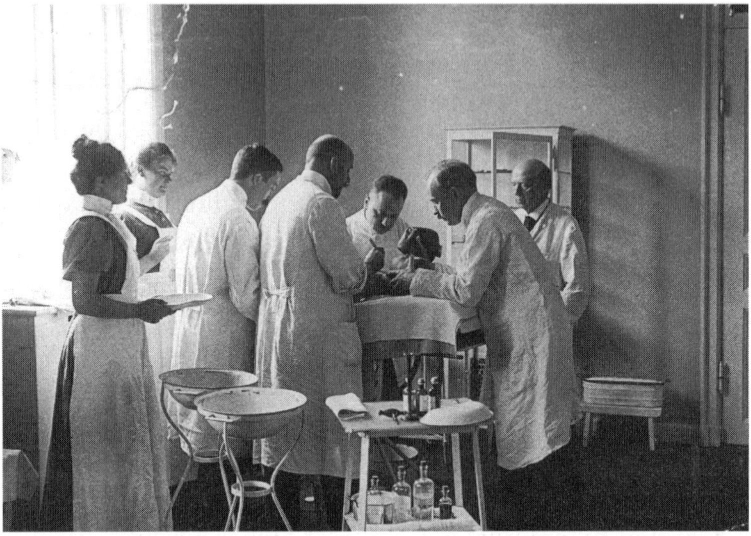

Fig. 2. Photo from the operation theatre of Queen Louise's Children's Hospital 1904. Harald Hirschsprung is standing to the right of the anaesthetist, watching the operation.

Three days later the boy was still vomiting and had lost weight — down to 3490 g. Now even the paediatrician advocated operation, so on day 11 the boy was operated in ether anaesthesia. The atresia was not visualised, but it was noted that the rest of the intestine was totally empty. A duodeno-jejunostomy was made antecolically in two layers with no. 1 silk (!). Oral nutrition was started on the day of operation, and no parenteral fluids were administered. There were still vomiting the first three days after surgery, but the patient was dismissed in good condition five days post-operatively.[6]

He was readmitted when he was six years old with an inguinal hernia, and it was noted that he had been well and thrived normally. This patient was also seen in 1975, when he was 60 years old, by the paediatric surgeon C. M. Madsen.[7] He had been in good health always. He was 182 cm tall and weighed 92 kg. This seems to be a world record in terms of the length of follow-up in duodenal atresia. And the surgical result is honourable, considering the conditions of fluid and electrolyte regulation, diagnostic tools, anaesthesia, pathophysiological understanding and surgical instruments at the time.

After 1945

The development of the specialty of paediatric surgery started in the period after the second world war, when reports of successful neonatal surgery began to appear. Paediatricians and surgeons in the western world soon became interested, because it now seemed possible to salvage babies with congenital anomalies which had until now been fatal. Each of the Scandinavian countries developed in rather different patterns.

The Crown Princess Lovisa's Hospital for Sick Children in Stockholm had 150 beds in 1945; 75 of these were surgical but were served only by an external consultant, **Gunnar Ekström**. In 1945 he was appointed as internal paediatric surgical consultant. In 1950 a large paediatric unit was erected in the Karolinska University Hospital, and **N. O. Ericsson** was appointed as chief of the paediatric surgical department. He went on to become the father of Scandinavian paediatric urology. Later, departments were opened in the cities of Gothenburg, Uppsala and Lund, and in a few provincial hospitals paediatric surgeons were appointed.

In Helsinki a large paediatric centre was instituted at the University Hospital in 1946, and **Matti Sulamaa** was appointed as chief of paediatric surgery. (He is considered the father of Finnish paediatric surgery and was also one of the BAPS founders). In 1962 Mikko Pasila and Kaarlo Parkkulainen were appointed and went on to develop paediatric thoracic surgery and paediatric urology, respectively. A municipal department was opened in the Aurora Hospital in 1957 with Lars Gripenberg as chief. Between 1961 and 1973, departments were opened in the University Hospitals of Turku, Tampere, Oulu and Kuopio. In many of the larger provincial hospitals a paediatric surgeon was appointed.

In Oslo, **Ola Knutrud** began operating on neonates in the surgical department of the University Hospital, and in 1962 a department of paediatric surgery was instituted with him as chief. Later a municipal department was opened in Ullevål Hospital, and a department was opened in the University Hospital of Trondheim 1975 with Torbjørn Kufaas as chief.

In Copenhagen **C. C. Winkel Smith** (1907–1962) began performing neonatal and other paediatric surgery in the surgical department of the University Hospital. The children were admitted in the department of paediatrics, and in 1949 Winkel Smith was formally appointed as surgical consultant at the paediatric department. He began introducing the current procedures of neonatal and infantile surgery. In 1959, an independent surgical unit was established in the department of paediatrics with Winkel Smith as chief. His wife was a descendant of Harald Hirschsprung, which might explain his enthusiastic interest in paediatric surgery. He was a BAPS member since 1954 and was well known among members for his extrovert personality and his occasional entertainment at the piano. But he also had a depressive streak, and in 1962 he suddenly disappeared. His document case was discovered in 1968 in a shrubbery at a forest lake in North Sealand.

He developed paediatric surgery in cooperation with Tyge Gertz (1913–1998) (Fig. 3), who was the operator of the first Danish neonate with TOF to survive in 1949.[8] Two years earlier the thoracic

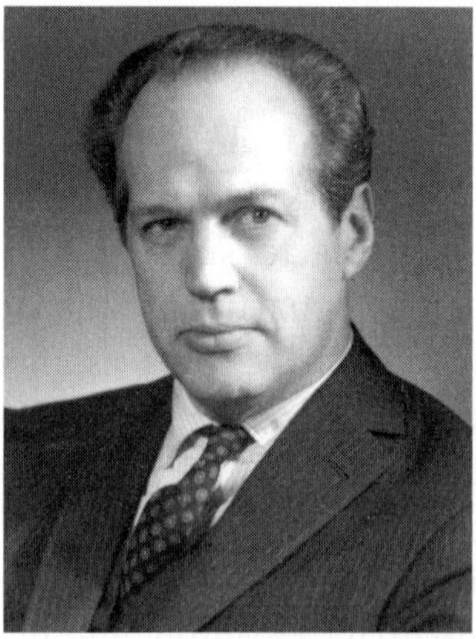

Fig. 3. Photo of Tyge Gertz, about 1955.

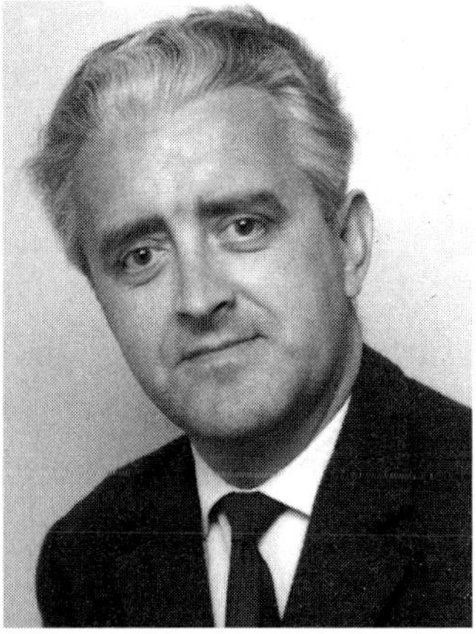

Fig. 4. Photo of Carl Martin Madsen, about 1965.

surgeon Erik Husfeldt (1901–1984) had operated on a neonate, adopting the Haight procedure, but the baby died three hours post-operatively. He also trained C. M. Madsen (1923–1995) (Fig. 4), who went on to become a consultant surgeon at Odense University Hospital, where he also continued to cultivate paediatric surgery. His doctoral thesis was about Hirschsprung's disease. From 1962 Winkel Smith's vacant consultant post was held by various *locum tenentes* until he was officially declared deceased in 1968. Knud Mauritzen was then appointed, and after him, **Ole Nielsen and Jørgen**. Their main research has been in paediatric urology, neonatal surgery and pre-natal diagnosis. Ole Henrik Nielsen has been engaged in international matters and has served office in both EUPSA and UEMS.

The Copenhagen department serves the eastern part of Denmark with specialised paediatric surgery (not including orthopaedic surgery and heart surgery), and has achieved good results measured with an international standard. There is not yet any other department of paediatric surgery in the country, but neonates and children with surgical diseases are operated within the frames of adult surgery or urology in the University Hospitals of Odense and Århus.

Paediatric surgery was recognised as a specialty in Sweden 1947, in Finland 1951, in Denmark as a surgical sub-specialty 1958 and in

Norway 1963. At the revision of the Danish specialty rules in 1971 the sub-specialty of paediatric surgery was cancelled, and it has not yet been reinstated. This is certainly due to ignorance within the authorities, and ignorance combined with misguided animosity within the specialties of surgery and paediatrics. The result is the above mentioned lack of specialised departments outside Copenhagen with the further consequence that the surgeons operating on children in other parts of the country must do so without proper training and professional infrastructure.

Professional Societies

A national association of paediatric surgeons was founded in Sweden 1963 (The Scandinavian Association of Paediatric Surgeons — q.v.) with other Scandinavian paediatric surgeons present. In Finland and Norway an Association was founded in 1973, in Denmark 1986.

Acknowledgement

The figures are from the archives of the Medical Museum of Copenhagen and thanks to them for the provision of these records.

References

1. Roed–Petersen K, Madsen CM. *Harald Hirschsprung (1830–1916).* Dansk Medicinskhistorisk Årbog 1980; p. 182–199.
2. Hirschsprung H. Den medfødte Tillukning af Spiserøret samt Bidrag til Kundskaber om den medfødte Tyndtarmstillukning. Thesis, S. Trier, Copenhagen 1861.
3. Hirschsprung H. *107 Fälle von Darminvagination bei Kindern, behandelt in Köningin Louisen-Kinderhospital in Kopenhagen während der Jahre 1871–1904*. Grenzgebiete der Medizin und Chirurgie 1905; p. 555.

4. Hirschsprung H. Stuhlträgheit Neugeborener in Folge von Dilation und Hypertrophie des Colons. *Jahrbuch für Kinderheilkunde* 1888; 27:1.
5. Hirschsprung H. Tilfælde af medfødt Pylorusstenose iagttaget hos Pattebørn. *Hospitalstidende* 1895; 31:125.
6. Ernst NP, *Brit Med J* 1916; 1:644.
7. Madsen CM. Duodenal atresi. *Dansk Medicinskhistorisk Årbog* 1977; 117:121.
8. Gertz TC. *Acta Pædiatr* 1950; 37:391–401.

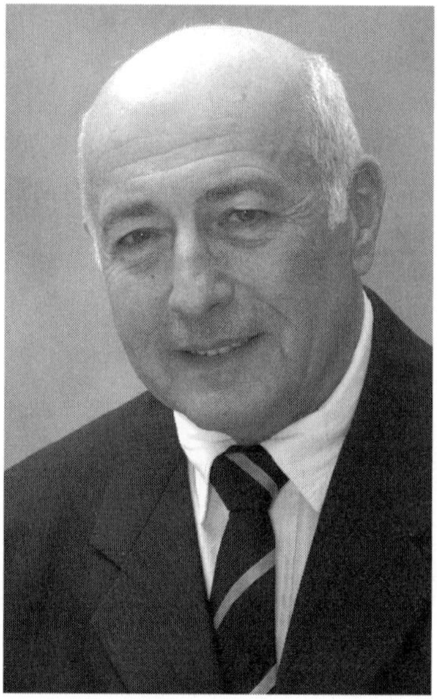

Andras W. Pinter

EASTERN EUROPE

Andras W. Pinter

Introduction

Having been asked to give an outline of the development of paediatric surgery in the previously known eastern block of European countries, I had elicited the help of many colleagues in the East and have recorded many of the facts given by them on the development in their area. It is not fully comprehensive as there has been some difficulty in getting details from all sources tapped, but the following is an outline of the development and the experience on development which have been commanded by factors completely outside the medical field.

Belarus

Before 1955 general surgeons took care of surgically ill children in Belarus despite the fact that the first textbook of paediatric surgery in Belarus was already written by Prof A.E. Mangeim in 1933. The first paediatric surgical department for 25 children was opened in November, 1955 in Molodechno and the second one in 1956 in Minsk for 30 children. In 1963 Prof S.L. Lybov founded the second paediatric surgical department for 40 children in Minsk and began the epoch of paediatric chest and cardiac surgery in Belarus.

In 1970 the centre of Paediatric Surgery for 240 children was built in Minsk for taking care of children with a wide spectrum of urgent and elective surgical pathology. Prof O.S. Misharev was the first medical director of this department. He established the very first paediatric ICU (1971) and had special interest in laboratory aspects of homeostasis in children with septic disorders (1975). Some years later departments of paediatric surgery were opened in Grodno, Vitebsk (1964), Mogylev (1965), Brest (1968) and in other cities of Belarus. Now approximately 100 paediatric surgeons work in Belarus.

Bosnia–Herzegovina

In 1956 paediatric surgery separated from general surgery and the first department of paediatric surgery was founded as a part of general surgery in Sarajevo. By 1979 paediatric surgery had developed and was recognised as an independent speciality.

The paediatric surgical department in Sarajevo had six units. This department was the basis of the professional and scientific education for students, residents, specialists, and different subspecialists. Paediatric surgery gradually developed in other cities in Bosnia and Herzegovina (Tuzla, Banja Luka, Zenica, and Mostar). Prof Ivan Kafka (1923–1985) played an important role in the establishment of paediatric surgery in Bosnia–Herzegovina. He was educated in Great Britain and after that he started to develop paediatric surgery in Bosnia cand Herzegovina. Beside the operations in the field of general paediatric surgery, he introduced neonatal surgery, operative procedure of congenital megacolon by Swenson technique and operative procedure of hypospadias by Ombredane and Denis Browne.

Bulgaria

The first Department of paediatric surgery in Bulgaria was founded in 1952 at the Medical University of Plovdiv by Dr Jury Toshev. At the same time the Emergency Hospital "N. I. Pirogov" in Sofia was founded as the first paediatric surgical emergency unit, created by Dr Boris Raponski. Later, in 1964 this unit was structured as the University Department under the leadership of Prof Dimitar Arnaudov. It consisted of three units containing 120 beds: the first abdominal surgical unit, second unit for neonatal and thoracic surgery, and the third Anaesthesiology and Intensive Care Unit. Under the leadership of Prof Ivan Ivantchev (1977–1989) and Prof Angel Bojanov (1990–2000) the Bulgarian paediatric surgery reached a European level in the field of neonatal, thoracic and abdominal surgery. There are 82 board-certificate paediatric surgeons in Bulgaria. There are University departments for paediatric surgery in Sofia Plovdiv, Varna, Pleven and Stara Zagora.

Czech Republic

In 1902 a new building of Czech Paediatric Hospital was built in Prague with the first independent department of paediatric surgery. It was headed by Dr Václav Kafka sen. (1869–1946) till his retirement in 1939 (Fig. 1). His performance included the whole spectrum of paediatric surgery of those times. He was interested in plastic and reconstructive surgery, and urological anomalies. He was a master in diagnosing acute abdominal illnesses and also active in paediatric orthopaedic surgery.

In 1956 this independent department of paediatric surgery was upgraded as a teaching institution of Charles University in Prague. It was then headed by Prof Václav Kafka jun. for 12 years

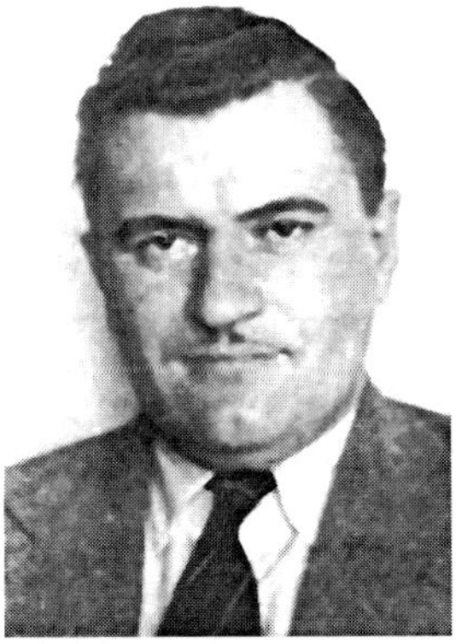

Fig. 1. Václav KAFKA sen./Czech Rep.

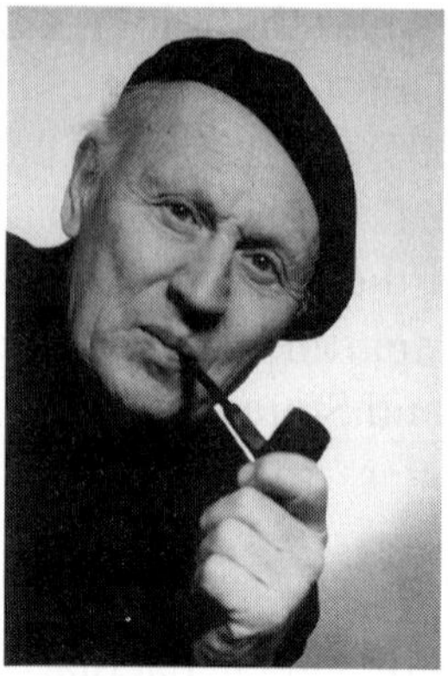

Fig. 2. Václav KAFKA jun./Czech Rep.

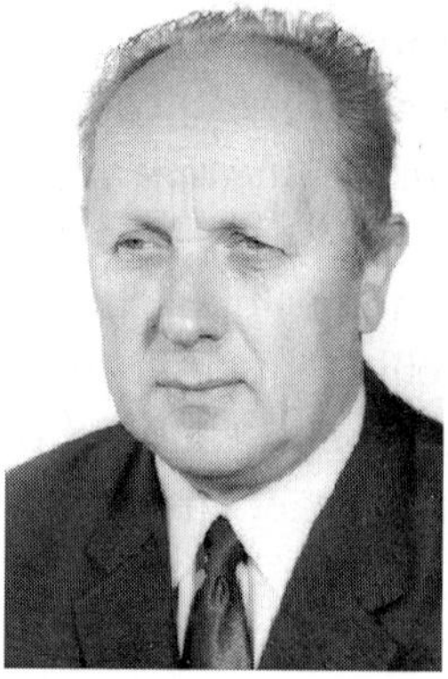

Fig. 3. Václav TOŠOVSKÝ/Czech Rep.

till 1968 (Fig. 2). Václav Kafka jun was a very well-known member of the BAPS and internationally highly respected. He developed and maintained active contacts with many University centres in Western Europe. In 1960 the 1st congress of paediatric surgery with international participation was organised in Prague. A successor to Prof Kafka was Prof Vclav Tošovský whose interests were inborn malformations of the gastrointestinal tract and traumatology (Fig. 3). Another important personality in paediatric surgery was Prof Miroslav Kabelka who was an expert in paediatric thoracic surgery.

In 1990 the independent Czech Association of Paediatric Surgeons was established.

Estonia

The first person acquiring recognition in the specialty of paediatric surgery in Estonia was Inga Freiberg who specialised in this field in the Leningrad (now St. Petersburg) Institute of Paediatrics in 1952. Later, special wards for surgical treatment of children were set up at the departments of general surgery in Tallinn and in Tartu. Subsequently, specialised departments were established both in Tallinn and Tartu in 1962. The department of paediatric surgery in Tartu University Clinic serves as a study base for the University of Tartu, which was headed by Docent Uudo Reino from 1966 to 2000. The departments of paediatric surgery in Tartu and Tallinn serve paediatric patients with general paediatric surgical, urological and orthopaedic pathologies from birth up to the age of 15 years.

Georgia

Paediatric surgery as an independent specialty started its development in 1913, when the first paediatric surgical department was created in Tbilisi. In 1933, the Paediatric Surgical Faculty was opened and a chair of Paediatric surgery and orthopaedics was founded in Tbilisi, headed by Prof M. Kokochashvili (1933–1964) (Fig. 4). During that period further paediatric surgical departments were opened in major cities of Georgia (Batumi, Sokhumi, Kutaisi, Telavi).

The Georgian Paediatric Surgery Association was founded in 1996. Over the last 15 years, the following operations were successfully implemented: neonatal congenital malformations (esophageal atresia, pulmonary cysts, atelectasis, small and large bowel atresia), correction of orthopaedic, neurosurgical pathologies, and advanced endoscopy (bronchoscopy, video-gastro-duodeno-colonoscopy, urethrocystoscopy). Ultrasound, CT and MRI are routinely used for diagnosis and treatment. Also endoscopic surgery is performed on GI tract.

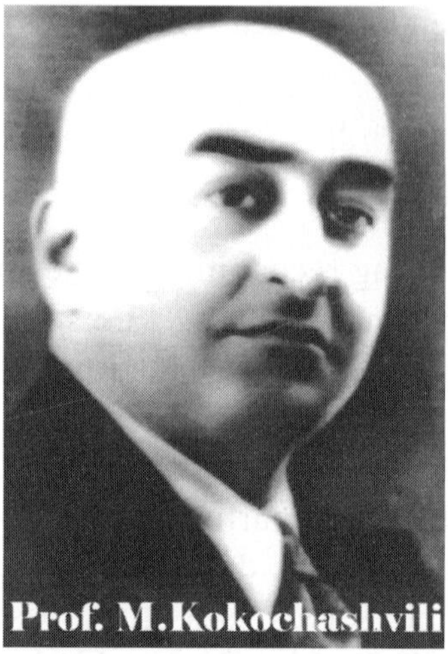

Fig. 4. Michael KOKOCHASHVILI/Georgia.

Hungary

In Hungary, paediatric surgery has been officially acknowledged as an independent speciality, like general surgery or internal medicine, since 1965. However, there is no university chair for paediatric surgery yet. Initially, the speciality exam was allowed only for those who had undertaken specialisation in general surgery. Fortunately, since 1990 the paediatric surgical exit examination can be given without the prerequisite of passing the examination in general surgery, which consists of six years of training.

The 1st Paediatric Department was established in Budapest on the 15 August 1839. Between 1871–1914 László Verebély, as a general surgeon, led a paediatric surgical outpatient unit in the Department. In the year 1914, Aurel Koós was the person who organised the first Paediatric Surgical Ward with a separate operating theatre. He was the "father" of Hungarian paediatric surgeons (Fig. 5). His delicate surgical technique allowed him to not only perform many cases of cleft lip and palate, but some on neonates as well. Many doctors, both from Hungary and abroad, were trained under him. He worked for several decades, till 1957.

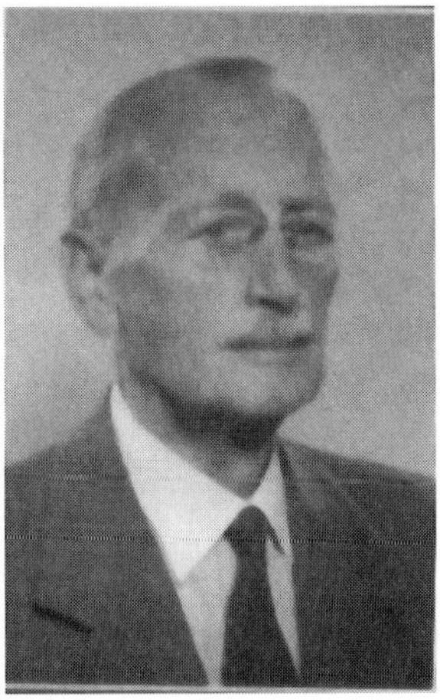

Fig. 5. Aurel KOÓS/Hungary.

Besides Budapest, the other Hungarian cities with a Medical University have units with many sub-specialities for the past several decades. Their chiefs János Dénes (Budapest), István Altorjay (Szeged), Imre Pilaszanovich (Pécs) established paediatric surgery in Hungary.

Latvia

In Latvia, up to the end of the 19th century, surgical care to children was provided by general surgeons. Paediatric surgery in Latvia originated in 1899 when the first children's hospital was founded in Riga (Fig. 6). The hospital was financially supported by the patron of British origin James Armsteadt. The first principal of Latvian Paediatric Surgery Department was Paul Klemm, a doctor of German origin.

In 1915 Reinchold Girgenson, who was of Baltic–German origin, became head of the Surgical Department in the Children's Hospital. After him the paediatric surgeon of Latvian origin Aleksandrs Biezins took up the leadership of the Paediatric Surgery Department (Fig. 7), having had training in Germany, Austria and

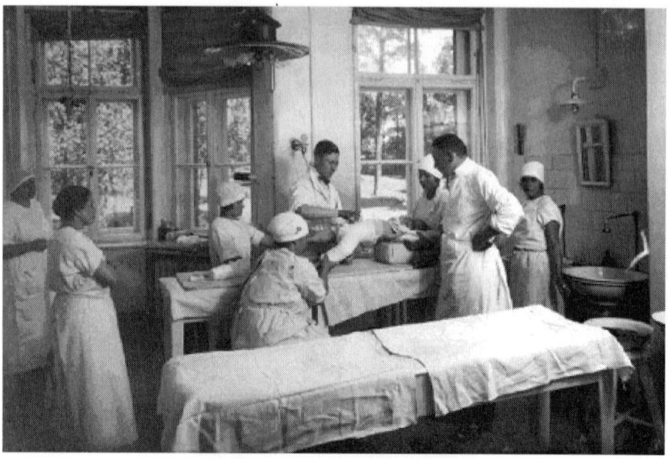

Fig. 6. Latvian Hospital.

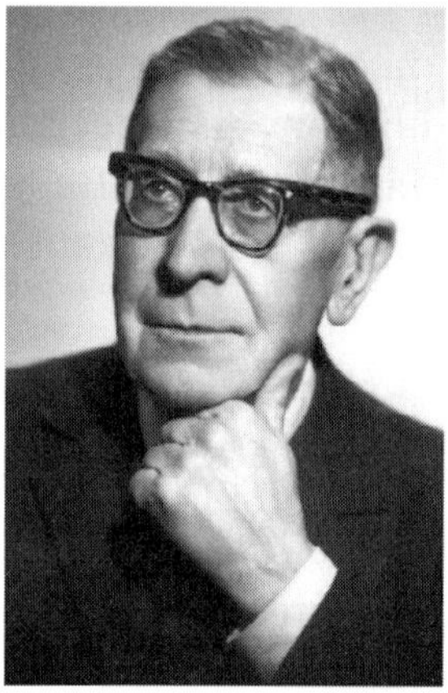

Fig. 7. Alexander BIEZINS/Latvia.

France. From 1972 the paediatric surgery clinic was headed by Prof Janis Gaujens.

The Department of Paediatric Surgery of the Children's University Hospital of Riga has become an up-to-date European Union medical centre of the 21st century, where about 4500 operations are performed annually.

Lithuania

The beginning of Lithuanian Paediatric Surgery as a separate field of surgery dated back to 1895, when the first Department of Paediatric Surgery was established in the Vilnius Red Cross Hospital. More than 40 years later with 16 beds, another unit for paediatric surgery was opened in the Department of Surgery of Kaunas University. Now, the paediatric surgeons are trained in the Medical Faculty of Vilnius University and Kaunas Medical University.

In 1989 Prof Jonas Gradauskas (Vilnius) issued his first book on "*Paediatric Surgery*". In 1990, the possibilities for cooperation arise between the leading paediatric surgical units in Europe and the Lithuanian paediatric surgical wards and Lithuanian paediatric surgeons. The equipment in the departments are constantly improving, and innovations, especially minimal surgical intervention, are being introduced in Lithuania.

The 3 Baltic States — Lithuania, Latvia and Estonia — have been organising their biannual international congresses, which are very successful and well-attended meetings over two decades.

Romania

The first children's hospital in **Romania** and also in the Balkans was founded in **Bucharest** in 1858. "Grigore Alexandrescu" Children's Emergency Hospital was divided into two departments: Paediatrics and Paediatric Surgery. Children up to 14 years of age were admitted. In 1914 a new Department of Paediatric Surgery and Orthopaedics was opened. By 1966 it had 90 surgical, 64 orthopaedic, 50 urological and 30 intensive care beds with 8 operating theatres. The surgeons who led this department were: Prof Iacob Iacobovici (1879–1959), Prof Alexandru Cosacescu (1888–1951), Prof Filip Gottlieb (1897–1966), Prof Dimitrie Vereranu (1909–1994), Prof Mircea Socolescu (1925–2006) and Prof Tudor Zamfir (born 1936) (Fig. 8).

Prof Tudor Zamfir was a good surgeon, teacher and academic. He wrote a textbook of Paediatric Surgery and developed an original procedure "Detachment of the triceps in the treatment of elbow

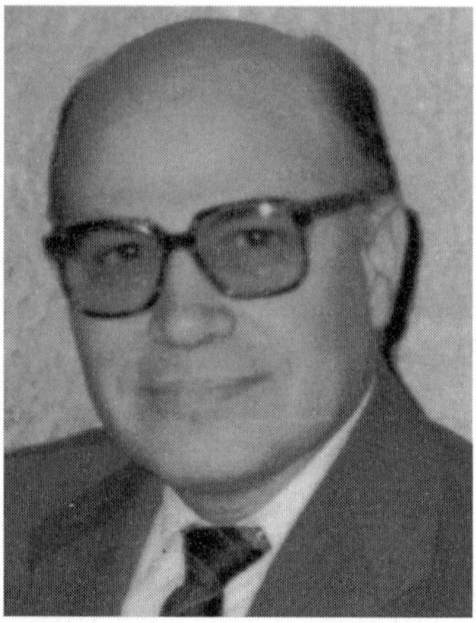

Fig. 8. Tudor ZAMFIR/Romania.

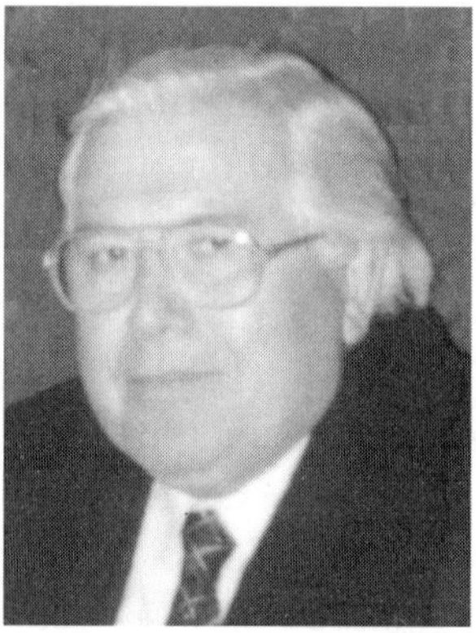

Fig. 9. Alexandru PESAMOSCA/Romania.

stiffness in extension in children". This technique is mentioned in Campbell's "*Operative Orthopaedics*" textbook.

In 1984 in **Bucharest**, a completely new hospital was inaugurated, "Maria Sklodowska Curie" Emergency Children's Hospital. The chief of the Department of Paediatric Surgery was Prof Alexandru Pesamosca (Fig. 9). The modern history of Romanian Paediatric Surgery began with the Prof Alexandru

Pesamosca. He was a very skilled surgeon and he had a very long and successful career.

In **Romania**, paediatric surgery is taught and performed in 9 university cities: **Bucharest**, Lasi, Timisoara, Cluj, Craiova, **Tirgu Mures**, Constanta, **Brasov** and Arad. One of the prominent paediatric surgeons who headed these centres was Prof Vasile Fufezan (1928–2000, in Timisoara). He developed two personal techniques. One of them was adding a patch of azygos vein over the end-to-end anastomosis of the oesophageal pouches in esophageal atresia, as a security measure for preventing leakage. His second technique concerned the omphalocele. Due to the lack of synthetic materials, he used the omphalocele membrane, excising the borders and, after reintroduction of the viscera into the abdominal cavity, suturing the membrane to the muscular fascia to close the defect.

Serbia

Pioneer steps in the development of surgical paediatrics in Serbia are closely intertwined with the name of Dr Dimitrije Jovcic. He was trained in Paris and after the end of the 1st World War, he returned from Paris to Serbia as the first faculty educated paediatric surgeon. In 1921 the 1st Department of Child Surgery, headed by Dr Dimitrije Jovcic, was opened at the General State Hospital of Belgrade.

The second person who bears merits for the development of surgical paediatrics in Serbia is Dr Matija Abrozic. It was because of him that the construction of a new children's hospital building was begun with 180 hospital beds, of which 80 were to be used for surgical paediatrics. The new building, today's University Children's Hospital of Belgrade, was constructed according to the strictest European criteria for a children's hospital. In the period between the 1st and the 2nd World Wars, paediatric surgeons were mainly preoccupied with emergency states and orthopaedic diseases.

A rapid development of surgical paediatrics, as a surgical discipline, occurred in 1947, when paediatric surgery became acknowledged as an obligatory subject in the Belgrade Medical School's curriculum and also became a subspecialisation in Serbia. Consequently, the Belgrade Hospital became capable of covering the whole surgical pathology of children, from the neonatal to the teenage period. At the University Children's Hospital of Belgrade Dr M. Mitrovic (Nis), Dr J. Dzokovic (Novi Sad), Prof Dr D. Jovanovic (Belgrade), Prof Dr D. Bajec, Dr Jelenic and many others completed their paediatric surgical training.

Today Serbia has 152 paediatric surgeons, who, based on the regional principle within secondary and tertiary health protection, cover the whole territory of Serbia. Today there are two paediatric cardio-surgical centres (Institute for Mother and Child and University Children's Hospital), one Paediatric Centre for Hemodialysis and Kidney Transplantation (UCH) and one Centre for Bone Transplantation (IMCH).

Russia

It is difficult to separate the history of paediatric surgery of the previous Soviet Union from that of present. Five leading paediatric surgeons whose work hallmarked and determined the development of paediatric surgery both in the Soviet Union and Russia in the 20th century have contributed to this synopsis and their contributions are presented.

Ternovsky Sergey Dmitrievich (1896–1960) was a scientist, a surgeon and a teacher. He was one of the founders of paediatric surgery in the USSR. He led the paediatric surgery and orthopaedics of Pirogov's 2nd Medical Institute in Moscow from 1943 till he passed away. He was author of 75 scientific workpieces, including three monographs and textbooks on acute thoracic, abdominal and neonatal surgery, surgery of osseous-articular tuberculosis, harelip and corrosive strictures of oesophagus. His textbook was re-printed three times and translated into a many languages.

Isakov Yury Fedorovitch (1923–present) was a most outstanding paediatric surgeon and teacher and public figure. Isakov was first engaged by general surgery and later became a paediatric surgeon under the supervision of Prof Ternovsky. In 1966 he was elected to the chair of paediatric surgery of Pirogov's 2nd Medical Institute in Moscow.

Isakov has written over 400 scientific publications, including 20 monographs, seven textbooks and manuals on subjects of surgery of newborns and children. His courses for thoracic and abdominal surgeries in infants and young children and paediatric endosurgery were well-attended by participants from all over the country.

Stepanov Eduard Alexandrovich (1929–2007) served as Professor of Paediatric Surgery of Pirogov's in the 2nd Moscow Medical Institute for many years. Stepanov published over 330 scientific works, including seven monographs and two manuals on childrens' chest surgery, plastic, abdominal and emergency surgery, permanent magnets application for the closure of intestinal fistulas and proctology.

Bairov Girey Alievitch (1922–1999) was one of the most widely known Soviet and Russian paediatric surgeons. In 1951 he was promoted as head of the Institute of Paediatric Surgery in Leningrad (now, St. Petersburg). He published over 380 scientific works, including 17 monographs regarding diagnostic, clinical and surgical treatment of developmental anomalies in children, traumatic shock, purulent-septic and urgent surgery, paediatric reanimation, surgery of the prematures, proctology, orthopaedics and traumatology.

Dolecky Stanislav Jakovlevich (1919–1994) was probably the most widely known Soviet and Russian childrens' surgeon internationally. He was one of the organizers of paediatric surgical service in the Soviet Union. In 1958 he was elected to the chair of paediatric surgery of Leningrad Medical Paediatric Institute. Later, he moved from Leningrad to Moscow. In 1959 he became the managing director of paediatric surgery of Central Institute of Postgraduate Education in Moscow. Dolecky has published over 500 scientific works, including 25 monographs (diaphragmatic hernia, obstructions of colon in first month of life, and portal hypertension). Not only an outstanding surgeon he was also a skilled pianist who entertained many groups of paediatric surgeons to highly entertaining evenings after dinner.

Slovakia

Slovakian paediatric surgery began as a speciality in 1894, when a new hospital building was built in Bratislava. In 1939, Prof Žucha (Fig. 10) arrived in Slovakia. He was a neurosurgeon, but since his early beginnings in the Children hospital he paid intensive attention to paediatric surgery and its development. Since January 1950, Paediatric Surgery became a separate ward in Bratislava. Three years later it became an independent University Department, where neonatal and abdominal surgery, traumatology and orthopaedic procedures were performed in large numbers.

In 1962 Prof Žucha was followed by Prof Kratochvil, who enriched the surgical palette with lung and portal hypertension surgery. He founded a laboratory of surgical pathophysiology to solve various problems of paediatric surgery on an experimental basis; furthermore he established an advanced level of anaesthesiology and resuscitation in his institute.

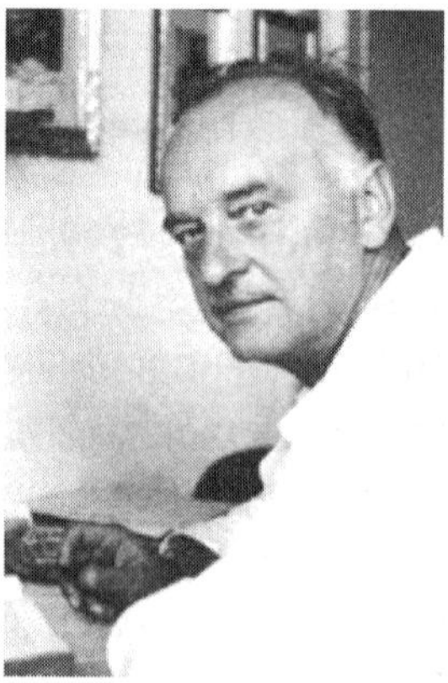

Fig. 10. Josef ŽUCHA/Slovakia.

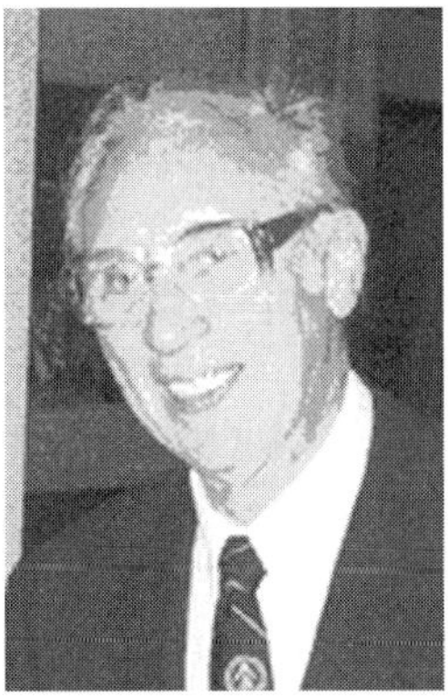

Fig. 11. Eduard PEKAROVIČ/Slovakia.

In 1990, Prof Dr Eduard Pekarovič became the head of the department (Fig. 11). He was a world-acclaimed paediatric surgeon, and has been well-received both in the American and European paediatric surgical communities, where he was well-known as "Eddie". Prof Pekarovič remains forever a respectable example for being not only a highly knowledgeable, theoretically sound, but also manually skilful surgeon.

Ukraine

In 19th century paediatric surgical cases were treated in general hospitals in Ukraine. First department of paediatrics was established in Kiev in 1899, which had a paediatric surgical ward. In 1900 a "Society of Hospitals" was founded, also in Kiev, where mainly children were treated with diseases of bones and joints. Vira Gedroitz, a student of Caesar Roux of Lausanne, Switzerland, was the first female professor of surgery in Ukraine to have had courses of paediatric surgery in Kiev from 1927 to 1929. The teaching departments of paediatric surgery in Ukraine were established in Kiev (1935), Kharkov (1935), Odessa (1938), and Dnepropetrovsk (1938).

The first operation in a child with Hirschsprung's disease, which was performed by professor Andrey Shurinok in 1959, gave impetus for foundation of endotracheal anaesthesia in children. In his article in 1963 he made conclusion that "children have to be operated for Hirschsprung's disease earlier then two to three years of age", and that "intratracheal anesthesia allowed for absence of pneumonia and atelectasis cases in post-operative period". The speciality of paediatric thoracic surgery was founded in Ukraine in 1964. By 1960, seven teaching departments of paediatric surgery were already running in Kiev, Kharkov, Odessa, Dnepropetrovsk, Lviv, Donetsk, and Simferopol.

The first conference of Ukrainian paediatric surgeons was held in 1960 in Odessa and attended by 243 delegates from Ukraine.

Acknowledgement

Numerous paediatric surgeons past and present have assisted in the preparation of this manuscript and to them I extend my thanks. For current assistance in this manuscript I wish to extend special thanks to the following who have contributed:-

Vasiliy AVERIN (Belarus), Vidmantas BARAUSKAS (Lithuania), Ognjan BRANKOV (Bulgaria), Merab BUADZE (Georgia), Salahudin DIZDAREVIC (Bosnia Herzegovina), Kristof FUZESI (Hungary), Vladimir KHURSIN (Ukraine), Zoran KRISTIC (Serbia), Sergey MINAEV (Russia), Aigars PETERSONS (Latvia), Jiri SNAJDAUF (Czech Republic), Karin VARIK (Estonia), Tibor VEREBELY (Hungary), Marian VIDISCAK (Slovakia) and Corina ZAMFIR (Romania).

Footnote from the Editors

The editors would add to the content of this chapter, collected and written modestly by a Hungarian surgeon, an appreciation of the marked development of the specialty which has been advanced by the next generation of Hungarian surgeons who have followed the instigators mentioned in the Hungarian section. Andras Pinter (Pecs), Kristof Fuzesi (Szeged), Tibor Verebly (Budapest) and Akos Kiss (Miskolc) (Figs. 12(a)–(d)), three recently retired but

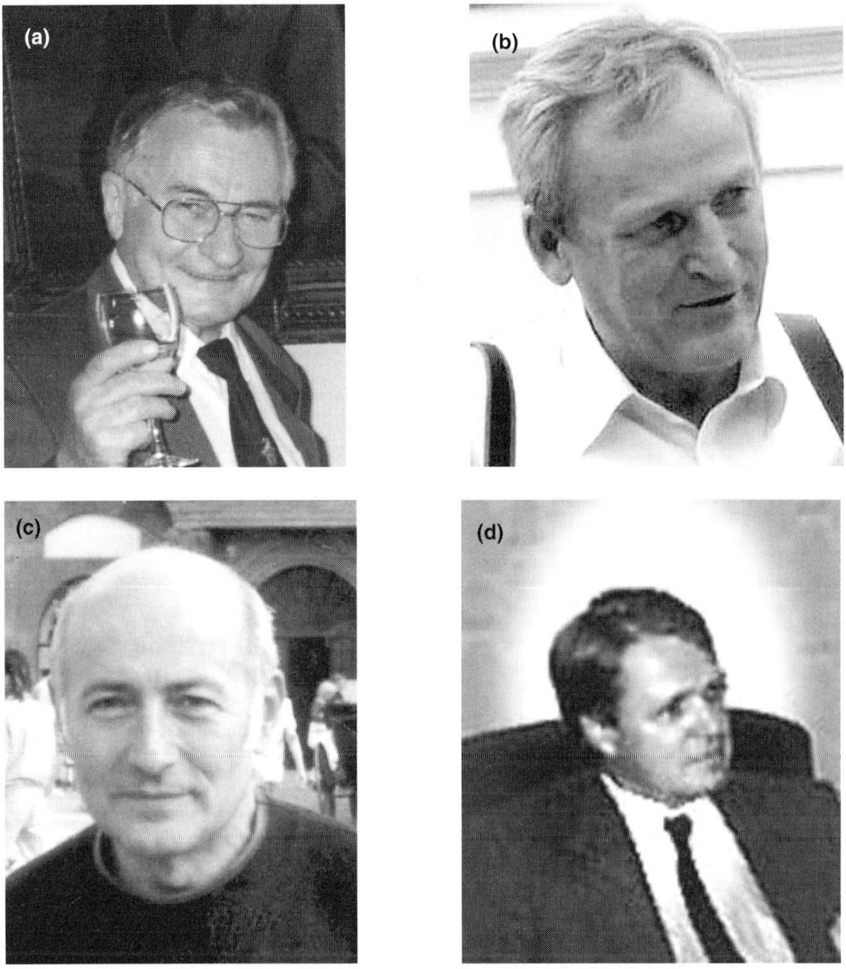

Fig. 12. (a) Fusezi, (b) Kiss, (c) Pinter, (d) Verebly.

Tibor Verebly remains in active clinical practice, with their colleagues have provided rapid and planned developments in the training of paediatric surgeons. With their Hungarian colleagues they have been very successful in advancing paediatric surgical standards and particularly in organising structured training of their junior staff. By their efforts in maintaining active communications with paediatric surgeons in many countries round the world they have contributed sustantially to the development of the specialty and have conducted the European Paediatric Surgical examination now functioning in EEC countries. The very high performance by the Hungarian candidates was recorded by the examiners. Their substantial contribution in Europe has to be acknowledged.

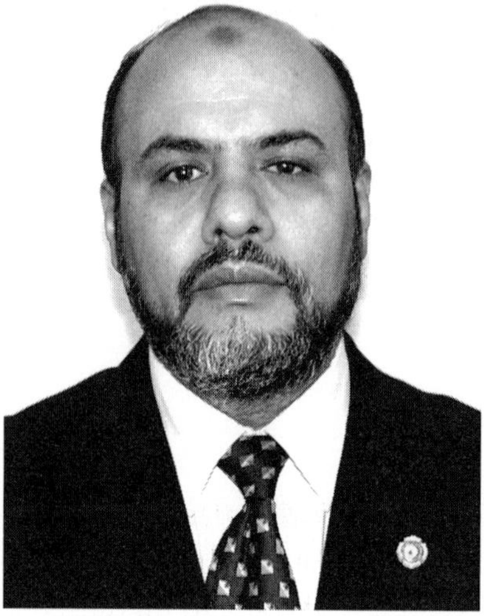

Essam A. Elhalaby

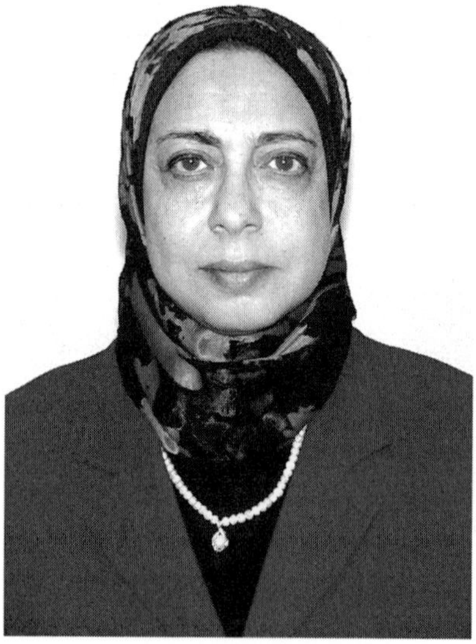

Amel A. Hashish

EGYPT

Essam A. Elhalaby
Amel A. Hashish

Surgery in Ancient Egypt

The ancient Egyptian surgical literature. In 1862, Edwin Smith, an American dealer and collector of antiquities, was sold an ancient roll of papyrus, 15 ft long and one ft wide. Incomplete and missing on its outer portions but with unusual content, the papyrus was surely a good buy. Two months later, on another tour in the city of Luxor, Egypt, the same dealer offered him a second papyrus, which turned out to be the missing parts of the first one, glued to another roll. Smith recognized it immediately and bought the new one. Later, he reconstructed the papyrus. He even made some efforts at translation, but never published it. It was not until 1920, when James H. Breasted, the famous archaeologist and historian, was asked by the New York historical society to translate the papyrus. This mission that took ten years to be completed. What Breasted found was utterly remarkable.

The papyrus turned out to be an ancient copy of a manuscript (written around 1700 B.C.) that contained 48 case histories on the topic of "Trauma." They were arranged starting up at the head, and going down the body. The manuscript went as far down as the thorax and the spine, after which it cuts off. The manuscript went through what should be done in the instance of certain injuries (i.e. a protocol of management). The Papyrus opens with eight paragraphs concerning head wounds, followed by nineteen paragraphs on treatment of wounds of the face (forehead, eyebrows, nose, cheeks, temples, mouth, and chin), six descriptions of how to deal with injuries of the throat and neck, five dealing with collar-bones and arms, and seven on chest complaints. It describes how to stitch a gaping wound with acacia thorns used as needles and pieces of flax as suturing material; it describes also the after management of sutured wounds: "hast it stitched, thou shouldst lay fresh meat upon his wound the first day. Thou shouldst not bind it. More as his injury passes by. Thou shouldst treat it afterward with grease, honey, and lint everyday, until he recovers". For "pus-filled tumors" (abscesses), it recommends cauterization, in which a very hot copper instrument would be used, not only to cut away the damaged tissue but also to seal all the blood vessels. The papyrus also contains the first description of the meninges (the membranes covering the brain), the external surface of the brain and the cerebrospinal fluid. It also notes that brain injuries are associated with changes in the function of other parts of the body, especially the lower limbs.[1]

The Edwin Smith papyrus, now at the New York Medical Academy, is currently considered the first surgical textbook *per se*. The earliest textbook that is almost devoid of magical thinking and describes in exquisite scientific manner the examination, diagnosis, treatment, and prognosis of numerous ailments.[2]

Approximately, a dozen other papyri on ancient Egyptian medicine and surgery have survived and act today as our primary source of their medical knowledge. Most of these were written between 2000 B.C and 1200 B.C., but some templates dates as far back as 2500 B.C. The most popular and well known papyri are: The Kahun Gynecological Papyrus, The Ebers, The Hearst, The Chester, The Berlin, and The London papyri, in addition to the Edwin Smith manuscript.

The Ebers concentrates on diseases of the eye, the digestive system, the head, the skin and disease of the urinary tract. This papyrus also provides our earliest possible documentation of ancient awareness of tumors. It also mentions treatment of volvulus "if he does not evacuate it for a twist in the bowel and if the phlegm does not find a way out, it shall rot in the belly."[3]

The ancient Egyptians medical knowledge was valuable enough to be engraved on tombs' walls as well. One of the best solid evidence of practice of surgery in ancient Egypt was discovered written on the wall of a tomb of Ankh-Mahor (2000 B.C.) at Saqqara (about 19 miles south of Cairo).[4]

Open wounds were often treated with honey. A freshly peeled clove of raw garlic wrapped in muslin or cheesecloth and pinned to the undergarment is hoped to protect against infectious diseases. Powdered cumin mixed with grease or lard was inserted as an anal suppository to disperse heat from the anus and stop itching. Leaves from many plants, such as willow, sycamore, acacia, were used in poultices and the like. Tannic acid derived from acacia nuts commonly helped heal burns. Castor oil, combined with figs and dates, was used as a laxative. Yeast was recognized for its healing qualities and was applied to leg ulcers and swellings. Yeast's were also taken internally for digestive disorders and were an effective cure for ulcers.

The ancient Egyptians had advanced medical practice for their times. They were masters in human anatomy and in the art of healing. This is probably due to the extensive mummification ceremonies which involved removing most of the internal organs including; the brain, lungs, pancreas, liver, spleen, heart and intestine. Ancient Egyptian physicians were actually treated "in a way" like celebrities and were even worshiped by the public. Imhotep (Fig. 1) was the physician and advisor of King Zoser, of the 3rd dynasty. He was worshiped after his death as the "God of Healing and Medicine." Imhotep (Fig. 1) in fact was a living genius, an astronomer, architect and a physician too. Not only considered the original author of the Edwin Smith papyrus, but the builder of the Stepped Pyramid at Saqqara as well. The Greeks later identified him with their own humanized god of healing, Asclepias. His statue stands today in the Hall of Immortals at the International College of Surgeons in Chicago.

The fame of the Ancient Egyptian physicians travelled far and it was not uncommon in both the early and the late dynasties for scholars from ancient Greece and other parts of the Mediterranean to

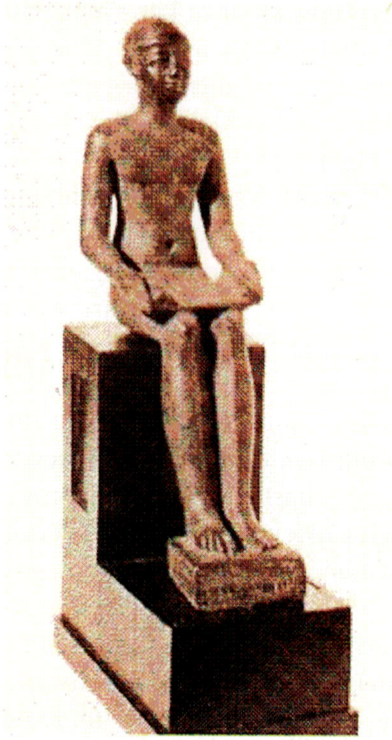

Fig. 1. Imhotep, the "God of Healing".

study medicine on the Egyptian masters. Herodotus and Pliny, whose contributions to the art of medicine are well known, were in fact travelling scholars in Egypt.

The ancient surgical instruments. The surgical tools in ancient Egypt were different from our modern times tools. Theirs included knives, drills, saws, hooks, forceps and pinchers, scales, spoons, and a vase with burning incense. Knives had stone blades with edges sharper than modern surgical steel. Blades made of iron and bronze came relatively late to Egypt. By that time, metal instruments were used to cut and cauterize. In some procedures, the blade was heated until it glowed red, and then used to make incisions.[5]

In the temple of Sobek, there are reliefs of medical instruments: bone saws, suction cups, knives and scalpels, retractors, scales, lances, chisels and dental tools. At the temple of Kom Ombo, a box of surgical instruments has been carved into the outer corridor wall. The box contains thirty-seven instruments, including metal shears, knives, saws, probes, spatulas and spoons.

Surgical procedures. Details of their practiced surgical procedures were depicted on the wall of the tombs. On the wall of Ankh–Mahor tomb, there is a picture of a circumcision of an adolescent with an hieroglyphs manuscript saying: "The ointment is used to make it acceptable," in another words, a local anesthetic has being used, though this reading is not bulletproof, as happens often in such inscriptions (Fig. 2).

Trepanation, practiced in many early cultures for a number of reasons, was not mentioned in any of their papyri or in the tombs. However, it seems to have been performed occasionally using a mallet and a chisel. Fourteen skulls with trephine holes, some healed or partially healed, have been found. Limb amputations were also performed as observed in the mummies.

Egyptians practiced surgery on the dead as well. The mummy of the great pharaoh Rameses II, now in Cairo museum, was surgically amended by inserting a small bone and a quantity of seeds into his nose. During his lifetime, Rameses' nose had been his most prominent

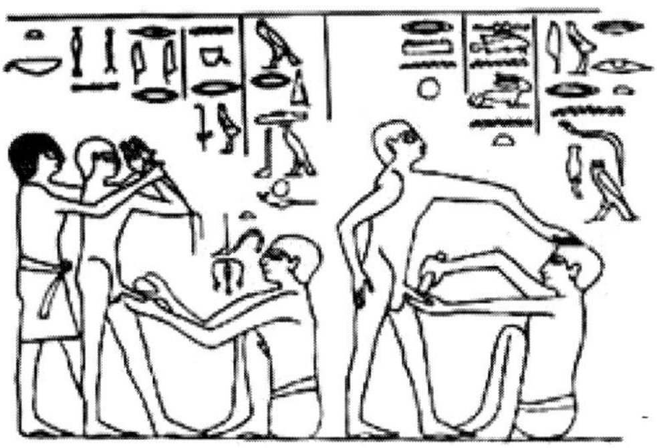

Fig. 2. First circumcision scene shown carved on the wall of 6th Dynasty painting.

feature, and the Egyptian surgeons ensured that in death, it remained just as prominent.

Medical education. Nothing certain is known about the way physicians acquired their medical knowledge, but one surmises that after their formation as scribes they were apprenticed to practicing healers. When Harsiese, the fictional physician in the prologue "the Instructions of Ankhsheshonq" was summoned to the royal court, he underwent some quizzing by the king himself and then became a member of the medical team looking after the pharaoh.[6]

Although there were no medical schools, doctors and some priests were taught medicine through years of training at the temples. Their knowledge, as mentioned before, came primarily through the process of mummification, in which they removed and examined different parts of the body after death.

The Egyptian physicians were much sought after in the Ancient World. Ramses II sent physicians to the king of Hatti. Many rulers, the Persian Achaemenids among them, had Egyptian doctors in attendance. Egyptian theories and practices influenced the Greeks, who furnished medical thinking for centuries to come.

In summary, the medicinal skills of ancient Egyptians were far beyond their time. With the writing of the first medical texts, performance of the first surgical techniques, use of the first splints and bandages, the first drug therapies, and the first medical dictionary (Fig. 3), the ancient Egyptians revolutionized the world of medicine and laid a path and framework for the advances in medicine that exist in our world today.

Surgery in the Alexandrian Era

Alexandria was founded in 331 BC by Alexander the Great and governed by a dynasty stemming from his general Ptolemy. The Ptolemaic rulers gave lavish financial support to the library and museum at Alexandria, which consequently attracted researchers in all fields. The study of anatomy in Egypt reached its peak in the Greek era as two senior physicians, Herovel and Erasystran, came to

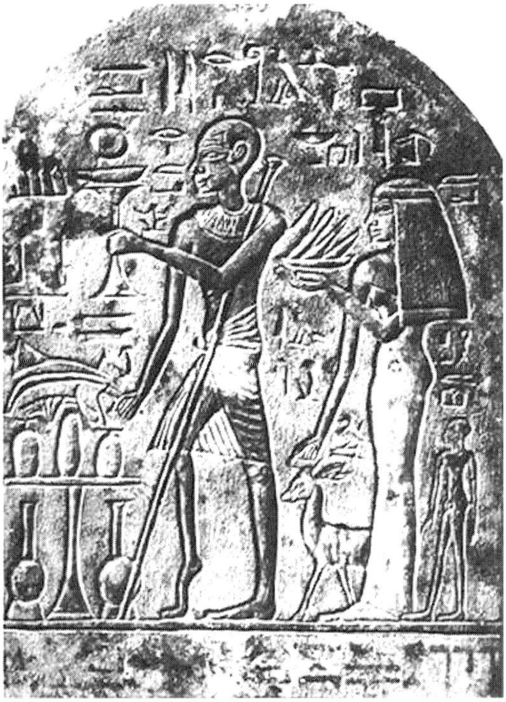

Fig. 3. Young man with withered leg characteristic of polio (1500–1350 B.C.).

Alexandria to gain a detailed knowledge of the anatomy of the human body to be able to treat all pathological cases. Physicians from all over the world came to Alexandria to be trained in anatomy.

Around 200 A.D., Flavius Clemens Alexandrinus, founder of a Christian school in Alexandria, reported six complete Egyptian medical books, in which the subject was systematically handled, one of which was "about the construction of the body." According to Flavius, these six books were part of a series of 42 holy books, which have been ascribed to Thoth (Hermes Trismegistos). Sadly, the 42 Hermetic books have been lost.

The surviving medical texts are not textbooks, as we understand them today, but rather descriptions of cases and instructions for treatment. A few technical and philological commentaries exist, describing the position or normal function of certain organs or parts of the body.

Whilst making this assessment, following points should, however, be considered: firstly, the Egyptian meaning is exceptionally difficult to translate: secondly, some terms are ambiguous. One word is, for example, used for muscles as well as tendons, veins or nerves. Another word is used for both "body" and "flesh." A final point being that it is not possible to distinguish to what extent the physical is fused with the spiritual in a symbolic or analogous manner.

Recovered surgical instruments used during that period indicate that the art of surgery progressed and proliferated greatly during this time. Most instruments were made of bronze, or occasionally of silver. Iron was rarely used because, as in most ancient cultures, it was considered a religious taboo. The full repertoire of Roman surgical equipment is still far from completely known.

Archaeological remains of what appear to be surgeons' "shops" are common enough to indicate that some physicians specialized in surgery. Philological evidence seems to support the idea that there was at least some distinction, even if not a rigid one, between a general practitioner and a surgeon.

In Alexandria, the dissection of corpses was a regular practice, whereas before the fourth century BC it had been condemned and outlawed on religious principles. Celsus had also publicized a rumor that the anatomists used living people, most likely condemned criminals, in vivisection.

In Roman Egypt circumcision of men and women was widespread. Even the total removal of a woman's clitoris was common, as a Greek text of Aëtius tells us. In order to stop the bleeding after this surgery a kind of pad was used made from a compress with a sponge on top. Similar designs might have been also utilized to absorb menstrual blood. Interestingly, both the ancient Greek doctor Hippocrates and the Roman scholar Galen reported having seen Imhotep's works in a temple in Memphis, Egypt.[7]

Surgery in the Islamic Era

The world owes the development of the concept of the "hospital" to Islamic medicine. Much thought was given to the concept and to the technical details. They even went as far as testing the soil for germs before picking the hospital sites, as described by Abu Bakr Al-Razi, but perhaps the most impressive aspect of this invention was its mission: treatment for all who need it, regardless of their status.

In 872 A.D., Ahmed Ibn-Tulun, governor of Egypt, built Al-Fustat hospital in the city of Al-Fustat, which lies now in the old district of Cairo. It served the growing Cairo population well for six centuries. It was divided into separate wards. On admission, the patients were given special apparel while their clothes, money, and valuables were stored until the time of their discharge.

In 1284 A.D., King Al-Mansur Qalawun built Al-Mansuri Hospital, one of the largest hospitals ever built, as mentioned by Ibn-Battota and El-Kalkashandi, the great historians. The hospital had different wards for different diseases e.g. for surgery, fevers and eye diseases. The Hospital had its own pharmacy, library and lecture halls. There was also a mosque for the Muslims, as well as a chapel for the Christians. The hospital had unusual methods of treatment and music was used as a line of treatment for psychiatric patients. On discharge; the patient was given food and money as compensation for his off-work time. Al-Mansuri Hospital served 4000 patients daily and has served Cairo for seven centuries since it has been built. It is now used for ophthalmology and is called Mustashfa Qalawun. Its ancient door is kept in the Islamic Museum of Cairo.

In that period, when Arab civilization flourished, many of the famous physicians emerged, like Abu Ali al-Hussain, Ibn Abdallah, Ibn Sina, and Ibn Al-Nafees. The latter described the pulmonary blood circulatory system for the first time in the history of medicine.

The biggest contributor in the field of surgery is perhaps Abu-Al-Qasim Khalaf Ibn'Abbas Al-Zahrawi (930–1013 A.D.). He had been known in the western world as Abulcasis, Bucasis or Alzahravius. Al-Zahrawi spent a productive life in practicing medicine, especially in surgery and medical writings. He died at the age of 83. He wrote four books; the most famous of them all is "Al-Tastif Liman Ajiz'an Al-Ta'lif," which is by for the best medieval surgical encyclopedia ever written.[8] It was used in Europe until the 17th century.

Al-Zahrawi mentioned the techniques of various pediatric surgical procedures, besides he created instruments for pediatric operations. Probably he was one the first who described the pediatric operations with pictures and drawn the pediatric surgical instruments. Besides his book has been shown as a guide for the 15th century surgeon Serfadeddin Sabuncuoglu from Turkey.

In his books, he stressed the importance of the basic sciences: "... Before practicing, one should be familiar with the science of anatomy and the functions of organs.... Also he should know the bones, nerves, and muscles, their numbers, their origin and insertions, the arteries and the veins, their start and end.... If one does not comprehend the anatomy and physiology, he may commit a mistake that can kill the patient. I have seen someone, who pretended to be a surgeon, incising an aneurysm in the neck of a woman, mistaking it for an abscess. The woman bled to death."

Heller stated that Al-Zahrawi described the ligature of arteries long before Ambrose Pare.[9] He also used cautery to control bleeding and used wax and alcohol to stop bleeding from the skull during cranial surgery. Al-Zahrawi also described the tracheotomy operation and was the first to write on orthodontia. He showed evidence of great experience from details of clinical picture and surgical procedures e.g. his description of varicose veins stripping, even after ten centuries, is almost like modern surgery. He also wrote about fracture of the skull.[10,11]

As he once wrote "... Choose your instruments carefully beforehand according to the operation. However, you should design other devices if needed." Thus he encouraged the physician to be innovative. During the time of Al-Zahrawi, surgery in the Islamic world and in Egypt became a well-respected specialty, practiced by reputable physicians.

Pediatric Surgery in Modern Egypt

Pediatric surgery units. Modern pediatric surgery in Egypt can be traced back to the early 20th century. In 1934, during the first year of King Farouk reign, a charity organization named "healthy child organization" built a specialized hospital dedicated only for sick children — the "Abou Elrish Hospital." This could come true due to the efforts of an eminent Egyptian pediatrician, Dr Sami Kamal. Three years later, the building was donated to the University of Cairo (known as king Fouad University at that time) to be the first University Children's Hospital. Dr Ibraheem Shawky Bek, a pediatrician and head of the hospital, allocated four beds, for the first time, to the surgical patients. In the beginning, a house officer carried the duties of the surgical registrar. Two years later, Dr Sebaay Alzenfaly was assigned the first registrar job in the pediatric surgery unit followed by Dr Aly Ibraheem (later Aly Pasha Ibraheem) a pioneer of modern surgery in Egypt.

The unit remained under the supervision of pediatricians until 1961, when control came finally to a pediatric surgeon. The credit goes to Prof Dr Ismail Mehrez, Professor of General Surgery, who decided that the unit should be supervised by a pediatric surgeon.

As the time went by, Abou Elrish Children's Hospital turned to be perhaps the largest and most famous children's hospital in the Middle East and Africa. The old Abou Elrish Children's Hospital (1937–1991) has been replaced by two newer children's hospitals. The first is Cairo University Specialized Pediatric Hospital, which was established in July 1983 with the financial help of the Japanese government. It includes 176 beds, five operating rooms (OR), and two neonatal and pediatric intensive care units (NICU, PICU), in addition to a large outpatient clinic for all pediatric sub-specialties. The second and more recent hospital is the Moniera Children's Hospital, which is even larger (320 beds and 32 incubators at the NICU). Both hospitals are part of the Cairo University Hospitals and are level 3, tertiary referral pediatric surgical centers.[12]

The second oldest children's hospital in Egypt, "Al Shatby Hospital for Women and Children," was established in Alexandria in 1954. These were followed by pediatric surgical units in Tanta, Ain Shams, Assuit, Maudi Milding Hospital, Alazhar, Almansoura, Zagazig, Ismailia, Benha, and in Sohag. Many of these units have progressed to a full Children's hospital. Currently there are nine children's hospitals in Egypt serving more than 30 million children.

Egyptian Pediatric Surgical Association (EPSA) (Figs. 4, 5). The Egyptian Pediatric Surgical Association has been established in

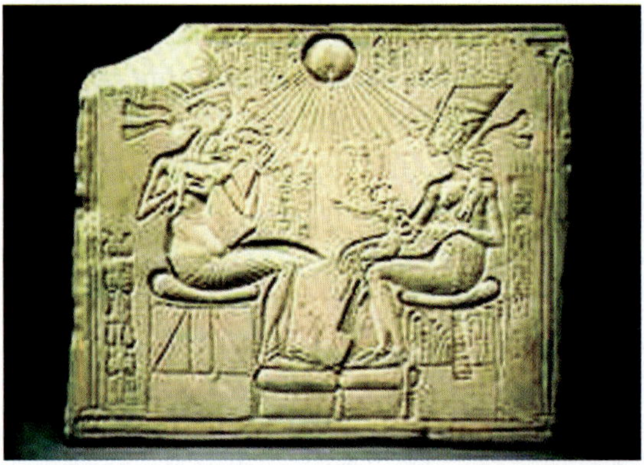

Fig. 4. King Akhenaton and his beautiful wife Nefertiti carrying their royal children. Artists were allowed for the first time to portray the pharaoh and his wife carrying their children.

Fig. 5. EPSA Logo.

1980. Today, 265 of Egyptian finest surgeons in more than 12 specialized pediatric surgical centers form the core of EPSA. Almost half of them are full members and the remaining are associate members who are still in training or affiliated members who are working in other specialties but have major interest in pediatric sub-specialties, such as pediatric plastic surgery and pediatric urology.

The EPSA offers a lot of scientific and social services to its members. The annual meeting of EPSA is considered the largest and most important pediatric surgical scientific event in the Middle East and North Africa. It grasps the attention of many pediatric surgeons from various parts of the world. Every year, some of world leaders in pediatric surgery are invited to participate in this meeting (Fig. 6). The EPSA have established an Akkary Lecture in memory of man having established the Children's Hospital in Alexandria (1958).

It is interesting to note that almost one half of the Egyptian pediatric surgeons are working temporary outside Egypt in the Arab Gulf countries and other Arab and non-Arab countries in Africa, Europe and North America. It is an honor for the Egyptian pediatric

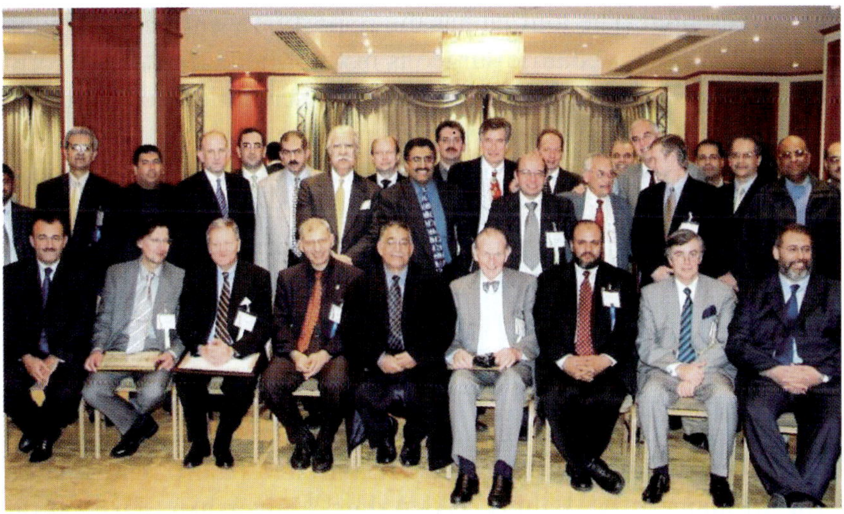

Fig. 6. Photo taken during the 20th Annual Meeting of EPSA, December 2004, Cairo.

surgical community that many regional pediatric surgical centers in the Arab countries were established by members of EPSA.

The commitment of Egyptian pediatric surgeons to improving pediatric surgical practiced in other regional countries in Africa is remarkable. During the past three decades, many Egyptian pediatric surgeons have worked in African countries, and three of the six meetings of the Pan African Pediatric Surgical Association (PAPSA) were held in Cairo and Alexandria and were sponsored and organized by EPSA.

Egyptian pediatric surgeons have been always in contact with pediatric surgeons in various parts of the world. Most of the recent updates in pediatric surgical field were quickly and efficiently brought to the country.

Annals of pediatric surgery. The latest achievement of EPSA is the establishment of "*Annals of Pediatric Surgery*." An international pear reviewed journal. Almost 2.5 years have passed since the publishing of the first issue of the journal, which is published quarterly. The "*Annals of Pediatric Surgery*" is striving to fill an important niche that provides focus to clinical care, technical innovation and clinical research. The journal has the opportunity and responsibility to serve not only pediatric surgeons in the Middle East and North Africa but is also an important conduit for scientific information on a very broad international level.[13] During the past year the Journal was approved to be the official Journal of the Mediterranean Association of Pediatric Surgeons (MAPS) and was also endorsed by the Pan African Pediatric Surgical Association (PAPSA).

Acknowledgment

The authors would like to thanks all colleagues, who offered some of the scientific material and data used in the preparation of this chapter especially Prof Mohamed Elbarbary (Cairo University), Prof Mohamed A. Fahmy (Al-Azhar University), Dr Ashraf Al-Atar (Tanta University), and Dr Marium Frham (South Valley University).

References

1. Breasted JH. *The Edwin Smith Surgical Papyrus*, University of Chicago Press, 1930.
2. Ebbell B, tr. The Papyrus Ebers: The Greatest Egyptian Medical Document. Oxford University Press, Levin & Munksgaard, Copenhagen, H. Milford, London, 1937.
3. Bryan PW. *The Papyrus Ebers.* Geoffrey Bles, London, 1930.
4. Joachim H. *Translation of Papyrus Ebers*, Berlin, 1973, p. 171.
5. Ebeid NI. *Egyptian Medicine in the Days of the Pharaohs.* General Egyptian Book Organization Cairo, 1999.
6. Majno G. *The Healing Hand: Man and Wound in the Ancient World.* Harvard University Press, Cambridge, 1982, p. 86–121.
7. Brunner-Traut, *Die alten Ägypter*, Stuttgart, 1974, p. 145.
8. Hitti PK. *History of the Arabs*, 10th ed. St. Martin's Press, New York, 1977, 602–614.
9. Khairallah AA. Arabic contributions to anatomy and surgery: *Ann Med Hist* 1942;3(4):409–415.
10. Al-Okbi. Lights on History of Science: Abu Al- Khasim Al- Zahrawi, the pioneer in surgery. *Hospit Med Prac* 1971;1:14–29.
11. Elgohary MA. Al Zahrawi: The Father of Modern Surgery. *Ann Ped Surg* 2006;2:82–87.
12. Elbarbary M. EPSA Presidential address Pediatric Surgery in Egypt: Past, present and future. Presented at 19th Annual Meeting of Egyptian Pediatric Surgical Association (EPSA), 10–12 December 2003. Cairo, Egypt.
13. Azizkhan R. Preface. *Ann Ped Surg* 2006;2:1.

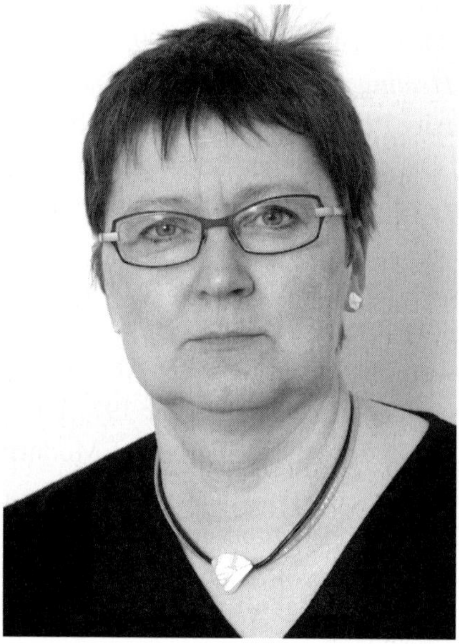

Salminen Päivi

FINLAND

Salminen Päivi

Early History

In Finland the first general hospital was established in 1759; in the 18th century there were five District Hospitals in Finland overall. An organisation of District Physicians to run community healthcare was also established in the eighteenth century. The first surgical hospital started in 1888 and the first paediatric hospital in 1893. In the paediatric hospital there were no surgical beds; surgical paediatric patients were transferred to the adult surgical hospital for surgery.

The number of disabled children was high in the 1800's. They were mainly crippled as a result of congenital anomalies, scurvy, rickets, tuberculosis, osteomyelitis and trauma. These children were generally treated in District Hospitals, usually with bad outcome. In 1889 a primary school teacher Vera Hjeltin established the Society of Aid for Cripples. The Society maintained a children's home, which specialised in taking 4–12-year-old children with orthopaedic needs. In 1900 the Society established an orthopaedic out-patient clinic for poor people in connection with a sheltered workshop. Spinal defects were treated by cast and braces and other body disabilities with bandages and special shoes. Operations to correct orthopaedic problems were started in the year 1905. In autumn 1927 the Society opened an orthopaedic hospital with 20 beds and an out-patient clinic. A workshop for the production of prostheses and support bandages was built within the Orthopaedic Hospital.

The Helsinki Deaconess Institute was founded in 1867 at the initiative of, and with financial support from, Aurora Karamzin, a Finnish wealthy wife of Prince Karamzin who was a Russian Army colonel. The model for this establishment was obtained from Germany. In accordance with the German model, this, Finland's first deaconess institute, provided care for the sick and training for women to become deaconesses. Assistance was given to the poor, and homeless children were given shelter. Crop failure years, famine and epidemics went hand in hand, and the small 8-bed hospital was sorely needed. In early 1900's during tuberculosis epidemics there were several sanatoriums which had wards specialised in "surgical tuberculosis" of children.

Before the Second World War general surgeons operated on children and paediatric surgical patients were usually placed in separate rooms in women's wards. At that time paediatric surgery was mainly concerned with the treatment of infection complications, some orthopaedic conditions and cleft palate and lip surgery. Repair of cleft lips was one of the first specialist fields of surgery for children.

Matti Sulamaa's Time

A new Children's Hospital was completed in 1946 but surgical activities were not included in the plans of the new building. During construction, the lack of paediatric surgery was noticed by Arvo Ylppö (Professor of Paediatrics) and Fabian Langenskóld (Professor of Surgery). The architect was advised to plan operating theatres and surgical wards. Professor Ylppö was an enthusiastic card player and during a game of whist he asked a young orthopaedic registrar, Matti Sulamaa (Fig. 1), if he was interested in starting to work in the new Children's Hospital. This is how Matti Sulamaa become the father of paediatric surgery in Finland. The first paediatric surgical ward and operating theatre were opened on October 15th, 1946. One year later Matti Sulamaa got the first paediatric surgical registrar to work with him. It was not until 1962 when the next two permanent Paediatric Surgical specialists, Mikko Pasila and Kaarlo Parkkulainen, were appointed.

According to his first registrar, the dominant feature of Sulamaa was the confidence he placed on his staff. He expected a lot from

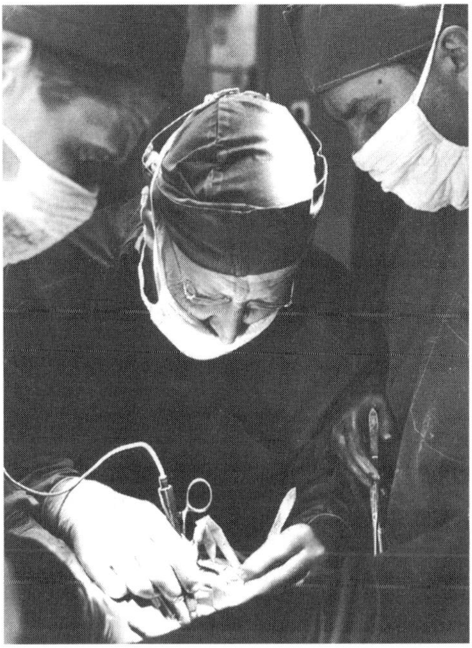

Fig. 1. Prof Sulamaa with on his right Ilmari Viitanen and Mikko Pasila on his left (photo by Caj Bremer).

them but gave them freedom to work; challenged their ideas but never fell out with them as individuals. They were encouraged to use new methods and techniques provided they could convince him of their efficacy. One of the first surgical nurses said: 'We were all learning, even Sulamaa. Almost everything we did, was being done for the first time in Finland.' From the beginning Sulamaa understood the value of international co-operation. He was active in building international bridges in Paediatric Surgery. He had good connections to centres and Paediatric Surgeons abroad. He visited Sweden, Denmark, Germany and different units in Britain and USA. He arranged visits abroad also for his registrars. He especially respected the Boston Children's Hospital and stated that Professors Ladd and Gross had clearly defined the realm of paediatric surgery. He valued the treatment of children in specialised

Paediatric Hospitals that had staff dedicated and trained to treat children.

Sulamaa was one of the founding members and the first "Overseas member" of British Association of Paediatric Surgeons (BAPS). BAPS-meetings became a yearly tradition for Matti Sulamaa. He usually travelled together with his registrar. In 1962 he was invited as honorary member of the Scottish Paediatric Surgical Association. In 1973 he received the Denis Browne Gold Medal, and in 1978, was granted honorary membership of the Royal College of Surgeons in Edinburgh.

Matti Sulamaa was a very innovative surgeon. He described his own modifications of the correction of oesophageal atresia and Hirschprung disease. The first patient to survive an operation for oesophageal atresia was treated in 1949. Because Matti Sulamaa was the first full-time paediatric surgeon and the surgical ward of Children's Hospital of Helsinki the only Paediatric Surgical Department in the country, cases were sent to him from all over Finland. In 1946 and 1947 the number of surgical cases treated was 32 and 1023, respectively. The operations increased dramatically over the following years rising to 3000 by 1966. By 1956 Matti Sulamaa was able to report correction of 159 anorectal anomalies, 99 patients with Hirschprungs disease and 134 oesophageal atresias. In 1953 cardiac surgery was commenced by ligating PDA. Open heart surgery was inaugurated in 1961 and the 1000th cardiac operation was reached by 1966. He gained wide experience in the treatment of skeletal abnormalities and developed his own technique for funnel chest. His innovative clavicular transposition for phocomelia of the upper limb earned him invitations from many countries.

Sulamaa found it important to evaluate his own patients and publish his results. He encouraged his residents to undertake scientific work and he understood early the importance of specialising in Paediatric Surgery. His first two full-time consultant surgeons, Mikko Pasila and Kaarlo Parkkulainen, developed Paediatric Surgery within their own fields. Dr Pasila developed paediatric thoracic and cardiac surgery and Dr Parkkulainen paediatric urological surgery, thus creating Finnish paediatric surgical standards that reached high international levels.

Paediatric Anaesthesiology and ICU

In the 1940's and 50's only ether and local anaesthetic were available for paediatric anaesthesia. The first Paediatric Anaesthetist (who had studied in the US) was appointed in 1953. When he left in 1957 a local replacement was very difficult to find. Anxious to improve surgical care Sulamaa put an announcement in the British Medical Journal to find an anaesthetist who would work only with children. As a consequence, a British anaesthetist Neville Hicks, came to work in Helsinki. The true father of Finnish Paediatric Anaesthesiolgy, Toivo Suutarinen, who had also studied in the US, was appointed in 1957. He assumed responsibility for the systematic development of Paediatric Anaesthesiology throughout Finland. Together with Matti Sulamaa, they established the first ICU in Finland (1963) and this was for children. This elevated neonatal care to a new, higher, level; post-operative care being such a critical element. Simultaneously Toivo Suutarinen was one of the pioneers in anaesthesia for thoracic and cardiac surgery in Finland.

Expanding of Paediatric Surgery in Finland

Helsinki city set up a unit of paediatric surgery in 1955 in Aurora Hospital. The first head of paediatric surgery in Aurora hospital was Lars Gripenperg, who had been Sulamaas' first registrar in paediatric surgery. Later Aurora hospital specialised particularly in paediatric trauma surgery. It was merged with Helsinki University Children's Hospital in 1995. Between 1961 and 1971 Paediatric Surgical units were established in all of the four University Hospitals in addition to Helsinki. In Helsinki, Turku and Oulu the paeditric surgical units are a part of the Children's Hospital, whereas in Tampere and Kuopio they are part of the Department of Surgery. Paediatric Surgery was started in Turku by Dr Kaleva Korttila in 1952, and in Tampere by him in 1963. In Kuopio, paediatric surgery was started by Leena Lindell–Iwan in 1970, and in Oulu by Erkki Heikkinen in 1971. All five University Hospitals now train paediatric surgeons. In addition to five University Hospitals a significant number of trained paediatric surgeons have worked in district general hospitals since 1963.

Professors of Paediatric Surgery

In 1965 Sulamaa was awarded the honorary Professorship. He retired in 1973. Sulamaa's successor as the chief of the Department of Paediatric Surgery in the Helsinki University Children's Hospital was Ilmo Louhimo who was nominated the first full Professor of Paediatric Surgery in Finland in 1992. He continued to develop the specialisation of surgeons within paediatric surgery. Prof Louhimo initiated the systematic evaluation of neonatal surgical patients, which continues to this day and has produced valuable scientific results.

After Ilmo Louhimo, Risto Rintala was appointed to the Chair of Paediatric Surgery in 1998. He has continued to develop strong scientific programmes especially in the field of clinical research and maintained strong international links. For example he initiated a registrar exchange programme between Finland and a number of other countries and continued transfer of knowledge regarding methods and techniques between paediatric and adult specialties.

Finnish Association of Paediatric Surgeons

Prof Sulamaa having retired on May 30, 1973, his colleagues honored him by founding the Finnish Association of Paediatric Surgeons — Sulamaa Society the same day. The first president was Lars Gripenberg. For Sulamaas 70th birthday the society decided to commemorate his work by commissioning a medal. The artist was the famous Finnish sculptor Prof Terho Sakki. The medal shows Prof Sulamaa on its face, and on its back a child who had been operated on for pectus excavatum. A special method to repair pectus excavatum was one of Professor Sulamaas innovations. Surplus money from the medal production was used to create the Matti Sulamaa fund. From the initiative of Prof Ilmo Louhimo, the Sulamaa Lectures started in 10th anniversary of the society and the fund was used to cover the travelling fees of invited speakers. Every fifth year the Sulamaa Society invites a visiting expert to give a Sulamaa lecture. Sulamaa lecturers included James Lister, Hardy Hendren, Lewis Spitz, David Lloyd, Paul Losty and Klaas Bax. The Sulamaa Society had 115 members in 2007.

Milestones in Finnish Paediatric Surgery

Traditionally Finland paediatric surgery has consisted of general paediatric surgery, paediatric urology, paediatric cardiac surgery and major part of paediatric traumatology and orthopaedics. During the last decades there has been increasing specialisation within paediatric surgery and different sectors of paediatric surgery are today run by experts in each field. In the following paragraphs we aim to delineate some significant milestones in Finnish Paediatric Surgery.

1940's. Start of modern paediatric surgery in Finland. Even though paediatric anaesthesia services were undeveloped, first oesophageal atresia patient survived operative repair in 1949.

1950's. Development of neonatal surgery continued. First Swenson operation in Hirschprung's disease was performed. Hydrocephalus was treated by various drainage systems of the spinal canal. Closed heart surgery started in 1953. Systematic early diagnostics of congenital dislocation of hips was started. Early operations of club-foot started. First paediatric cardiac operation in hypothermia was performed in Aurora hospital in 1959.

1960's. First cardiac operations in cardiopulmonary bypass were performed in Turku 1960 and in Helsinki 1961. Sub-specialisation in paediatric surgery started. First colonic replacements of oesophagus were performed. Urethrocystoscopies and electrical resections of urethral valves were started.

Hydrocephalus shunt-operations and phocomelia operations were started. Finland's first intensive care unit was established in Helsinki University Children's Hospital in 1963. There was rapid progress in the development of ventilators suitable also for children, leading to more effective post-operative care.

1970's. Development of parenteral nutrition and establishment of intensive care unit created a ground for successful neonatal surgery. Mortality of oesophageal atresia decreased under 15%. Operative treatment of Perthés disease was started in Oulu. In Helsinki systematic neuro-orthopedy, lengthening of lower extremities, prophylactic intramedullary nailing of long bones in osteogenesis imperfecta, cervical spinal fusions and pelvic osteotomies were started. The first infant and neonatal heart operations were performed. Conjoined twins were separated successfully.

1980's. Echography and computed tomography revolutionised diagnostic imaging. Prostaglandins and advanced intensive care improved results of heart surgery. First arterial switch operations in transposition of great vessels were performed. PSARP operations for anorectal anomalies were started. Operative management of neuromuscular scoliosis was initiated. Development of paediatric applications in microsurgery and craniofacial surgery were started in Oulu. Paediatric transplantation surgery program started in cooperation with adult transplantation unit and first paediatric liver and kidney transplantations were performed. Fiberoptic endoscopies became routine in paediatric gastroenterological diagnostic work; in Helsinki fiberoptic endoscopies have been performed by surgeons since early 1980's. There were advances in the surgery of prematures; surgery for necrotising enterocolitis and closure of persistent ductus arteriosus were common procedures. Urodynamics became a routine investigations in paediatric urology.

1990's. Day case surgery became a routine approach for general paediatric surgical problems. Magnetic imaging changed diagnostic imaging. Perfusion operations of premature babies started; ECMO, heart transplantations and operations of hypoplastic left heart started. Bladder augmentation became a routine procedure in the management of severe neurogenic bladder. Mini-invasive surgical approaches, mainly laparoscopic procedures, were developed. The first EXIT (ex-utero intrapartum treatment) procedure was performed.

2000's. Position of laparoscopic and thoracoscopic surgery became established. First paediatric lung transplantation was performed. Nationwide management programme of short bowel syndrome — nutrition and surgery — was developed. Intestinal transplantation programme started.

Acknowledgement

My thanks to Prof Risto Rintala who has checked the content of this document.

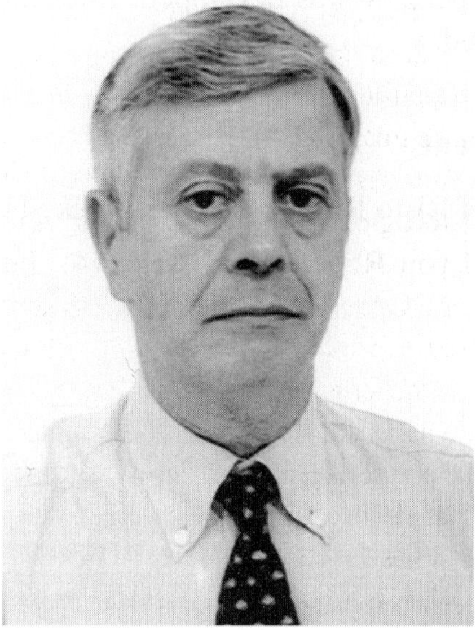

Lionel Coupris

FRANCE

Lionel Coupris

From 1614, King Louis XIII ordered that children and adults in the Lyon City Hospital should be separated. A surgeon named **Mosnier** was assigned to the children. This decision of separation remained unchanged in France until the end of 18th century.

At the same time, certain physicians started to show an interest in paediatric pathologies, such as **Nicolas Andry** (1658–1742), Professor at the Lyon Royal College. In 1741, he coined the term "***Orthopédie***" (from Greek "ortho" meaning straight and "paido" meaning child) in the book published in Lyon: "*L'Orthopédie ou l'Art de prévenir et de corriger dans les enfants les difformités du corps*". This book was a real success; it was translated into English in 1743 ("Orthopedia or the Art of correcting and preventing deformities in children") and into German in 1744. Nicolas ANDRY is widely regarded as "the father of orthopaedics".

Shortly after the French Revolution, during the Consulate Period (when Bonaparte, who would become Napoleon the first, was the prime consul) it was decided to create a specific hospital for children of both sexes aged fifteen and under, which opened on May 8th, 1802. It was **the first independent paediatric hospital in the world**. It was built on the site of the former convent of "*Dames Hospitalières de Saint Thomas de Villeneuve*", which in 1764 became "*La Maison de l'Enfant Jésus*" and in 1795 "*La Maison Nationale des Orphelines*". It is located in Sèvres street, in Paris. Its name: "***Hôpital des Enfants Malades***" has become famous all around the world and been copied in a number of countries ("Sick Children Hospital"). Its first medical team included two physicians, one surgeon

(**Petitbau**, an unknown but tireless worker), a pharmacologist and eight students.

In 1844, **Paul Guersant** (1800–1869) set up in the Hôpital des Enfants Malades **the first paediatric surgical care unit**. At the same time, he wrote a book called "*Notices sur la Chirurgie des Enfants*" ("Notes on Children's Surgery"), which was the first specific book about paediatric surgery, promptly translated into English and German. **Guersant can also be considered as one of the pioneers of paediatric surgery**.

In the second part of nineteenth century, two more paediatric hospitals were opened in Paris: "*Hôpital Saint Eugénie*" (1854) (which became "*Hôpital Trousseau*" in 1880) and "Assisted Children Hospital" (which became "Hospital Saint Vincent de Paul"). It was here that a specific surgery unit was created in 1893, with **Edouard Kirmisson** (1848–1927) as supervisor.

In 1899, The City of Paris decided to create at the "*Hôpital des Enfants Malades*", **the first university department of paediatric surgery in France**, called "*Clinique Chirurgicale Infantile et Orthopédique*", with Prof Kirmisson as the first titular surgeon in 1901. Many famous paediatric surgeons succeeded him: Profs **Louis Ombredanne** (1871–1956), **Auguste Broca** (1859–1924), **Jacques Leveuf** (1885–1948), **Marcel Fevre** (1897–1978) and lastly, our mentor, Prof **Denys Pellerin**. Prof Denys Pellerin, one of the most respected voices in French paediatric surgery around the world.

Outside Paris, a similar revolution was starting. A University Department of Paediatric Surgery was created both in Bordeaux and Lille (1907), Montpellier (1909), Nancy (1910), Lyon (1921) and a little later in Marseille, Nantes and Strasbourg. The departments' names differed according to the places where they were created.

At the same time, **Pierre Fredet** (1870–1946) successfully performed the first extramucosal pyloromyotomy for infant pyloric stenosis, on October 12th, 1907, four years before Conrad Ramstedt (a German surgeon in Munster). This procedure saved more babies than any other in the last century.

While the first quarter of the 20th century saw the influence of French paediatric surgery worldwide, the period between the two

World Wars was much less brilliant. There was one exception: **Victor Veau** (1871–1949) who had great experience in labial and palate clefts and who published anatomical (1928), clinical and technical articles (1938) on that subject. Millard (Cleft Craft, Vol 1, p. 94), said that "Victor Veau, a general surgeon from Paris, was one of the greatest cleft surgeons of all times".

During the Second World War, German occupation in France did not allow true French contributions to international progress in surgery, especially in paediatric surgery development. After the War, several young and brilliant surgeons worked hard to make up for lost time especially in surgery for newborn babies.

Pierre Petit (1905–2002) was the first French surgeon who successfully operated on an esophageal atresia with distal tracheoesophageal fistula, in 1949, at Hôpital Saint Vincent de Paul (eight years after the world's first success carried out by Cameron Haight).

In 1960, **Bernard Duhamel** described his own procedure for Hirschsprung's disease. This operation was used widely around the world. He was also a famous "embryologist", well-known for his books in connection with the genesis of malformations. At the same time, **Dr Odile Schweisgut** (Villejuif) set up and developed French paediatric oncology.

For a long time, paediatric surgery was, in France, a form of surgical activity but not an official surgical speciality as it is now. For years, French Universities only recognised general surgery. Surgeons had a part-time public hospital paediatric practice, associated with a private practice, even for both adults and children. In 1958, a major hospital reform set up the University Hospital Centres (CHU) with an obligatory full-time practice for all their physicians.

Professor **Michel Carcassonne** was the first French paediatric surgeon who was employed (1962) in the new hospital and university organisation in Marseille. According to this new organisation (CHU), in the nineteen seventies, quite a lot of new paediatric surgery units were created in smaller towns, elsewhere in France. The paediatric surgeons had previously been trained in the major paediatric surgery departments.

Today, the French population is estimated at about 66 million people. There are 27 CHUs, with at least one university team for paediatric surgery, ten to fifteen hospitals with no university team and few exclusive private paediatric surgery centres. In 2007, in France there were about 250 senior paediatric surgeons and 80 senior paediatric orthopaedic surgeons.

In December 1959 the "*Société Française de Chirurgie Infantile*" was founded, which subsequently became (1983) the "***Société Française de Chirurgie Pédiatrique***" (French Society of Paediatric Surgery — SFCP). The founder members were Barcat, Beau Chigot, Duhamel, Etienne, Fevre, Fourrier, Guillemet, Ingelhrans, Lagrot, Laurence, Marion, Pellerin, Petit, Salmon, and Virenque. Prof M. Fevre was its first President.

The first scientific meeting was held at the "*Hôpital des Enfants Malades*" in Paris on March 12th, 1960. Very soon after, in 1960, paediatric radiologists (Profs J. Lefevre and J. Sauvegrain), and paediatric anaesthesiologists (Mrs Doctors Delegue, who later became a professor) and Languepin were elected as associated members.

For 30 years, the SFCP had its own review, written in French; "*Annales de Chirurgie Infantile*" (1960–1978) and then "*Chirurgie Pédiatrique*" (1978–1989). Since 1989, the "*European Journal of Paediatric Surgery*" has been published in collaboration with many European Associations or Societies, and is, now, the official review of the SFCP.

Prof Beau, Dean of the Medical Unit at Nancy University, has worked hard to promote paediatric surgery in France. Paediatric Surgery became a university discipline in 1969 and a specialised surgery skill for general surgeons, recognised by the French Medical Council in 1976. It only became a true surgical speciality in 1984, with official specific training and an exclusive paediatric practice for specialised surgeons. In France, this speciality covers all childhood surgical pathologies except otorhinolaryngology, ophthalmology, cardiac surgery and neurosurgery. Gradually, through the development of adult care, orthopaedia lost its original sense, and the mixed orthopaedic and paediatric surgery departments were split for the first time in the 1960's in adult orthopaedic, paediatric surgery and paediatric orthopaedics. Today these two aspects of paediatric surgery are usually separated in distinct units in the bigger centres.

Prof **Jacques Valayer** (Kremlin–Bicêtre hôspital, Paris), has developed a reputed centre for children's liver surgery and liver transplantation (a reference in France).

Prof **Paul Mitrofanoff** (Rouen) published his outstanding operation procedure for continent trans-appendico-cystostomy for neurologic bladders in 1980. This procedure was extended to neurogenous non-neurologic bladders or derivatives and has provided a better quality of life for children.

Mrs **Claire Nihoul–Fekete** was the **first French woman to obtain the title of Professor of Paediatric surgery**. She is well-known for her particular interest for antenatal diagnosis, sexual differentiation anomalies and endocrinal surgery. She succeeded Prof Denys Pellerin in 1990, as the head of the paediatric surgery department of the *Hôpital des Enfants Malades* in Paris.

Prof **Yann Revillon**, the current chief of the paediatric surgery department of the *Hôpital des Enfants Maladies* performed in 1994 the first small bowel transplantation on a child in France.

Laparoscopic surgery was invented in France. French paediatric surgeons rapidly adopted these procedures on children. In 1990, Prof **Jean-Luc Alain** and Dr **Grousseau** from Limoges did **the first laparoscopic extramucosal pyloromyotomy for infant pyloric stenosis in the world**. Now, laparoscopic surgery is practiced in all French paediatric surgery centres using a number of innovations. Professor **Jean-Stephane Valla** from Nice is the President of The International Paediatric Endoscopic Group (IPEG) for 2007/2008.

On account of these renowned surgeons, the story of French pediatric surgery was written, day after day, by all French pediatric surgeons and their surgical teams culminating in the current excellent results for paediatric health care.

Meanwhile, in the near future, French pediatric surgery would be harmonised with European recommendations in matters of training and care unit organisations.

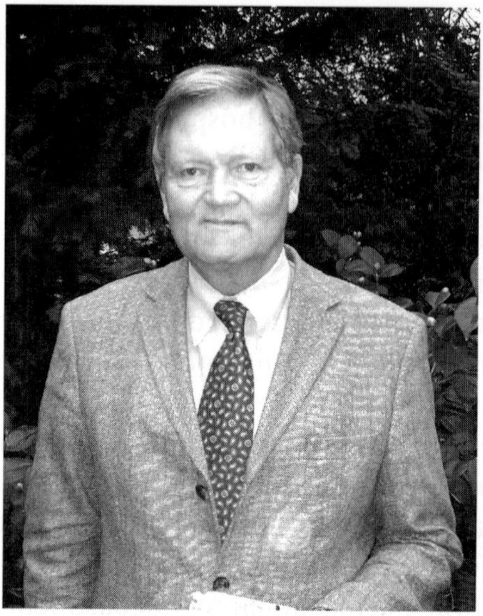

Alexander Holschneider

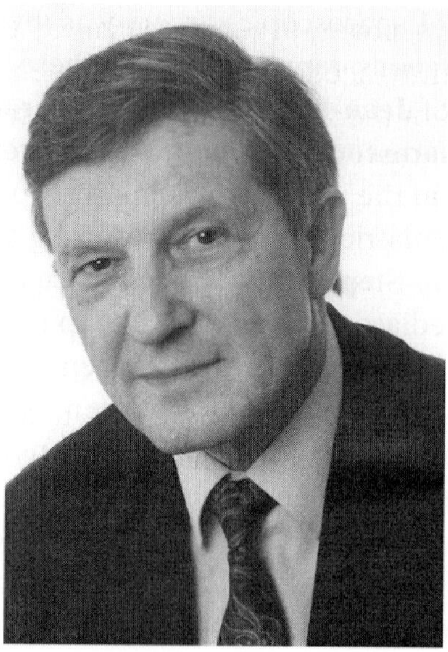

Kurt Gdanietz

GERMANY

Alexander Holschneider
Kurt Gdanietz

General Historical Tradition

In general, the beginning of the specialisation paediatric surgery started at the end of the 18th and the first half of the 19th century, and followed the same steps as the development of Paediatrics. In those old days, sick children were treated usually at home and according the rules known for the treatment of adults. However, accidents, tumours, complications from infectious diseases and congenital malformations needed surgical therapy. Besides, poor children and orphans, living in special founding hospitals and orphanages frequently needed medical treatment too. However, it was only at the end of the 18th century and in a few big cities in Europe that special paediatric units were founded, such as like the "Dispensary for Sick Children" (1769) in London, the "*Öffentliche Kinderkrankeninstitut*" (1787) in Vienna, or the "*Institut für arme Kinder*" (1793) in Breslau. Many of these institutes were especially founded for poor children, as the name of the children's hospital in Breslau indicates. Unfortunately, due to the poor knowledge of physiology and pathophysiology in that time and without adequate anaesthesia, the treatment had more charitable than curative character.[1]

Books

A first indicator for the development of a medical speciality are books dedicated to special issues. The first paediatric textbooks appeared at the end of the 18th century, e.g. Friedrich Hoffmann's

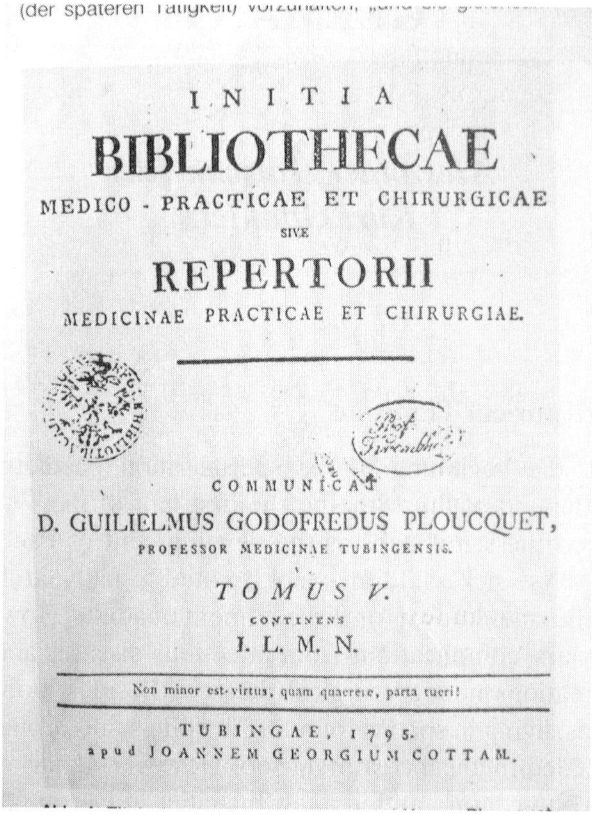

I N I T I A

BIBLIOTHECAE

MEDICO - PRACTICAE ET CHIRURGICAE

SIVE

REPERTORII

MEDICINAE PRACTICAE ET CHIRURGIAE.

COMMUNICAT

D. GUILIELMUS GODOFREDUS PLOUCQUET,

PROFESSOR MEDICINAE TUBINGENSIS.

TOMUS V.

CONTINENS

I. L. M. N.

Non minor est virtus, quam quaerere, parta tueri!

TUBINGAE, 1795.

apud JOANNEM GEORGIUM COTTAM.

Fig. 1. D. G. G. Ploucquet: Repertorii Mecinae Practicae et Chirurgiae, 1795.[2,3]

"*Vernünftige and gründliche Abhandlungen von den fürnehmsten Kinderkrankheiten*" (1741) or D. G. G. Ploucquet's "*Repertorii Medicinae et Chirurgiae*" (1795) entitled. The second volume of "*Thesauri Sanitas or Schatzes Menschlicher Gesundheit*" (Fig. 1), published after the death of the author, dealt especially with medical and surgical problems and was targeted for students.[2,3] Other books with special paediatric and surgical contents were, for example, Joh. Jacob Bräuner's "*Kern Außerlesenster Arzney-Mittel, Vol 7: Thesaurus Sanitatis: Operationes et Experimenta Chirurgica*" (1725), M. Underwood's "Treatise on the Diseases of Children" (1784), J. A. Murray's "*Die Anweisungen zu Kenntnis und Kur der Kinderkrankheiten*", published in 1764 in

Swedish and 1766 in German language, or Zwinger's Monograph, published 1722 in Latin "*Paedojatreja Practica*".

In all these books, paediatric but also surgical subjects were discussed like hydrocephalus, a frequent disease after meningitis, especially the basal meningitis by tuberculosis, surgical problems after croupy diphtheria, wound treatment, tumours and congenital malformations called in that time "*Abweichungen*". However in some books, like the publication of Christoph Girtanner (1760–1800), "*Abbhandlungen über die Krankheiten der Kinder und über die physische Erziehung derselben*", more surgical topics were discussed, such as frenulum of the tongue, hydrocele, inguinal hernia, testicular tumours, undescended testicles, hydrocephalus, myelomeningocele, cleft lips and palate, cephalhematoma, ranula, imperforate anus, urethral atresia, vaginal atresia, birth traumata, bone fractures and luxations, contused wounds, and trismus as an important manifestation of tetanus.

The first German textbook of paediatric surgery was published in 1783 by Karl Joseph Oehme, a medical doctor from Dresden, entitled "*De morbis recens natorum chirurgicis*". In 1860 a "*Handbuch für Kinderheilkunde*" was published by Gerhard and contained many chapters dedicated to surgical diseases. In 1894 Ferdinand Karewsky[4] published in Berlin the first comprehensive paediatric surgical textbook entitled "*Die chirurgischen Krankheiten des Kindesalters*". The main topics of its 762 pages were: Examination of the child, Anaesthesia (Chloroform, Aether, Bromäthyl, Pental), Antisepsis, Wound treatment and special surgical problems arising from infectious diseases like tuberculosis, diphtheria, poliomyelitis. Special chapters were dedicated to traumatology, congenital malformations, orthopaedic problems and tumours. A chapter called "*Varia*" discussed intussusception, prolapsus ani and recti, perityphlitis, fissura ani, fistula ani and bladder and urethral stones.[5,6]

During the following decades many important German textbooks were published. The most important of them were the book of Fritz Lange and Hans Spitz (1910) and the textbook of Gohrbandt, Karger and Bergmann (1928). In 1930 R. Drachter and J. R. Gossmann[7] published in Pfaundlers and Schloßmanns' Handbook for Paediatrics

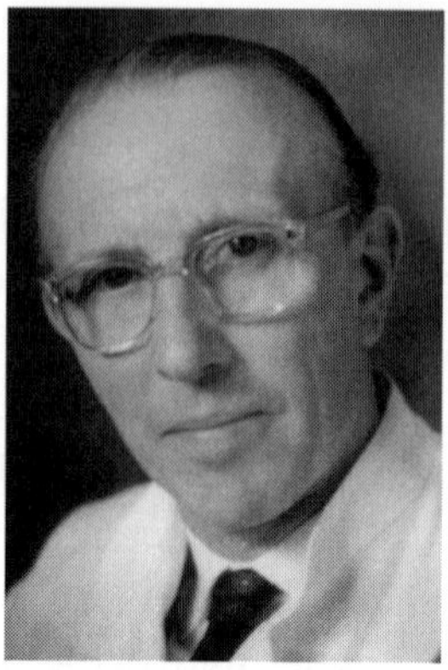

Fig. 2. Prof Anton Oberniedermayr.

a large chapter on "*Chirurgie des Kindesalters*". After the second world war, in 1959, Anton Oberniedermayr (Fig. 2), a pupil of Drachter, and co-workers published the most extensive book ever written about paediatric surgery, the "*Lehrbuch der Chirurgie and Orthopädie des Kindesalters.*"[8] In its three volumes, the surgical diseases of children were presented as a whole without taking care of the ongoing specialisation of surgery in urology, orthopaedic surgery, neurosurgery, cardiac surgery and oral surgery, it was a textbook and atlas together.

Other important German books, which were widely distributed, were an atlas for paediatric surgery edited by H. Kunz and co-workers in two volumes, entitled "*Operationen im Kindesalter*" (1973)[9] and Hecker, Daum and Maier's chapter in "*Breitner's Chirurgische Operatonslehre*" (1970) called "*Die Eingriffe im Säuglings- und Kindesalter*".[10] This was an atlas and textbook of the most frequently performed surgical procedures in childhood. Finally the textbook of Fritz Meißner[11] should be mentioned. It became widely distributed in and outside the former German Democratic Republic.

From the huge number of further books written by German authors and dealing with paediatric surgical topics, a few should be mentioned because they have profoundly influenced the development of paediatric surgery in Germany like Fritz Rehbein's

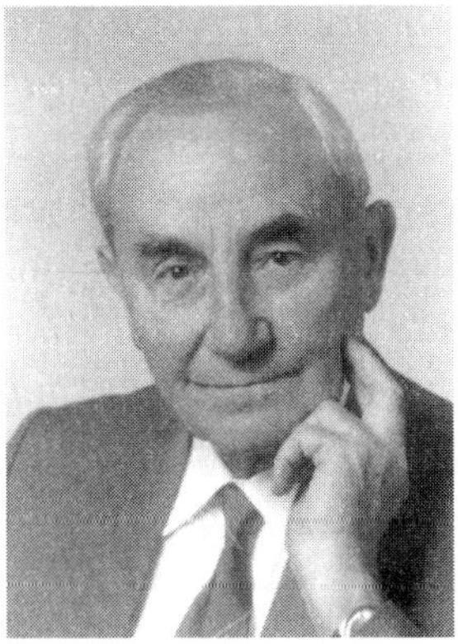

Fig. 3. Prof Fritz Rehbein.

"*Kinderchirurgische Operationen*" (1976).[12] In this book, published at the end of his carreer, Rehbein (Fig. 3) summarised all his life-long experiences and demonstrated step-by-step the techniques of the most important surgical procedures which he has introduced himself for the treatment of Funnel chests, Imperforate anus, Hirschsprung's disease, small bowel and colon atresia, and others.

In the last decades of the 20th century paediatric surgery changed from a speciality, covering in general every kind of surgery in infancy and childhood, to a discipline concentrating on congenital malformations and diseases of the abdomen and thorax. It was especially at universities that this development took place, whereas in the larger city hospitals the much broader, original spectrum of surgical diseases in childhood was treated. These centres continued to perform paediatric urology, traumatology, oral surgery such as reconstruction of cleft lips and palates and operations for hydrocephalus and myelomeningoceles.

The cooperation with adult surgery and other medical specialties however, became more and more important and sub-specialisation took place in paediatric surgery as well. Therefore, some paediatric surgeons wrote important and widely distributed books dedicated to a special, important topic such as Lutz von Laer *et al.*'s "*Frakturen und Luxationen im Wachstumsalter*", which got its 5th edition in 2007,[13]

Dietz *et al.*'s "*Intramedulläre Osteosynthese im Waschtumsalter*",[14] Berlien and Müller's "*Angewandte Lasermedizin — Lehr- und Handbuch für Praxis und Klinik*" (1989).[15] Other German authors brought together the whole knowledge of special diseases in very comprehensive and internationally well-known monographies like Jürgen Waldschmidt's "*Das akute Abdomen im Kindesalter*",[16] P. Schweizer and F. Schier's "*Hepatobiliary Surgery in Childhood*",[17] Holschneider and Puri's "*Hirschsprung's Disease and Allied Disorders, 3rd ed.*"[18] and Holschneider and Hutson's "*Anorectal Malformations in Children*".[19] This multi-authored book is the fourth edition of D. Stephens and D. Smith's famous book on "*Anorectal Malformtions*" from 1963.[20] Finally, Ahmed Hadidi's book on hypospadias,[21] which he recently published in cooperation with A. F. Azmy should be mentioned as a further example of an excellent specified publication on a special paediatric surgical subject.

Hospitals

In Table 1, the General Hospitals in German language countries from 70 A.C. to 1829 are listed. However these hospitals were not hospitals in a modern sense. They were in general dedicated to the Holy Spirit and are similar to hospices in our days. The Hospital in Beaune/France and the Hospital of Saint Jans in Brügge/Belgium are good examples for this early type of hospital and can be visited even today.

French Roots

For special Paediatric Surgical hospitals however, the roots lay in France. An important step forward to specialisation in paediatric surgery came by the French revolution and the disappropriation of monasteries in 1803 during the "*Säkularisation*" by Napoleon, where the goods of the churches were confiscated and sold by the governments. It can be suggested that the first paediatric and paediatric surgical hospital in a modern sense was the "*Hôspital des Enfants Malades*" in Paris. In May 8th, 1802, as Consul of the new French

Table 1. Hospitals in German Language countries from 70 A.C.–1829, modified from Jetter.[22]

About 70 AC	Vetera/Xanten, "Valetudinarium" in a Roman camp
About 820	St Gallen; Hospital in the "Klosterplan"
About 1220	Eberbach; "Zisterzienser Infirmarium"
Before 1287	Lübeck; Holy Spirit Hospital
Before 1300	Lübeck-Gronau; "Hospital St Jürgen" for leprosy patients
1319	Basel; "St Jacob an der Birs", for leprosy patients
1326	Goslar; Major Holy Cross Hospital
1327–1350	Salzburg; "Bürgerspital" of the bishop
1332	Nürnberg; Holy Spirit Hospital
1417	Braunau; "Bürgerhospital"
1451–1458	Bernkastel-Kues; "Nikolaushospital" of the Cardinal
1535	Hofheim and Haina; "Hohe Hessische Landeshospitäler"
1554	Nürnber; Pesthouse St. Sebastian
1556–1562	Salzburg; "Bürgerhospital, Arkadienflügel"
1576–1580	Würzburg; "Juliusspital"
1601 and 1625	München; "Herzogsspital"
1614	Graz; "Spital der Barmherzigen Brüder"
1625–1630	Augsburg; Holy Spirit Hospital
1692–1705	Salzburg; "St Johannes Hospital"
1693	Wien; "Großes Armenhaus"
1697–1702	Berlin; "Großes Friedrichs Hospital"
1700–1714	Würzburg; "Julius Spital Nordflugel"
1710–1732	Celle; "Zucht- Werk- und Tollhaus"
1710	Berlin; "Großes Lazarett", later on called "Charité"
1818–1724	Bern; "Inselspital"
1745–1753	Münster; "Clemenshospital"
1746–1748	Berlin; "Kgl. Invalidenhaus"
1746–1749	Ludwigsburg; Doll-Haus
1771	Frankfurt; "Senckenbergisches Bürgerhospital"
1793	Breslau; "Institut für arme Kinder"
1829	Berlin; "Charité", first German Hospital for Sick Children

Republic, Napoleon ordered to use the expropriated former cloister of the "*Dames Hopspitalières de Saint Thomas de Villeneufe*" as a hospital for sick children. It was called first "*Hôspital des Enfants Jesus*", later "*Hôspital des Enfants Malades*". But Napoleon not only ordered the transformation of the cloister in a hospital, but also the

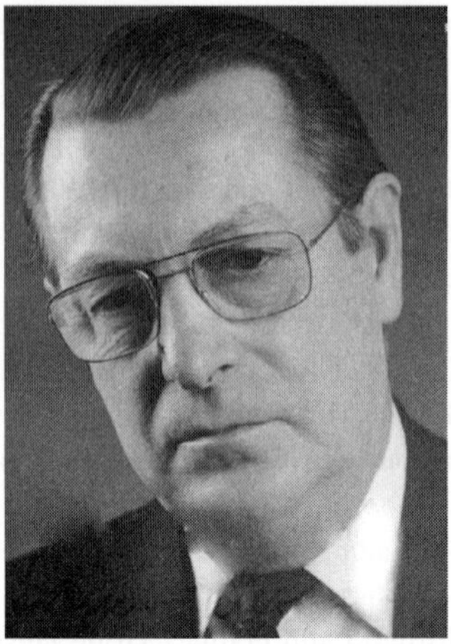

Fig. 4. Prof Waldemar Hecker.

establishment two different departments: one for Paediatrics and another one with 14 beds for Paediatric Surgery. This is important to mention, because the compilation of cloisters into hospitals became an important stimulus in Germany too for the foundation of new hospitals, for further medical specialisation and for the creation of special surgical units in hospitals for sick children. The first chief of the surgical unit at the *Hôspital des Enfants Malades* in Paris was Dr Petit Beau, and from 1814 on, Dr Baffos. Baffos was one of the most important personalities in Paris of that time, a friend of Châtaubriand, of Madame de Berry and of Cardinal Fesch, an uncle of Napoleon. His successor, Guersant, wrote the first modern textbook of paediatric surgery (1861) entitled "*Notices sur la chirurgie des enfants*", which was translated three years later into English and became important for Germany too.[5,6]

Paediatric Surgery in Germany

Concerning the development of paediatric surgery in Germany, five steps of progression can be distinguished (Table 2).[24,25] The *first step* of development was the founding of children's hospitals. These

Table 2. General steps of the development of paediatric surgery in Germany modified according to Hecker.[24,25]

Up to 1802	No special Paediatric or Paediatric Surgical units. The Hospitals were usually dedicated to the holy spirit and more hospices than hospitals in the modern sense
1802–the second half of the 19th century	Children's hospitals with a Practitioner operating himself
From the second — last third of 19th century	General Surgeon as consultant
End of the 19th century — beginning of the 20th century	Children's hospitals with two independent departments for Paediatric and Paediatric Surgery especially in big Municipal hospitals
First half of the 20th century	Paediatric Surgical departments at universities

units concentrated in particular on children with infectious diseases and of those who needed surgical treatment for the incision of abscesses, phlegmons, gangrenes, traumata's, evolvements of contractures after poliomyelitis, tracheotomies after diphtherias croup, correction of simple congenital malformations, treatment of fractures, distortions, orthopaedic problems excision of tumours and others. The Greek word "*orthos*" means upright and "*paideia*" to educate. "*Orthopaedic*" stands therefore to help (deformed) children to stand upright.

In the first modern children's hospital of the 19th century, the chief of the hospital, usually a practitioner with medical and surgical experience, performed the surgical procedures himself. The increasing number of surgical procedures however, made it necessary to employ a surgical consultant (*second step*). These surgeons specialised in paediatric surgery (*third step*) and finally, established an independent general surgical department Inside the children's hospital (*fourth step*). In a few cases, this paediatric surgical unit became later, in the 20th century, a chair of a medical faculty of a university (*fifth step*) (Table 2).

In detail, the development of paediatric surgery in Germany was similar to the development in France. Under the influence of

Napoleon or may be just to use the empty rooms of the cloisters, the so-called "*Bürgerhospitäler*", or hospitals for citizens, were established. The patients were separated according to their sexes, and old people and children with infectious eruptions were brought apart from the others. In the second half of the 19th century the foundation of special department for sick children increased, mainly by support of private sponsors. The rapid development of surgery at the end of the 19th century made this development possible.

Hecker and Locher gave a nice example of these steps of development by the illustrating the history of the "*Dr von Haunersches Kinderspital*" in Munich (Fig. 5).[25,26] Dr von Hauner, a medical practitioner, founded this hospital in 1846 and personally performed during the founding year 46 surgical procedures such as incisions of abscesses, incarcerated inguinal hernias, prolapsed anus, contusions, and wound treatments. Later the numbers of operations and the

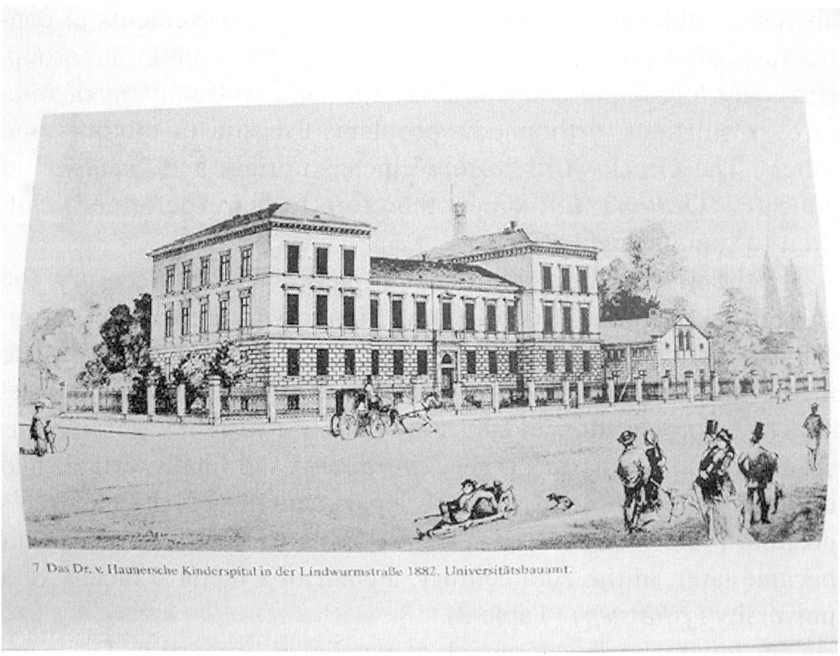
7 Das Dr. v. Haunersche Kinderspital in der Lindwurmstraße 1882. Universitätsbauamt.

Fig. 5. The Doctor von Hauner'sche Children's Hospital 1882, taken from Locher.[26]

complexity of the surgical procedures increased so much that Dr Hauner was forced to ask a surgeon from the neighboured surgical hospital to perform the operations in his paediatric unit. The first surgical consultant in Munich was Prof Karl Thiersch, who introduced the Thiersch ring against anal-and rectal prolapse and the transplantation of skin flaps in burned patients. Both procedures bear his name. He was followed by Prof Johann Nepomuk Ritter von Nußbaum, who worked 32 years in this children's hospital. A pupil of Nussbaum, Dr Castenholz became the chief of the first surgical unit of the children's Hospital "In der Buschgasse" in Cologne in 1883 (Fig. 6).[28] In 1850, 114 surgical procedures were performed in the "*Dr von Haunersche's Kinderspital*", among them strumectomies, cleft lips and palates, anal atresias, and spinae ventosae. In 1886, Prof Otmar von Angerer established the first self-dependent

Bürgerhospital der Stadt Köln

Asklepios, Hygieia, die 3 Parzen.

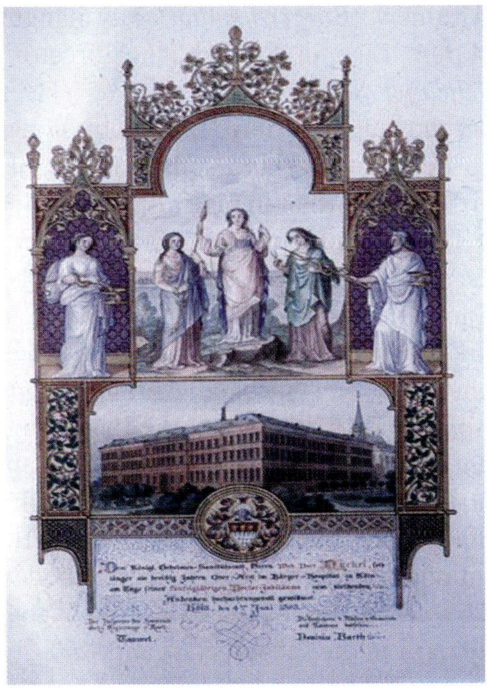

Fig. 6. Honorary certificate for Dr. Benedict Daniel Nückel.

unit for Paediatric Surgery in Munich. In 1891, Prof Herzog took over and became "*ausserordentlicher*", which means Associate Professor for Paediatric Surgery of the Maximilians University of Munich in 1910. He was followed by Richard Drachter in 1914, who wrote together with his co-worker J. Gossmann in 1930, a contribution in von Pfaundlers and Schloßmanns' Handbook of Paediatrics, entitled "*Chirurgie des Kindesalters*", which became widely distributed.[7] Unfortunately, Drachter died from an undiagnosed appendicitis. From 1936 to 1969 Prof Anton Oberniedermayr became chief of the hospital and got, at the end of his career, as a personal honour, a personal Professorship for Paediatric Surgery of the medical faculty. He was followed by Prof Waldemar Hecker (Fig. 4) in 1969. He was the first Professor for Paediatric Surgery in the Federal Republic of Germany.

The situation in Cologne was similar. The former cloisters St Cécile and St Michael were converted to hospitals and St Cécile was renamed "*Cecilienhospital*" and later "*Bürgerhospital*".[27] In 1847 a new "*Bürgerhospital*" was inaugurated with 83 beds for sick children. Like in Munich, the director was a practitioner called "*Geheimer Sanitätsrat Dr Nückel*". He too had a surgical advisor from the neighbouring department of general surgery. The relationship between bed and square meter of the room was 7.5m^2/bed, which is more than in many of our modern hospitals.[28]

The first independent paediatric and paediatric surgical children's hospital in Cologne was opened November 10th, 1883. It was a foundation of Charlotte von Oppenheim who gave 1 million goldmark to build the "*Abraham von Oppenheim'sche Kinderspital*" to memorialise her husband Abraham von Oppenheim (Fig. 7). This hospital was divided from the beginning into a paediatric departement (Chief Prof Ferdinand Siegert from Halle/Saale) and in a paediatric surgical unit (Chief Dr Kastenholz from Munich[29]). In his first annual report in 1888, Kastenholz described his unit in detail.[30] The relationship of room square meters/bed was 6 m^2, and 24.4 m^3. From 1924 to 1936, the fee per day was 4–7 goldmark in the first class, 3–4 goldmark in the second class and 1.50–2 goldmark in the third class. The surgical unit had 24 beds and one theatre. In the founding year 1883/84, 112 children were treated; and in 1886/87, 224 patients. Two

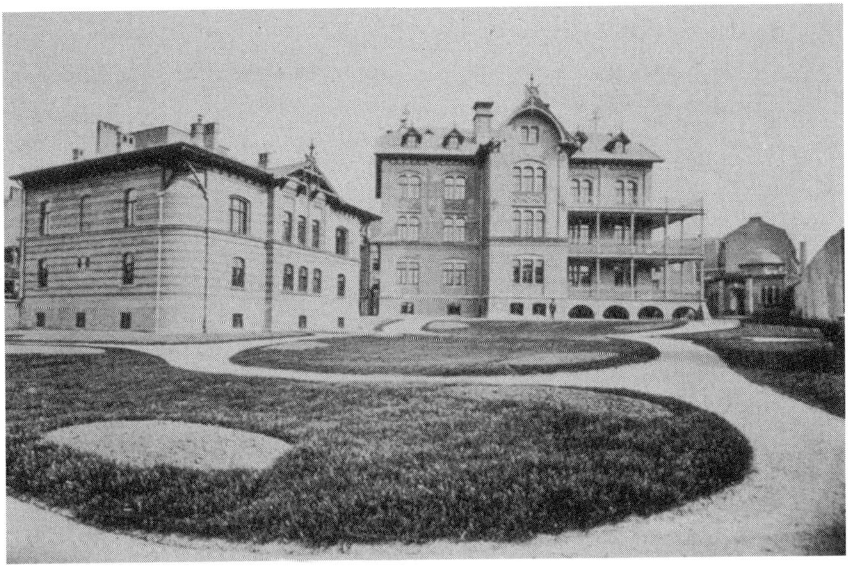

Das Kinderkrankenhaus der A. von Oppenheim Stiftung 1881 von der Gartenseite

Fig. 7. The first hospital for Sick Children in Cologne "In der Buschgasse" 1883.

thirds of the patients of the hospital suffered from surgical diseases. Figure 6 shows the "*New Bürgerhospital*" from 1863 on a certificate to honour Dr Nückel, (Fig. 6) the first hospital for Sick Children in Cologne, 1883. The following Figs. 8 to 11 give impressions of other surgical departments of that time.[32,23] During the Second World War the Children's hospital of the City of Cologne was completely destroyed. A new building was opened in 1964 by Prof Helbig.[31]

In other hospitals in Germany the development of paediatric surgery was similar. In *Berlin — Wedding*, former "*Kaiser und Kaiserin — Friedrich–Kinderkrankenhaus*", a paediatric surgical department was founded in 1890 and managed by Prof Gluck, a pupil of the surgeons v. Bergmann and Langenbeck. Later, in 1972 Prof Haße became chief of this department.[32]

In *Heidelberg*, the founder of the "*Luisenheilanstalt Kinderklinik*" in 1860 was Prof Dusch, a practitioner who also personally operated

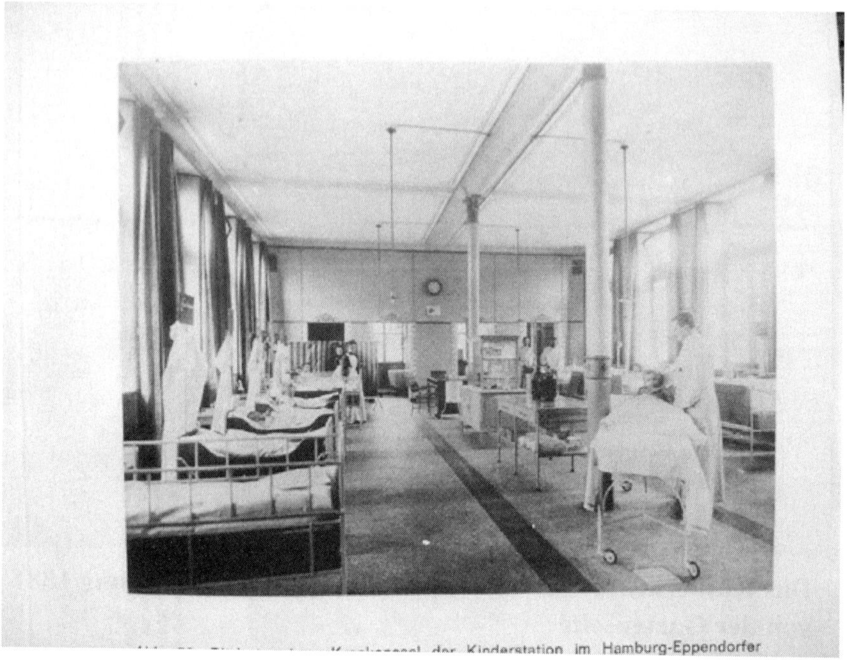

Fig. 8. Ward of the Children's hospital Berlin-Wedding 1890, from Haße.

during the founding years. However, he was trained before for two years in the surgical department of the university by Prof Chelius. In 1864 Prof Herrmann Lossen became surgical consultant. In 1884 the unit became independent. Prof Dusch was followed by Prof Benno Schmidt, later by Prof Waldemar Hecker and Prof Roland Daum. Today, this old paediatric surgical unit is part of the chair of Paediatric Surgery of the University of Mannheim (Chief: Prof Karl Ludwig Waag).

The beginning of paediatric surgery in the Children's Hospital in *Hamburg–Altona* (built 1859–1861) followed the same steps. The founders of this Children's hospital a "*Bürgerverein*" asked a practitioner, Dr Grünberg, to become the chief of the hospital. He too performed the first operations himself. Later, the surgical consultant was Dr Süßenguth, followed by Dr Kluth, Dr Marwege, Dr Reifferscheid, and until recently, by Prof Lambrecht, who was also chief of the chair of Paediatric Surgery at the university

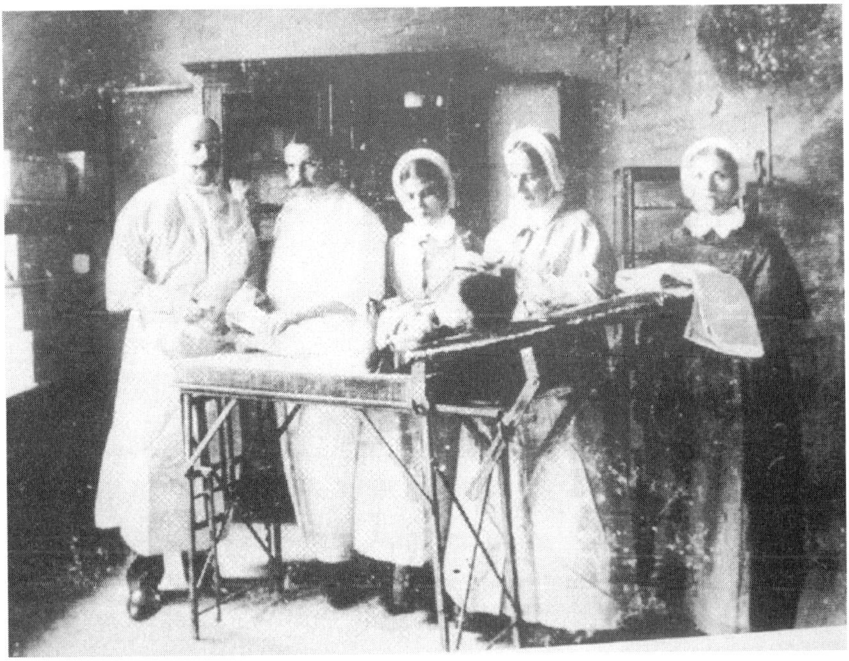

Fig. 9. Operation Theatre of the Children's hospital Berlin-Wedding 1890, from Haße.

Hamburg — Eppendorf, which has been set up for him just a few decades ago.

The children's hospital in Stuttgart, called "*Kinderheilanstalt Stuttgart*" (Fig. 11), was founded in 1842 in a four rooms apartment by two practitioners, Dr Georg von Cleß (1815–1884), a practitioner and surgeon, and by Dr Otto Elben. In 1847, after her wedding with the king of Württemberg, Olga Nikolajewna, a daughter of Zar Niklolaus I from Russia and princess Alexandra of Prussia became the patroness of the hospital. It is called since that time "Olga-Hospital". Surgical procedures were performed by the two founders and 2 consultants, especially for orthopaedic diseases. In 1882 a new hospital was opened to the public and a special surgical-orthopaedic department was now established. Its chief was Prof Heinrich von Köstlin, a pupil of von Bergmann and Volkmann.[33]

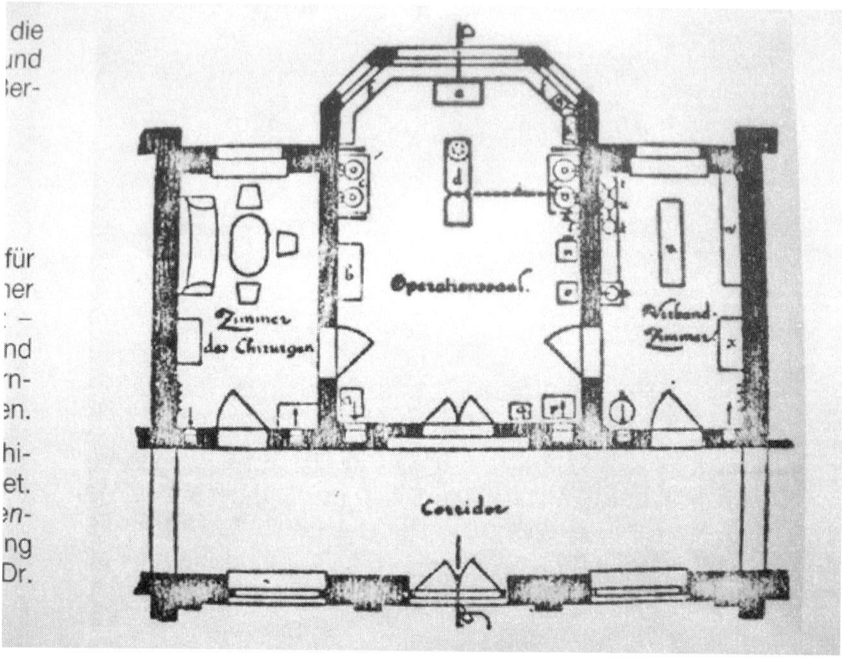

Fig 10. Floor plan of the operation theatre of the Chidren's hospital Berlin-Wedding. Note the surgeons room on the left, a room for wound dressings at the right (1890) from Haße 1990.

One of the oldest hospitals in Germany, the "*Charité*" in Berlin was founded in 1710 in expectation of a pest epidemic. In 1727 it became a military hospital called "*Königliches* (*Friedrich Wilhem I*) *Charité — Krankenhaus*", in the so-called "Pépinière" lessons were given for students. Many famous scientist arose later on from this institute like Rudolf Virchow, Hermann von Helmholtz, Emil von Behring, Robert Koch. In 1810 the University from Berlin was founded and took over the hospital, which in the meantime was united with the botanical garden and the anatomical theater to a "Collegium medico-chirurgicum". The children's hospital of the Charité was built in 1830 and was the first children's hospital in Germany (Fig. 12). The recent well-known building in red bricks was built 1896 to 1917. In 1906 the Rudol Virchow hospital was opened

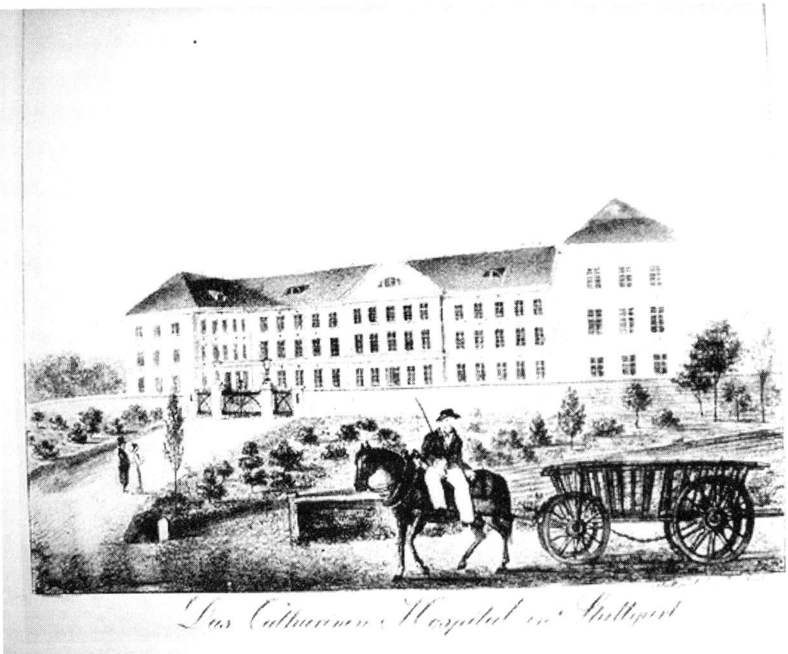

Fig 11. Das Katharinen Hospital in Stuttgart, 1830, from Murken.

and in 1968 the University Steglitz in West-Berlin which became from 1994 on the Bejamin Franklin University of Berlin. Chief of the paediatric surgical unit there was Prof Jürgen Waldschmidt. In 1986 the Rudolf Virchow Krankenhaus became a University Hospital too ("*Freie Universität Berlin*") and amalgamated in 1997–1998 with the Charité and in 2003 with the Benjamin Franklin University to one of the biggest hospital centers in Europe called now "*Charité — Universitätsmedizin Berlin*". Up until now the chief of the department of Paediatric Surgery is Prof Harald Mau. Other children's hospitals in Berlin were the "*Elisabeth-Kinderhospital*" (1843), the "*Luisen-Kinderheilanstalt*" (1844) and the "*Kaiserin-Auguste Viktoria-Haus*" (1909).

The department of Paediatric Surgery in *Leipzig* was established in 1889 and like in Cologne there was a separate paediatric and paediatric surgical from the beginning. The Chief was Prof Herrmann

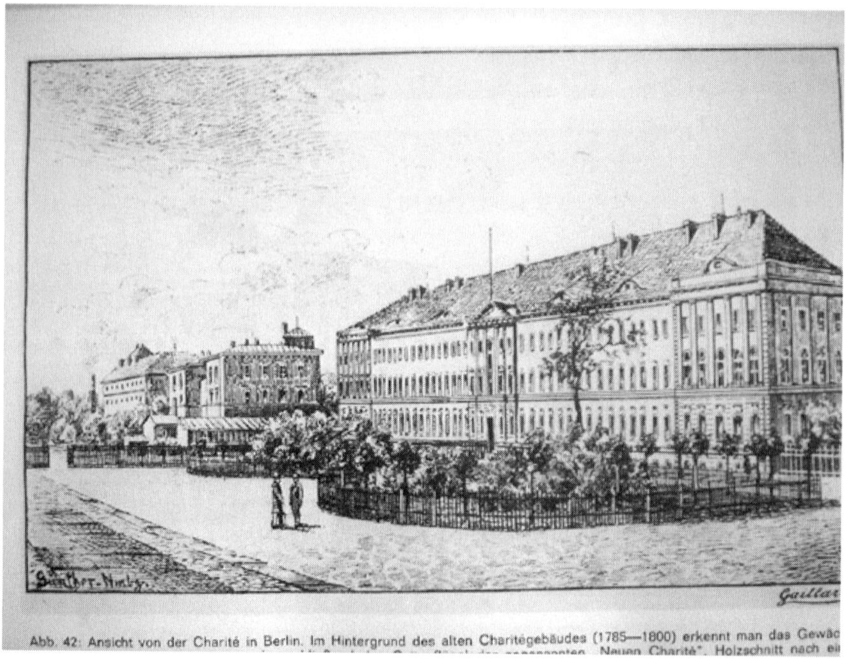
Abb. 42: Ansicht von der Charité in Berlin. Im Hintergrund des alten Charitégebäudes (1785—1800) erkennt man das

Fig. 12. Wood carving from Charité Berlin 1885, in the back the old building from Murken 1978.

Tillmanns and from 1920 on Prof Roderich Sievers.[34,35] In 1958 an independent clinic and out-patient department for Paediatric Surgery was founded and in 1959 Prof Fritz Meißner became its chief. In 1961 he got a chair at the University of Leipzig. His successors from 1986 on were Prof Wolfram Tischer, Prof Joachim Bennek and recently Prof Holger Till.

It is impossible to mention the development of all paediatric surgical units in Germany, but one can summarise that some units followed the above mentioned development of four or five steps, in other hospitals like in *Heidelberg, Hannover-, Hamburg-Eppendorf* paediatric surgery was established as part of and inside departments of adult surgery. A paediatric surgical unit could therefore be situated inside a surgical center like in *Mannheim* or *Krefeld*, or be part of a children's hospital like in *Bremen, Stuttgart, Hannover-Bult, Dortmund, Köln, München-Schwabing, Kassel-Park Schönfeld,*

Bonn-St Augustin, Karlsruhe, Kinderheilanstalt (today: Hannober Bult, founded 1863), and *Berlin Buch*. Most of these departments are attached at an university with students and teaching responsibilities (Academic Teaching Hospitals). Much rarer (18 out of 64 Departments) are chairs for paediatric surgery such as: *Mannheim, Mainz, Munich-Haunersches Kinderspital, Bochum-Herne, Lübeck, Hannover, Tübingen, Greifswald, Dresden, Erfurth, Leipzig, Jena, Magdeburg, Berlin-Charité, Hamburg-Eppendorf*, and *Halle*.

Most of the departments of paediatric surgery date from the 19th century, some are more modern foundations. One of the most modern is the department of Paediatric Surgery in *Berlin-Neucölln*, dating from the end of the 20th century.

In *Bremen* an independent Paediatric surgical Unit was established after the First World War. In *Würzburg*, which got one of the oldest chairs for Paediatrics in the 19th century, paediatric surgery became an independent unit only a few decades ago.

Development of Surgical Procedures

Being a sub-specialisation of surgery, the surgical roots of paediatric surgery came of course from adult surgery. Most of the procedures still used today, were invented by adult surgeons and first used for adults and only later on for children. Tables 3 and 4 summarise some of the most important steps of this development with special regard to paediatric surgery.

The mortality in those days was very high. During the four years from 1874 to 1878, about 80% of the babies under six month of age admitted in the *Charité* died, about 70% of the infants under two years and 19% of the children under four years, therefore, in some hospitals babies were even not allowed to be admited.[38] As mentioned before, the first chief of a children's hospital was usually a practitioner who was trained in medicine and surgery for some years and he was able to operate himself. But with the rapid development of surgery, especially with the progress in anaesthesia (chloroform, ether) mayor surgical procedures became possible. The surgical problems of sick children were treated more and more by

Table 3. Periods of development of modern medicine with special regard to surgery; according to Aschoff *et al.*[36]

Time	Periods	Important steps for Surgery
~1500–~1700	**First Period of Natural Sciences** *Modern anatomical and physiological thinking* From Theophrastus von Hohenheim (1494–1541) and Andreas Vesal (1514–1564) to William Harvey (1578–1657) and Giovanni Battista Morgagni (1682–1771)	Ambroise Paré (1510–1590; France: Wound treatment Pierro Franco (+1500–1570/80?); Bladder stone extirpation
~1750–~1838	**Second Period of Natural Sciences** *Influence of Philosophy on Medicine* Gottfried Wilhelm Leibnitz (1646–1716), Wilhem Schelling (1775–1854), Immanuel Kant (1724–1804) Lorenz Oken (1779–1851); *Periode of Physiological sciences*: Albert von Haller (1708–1777) Systematics: Carl von Linné (1707–1778)	Jean Louis Petit (1674–1760), Pathologic Anatomy Nicolas Andry (1658–1742): introduced the word Orthopedia for the treatment of deformities in children Lorenz Heister (1683–1758) first important textbook for surgery, translated in many languages First reliable suture at the bowel by Antoine Lembert (1802–1851)
1838–1918	**Third Period of Natural Sciences** *Cell pathology* Virchow (1821–1902): Cell pathology: omnis cellula e cellula *Infectious Contaminations*: Igaz Philipp Semmelweis (1818–1865) Louis Pasteur (1822–1895) Robert Koch (1843–1910) Tuberculosis (1882) 1867 First use of a gastric probe for eternal nutrition by Adolf Kussmaul (1822–1902)	Henry Hancock (1809–1880): First appendectomy; Friedrich Esmarch (1823–1908) operation in exsanguinations (1873) Alexander Watson?–1902): First Extirpation of larynx; Jacques Reverdin (1842–1929) and Karl Thiersch (1822–1895) Skin Transplantations; 1872 Theodor Billroth (1829–1894) First resection of an esophagus at a dog 1880 First thyreoidectomy

(*Continued*)

Table 3. *(Continued)*

Time	Periods	Important steps for Surgery
	Anesthesia Eugène Soubeiran (1797–1858), Justus Liebig (1803–1873), and Samuel Guthry (1782–1848): discovery of Chloroform Charles Jackson (1805–1880) and William Morton (1819–1869) discovery of Aether-Anesthesia Joseph Lister (1827–1912) Introduction of *Antisepsis* 1882 Introduction of the first Sterilisation apparat for surgical instruments in Bonn by Friedrich Trendelenburg (1844–1924) 1890 introduction of guns into surgery by William Steward Halsted (1852–1922) 1894 *Paediatrics* became an independent speciality (Otto Heubner got a chair for Paediatrics in Berlin/ Charité) 1881 First instrument for esophago- and gastroskopy by Johann Mikulicz-Radecki (1850–1905) 1895 discopvery og X Ray radiation by William Conrad Röntgen (1845–1923) in Würzburg	by Ludwig Rehn 1877 Resection of Colon in Patients with cancer by Carl Gussenbauer (1842–1903) 1886 Description of Megacolon congenitum by Harald Hirschsprung (1830–1916) 1881 First incubator for newborns 1885 First Endolaryngeal intubation Stéphane Tannier 1882 First extirpation of a gallbladder by Karl Langenbuch (1846–1901) 1884 Trendelenburg's position published 1884 First Posterior Sagittal Approach for resection of a high rectal cancer by Paul Kraske (1851–1930) 1885 First Choledochotomy by Hermann Kümmel (1852–1937) 1887 Improved technique of inguinal hernia repair by Eduardo Bassini (1844–1924) 1896 First heart suture by Ludwig Rehn (1849–1930) 1897 First total gastrectomy by Carl Schlatter (1864–1934)
1918–1950	**Newest Time**	
	1929 First Heart catheterisation by Werner Forssmann (Nobel Prize) 1932 Flexible Gastroscopy by R. Schindler and Norbert Henning 1929 Development Penicillin by Alexander Fleming (1881–1955) 1940 Development of Sulfathiazole against Tbc by G. Domagk	1914 Myotomie of the cardia by E. Heller 1956 Fundoplicatio by Rudolf Nissen, 1966 modified by Rossetti.

Table 4. Further important surgical procedures influenced the specialisation in surgery.

1869	First Extirpation of a kidney by Gustav Simon (1824–1876)
1881	First Resection of a stomach by Theodor Billroth (1821–1894)
1883	First Pancreas operation by Karl Gussenbauer (1842–1903)
1896	First operation at the thyroid in a patient with M. Basedow by Ludwig Rehn (1849–1930)
1903	Thorax operation in a gauge presser equalizing chamber by Ferdinand Sauerbruch (1875–1951)
from 1905 on	Development of Neurosurgery by Harvey W. Cushing (1869–1923)
1879	Introduction of Cystoskopy by Max Nitze (1848–1906) and beginning of modern Urology
1907	First successful lobectomy by Werner Körte (1850–1923) and beginning of Thoraxsurgery
1910	Beginning of Reconstructive and Plastic surgery by Erich Lexer (1867–1937)
From 1924 on	Development of Traumatology by Lorenz Böhler (1885–1973) war and start of an special discipline oral surgery and operative dentistry
From 1938 on	Progresses in heart surgery by Alfred Blalok, Helen Taussig, Robert E. Gross and Clarence Crafoord

surgeons, first by surgical consultants. Later these consultants began to specialise. The first pyloromyotomie was done by the surgeon Conrad Ramstedt (1867–1963) in Münster 1911. Max Wilms (1867–1918) was a surgeon too, working in Leipzig under Trendelenburg (Friedrich Trendelenburg, 1844–1924) between 1897 and 1899, when his book on what has come to be known as Wilms' tumour was published. Later he got a chair for adult surgery in Heidelberg.

The definitive development of paediatric surgery started in Germany only after 1950. It was mainly influenced by the first successful end to-end anastomosis in 1941 by Haight in the United States, the textbook and the atlas by Robert E. Gross[39,40] and the publications by Denis Browne[41] which were now available in Germany too. One can say that the pioneer operation by Haight was the birthday for paediatric surgery in Germany. A very nice review of timelines in the international history of paediatric surgery was given in 1986 by Chang.[42]

In the Federal Republic of Germany it took however, another ten years until, from 1951 on, *esophageal atresia* could be treated successfully.[43] For the approach a 2 cm long part of the 2nd to 6th rib was resected, and by Rehbein an extrapleural, by Hecker an intrapleural approach to the esophagus was performed. For many years a simultaneous gastrostomy was established. Many children suffered post-operatively from severe anastomotic strictures and different types of bouginage had to be invented. The most common one was the bouginage with a transesophageal, nasal thread coming out at the gastostomy site. For long segments colon interpositions were used until Howard and Myers, in 1965, introduced the systematic bouginage of the upper pouch which led in many cases to a significant elongation and allowed a secondary anastomosis without any interposition.

In the 50's and 60's, many children suffered from a distal esophageal stenosis due to massive *Gastroesophageal Reflux Disease* (*GERD*). The generous introduction of Nissen's fundoplication or of a retroesophageal hiatusplastique with gastropexy after conservative treatment has eliminated this complication today almost completely. In addition, the fundoplication is performed today in most of the cases laparascopically.

The treatment of duodenal obstruction changed after the first successfull adhesiolysis perfomed by Ladd in 1932 and in Germany too. However the understanding of bowel rotation and volvulus came only after its detailed description by Max Grob[44] in **1953**, in a founding monography. In *atresias of the small bowel*, usually a double loop enterostomy was created and a secondary anastomosis performed some weeks later.

The first resection of *congenital Megacolon* was performed by Ovar Swenson in 1948 in USA. In the 1950's, his proposed type of extraanal anastomosis after the resection of the narrow segment was adopted by only a few surgeons in Germany. Many authors favored Soaves technique from 1964, or Rehbein's deep intrapelvic, anterior resection from 1963 which was a modification from States high rectectomy. The treatment of *anal and rectal atresias* was modified by Rehbein too, using a sacral approach according to Stephens and Smith for intermediate anomalies, but a rectal mucosectomy and abdomino-perineal transrectal pullthrough for high types of imperforate anus. Many modifications according to the different conditions of these diseases were introduced by Rehbein and described in detail in his book.[12]

For *biliary atresias* the hepatoportoenterostomy seemed to be the treatment of choice after its introduction by Kasai, Japan, in 1959, but an additional lymphatic drainage was introduced by Schweizer in 1972 to improve the results.

Funnel Chests were treated with special metallic stents which have been invented by Rehbein in 1957. Other paediatric surgeons preferred Ravich's technique. Today both techniques are replaced by the minimal invasive technique of Nuss.

The names of Paul-Gerhard Hecker (1897–1980) and his son Waldemar Hecker are connected with an elegant technique for the treatment of *anal-* and *rectal prolapse* by a sacral approach and the placation and fixation of the rectum at the sacrum.[10,47]

The Development of Paediatric Surgery in the German Democratic Republic (GDR, East Germany)

After the Second World War Germany was separated into four occupied zones, three west of the Elbe-Werra-Linie, the American, British, French and one East of the Linie, the Soviet Occupied zone. The western zone became the BRD (*Bundesrepublik Deutschland*), the eastern zone the DDR subdivided into 16 areas. In the middle was Berlin with three western and one eastern sector which was the capital of DDR. Country and people were governed according to the politic and economic needs of the Soviet Republic. The Health System was state ruled/owned. The DDR existed between October 7, 1949 to November 2, 1990. On the October 3, 1990, Germany was reunited.[48]

The DDR and its health system. In the territory of the DDR after 1945, the former political system and living conditions were broken down. Famine and epidemics were a threat to the people. However, within the first years after the war the worst effects were overcome. Particular attention was paid to developing measures for mothers, teenagers and children. The mainstay of the Health System was its communistic character, meaning that institutions and its employees were governed and controlled by the State. However, every person/citizen was entitled to free medical care. The Health System was aimed at prevention of illnesses. Of the 18 million inhabitants, the proportion of children was 20%.

Paediatric surgery in the DDR. As mentioned above, paediatric surgery found its true scope after the Second World War. In the former DDR too, this happened only in 1960 when it was decided to create new, specific Societies, Sections and Working Groups of Paediatric Surgery. The paediatric surgical institutions of the University of Leipzig and the one of the City Hospital Berlin-Buch were the first paediatric surgical institutions of the DDR. In 1961, the Berlin Wall completely separated the DDR from the BRD and East from West Berlin. At that point four paediatric surgical institutions existed in the DDR: Leipzig, Berlin-Buch, Karl-Marx-Stadt (former Chemnitz) and Rostock. Further institutions followed and can be described in three steps: working group, section, society (Table 5).

Working groups and section (1964–1968). In 1958 the qualification (speciality) of paediatric surgery already existed as well as four paediatric surgical institutions with specialists and trainees. In 1964 it therefore seemed reasonable to create a working group. The founding members were Prof Dr Fritz Meissner of the University of Leipzig (Fig. 13), and Dr Ilse Krause of the Hospital Berlin-Buch (Fig. 14). General surgeons observed this development with suspicion. Professor Meisner wrote "we will need much more discussions to convince the General Surgeons of the advantages of an independent surgical speciality: Paediatric Surgery". However the development went well.

Table 5. Founding years of paediatric surgical institutions in the GDR.*

Founding years	Place and kind of the institutions
1889	Leipzig, Karl-Marx Universität
1956	Berlin-Buch, Städtisches Klinikum
1958	Karl-Marx-Stadt (Chemnitz) Bezirkskrankenhaus
1959	Rostock, Wilhelm Pieck-Universität
1966	Dresden, Medizinische Akademie
1967	Potsdam, Bezirkskrankenhaus
1968	Halle, Martin-Luther-Universität
1969	Greifswald, Ernst-Moritz-Arndt-Universität
1969	Stralsund
1970	Magdeburg, Medizinische Akademie
1972	Burg, Kreiskrankenhaus
1972	Suhl, Bezirkskrankenhaus
1972	Wismar
1973	Altenburg, Kreiskrankenhaus
1973	Aue
1973	Erfurt, Medizinische Akademie
1973	Jena, Friedrich- Schiller-Universität
1974	Schwerin, Bezirkskrankenhaus
1974	Zwickau
1976	Berlin-Köpenick, Bezirkskrankenhaus
1976	Frankfurt/Oder, Bezirkskrankenhaus
1976	Hoyerswerda, Bezirkskrankenhaus
1977	Halle/Saale, St. Barbara-Krankenhaus
1977	Neubrandenburg, Bezirkskrankenhaus
1977	Wermersdorf, Kreiskrankenhaus
1979	Berlin-Charité, Universitätklinik
1980	Dresden-Neustadt
1984	Brandenburg

* In Güstrow, Wittenberg, Pritzwalk, Berlin-Friedrichshain, Cottbus additional paediatric surgeons, but no institutions.

Within the Working Groups there were separate working parties for certain areas such as: prognosis, bacterial colonisation, tumours in the paediatric age group, paediatric urology, paediatric trauma, and maintaining traditions. Paediatric trauma merged with the interest group Paediatric Trauma in the Adult in 1973 to form a joint

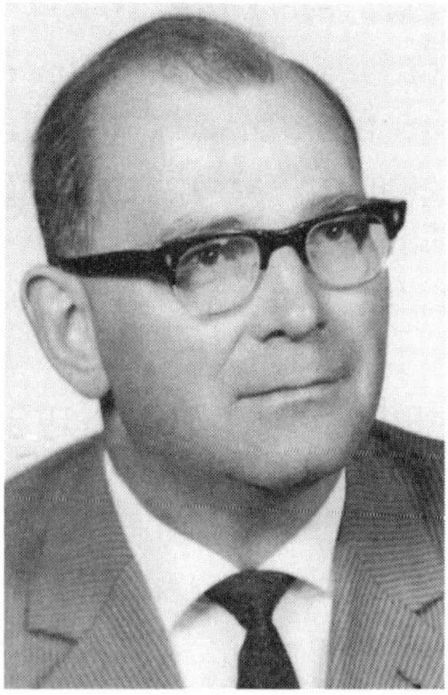

Fig. 13. Prof Meisner.

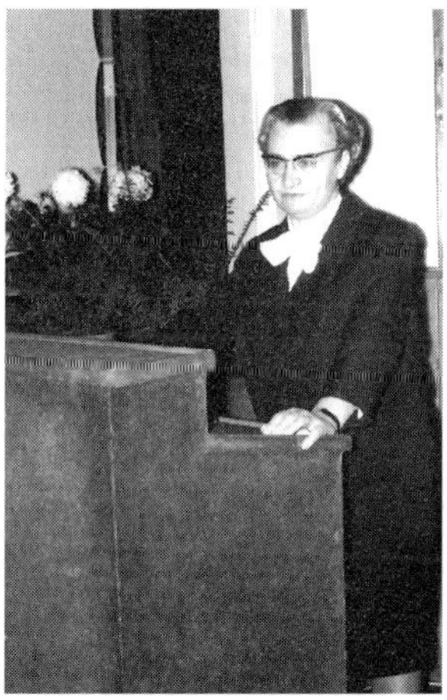

Fig. 14. Dr Ilse Krause.

working group of "Paediatric Trauma". The executive was equally shaped by the Paediatric Surgeons and Adult Trauma Surgeons. The number of Paediatric Surgeons increased. In 1968 the Society of Surgery in the DDR was created and Paediatric Surgery became an independent surgical Section of the Society of General Surgery.

Society of paediatric surgery (1968–1990). On 1968, November 22, a meeting of representatives of the Ministry of Health, the Society of Surgery and Paediatrics took place. The Ministry was interested in having a qualified surgical provision for surgeons to provide specific surgery for children. The Society of Surgery itself demanded to create specific paediatric surgical units at Universities, Academic and District General Hospitals, which should be staffed by qualified paediatric surgeons and which should provide special Paediatric Surgical care everywhere in the DDR. The departments included also polyclinic care. This enabled a close coordination of surgical procedures, prophylaxis, diagnoses, post-operative and conservative therapy as well as rehabilitation.

An independent Society of Paediatric Surgery of the DDR was finally created on October 19, 1985.

Training and CPD. The training in the former DDR used to take five years. The trainee was involved in shaping the process. Leading clinicians were allowed to send trainees on other training centers to intensify their training. However the original job was maintained and the salary continued to be paid. Courses were part of the training. They were organised once a year and every trainee would take them to an appropriate level of their training. Course material was selected in a way that it nearly covered the whole curriculum of paediatric surgery. Courses tended to last a week. They were free of charge. Trainees were exempt from their clinical duties, overnight and travel expenses were paid. Lecturers offered their services for free. A different way of training was the consultation forum initiated by Prof Meisner in 1972. The challenging problems were presented and discussed to find the best possible treatment for the patient. These meetings happened once a year. The paediatric surgical training finished with an exit examination taken by the "Central Expert Commission for Paediatric Surgery".

Quality control. In 1949 commissions were created to deal with paediatric mortality. Neonatologists, paediatricians, paediatric surgeons, radiologists and pathologists were part of those. Since 1953 medical review commissions existed for the whole of medicine. Every injury from medical treatment, small or large, every death had to be notified and was analysed by the commission and classified as avoidable, partially avoidable or unavoidable. Institutions where the injury happened were given the decision of the commission to review it and initiate changes to avoid similar incidents in the future. The review of such an accident with the associated remarks and proposals by the commission was more effective than any theorctical discussion about quality control.

Scientific activities. Beside many scientific articles, the most important books published in the DDR were: F. Meissner's "*Kinderchirurgische Erkrankungen*,[11] W. Tischer and K. Gdanietz's "*Paediatric Surgery in Practice*[49]; and V. Hofmann's "*Sonographic Diagnosis in Paediatrics and Paediatric Surgery* (1st ed.).[46]

Epilogue. Paediatric Surgery in the DDR began with F. Meissner and Ilse Krause (Fig. 14). Ilse Krause died in 1984. In memory of this great paediatric surgeon the Academy of Paediatric Surgery of the German Society of Paediatric Surgery created a prize to support Paediatric Surgical Trainees/Junior. It is named "*Ilse-Krause-Nachwuchs-Preis*". Prof Meissner became Honorary President of the German Society for Paediatric Surgery. After the German unification on October 3, 1990, the members of the 33 Paediatric Surgical Units of the Society of Paediatric Surgery of the DDR joined the German Society for Paediatric Surgery on November 17, 1990.

Future

The future of paediatric surgery is uncertain. The new training conditions of the European Union and its consequences have led to a reduction in training time and numbers of operations. Besides, the conditions to become a paediatric surgeon differ a lot among European countries, but there is a trend by the EU to allow free cross-border exchange of doctors and to equalise the training standards. This will not increase the quality of doctors. Surgical sub-specialties reclaim children to be part of their own individual speciality and paediatricians reclaim in general children for their own departments. Finally, the birth-rate is decreasing in many European countries in contrast to the high number of doctors in training.[45]

Therefore, we can only cite the last two lines of a poem by W. H. Auden:

"If I Could Tell You:
Will Time say nothing but I told you so?
If I could tell you I would let you know."

References

1. Oehme J. *Medizin in der Zeit Aufklärung unter besonderer Berücksichtigung von Kinderkrankheiten.* Hansisches Verlagskontor, Lübeck, 1986.
2. Oehme J. Arzt im 18ten Jahrhundert. *Der Kinderarzt* 1986;17:411–416.
3. Oehme J. Pädiatrie-historische Schriften unter besonderer Berücksichtigung von Albrecht Peipers. "Chronik der Kinderheilkunde." *Der Kinderarzt* 1991;22:902–910.
4. Karewski F. *Die Chirurgischen Krankheiten des Kindesalters.* Berlin, 1894.
5. Holschneider AM. Tradition und Zukunft der Kinderchirurgie Teil I. *Der Kinderarzt* 1989;20:241–245.
6. Holschneider AM. Tradition und Zukunft der Kinderchirurgie Teil II. *Der Kinderarzt* 1989;20:408–410.
7. Drachter R, Gossmann JR. Chirurgie des Kindesalters. In: v. Pfaundler M, Schloßmann A (hrsg.) *Handbuch der Kinderheilkunde* bd IX, Springer: Berlin, 1930.
8. Oberniedermayr A. *Lehrbuch der Chirurgie und Orthopädie des Kindesalters.* Springer: Berlin, Göttingen, Heidelberg, 1959.
9. Kunz H. *Operationen im Kindesalter.* Ein Atlas in 2 Bänden, Georg Thieme Stuttgart, 1973.

10. Hecker WCh, Daum R, Maier WA. Die Eingriffe in Säuglings- und Kindesalter. In: Breitner B, Zukschwerdt L, Kraus H (hrsg.) *Chirurgische Operationslehre.* Urban and Schwarzenberg München Berlin Wien Bd II, S1–171, 1970.
11. Meißner F. *Kinderchirurgische Erkrankungen Band I.* VEB Georg Thieme, Leipzig, 1965.
12. Rehbein F. *Kinderchirurgische Operationen.* Hippokrates Verlag, Stuttgart, 1976.
13. von Laer L, Kraus R, Linhart WE. *Frakturen und Luxationen im Wachstumsalter.* Thieme Stuttgart, Auflage, 2007.
14. Dietz HG, Schmittenbecher PP, Illing P. *Intramedulläre Osteosynthese im Wachsstumsalter.* Urban&Schwarzenberg, München Wien Baltimore, 1996.
15. Berlien H-P, Müller G. *Angewandte Lasermedizin. Lehr- und Handbuch für Praxis und Klinik.* Ecomed Verlag Landsberg München Zürich, 1989.
16. Waldschmidt J. *Das Akute Abdomen im Kindesalter.* Edition Medizin VCH Verlagsgesellschaft Weinheim, 1990.
17. Schweizer P, Schier F. *Hepatobiliary Surgery in Childhood.* Schattauer Verlag, Stuttgart, New York, 1991.
18. Holschneider AM, Hutson J. *Anorectal Malformations in Children.* Springer, Heidelberg, 2007.
19. Holschneider AM, Puri P. *Hirschsprung's Disease and Allied Disorders* Springer, Heidelberg, 2008.
20. Stephens D, Smith D. *Congenital Malformations of the Rectum, Anus and Genito-Urinary Tracts.* E & S Livingstone LTD, Edinburgh and London, 1963.
21. Hadidi AT, Azmy AE. *Hypospadias Surgery.* Springer Heidelberg, 2004.
22. Jetter D. *Das europäische Hospital.* Von der Spätantike bis 1800. DuMont Buchverlag, Köln, 1986.
23. Murken AH. *Das Bild des Deutschen Krankenhauses.* Verlag Murken-Altrogge, F Coppenrath Verlag, Münster, 1978.
24. Hecker WCh. Kurzer Abriß zur Geschichte der deutschen Kinderchirurgie. *Der Kinderarzt* 1985;16:1417–1420.

25. Hecker WCh. The History of Pediatric Surgery in Germany. *Progr Pediatr Surg* 1986;20:1–8.
26. Locher W. 150 *Jahre Doktor von Hauner'sches Kinderspital 1846–1996*. Von der Mietwohnung zur Universitätsklinik. Cygnus Verlag München, 1996.
27. Leichtenstern D, Schwartz O. *Generalbericht für das öffentliche Gesundheitswesen aus dem Jahre* 1880, S.6ff, 1881.
28. Siegert F. Das Freiherr Abraham von Oppenheim'sche Kinderspital. In: Bachem JP (ed.) *Naturwissenschaft und Gesundheitswesen in Köln*. Festschrift für die Teilnehmer an der 80sten Versammlung der Gesellschaft für Naturforscher und Ärzte in Köln. Verlag S, 1908, pp. 404–408.
29. Hoyme H. *Die Entwicklung der Kölner Universitätskinderklinik bis zum Ende des zweiten Weltkrieges*. Inaug. Diss. Köln, 1983.
30. Kastenholz. Das Freiherr Abraham von Opppenheim'sche Kinderspital. In: *Festschrift für Mitglieder und Teilnehmer der 61. Versammlung Deutscher Naturforscher und Ärzte*. Dumont Schauberg Verlag, Köln S, 1888, pp. 280–288.
31. Haße W. 100Jahre Kinderchirurgie Berlin-Wedding. *Der Kinderarzt* 1990;21:1485–1489.
32. Helbig D. Die Kinderchirurgische Klinik im Kinderkrankenhaus der Stadt Köln. *Z Kinderchir* 1973;12:1–2.
33. Köhler B. Das Olgahospital in Stuttgart. Von der Etagenwohnung zum Pädiatrischen Zentrum. *Der Kinderarzt* 1988;19:557–565.
34. Meißner F. Klinik und Ambulanz für Kinderchirurgie. In: 550 Jahre Medizinische Fakultät. Hrsg. Medizinische Fakultät der Universität Leipzig. *Mathematisch-Naturwissenschaftliche Reihe* 1965;14:173–175.
35. Weingärtner L. Erinnerungen an die Leipziger Kinderchirurgie. *Der Kinderarzt* 1986;17:1197–1202.
36. Aschoff/Diepgen/Goerke. *Kurze Übersichtstabelle zur Geschichte der Medizin*. 7. Auflg. Springer Verlag Berlin Göttingen Heidelberg, 1960.
37. Gölis LA. *Praktische Abhandlungen über die vorzüglicheren Krankheiten des kindlichen Alters. Wien 1815 und 1818*; 2. Auflg. 1820, Darin: Geschichte des Wiener Krankeninstituts I, p. 294, 1818.
38. Peiper A. Chronik der Kinderheilkunde. *Georg Thieme Leipzig*, 1992.

39. Gross RE. *The Surgery of Infancy and Childhood. Its Principles and Techniques*. WB Saunders Company, Philadelphia London, 1953.
40. Gross RE. *An Atlas of Children's Surgery*. WB Saunders company, Philadelphia, London, Toronto, 1970.
41. Browne D. An Operation for Hypospadias. *Proc Roy Soc Med* 1949; 42:466.
42. Chang JHT. Timelines in the history of Pediatric Surgery. *J Ped Surg* 1986;21:1068–1072.
43. Rehbein F. Kinderchirurgie. In: Schreiber HW, Carstensen G (eds.) *Chirurgie im Wandel der Zeit 1945–1983*. Springer-Verlag Berlin Heidelberg New York, 1983.
44. Grob M. *Über Lageanomalien des Magendarmtractus infolge Störungen der fetalen Darmdrehung*. Basel, Benno Schabe Verlag & Co, 1953.
45. Holschneider AM. Pediatric surgical reality in Germany and visions for the future. *Eur J Pediatr Surg* 2001;11:75–81.
46. Hofmann V, Deeg KH, Hoyer PF. *Ultraschalldiagnostik in Pädiatrie und Kinderchirurgie. Lehrbuch und Atlas*. 2. völlig überarbeitete und erweiterte Auflage. Thieme Stuttgart, New York, 1996.
47. Gdanietz K, Borgwardt G. In: Zetkin M, Schaldach H (eds.): *Wörterbuch der Medizin, Fünfzehnte vollständig überarbeitete Auflage*. Ulstein Mosby S 886, 1992.
48. Gdanietz K. Die Entwicklung der Kinderchirurgie in der DDR — 1949 bis 1990. *Pädiatr Grenzgeb* 1997;36:95–106.

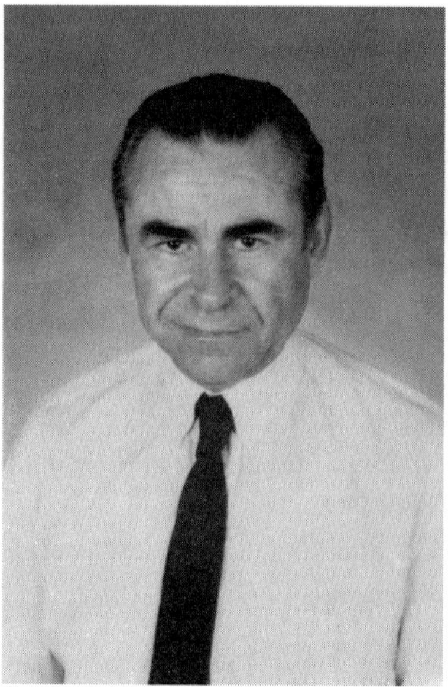

Demitris C. Keramidas

GREECE

Demitris C. Keramidas

The scientific activities of specific persons involved in paediatric surgery are interconnected with the establishment of training centres providing the appropriate subject material for training in neonatal and paediatric surgery. These centres, in chronological order are: Children's Hospitals; Departments of Paediatric Surgery in University Medical Schools; and Departments of Paediatric Surgery in General Hospitals.

It is in this context that the History of Surgical Paediatrics in Greece is presented and short references made to paediatric surgeons and their associates responsible for the organisation of these Departments.

Separate sections will follow in reference to:

(1) other Departments of Paediatric Surgery in General Hospitals,
(2) the recognition of Paediatric Surgery as speciality by the Greek State,
(3) the establishment of the Greek Association of Paediatric Surgeons (GAPS) and its activities and finally,
(4) the present status of Paediatric Surgery in Greece.

Children's Hospitals

There are four Children's Hospitals in Greece and two more are scheduled to open. Three of the existing hospitals, Aghia Sophia, Aglaia Kyriakou and Penteli, are located in Athens, and Karamandaneion is based in Patras. The Hospitals Aghia Sophia and Aglaia Kyriakou are affiliated with the Athens University by means of housing respectively the 1st and 2nd University Departments of Paediatrics. As regards the Karamandaneion Children's Hospital Department of Paediatric Surgery, it has a history of cooperation with the University of Patras Department of Paediatric Surgery.

Aghia Sophia Children's Hospital is the largest (750 beds) and oldest of its kind in Greece. There are Departments covering the entire spectrum of surgical paediatrics, i.e. general paediatric and neonatal surgery, paediatric urology, neurosurgery, cardiac surgery, orthopaedics, plastic and reconstructive surgery, ENT and eye surgery. Construction of the Hospital began in 1896 under the auspices of Princess Sophia of the Royal Family of that time. It was in that Hospital that a Department of Paediatric Surgery was established in 1901, in a nice building housing the administration offices of the hospital today. The Department was organised and directed by Dr Socrates Tsakonas. In 1911 Dr Tsakonas resigned from his post, having been elected Professor of Gynaecology at Athens University. He was succeeded by Dr Dimitris Kokkoris. He worked for 15 years until 1926, when the Department was unjustifiably abolished during a period of political instability. During the 25-year period (1901–1926) almost 2000 children were treated for the following diseases: appendicitis-peritonitis, empyema thoracis, herniae, injuries including intra-abdominal and burns, hydatid cysts of various localisations, stones of the bladder, and tuberculosis of lymph nodes and bones. No congenital anomalies of either the gastrointestinal tract or the genitourinary system could be found in the records of the Department.

In the following 27 years, children with surgical diseases were treated in general hospitals or in private clinics until 1953, when a Department of Paediatric Surgery was established in Aglaia Kyriakou Children's Hospital. Dr Basil Petropoulos, following his training in Prof's Fevre Unit of Paediatric Surgery and Orthopaedics in *Hôpital d'Enfants Malades* (Paris, France), was appointed Chief Surgeon. He organised a modern Department of Paediatric Surgery and Orthopaedics in Aglaia Kyriakou Children's Hospital, thus becoming the person with whom paediatric surgery began in Greece.

Aglaia Kyriakou Children's Hospital is a 350-bed hospital. Its construction started in 1934 on a site donated by the neighbouring Aghia Sophia Children's Hospital. The staff under Dr B Petropoulos was composed of young surgeons with a particular interest in Paediatric Surgery. Among them were Nicholas Voyatzis, Philip Hadjihaberis, Anthony Markantonatos, Emmanuel Miliaras, and later Alexander Vassilacopoulos, who after completion of their training in paediatric surgery constituted the nucleus of the first generation of paediatric surgeons involved in training young surgeons with a similar interest in paediatric surgery. Therefore, Dr B Petropoulos' Department in Aglaia Kyriakou Children's Hospital was the birthplace of Paediatric Surgery in Greece.

The Department started with 15 beds in 1953 and expanded gradually to 80 beds by the year 1961, when Dr B Petropoulos was elected Professor of a newly established Chair of Paediatric Surgery and Orthopaedics at the Aristotle University of Thessaloniki. During the seven-year period of his chairmanship in Aglaia Kyriakou Children's Hospital, 7162 operations were performed on neonates, infants, and children. With B Petropoulos' initiative in 1958, paediatric surgery was recognised by the Greek State Heath Authorities as a speciality, for which a four-year training in general surgery and a two-year training in paediatric surgery were required.

In 1962, after Prof B Petropoulos resigned to take up his duties at Thessaloniki University, Dr Nicholas Voyatzis was appointed Head of the **First Paediatric Surgery Department of Aglaia Kyriakou Children's Hospital**. Under his direction, orthopaedics was separated from paediatric surgery, forming a new independent department. Dr Voyatzis had returned from a fellowship in Great Ormond Street Children's Hospital and in the Karolinska where he was attached respectively to A. Wilkinson and Theodore Ehrenprens. Dr Voyatzis was an experienced surgeon, specialising in thoracic surgery and abdominal surgery. He was one of the first paediatric surgeons outside France to perform the Duhamel procedure. He designed a specific clamp for the Duhamel anastomosis and used this clamp in his operations. He presented his results in the 1st International Hedrologicum Conlegium in Cos, in 1961. Thereafter, several clamps for the Duhamel anastomosis were proposed by other paediatric surgeons such as Sulamaa, Bill and Ikeda.

In 1979, the **Second Department of Paediatric Surgery** was established at Aglaia Kyriakou Children's Hospital. Dr Christopher Moutsouris, paediatric surgeon and Associate Professor of Surgery in Athens University, was elected Head of this new Department, which he set up with the assistance of his associates Drs Maria Toumazani and Constantine Skondras who continued his duties as Chief Surgeon at the same hospital at a later stage. After completing his training in paediatric surgery, Dr Moutsouris continued his education in Sweden and Denmark. He successfully performed the entire spectrum of paediatric surgery including paediatric urology. Being interested in experimental surgery he also wrote papers, which were published abroad.

The reestablishment of the **Department of Paediatric Surgery** in 1962 saw the emergence of another training hub in paediatric surgery in **Aghia Sophia Children's Hospital**. Almost 37 years had passed since the abolishment of the Department in 1926. The Department was organised by Dr Elephtherios Tsakayannis, an experienced surgeon who, prior to his assignment as Head of the Department of Paediatric Surgery, was granted fellowships (1958–1959) to the Children's Hospital in Great Ormond Street (A. Wilkinson) and Boston Children's Hospital (R. Gross), and had worked in Great Ormond Street (1959–1960) under D. Waterston. Favourable factors for Dr Tsakayannis' newly-established Department were: the affiliation with the 1st Department of Paediatrics of Athens University, the large number of paediatric patients in Aghia Sophia Children's Hospital, and the tradition of the 1st University Department of Paediatrics as being the oldest, largest and best organised in Greece at that time.

Among Dr Tsakayannis' first associates, were those who became Heads of the Departments of Paediatric Surgery at the Children's Hospitals namely Christopher Moutsouris, Constantine Pappis, George Moussatos and, at a later stage, Emmanuel Adnroulakakis and they assumed responsibility for training young paediatric surgeons. Dr Moussatos had worked with W. Potts and O. Swenson in Children's Memorial Hospital, N. Western University in Chicago (1960–1962), having previously completed his internship in general surgery in the USA (1955–1960). He succeeded Dr Tsakayannis as Head of the Department at Aghia Sophia in 1980.

A **2nd Department of Paediatric Surgery** was established at **Aghia Sophia Children's Hospital** in 1985. Dr Dimitris Keramidas was elected Head of the Department, which was initiated with the assistance of his associates. Among them T. Aivazoglou, T. Dolatzas and M. Soutis continued their training duties in other Units and were later elected Chief Surgeons. Dr Keramidas had served as Associate to N. Voyatzis at Aglaia Kyriakou Children's Hospital during the previous 15 years. He was granted a fellowship with A. Coran in Los Angeles County-University of S. California (1973–1974). His interest in experimental surgery and surgical innovations led to relevant papers with clinical results being published in international journals.

With the inception of paediatric surgery in the curriculum of Patras University in 1997, Keramidas was elected Professor of Paediatric Surgery. He served as President of the Mediterranean Association of Paediatric Surgeons (2000–2002) and President of the Hellenic Surgical Society (2003). It was in his Department that two of his associates, Drs George Geroulanos who had trained at Boston Children's Hospital (1984–1987) and Evangelos Papandreou, initiated the diagnostic-interventional endoscopy (1988) and laparoscopic surgery (1996) respectively on a systematic and routine basis for the first time in Greek paediatric surgery. In 2003, Dr Geroulanos was elected Head of the Department, succeeding D. Keramidas.

Penteli Hospital, established in 1965, is the third Children's Hospital in Athens. The Department of Paediatric Surgery was set up in 1971 with a capacity of 30 beds. Dr Constantine Pappis was appointed Head of the Department. He organised the Department in which he worked until 1985 when he continued his career at Aghia Sophia Children's Hospital as Head of the 1st Department of

Paediatric Surgery till 1992. An active person, Dr Pappis organised meetings with foreign colleagues and it was with his initiative that the Greek Association of Paediatric Surgeons was formed in 1975.

In 1936, the **Karamandaneion Children's Hospital** was established in Patras. However, it was not fully operative until 1946 due to its occupation by the German and Italian armies for quartering purposes during the Second World War. The Department of Paediatric Surgery was established in 1976. Dr George Giannoulopoulos was the first Head of the Department involved in the organisation of the Department. He trained with Dr Tsakayannis at Aghia Sophia Children's Hospital and at Sheffield Children's Hospital with R. B. Zachary (1965–1966). Dr Yannoulopoulos succeeded C. Pappis as Head of the 1st Department of Paediatric Surgery at Aghia Sophia Children's Hospital.

University Departments of Paediatric Surgery

Paediatric surgery was subsequently included in the curriculum of Medical Faculties and relevant University Departments were established beginning in 1961 with Aristotle University of Thessaloniki.

There are 23 Universities in Greece but not all Universities include Medical Schools. There are seven Medical Schools with only four of them having paediatric surgery included in their curriculum. The four Universities in chronological order, are: Aristotle University of Thessaloniki, Macedonia; University of Crete in Heraklion, Crete; Democritus University in Alexandroupolis, Thrace; and University of Patras, Peloponnese. The topic of paediatric surgery is not included in the curriculum of Athens University at present time.

The **Aristotle University of Thessaloniki Department of Paediatric Surgery** was established in 1961 according to the French model of that time, that is paediatric surgery and orthopaedics. It was organised by Prof Basil Petropoulos in G. Gennimatas General Hospital. Among his associates, those who contributed to the teaching of medical students and training of young surgeons in paediatric surgery included: A. Markantonatos, E. Miliaras, G. Tryfonas,

C. Kotsianos, A. Petropoulos, N. Liolios, A. Zavitsanakis, D. Anagnostopoulos, A. Philippopoulos, and D. Kallergis. Following the retirement of Prof B. Petropoulos in 1982, the post was taken up by Prof A. Markantonatos. Orthopaedics was then separated thereby initiating an independent Department.

After Markantonatos' retirement in 1992, the University Department was divided in two Units under the direction of D. Anagnostopoulos and E. Miliaras, both Associate Professors of Paediatric Surgery. The Department of Paediatric Surgery at G. Gennimatas General Hospital has operated as the 1st University Department of Paediatric Surgery since 2005 under the direction of Prof Athanassios Zavitsanakis. The 2nd operative University Department of Paediatric Surgery, at N. Papageorgiou General Hospital, was organised by Prof Anastassios Petropoulos. He was trained in paediatric surgery at Prof Basil Petropoulos' Department and acquired further experience at Sheffield Children's Hospital under a fellowship with R. B. Zachary and L. Spitz (1975–1976). He was elected Professor of Paediatric Surgery in 2002. He showed a specific interest in neonatal surgery and organised a Neonatal Surgical Unit in 1994, now operating at N. Papageorgiou Hospital. In 2007, he edited a two-volume book titled "Neonatal Surgery", the first complete book of its kind to ever be edited in Greek.

The **Department of Paediatric Surgery of Crete University** was established in 1990 and is run at PEPAGNI University General Hospital, in Heraklion, the capital of Crete. It is a 26-bed Unit, serving the population of the largest Greek island and some neighbouring islands. The Department was organised by Prof George Harissis. He studied medicine at Freie Universität-Berlin, and was trained in paediatric surgery in Benjamin Franklin (former Steglitz) Free University of Berlin, under Prof W. J. Waldschmidt. In 1989, he was elected Associate Professor of Paediatric Surgery and Head of the Department of Paediatric Surgery of Crete University. In 2007 he was elected Professor of Paediatric Surgery. He had a special interest in minimally invasive paediatric surgery and organised the first pertinent workshop in Greece.

The **Democritus University in Alexandroupolis**, did not include paediatric surgery in its curriculum. Dr Helen Theocharous, Assistant Professor of Paediatric Surgery, was employed as Consultant Paediatric Surgeon in 1987. She organised paediatric surgery with the assistance of her associates (Drs A. Passalidis, C. Limas, and G. Soultanidis). In 2002 a small University Unit was established and Dr Stephen Gardikis, Assistant Professor of Paediatric Surgery, was assigned the duty of teaching the medical students as well as being responsible for the everyday practice in the Unit until 2007. In that year, Dr George Vaos was elected Professor of Paediatric Surgery. Dr Vaos was trained at Aglaia Kyriakou Children's Hospital and qualified in 1983. From 1983 to 1986 he worked with Prof Lister in Alder Hey Children's Hospital in Liverpool. During the period 2001–2007 he was Head of the Department of Paediatric Surgery in Penteli Children's Hospital. Among his duties at Democritus University are the establishment of the existing Unit as an independent Department and its expansion fulfilling its mission as a teaching and training centre.

The **Patras University** Administration decided in 1997 to create a new Chair of Paediatric Surgery in the Medical School. Dr Dimitris Keramidas was elected Professor of Paediatric Surgery. In 2000, Dr Keramidas resigned in favour of retaining his post of Head of the Department at Aghia Sophia Children's Hospital of Athens. As a result, Dr Christos Salakos was elected Assistant Professor responsible for surgical paediatrics. He was trained in Aglaia Kyriakou Children's Hospital. After qualifying as paediatric surgeon in 1990, he continued in France, in *Hôpital Necker* "*Enfant Malade*" as *Chef de Clinique Associé* with Prof Claire Nihoul–Fékété (1990–1992). He was assigned the post of *Chef de Clinique Assistant* in Tours (1992–1994), and the post of *Assistant a l'Hôpital Universitaire de Lill* (1994–1996). In 2000 he became *practicien Hôspitalier.* Dr Salakos is a general paediatric surgeon with experience in paediatric urology and laparoscopic surgery.

General Hospitals

The Department of Paediatric Surgery at **Hippocrates General Hospital** in Thessaloniki is run as a training centre covering the entire spectrum of paediatric surgery. Several University Units have been established at the same teaching hospital including paediatrics with which the Department is affiliated. It was established in 1978 with Dr Emmanuel Miliaras as Head of the Department. In 1979, Dr George Tryfonas was elected Head of the Department and proceeded to the organisation, which had began with Dr Miliaras. G. Tryfonas was trained at the University of Thessaloniki Department of Paediatric Surgery and qualified in 1967. He enriched his experience working at the Royal Hospital for Sick Children in Glasgow under Professor D. G. Young (1972–1973), at Westminster Children's Hospital in London with Lawson and Forrest, and later at the Royal Liverpool Alder Hey Children's Hospital with J. H. Johnston. Dr Tryfonas, in his capacity as Head of the Department till his retirement in 1997, was responsible for training young paediatric surgeons by imparting his experience in neonatal and paediatric surgery including paediatric urology.

In some hospitals the lack of appropriate material does not allow the application of the entire spectrum of paediatric surgery and international standards are not met for training in paediatric surgery. Hospitals including Paediatric Surgery Departments with the year of their establishment and the names of doctors responsible for their organization are listed below: **Tzaneion General Hospital, Piraeus** (1964, N. Tzemailas), **Aghios Panteleimon General Hospital, Piraeus** (1965, E. Moschakis), **Marika Heliadi Women's & General Hospital, Athens** (1971, P. Hadjihaberis), **Larissa General Hospital** (1986, A. Markou), **Tripolis General Hospital** (1989, G. Giannoulopoulos), **Rhodes General Hospital** (2001, P. Tsitouris).

Finally, consultant paediatric surgeons are employed in private children's or women's and children's hospitals, mainly in Athens and Thessaloniki.

Recognition of Paediatric Surgery as a Speciality and Establishment of the Greek Association of Paediatric Surgeons (GAPS)

Pediatric Surgery was recognised as a speciality by the Greek State in 1958. Requirements include three years training in general surgery followed by three years in paediatric surgery and two six-month periods respectively in urology, and either thoracic surgery, plastic surgery or ENT. After completing seven years training, each trainee participates in examinations conducted by the Speciality Examinations Committee in order to qualify. The Committee is made up of three Members, one Professor of Paediatric Surgery and two Chief Paediatric Surgeons, and is appointed for a 2-year term of office.

GAPS was established in 1976. It is governed by a Board of nine Members elected every two years. Greek paediatric surgeons are regular members of the Association, trainees are initiate members, and physicians of related specialities may become affiliate members. The seal of GAPS depicts Asclepios, the ancient Greek god of medicine and healing. The aim of the Association is the promotion of the speciality and improvement of the standing of paediatric surgeons. Scientific meetings are held throughout the year in various hospitals. Scientific events include the yearly spring meeting in Thessaloniki, and the biannual congresses with international participation. From 1976 till 2007, 27 congresses were organised of which the first 22 are held on an annual basis. Traditionally, an ancient coin representative of the area in which the congress takes place, is used as the congress symbol. The GAPS participates to the *European Journal of Paediatric Surgery* with an Associated Editor and the rest are elected delegates, representing GAPS on the international bodies: UEMS, EUPSA, WOFAPS.

Since 1970, the number of paediatric surgeons has increased almost 8-fold, to 160 members of the GAPS. This number is impressively high for a population of 11 million people having an extremely low birth rate. However the abundance of paediatric surgeons has created employment problems, incurring negative consequences to their scientific standard.

Acknowledgements

Data and valuable information for the writing of this text was provided by, among others, my colleagues in Greek Hospitals and University Departments. I would like to expend my thanks to the following in recognition of their constructive contribution: T. Dolatzas, S. Gardikis, G. Geroulanos, G. Giannoulopoulos, G. Hariss, E. Markou, G. Moussatos, A. Passalidis, A. Petropoulos, G. Salakos, M. Soutis, G. Tryfonas, D. Tsakayannis, P. Tsitouris, G. Vaos and A. Vassilakopoulos.

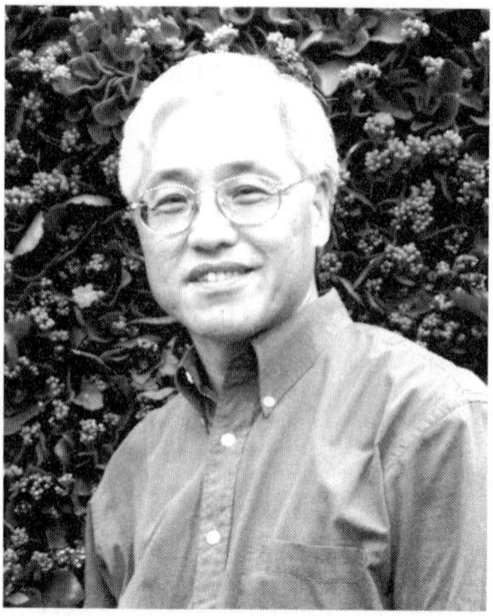

Paul K. H. Tam

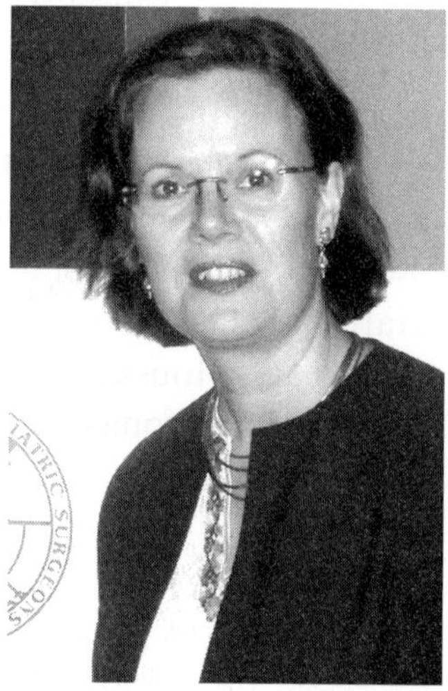

Anette S. Jacobsen

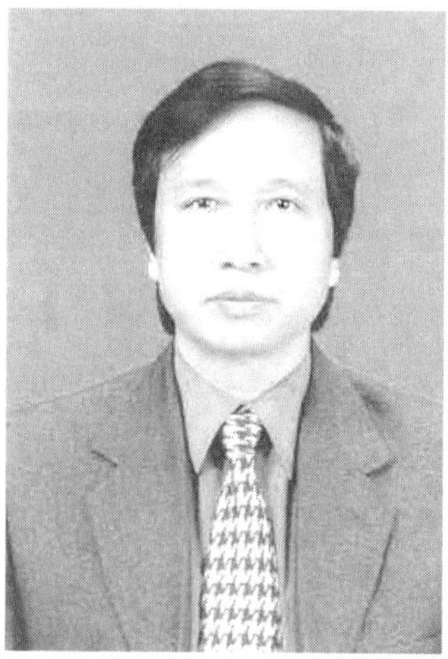

Nguyen Thanh Liem

HONG KONG, SINGAPORE AND VIETNAM

Paul K. H. Tam
Anette S. Jacobsen
Nguyen Thanh Liem

Hong Kong (Paul K. H. Tam)

Pre-specialisation. Paediatric surgery did not exist as a speciality in Hong Kong until 1967. Prior to this, neonates and children with major surgical problems were treated by general surgeons in different local hospitals, and "on the whole the result was uniformly disheartening".[1] Some notable exceptions were the first successful and primary repair of oesophageal atresia by Prof G. B. Ong, the doyen of General Surgery in the region, in 1963 at Kowloon Hospital,[1] and the first choledochal cyst excision in 1955 at Queen Mary Hospital.[2]

The first paediatric surgical centre. The first paediatric surgical unit in Hong Kong was established in 1967 at the Department of Surgery, University of Hong Kong, Queen Mary Hospital by Dr Paul C. K. Yue (Fig. 1) on his return from training in paediatric surgery in the United Kingdom. The unit consisted of a 22-bed children's ward and a eight-bed neonatal surgical unit, which was essentially an intensive care unit. Referrals increased steadily, and the number of neonatal surgical emergencies trebled within eight years; nevertheless, many neonates were still not referred to the new specialist unit.[3] As Reader in Paediatric Surgery at the University of Hong Kong, Dr Yue continued to develop the speciality, gaining both local and international recognition. He became President of Hong Kong

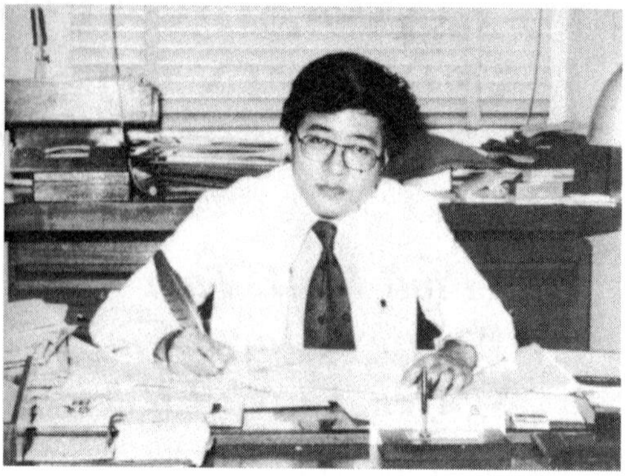

Fig. 1. Dr Paul CK Yue, first dedicated paediatric surgeon in Hong Kong.

Paediatric Society in 1977–1979 and was a founding member of the Asian Association of Paediatric Surgeons. Results of treatment of ***oesophageal atresia*** improved from 10% survival in 1951–1967 before the establishment of the neonatal surgical unit to 45% survival in 1968–1975.[3] In the latter period, overall survival rates neonates with ***intestinal obstruction*** and ***congenital diaphragmatic hernia*** reached 80% and 70% respectively. Complex procedures were increasingly performed, e.g. a series of 18 cases of ***choledochal cyst*** was reported in *British Journal of Surgery* in 1974 including ten cases of choledochal cyst excision without mortality.[2] The first Kasai operation for biliary atresia was introduced in 1975.[4] In 1978, Dr Yue left public service to become the first full-time paediatric surgeon in private practice. As health care in Hong Kong is primarily publicly funded, further development of paediatric surgery continued in the public hospitals.

In 1979, Dr H. Saing (Fig. 2), a paediatric surgeon from Rangoon, Burma, with training in the United Kingdom, was recruited to head the expanding Division of Paediatric Surgery at the University of Hong Kong, Queen Mary Hospital.[5] The unit was supported by two specialist surgeons, Dr James T. K. Lau and Dr K. C. Wong who had training in Australia and United Kingdom respectively. A training programme in paediatric surgery was established. The first trainee was Dr P. K. H. Tam (1980–1983), followed

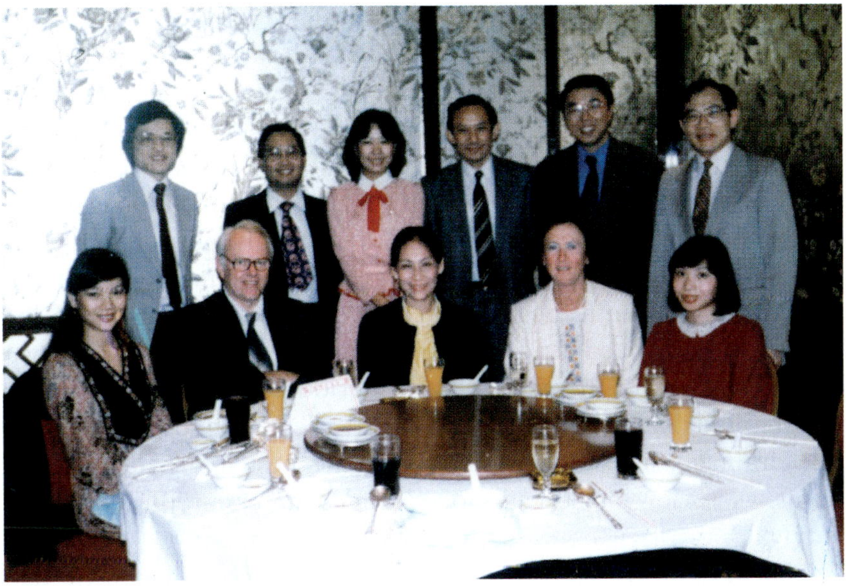

Fig. 2. Prof H Saing, first Chair of Paediatric Surgery in Hong Kong (third right, back), Dr James TK Lau (second left, back), Prof Paul KH Tam (first left, back) during a visit to Hong Kong by Prof James Lister (second left, front) in 1982.

by Dr C. K. Yeung (1986–1989), both of whom would later become Professors of Paediatric Surgery at the University of Hong Kong and the Chinese University of Hong Kong respectively and achieved international reputations in the field.

During this period, major improvements were made to equip the unit with modern facilities and 50 beds were added to the Division at the Duchess of Kent Children's Hospital nearby for simple elective surgery, and to provide convalescence cover for patients from the overcrowded unit at Queen Mary Hospital. In 1982, Prof James Lister, Prof of Paediatric Surgery, University of Liverpool was invited by the Committee for International Cooperation in Higher Education (CICHE) to advise on the academic development of paediatric surgery at Queen Mary Hospital. His report was enthusiastic and provided a blueprint for the expansion of the Queen Mary Unit into a regional centre of excellence, modelled after the regional/supraregional paediatric surgical units in the U.K. Emphasis on development of teaching both at undergraduate and postgraduate levels, and research was made alongside service improvements.

Surgery of increasing complexities was introduced. From 1980–1984, three pairs of ***conjoined twins*** (two omphalophagus; one thoracopagus) were separated and different clinical problems were overcome by a team approach with individualised management.[6]

The HKU Centre began to develop advancing expertise in the management of paediatric hepatobiliary conditions which are prevalent in this part of the world. In this period, 39 infants with ***biliary atersia*** had Kasai's portoenterostomy,[7] achieving 69% extended bile drainage, a result comparable to the best international standards. A review of 60 cases of ***choledochal cyst*** reported 91.4% survival.[8]

Paediatric GI endoscopy was introduced for diagnostic and therapeutic use in 1975, and the HKU Centre accumulated extensive experience in the procedure in this period reporting some 500 cases of upper GI endoscopy[9] and 65 cases of colonoscopy.[10] This would lay down the foundation for the development of paediatric endosurgery in later years.

Paediatric Urology was developed within the paediatric surgical unit. Results of paediatric pyelopasty[11] and new techniques in hypospadias surgery[12] were published in international journals, reflecting the rapid development of this sub-speciality in Hong Kong.

In 1980, plans were made to improve paediatric surgery services by constructing purpose-built facilities in a new children's block (K-Block) at Queen Mary Hospital. Re-location in 1990 resulted in a modern, well-equipped paediatric surgical unit.

A highly successful ***paediatric liver transplant*** programme was established in 1993 at QMH, led by Professor S. T. Fan, a world-renowned liver transplant surgeon, working closely with the paediatric surgical team.[13] While in early years, another liver transplant programme was developed at Prince of Wales Hospital, this was discontinued in 2003, and since then liver transplantation is undertaken only at the HKU-QMH Unit. Up to now, some 80 children have received liver transplants at HKU-QMH, the majority being living-related donor liver transplants, with 90% survival.

In 1996, Professor Paul K. H. Tam returned from the United Kingdom to succeed Prof H. Saing as Division Chief. The HKU-Queen Mary Hospital Centre has since then become increasingly recognised internationally for the excellence in research in addition to its high clinical standard. A state-of-the-art paediatric surgical laboratory staffed by surgeon-scientists (MD-PhDs) and full-time basic scientists was established for cutting edge research in ***genetic, genomics, stem cells, cancer biology and immunology.*** Examples of seminal contribution relevant to paediatric surgery include genetic dissection of Hirschsprung's disease[14] and other congenital anomalies. ***Minimal invasive surgery*** was introduced in 1990s and both HKU-Queen Mary Hospital and Prince of Wales Hospital (see below) have been at the forefront of development of the new technique. At HKU, Queen Mary Hospitals, most major paediatric surgical procedures are now performed laparoscopically/ thoracoscopically.[15] The HKU Centre had also been developing ***evidence-based surgery***, and reported the first prospective randomised control trial on laparoscopic repair of inguinal hernia.[16]

Expansion of speciality. In the 1980s, the number of specialist surgeons and hospitals providing paediatric surgical services increased. In 1984, the second paediatric surgical unit in Hong Kong was established at the Chinese University of Hong Kong, Prince of Wales Hospital (PWH) with Dr David W. K. Man as the first unit chief (1984–1988), followed by Dr Kelvin K. W. Liu (1988–1995), Prof C. K. Yeung (1995–2006) and Dr K. H. Lee (2006–present). Lack of central coordination and regulation initially resulted in paediatric surgery being carried out in most hospitals with acute paediatric services. A growing recognition that a high standard of care can only be achieved through concentration of cases and expertise resulted in a reorganisation of referral system in the public funded hospitals in 1999 and Queen Mary Hospital, Prince of Wales Hospital and Queen Elizabeth Hospital were designated as the only centres for major paediatric surgery.

Paediatric surgery became formally recognised as one of six surgical specialities at the College of Surgeons of Hong Kong and the Board of Paediatric Surgery was established in 1993. Prof H. Saing, Prof C. K. Yeung and Dr Kelvin Liu were successively elected Chairman of the Board. Training programmes, first established at Queen Mary Hospital (HKU Centre), were later developed at PWH, and in 1997 also at Queen Elizabeth Hospital. The first Exit Examination was held jointly by the College of Surgeons of Hong Kong and Royal College of Surgeons of Edinburgh in 1997.

Relationship with mainland and rest of the world. With Hong Kong's return of sovereignty to China under the "one-country, two-system" concept in 1997, Hong Kong while remaining autonomous, has developed closer with Mainland China. At HKU-Queen Mary Hospital, a train-the-trainers programme was established and in the past decades 17 surgeons from Mainland (including Beijing, Shanghai, Shenyang) have undergone training, many returning to take up positions of chief sub-speciality.

As a global city, Hong Kong has an international perspective. Hong Kong has hosted many international paediatric surgical meetings, including Congress of Pacific Association of Pediatric Surgeons, Asian Association of Paediatric Surgeons, etc. Examples of leadership include appointments as Presidents of Pacific Association of Pediatric Surgeons (Prof H. Saing in 1997, Prof P. Tam in 2008), Asian Association of Paediatric Surgeons (Prof H. Saing in 1996), International Paediatric Endosurgery Society (Prof C. K. Yeung in 2003).

Singapore (Dr Anette Jacobsen)

In Singapore, surgery in children was in the hands of general surgeons until very recently. In the 1950's and 1960's Prof Yeoh Ghim Seng and Dr Yahya Cohen headed 'A' and 'B' units respectively in the Singapore General Hospital. One of the early enthusiasts for a separate Paediatric Surgical Unit, Dr Christopher Thevatasen, was told by his boss that this request would only be allowed over his (the boss') dead body.[17] In 1974 Dr V. T. Joseph and Dr Chua W. H. became the first two trained paediatric surgeons. Still, Singapore had to wait until 1981 with the opening of the new General Hospital for a separate Paediatric Surgical Department headed by A/Prof V. T. Joseph.[18] Since 1997 this unit had been relocated to a dedicated children's hospital. Recently the Paediatric Surgical service at the National University Hospital has also developed into a separate Department of Pediatric Surgery.

The advanced training programme with the recognition of Pediatric Surgery as a separate speciality was started in the late 1980's. Currently the programme has four AST's in training, and the programme is a competency-based 3–4 year programme. As Singapore has only a population of 4 million, the incidence of some rare but (for paediatric surgeons) important clinical cases will be few and far between. Thus surgeons in training are encouraged to spend some time abroad to see a wider spectrum of clinical cases and their management. Sub-specialisation at consultant level in-line with what is practiced in the UK, Australia and the US was being developed.

The specialty has developed hand-in-hand with paediatric anaesthesia, neonatal and paediatric intensive care, allowing safe performance of life-saving surgery on babies as small as 5–600 g. Miniaturisation of instruments and supplies has gone hand-in-hand with the use of operating loupes and microscopes. Minimally invasive techniques are gaining ground and the number of procedures now done via a MIS approach are increasing by the day. Surgical conditions are in general diagnosed earlier, and definitive treatment is carried out as early as possible, e.g. the neonatal diagnosis of Hirschsprung's disease with neonatal laparoscopically assisted endorectal pullthrough.

In the late 1990's MIS was started, initially with viewing only and mainly for undescended testicles. In 1997 with the move to KK Hospital, the gynaecology colleagues encouraged the paediatric surgeons to venture into a broader range of MIS procedures. Dr Jacobsen started doing laparoscopic appendectomies in 1997.

Fundoplications followed in 1999, and splenectomies for hypersplenism in 2002. Now all the Registrars are trained in MIS and there is an established accreditation cum training programme.

Since 1992 the Postgraduate Medical School in Singapore has been overseeing paediatric surgical specialist training. Currently the programme is a four-year programme started on completion of the surgical MMED/MRCS III exam. The training duration is four years with one year spent overseas. The plan is to move to a competency-based seamless training programme as currently (as in many other countries) the training programme is seen as too long.

Vietnam (Prof Nguyen Thanh Liem)

Vietnam is a country in South-East Asia with an area of 330,000 km^2, a population is 84,16 million people (2006), of which 30% are children under 15 years old.

Since the first paediatric surgical departments were founded in 1957 there are now 13 departments throughout country, with over 100 professional paediatric surgeons.

Many new surgical techniques have been applied to improve the health care quality and reduce the mortality rate.

Hirschsprung's disease: Swenson, Duhamel, Soave, Rehbein

Modified posterior sagittal: 1998[19]
Transanal approach: 2002
No more mortality rate

Imperforate anus

Modified posterior sagittal approach: 1987
One stage modified PSAP in newborn: 1998

Esophageal atresia

First survivor: 1987
Present survivor rate: >90%
Transhiatal esophagoplasty for colon: 1998

Intestinal atresia:

Before 1994: mortality rate 55%
Current mortality rate: 2–5%

Choledochal cyst

First international publication: 1963
Cystectomy and Roux-en-Y: 1975
Cystectomy and replace the choledoque by an isolate intestinal segment and antireflux valve: 1997
Laparoscopic hepatico-jejunostomy: 2006
Laparoscopic cystectomy and hepatico-duodenostomy: 2007

Hypospadias

One stage Duckett procedure: 1987
Longitudinal flap: 1994
Onlay flap: 1994
Snoodgrass: 1999[20]

Fistula rate: 8%

Neurologic Bladder
Mitrofanoff: 1997
Bladder Augmentation with ureter: 1999

First laparoscopic operation: 1997

2006: Laparoscopic and thoracoscopic surgery carried out in 4 hospitals with over 1000 operations
Indications: 30 different diseases

Kidney transplantation (KT)

First Kt: 2004
Till 2007:11 KT in two hospitals

Liver transplantation (LT)

First LT: 2004
Till 2007: 9 LT in three hospitals

References

1. Yue PCK. Oesophageal atresia. *B Hong Kong Chinese Med Assoc* 1969;21:61–69.
2. Yue PCK. Choledochal cyst: a review of 18 cases. *Br J Surg* 1974; 61:896–900.
3. Yue PCK. *Paediatric Surgery — Its Development, Achievement and Role in the Delivery of Medical Care.* Elixir, 1976, p. 61–69.
4. Lau JTK, Ong GB. Biliary atresia before and after the introduction of the Kasai-type procedure. *Aust NZJ Surg* 1983;53:129–131.
5. Saing H. Paediatric surgery in Hong Kong: its birth, development and coming of age. In: *Hong Kong Paedaitric Society, the First 35 Years*, 1997, pp. 223–229.
6. Saing H, Mok CK, Tam PKH, Wong J. Problems in the surgery of conjoined twins. *Surg Rounds* 1987;81–94.
7. Saing H, Tam PKH. Biliary atresia: the Hong Kong experience. In: Ohi R (ed.) *Biliary Atresia.* Professional Postgraduate Services, Tokyo, Japan, 1987; pp. 141–144.
8. Saing H, Tam PKH, Lee JMH, Pe-Nyun. Surgical management of choledochal cysts: a review of 60 cases. *J Pediatr Surg* 1985; 20(4): 443–448.
9. Tam PKH, Saing H. Pediatric upper gastrointestinal endoscopy: a 13-year experience. *J Pediatr Surg* 1989;24(5):443–447.
10. Tam PKH, Saing H. Pediatric surgeons can and should perform colonoscopy. 1987;22(4):332–334.
11. Saing H, Chan FL, Yeung CK, Yeung DWC. Pediatric pyeloplasty: 50 patients with 59 hydronephrotic kidneys. *J Pediatr Surg* 1989;24(4): 346–349.
12. Lau JTK, Saing H, Tam PKH, Ong GB. Interposing fascial pedicle flap for the repair of urethral fistulae after hypospadias surgery. *Plast Reconstr Surg* 1982;70(2):206–208.
13. Saing H, Fan ST, Tam PKH, *et al.* Surgical complications and outcome of pediatric liver transplantation in Hong Kong. *J Pediat Surg* 2002;37(12):1673–1677.
14. Tam PKH, Garcia–Barcelo MM. Molecular genetics of Hirschsprung's disease. *Semin Pediatr Surg* 2004;13(4):236–248.

15. Wong KKY, Tam PKH. Recent advances in minimal access surgery for infants and children. *Curr Pediatr Reviews* 2006;2(2):177–186.
16. Chan KL, Hui TWC, Tam PKH. Prospective randomized, single-centre, single-blind comparison of laparoscopic versus open repair of pediatric inguinal hernia. *Surg Endoscopy* 2005;19:927–932.
17. Personal communication by Dr Thevatasen via Dr Earl Lu to author.
18. Tan, Bala, Nambiar (eds.), *Surgery and Surgeons in Singapore, a retrospective from 1819*, Academy of Medicine, Singapore, 1996.
19. Modified Soave procedure through the posterior sagittal approach for Hirschsprung's disease. *J Pediatr Surg* 2005;40(3):547–550.
20. Tubularized longitudinal island flap of the mucosa and skin on the dorsum of the penis in the treatment of hypospadias: Experience from 176 cases. *Asian J Surgery* 2006;29(3):185–187.

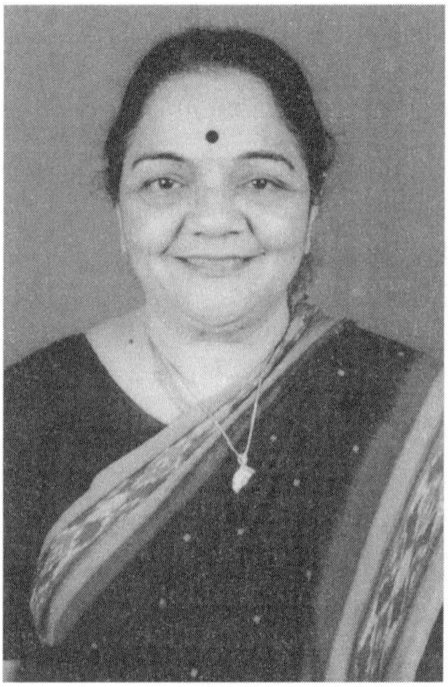

Snehalata S. Deshmukh

INDIA

Snehalata S. Deshmukh

In a country of the size of India, development of any specialty should be multicentric and necessitates coverage cross country.

Pediatric surgery in India had a very humble beginning and had to undergo trials and tribulations. It is a saga of sustained efforts by few committed, devoted and dedicated general surgeons. Human mind always resents a change. Similarly when the general surgeons, who were keenly interested in salvaging the neonates, the infants and the toddlers, got together; they faced tremendous resistance. After the initial resistance time was attenuation of the resistance and a growing appreciation of the results.

From **1963 till 1973** was a "period of establishment and recognition"of the specialty. From 1963 for about 10 years, there was a group whose sustained efforts in the children's hospital are to be appreciated. There were hardly five hospitals fully devoted to children. Most of the work was being done in general hospitals, in this period. There were four surgical teachers who were general surgeons, but who devoted time to pediatric surgery. They were Dr U. C. Chakrawarty at Calcutta Medical College, Dr Raman Nair at Trivendrum, Dr Anjanyela at Nilofer hospital Hyderabad and Dr Arthur Desa at Bombay. Dr Arthur Desa was attached to the children's hospital in Bombay and he really fostered pediatric surgery. Another person was Col R. Dr Ayyer at New Delhi. He actually managed to set up a department of pediatric surgery in the medical college.

In the early 1960's, some young surgeons returned to India after receiving training in pediatric surgery abroad. The initial activity was concentrated in Madras at the Government Medical College by Dr M. S. Ramakrishnan, in Bombay by Dr R. K. Gandhi and Dr S. S. Deshmukh, by Dr T. Dorairaian in Madurai, by Dr P. Upadhyaya in Delhi, Dr I. C. Pathak at P. G. I. Chandigarh, Dr K. C. Sogani at Jaipur and Dr Subir Chaterjee at Calcutta, Dr Meerabai at Hydrabad, Dr Singhal at Varanasi, Dr Taliat and K. K. Verma at Calicut followed suit.

There were sarcastic remarks by surgeons stating "what is so special about operating on a child" as to make a specialty. The child is just a miniature adult. Little did they realize that these tiny tots have to be handled carefully, monitored meticulously and required the tender loving care. The main attributes required to establish this age-based specialty were Patience, Perseverance and Pragmatism. Any one who reacted violently had a set-back.

The Pediatric Surgery Section of Association of Surgeons of India was born in 1964 and a postgraduate degree in pediatric surgery (MCH) was started in 1966 at Madras. It was during the Silver Jubilee conference of Association of Surgeons of India at Bombay in 1969 that surgeons who included only those devoting their work exclusively to pediatric surgery formed an association.

Though some people thought that such a move was premature, with strong support by Dr. Arthur Desa and Prof. P. K. Sen, the move to start pediatric surgical section was passed during the meeting. Dr. A. Venugopal, the President of the Association of Surgeons and Dr B. N. Sinha who was the President of Medical Council of India were also staunch supporters.

The Pediatric Surgical Association had an impact as it gave the opportunity for the pediatric surgeons to come together and work together. It also helped in persuading the universities to institute a postgraduate program. This Association was a national forum and hence could collaborate academically with international associations.

A main achievement was in 1972 when seven full fledged pediatric surgery postgraduate departments imparting teaching and training in pediatric surgery were started and there were also 15 service centres. The seven postgraduate departments were Madras Medical

College Madras, G. S. Medical College of Bombay, Madurai Medical College Madurai, All India Institute of Medical Sciences New Delhi, Post Graduate Institute Chandigarh and Medical College Trivendrum.

The "period of consolidation" as I would call it was **from 1973 to 1983**. During this period, many pediatric surgical centers were started. Many pediatric surgeons occupied the prestigious posts such as the chair of President of Association of Surgeons. Dr R. K. Gandhi, Dr Ramakrishna, and Dr Dorairajan were the Presidents in 1979, 1980 and 1981 respectively. Well over nine years later Dr S. S. Deshmukh was elected as a President of this august body. It is noteworthy that many pediatric surgeons also took part in the pediatric medical association, the Indian Academy of Pediatrics. They also participated in the academic affairs of National Academy of Medical Sciences, a prestigious body with the objective of promoting the growth of medical sciences.

During the international Pediatric Surgical Congress at Melbourne the delegates from the Asian countries had an informal meeting and decided to initiate the process of starting an Asian Association of Pediatric Surgery. Dr K. Suruga took the lead and the Asian pediatric surgeons met at Tokyo and elected office bearers. Two crucial offices were secured by two Indian pediatric surgeons Dr M. S. Ramakrishnan and Dr R. K. Gandhi.

The World Federation of Pediatric Surgeons was hosted in India in 1980. The World Federation elected a pediatric surgeon from India as the President.

From 1983 pediatric surgery was established firmly and was recognized as a specialty. A number of trainees obtained adequate experience and started departments in other states, like Andra Pradesh, Tamil Nadu, Kerala, Karnataka etc. Some of these achievements were:

In **Mumbai** from a very humble beginning, a fully fledged Department of Pediatric Surgery including a separate operating theatre and a pediatric surgical I.C.U. was started at G. S. Medical College. The Department worked in cooperation with others and organized the Asian Congress of Pediatric surgery. JJ Hospital, Bombay started the teaching department.

In **Calcutta**, Dr U. G. Chakrawarty and Dr Subir Chaterjee started a full unit.

(This is a dream city designed by a French architect). In the post-graduate institute at Chandigarh, Dr I. C. Pathak who was trained at Great Ormond Street in the UK came back in 1962 and started the department.

In **Delhi** 1963, Dr Purshottam Upadhyaya started the department with eight surgical beds. He was awarded a WHO fellowship and was then trained in pediatric surgery. He worked at Toronto and on return, devoted himself to pediatric surgery. At present this is a department at All India Institute of medical sciences which is known for their contribution in research headed by Professor D. Gupta.

Jaipur followed suit and in 1968 all pediatric surgical patients were admitted under Dr K. C. Sogani. He had taken training at Boston Children's Hospital and at Liverpool in the Alder Hey hospital.

In the South M.C.H. degree course started in 1966 the first one of its kind. A lion share of work goes to Dr M. S. Ramakrishna at **Madras**.

Hyderabad is the city with rich heritage which houses Salarjung museum. Dr Anjanayela, Dr Meerabai and T. V. M. Murty are the pioneers.

Madurai is a popular place for pilgrimage. Dr T. Dorairaian returned from Australia and started with ten pediatric surgical beds at Madurai and then shifted to Madras. The Madurai department was taken over by T. Subramaniam.

Trivendrum is the capital of Kerala. Kerala has the lowest infant mortality in India. Dr Raman Nair started the department at S. A. T. hospital and started MCH programme in 1971.

Varanasi is a city of temples and houses the most ancient university. It has an Institute of Medical Sciences. In 1965 Dr G. D. Singhal started pediatric surgery with 25 beds; he was trained in the U.K.

Vellore has a very reputed medical centre. Dr K E Mammen started the department in 1970 with a bed strength of five which was augmented to 25 and the department was recognized in 1977.

In **Vishakhapatnam** 1961, Dr S. S. Reddy was placed in charge. The department was started in 1978.

Most of the departments of pediatric surgery have started in medical colleges and hospitals attached to them. There are very few Institutes of child health which I feel is the need of the day.

The **Indian Association of Pediatric Surgeons** have over 800 members enrolled. However there are about 2000 surgeons practicing pediatric surgery in India.

The recognized training centres produce 40 pediatric surgeons per year. The concept of sub-specialization in super speciality is now gaining ground and there are pediatric urologists, pediatric oncosurgeons, and pediatric neurosurgeons. However fetal surgery has still to gain ground as has transplant surgery. Advanced facilities are being created and learning as well as research centres are on the way.

In near future we need to concentrate on the preventive aspect. We have a past full of patience and pragmatism, and we will certainly have a future when we will have the knowledge of 21st century and wisdom of the past.

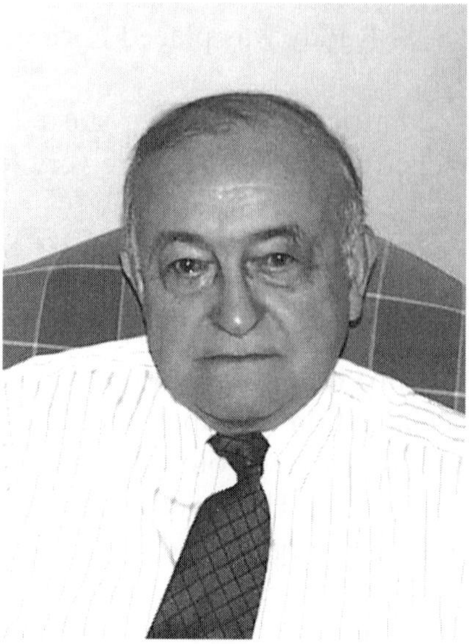

Edward J. Guiney

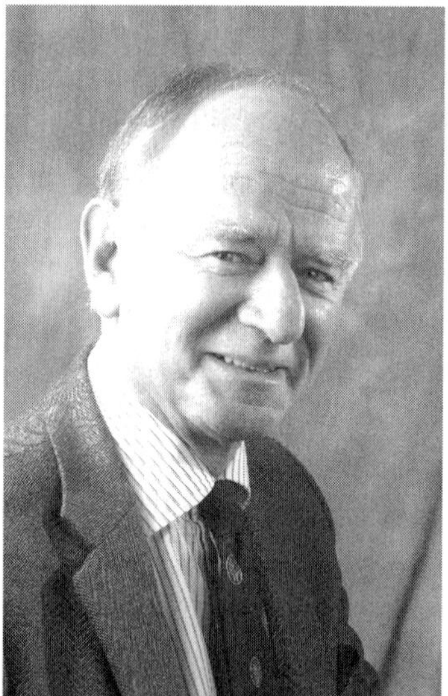

Ray Fitzgerald

IRELAND:
Southern Ireland

Republic of Ireland

Edward J. Guiney
Ray Fitzgerald

Dublin in the early 19th century had, like many other capital cities, a sharp contrast between rich and poor. It was, however, one of the first capitals in Europe to open a children's hospital. In 1821, a group of doctors and business men founded an establishment on the southside of the River Liffey which moved once or twice before eventually locating in Harcourt Street. It became the National Children's Hospital (NCH).[1] It was followed fifty years later in 1872 when a group of philanthropic women recognised the need for the care of children in the teeming tenements of crumbling northside Georgian Dublin. This started, in the capable hands of the Irish Sisters of Charity, in Buckingham Street as St. Joseph's but finally settled in Temple Street and now is known as the Children's University Hospital (CUH), but is still referred to colloquially as "Temple Street". Thus, Ireland's capital, by the turn of the century, had two hospitals, the role of which was solely focussed on the care of infants and children.

Ireland, an island nation of 32 counties, was, in 1922, divided into two political jurisdictions; six northern counties, known as Northern Ireland which has remained British, and 26 southern counties. This new political entity subsequently was recognised as the Republic of Ireland.

In the year following this political change John Shanley[2] was appointed to the children's hospital in Temple Street. He was an unsung pioneer of European paediatric surgery, devoting his considerable skills exclusively to the childhood age group. As was customary then, he treated all conditions, benefiting from major breakthroughs in medicine such as anaesthesia and antibiotics. He was an honorary member of the Scottish Surgical Paediatric Club, created in 1948, and was a founder member of the Irish Red Cross.[2] At the 1969 British Association of Paediatric Surgeons' Congress in Dublin he was made an honorary life member, in recognition of his then unique contribution.[3]

During the following thirty years there were huge worldwide advances. The realisation that up to 2% of all children born alive have a life-threatening congenital abnormality, many of which are amenable to correction, gave an irresistible impetus to the development of neonatal surgery with intensive care.

Around the country there were many hospitals where well-trained general surgeons with an interest in the problems of childhood provided neonatal and paediatric surgery. Temple Street itself was catered for by three general surgeons, James O'Neill, Kevin Maughan and Frank Duff, the latter particularly interested in urological and neonatal problems. Harcourt Street was covered by several surgeons, notably Stanley McCollum (Fig. 1) but also including the Professor of Surgery in Trinity College, Jack Henry. Indeed, Stanley McCollum carried out surgery at the famous maternity hospital, the Rotunda, in a neonatal operating theatre. It opened in 1956 with a trained theatre nurse in charge.[4] Paediatric surgery continued at the Rotunda until the early 1970's.

In 1956 a new institution, Our Lady's Hospital for Sick Children, (OLH) was opened on the edge of Dublin, in the western suburb of Crumlin, well-placed to serve most of rural Ireland. It was the brain-child of the then Roman Catholic Archbishop of Dublin, Dr John Charles McQuaid having been planned since the 1930s and was managed by the Daughters of Charity of St. Vincent de Paul. This was a large, well-equipped and staffed hospital with a full-time, fully-trained paediatric surgeon in the person of Barry O'Donnell

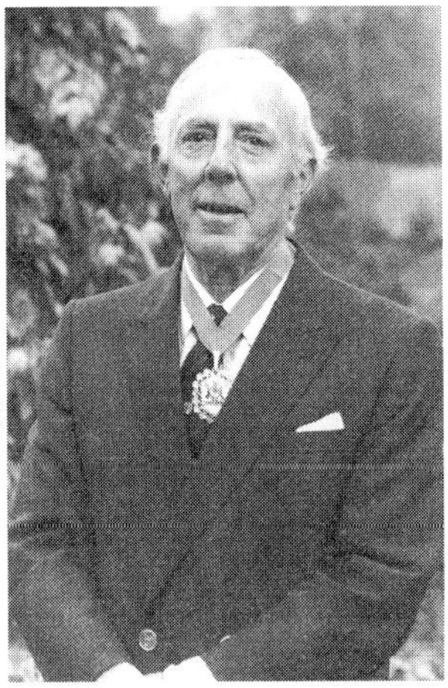

Fig. 1. Stanley McCollum.

(Fig. 2), supported by A. B. Cleary (a general surgeon). The three hospitals (NCH, CUH and OLH) continued to thrive, each with an independent academic affiliation, as Dublin was also in the unusual position, for a small city, of having three medical schools. The NCH undertook undergraduate and postgraduate teaching and training for Trinity College, Dublin University while CUH and OLH looked after students from the Royal College of Surgeons and University College, Dublin. The paediatric surgical staff was augmented in 1966 when Eddie Guiney (Fig. 2) was appointed to Our Lady's and shortly afterwards to Temple Street. In 1971, he also joined Stanley McCollum in the National Children's.

At that time the recommendation of the British Association of Paediatric Surgeons (BAPS) was that there should be one paediatric surgeon to 500,000 of population. (In 2008, the recommended BAPS figure is 1:250,000.) Because of its geographical and demographical status on an island nation thinly inhabited by a dispersed population of just over 4 million, these recommendations were not strictly applicable to the Republic.

With the appointment of Ray Fitzgerald in 1979, Prem Puri in 1991 and Martin Corbally in 1993 (Fig. 2), there were then four consultant paediatric surgeons in total who consequently had to spread

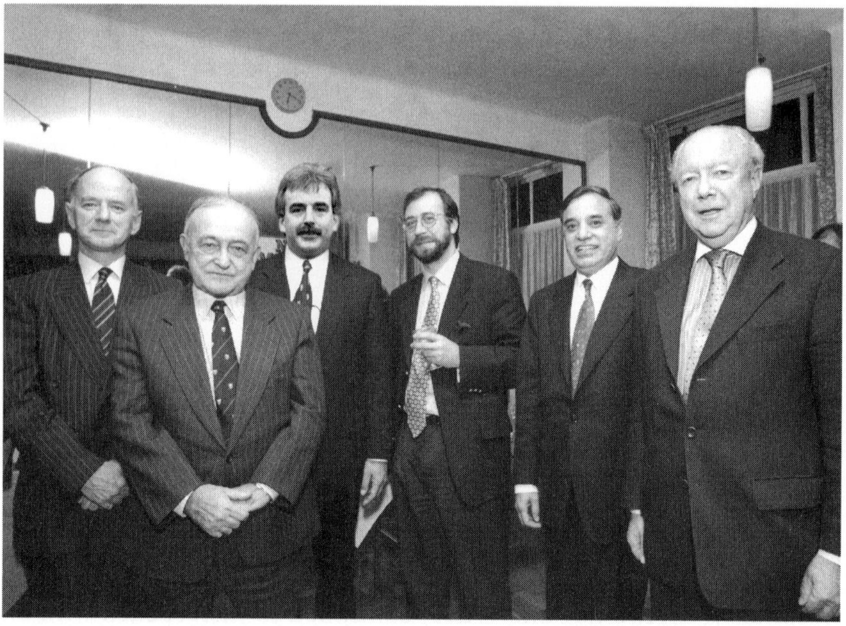

Fig. 2. Irish Group: Ray Fitzgerald, Eddie Guiney, Feargal Quinn, Martin Corbally, Prem Puri, and Barry O'Donnell.

themselves very thinly to cover the huge workload in all three units. Barry O'Donnell had retired in 1991.

Following Eddie Guiney's retirement in 1996, because of disagreement about the structure of his replacement, an unsatisfactory eight-year *locum* period ensued. The impasse was partially resolved by the full-time appointment of Feargal Quinn (Fig. 2) to OLH and the subsequent one of Sami Awadalla to CUH and NCH, following the retirement of Fitzgerald in 2005. This appointment brought the complement of trained paediatric surgeons in the Republic to five, one of which is a *locum*, well below the accepted norm. Both of these last appointments were made without Governmental approval.

In April 2004 the population was stated to be 4.04 million, which, based on the old recommendation, should suggest a quota of eight to nine surgeons. It can be predicted that in the Republic there will be approximately 100 neonates with major general paediatric surgical anomalies presenting in any given year (excluding, for example, cardiac). The challenge is how should these be shared between paediatric surgeons, in order to give them and the anaesthetic and nursing staff the chance to practice their skills. For a children's hospital, the ability to provide neonatal surgery to the community is a status symbol, reflecting necessarily the high quality service to be found in that institution. Furthermore, because a significant number of neonatal surgical anomalies have ongoing problems e.g. hydrocephalus and spina bifida or bladder extrophy which need attention during the whole of childhood, there is an ongoing service requirement from many departments, e.g. Radiology, which has a beneficial influence of service in the institution. Hospitals compete to acquire and treat these patients. Unfortunately, this has worked against progress in Dublin as it has proved very difficult to amalgamate services for the benefit of all. The failure in the 1980s, for sectarian reasons, to amalgamate the NCH and OLH on the site in Crumlin was a great disappointment. The former hospital eventually joined with two small hospitals, the Meath and the Adelaide, on a green field site in Tallaght, a western suburb in Co. Dublin. The political and social climate in Ireland having now changed, and with repeated recommendations for the centralisation of resources, a Government decision was made in 2006 to rationalise all three children's hospitals on the site of a major general hospital in north central Dublin (The Mater Misericordiae). There are grave reservations, however, about the choice of site and controversy will probably continue for some years.

Considering the few surgeons involved in providing a service over the years, many honours have been bestowed upon them. Barry O'Donnell was an international figure, both as a surgeon and raconteur. He achieved the unique honour of being made President of the three Medical Associations, British, Canadian and Irish simultaneously and he was the first full-time paediatric surgeon to become President of The Royal College of Surgeons in Ireland. He, Eddie Guiney and Ray Fitzgerald were, in turn, President of the British Association of Paediatric Surgeons. Eddie Guiney and Ray Fitzgerald have both been elected as President of the Society for Research into Hydrocephalus and Spina Bifida and of the Irish

Paediatric Association. Ray Fitzgerald was also President of the European Union of Paediatric Surgical Associations (EUPSA) and of IPSO, the International Society of Paediatric Surgical Oncology. Prem Puri is currently President of the World Federation of Associations of Paediatric Surgery.

Parallel to the growth of services in Our Lady's Hospital was the development of the Children's Research Centre on its campus. It was founded in 1971 and was totally funded from corporate and private donations.[5] The success of this establishment has been immense. It has worked in conjunction with the Faculty of Medicine in University College, Dublin where a statutory chair of Paediatric Research was founded, funded by the Research Centre. Eddie Guiney was appointed to this chair and as Director of the Research Centre in 1976. He was replaced by Prem Puri as Director. In the three decades of its existence, the quality of the research emanating from the Centre is relected in the numerous presentations and publications, relating to neonatal/paediatric immunology, oncology, medicine and surgery.

Probably the most significant contribution relating to paediatric surgery was that of the "Sting" procedure — the peri-ureteric injection of Teflon from inside the bladder. The original concept for this came from Barry O'Donnell, while Prem Puri worked out the practicalities of its clinical application. The importance of this work is reflected in the change it brought about worldwide in the management of the common paediatric urological condition of vesico-ureteric reflux, precluding the need for invasive surgery. For this work Professors O'Donnell and Puri were jointly presented with a "People of the Year" Award. They have both been recipients of the Denis Browne Medal (BAPS).

The Society of Irish Paediatric Surgeons (SIPS) was founded in 1985 in an endeavour to encourage cross-border co-operation and fellowship at a time of political upheaval. It also established a platform for young trainees north and south to present research and clinical papers in a friendly atmosphere and provides a forum for election of representatives to the European Union of Medical Specialists. It has had combined meetings with the Scottish Society of Paediatric Surgeons. Nevertheless, since its inception, Irish members have continued to be included in the Council of BAPS.

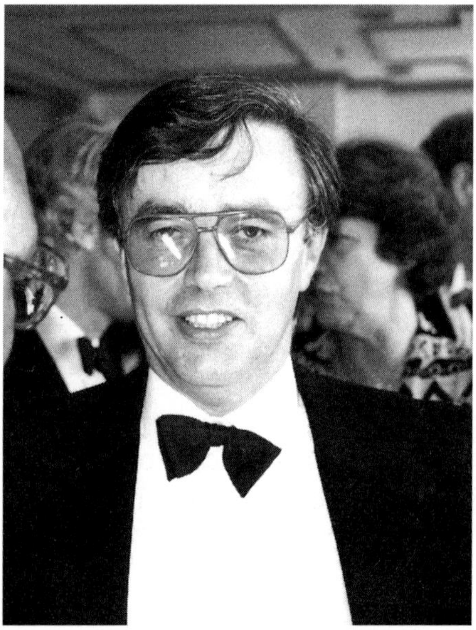

Victor E. Boston

IRELAND: Northern Ireland

Republic of Ireland

Victor E. Boston

Until 1959, the surgery of childhood in the province was undertaken by both general and specialist surgeons whose sessional commitment was to both adults and children. Prior to this time, there were no surgeons whose training was entirely dedicated to paediatrics. Outside Belfast, the capital of the province, all district general hospitals (DGH's) had paediatric wards where non-specialist surgical problems were treated. Specialist surgical conditions at that time were sometimes treated in these hospitals but usually these would be transferred to one of the three units in Belfast where more expertise existed for their safe treatment. In the capital, in and around the 1950's and 60's, children were treated in the Royal Belfast Hospital for Sick Children (RBHSC), the Ulster Hospital Dundonald (UHD) and the Belfast City Hospital (BCH). All three sites provided dedicated facilities for the medical and surgical treatment of children. At the Children's Hospital this was a free standing building on the site of the much larger Royal Victoria Hospital (RVH) in which most of the specialist surgical and medical services for Northern Ireland were concentrated. In the other two hospitals, the paediatric wards were part of the hospital as a whole, which is much the same arrangement as the other DGH's in Northern Ireland.

The speciality of Paediatric Surgery came into existence in Belfast due largely to the efforts of the late Sir Ian Frazer (Fig. 3),

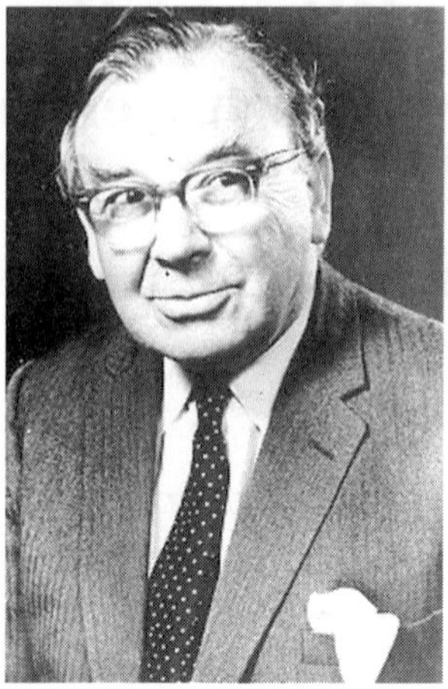

Fig. 3. Sir Ian Fraser.

past President of the Royal College of Surgeons in Ireland and the British Medical Association (BMA) and founder member of the British Association of Paediatric Surgeons (BAPS). Sir Ian, who was appointed to the staff of RBHSC and the RVH in 1927, had the foresight to understand the importance of specialist training in paediatric surgery as the way to achieve better outcomes. In 1952 the junior surgical staff rotated through the Children's Hospital as part of their general training, which at that time was coordinated by the Department of Surgery of the Queen's University of Belfast based in the RVH. This was largely organised by the then head of Department, the late Prof Harold Rogers, who himself has sessions in the RBHSC. In that year Sir Ian identified one such trainee, Brian Turbett Smyth (Fig. 4) who had developed a special interest in training as a Specialist Paediatric Surgeon, a speciality which at that time was in its infancy in the United Kingdom. He spend several years firstly at the Hospital for Sick Children Great Ormond Street with Sir Denis Browne, then at the Alder Hey Royal Liverpool Children's Hospital with Peter Paul Rickham and Isobella Forshall and lastly in Boston USA with Prof Ovar Swenson. He was appointed to the RBHSC and the UHD as the first Specialist Paediatric Surgeon in Northern Ireland in 1959.

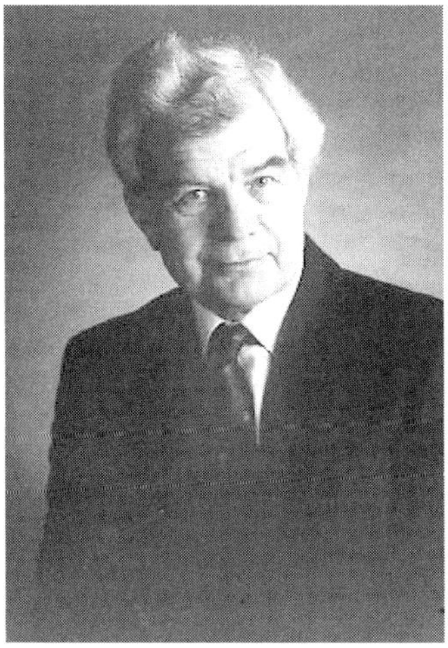

Fig. 4. Brian Smyth.

In that same year he was joined by the late Bill Cochran who had undertaken his paediatric surgical training in Edinburgh. Bill was appointed initially as a senior paediatric surgical registrar to both the RBHSC and the UHD and eventually in 1962 he was appointed as a Consultant Paediatric Surgeon to the Ulster Hospital. However, his appointment as a Consultant to the RBHSC was delayed by a further five years. This dreadful injustice was the result of the autocracy which existed at the time within the surgical community in Northern Ireland. This certainly could not have been justified on the basis of his work, which would by any standard, have deserved recognition by appointment as a Consultant. However, for Bill, this was a source of enormous disappointment and resentment. He returned to Glasgow and Scotland, the land of his birth in 1978 as a Consultant Paediatric Surgeon to the Yorkhill Children's Hospital.

The efforts of these two surgeons in promoting the specialist surgical care of children in Northern Ireland cannot be underestimated. New skills which had not previously existed were brought to the surgical treatment of children in Belfast in urology, oncology, gastroenterology, trauma and neonatal surgery. Brian Smyth who is alive and well, living in the South of England regularly keeps in touch with his colleagues. He still enquires about what is happening in the RBHSC and the UHD whose development through the years from 1959 to his retirement in 1986, was skilfully steered by him.

During the 1970's the Belfast City Hospital had indicated that they were interested in developing a Paediatric Surgical Department in their hospital. This fact is important in that they had the influence (as opposed to the RBHSC and the UHD) to generate the funding for a further post in Paediatric Surgery. It was generally recognised that there was sufficient work to justify the appointment of a further Consultant Surgeon to the Northern Ireland Paediatric Surgical Service. However, there was no funding available for the RBHSC and the UHD for such an appointment at that time. Brian Smyth and Bill Cochran recognised this opportunity and while in the long term, the development of three specialist paediatric surgical units in Belfast would not be appropriate, they understood that this might be the only way to secure the necessary funding for a third colleague.

In 1973 one of the surgical trainees in RBHSC, Victor Ernest Boston, having recently passed his FRCS examination, was approached to determine whether he was interested in training for such a position. He had during 1972, sought and secured a position as a Consultant General Surgeon in Alberta, Canada, but discovered that such a position required experience and training in Gynaecology; something which he had not undertaken except at an undergraduate level. The Canadian authorities had kept his appointment open while he attempted to secure the appropriate training in the UK, but unfortunately for them, there was a delay of six months before he could start this. As a stopgap arrangement, in August 1973, he secured a paediatric surgical registrar's post in the RBHSC and the rest is history. In his efforts to proceed with specialist paediatric surgical training as quickly as possible, he sought the advice of Prof Andrew Wilkinson, the then Chairman of the newly formed Specialist Advisory Committee (SAC) which was responsible for the organisation of paediatric surgical training in the UK and Ireland. Prof Wilkinson, who at that time was the Nuffield Professor of Paediatric Surgery in Great Ormond Street, recognised (because of his role on the SAC), the shortage of recognised appropriate training and Consultant posts in Great Britain.

His first advice was that, if unsure that paediatric surgery was his career choice, Victor Boston should seek specialist training in another speciality. Otherwise, there were two training posts coming up within the next year, the first in Newcastle Upon Tyne and the second in Dublin. John Scott, the senior surgeon in Newcastle remembers this young aspiring paediatric surgeon "interviewing" him when he came to inspect his department in 1973. By coincidence in Dublin, Victor Boston met the now Professor of Paediatric Surgery to the Universtiy College Dublin, Prem Puri, when he travelled to Dublin to enquire about the prospects of training there. Prem had spent some time in Newcastle Upon Tyne and had secured a training post in Our Lady's Children's Hospital Dublin the year before. It was clear to him following this conversation with Prem, that the position in Newcastle Upon Tyne would be appointed many months before Dublin and thus he decided to apply for the Newcastle training post. Had his decision been different and had he been appointed to Dublin he almost certainly would have become a consultant in that city. It is interesting to contemplate how this could have altered the development of paediatric surgical specialist services in Belfast and in Dublin.

He was successful in his appointment as a SAC recognised paediatric surgical senior registrar in Newcastle and spent 1975 and 1976 under the tutelage of John Scott and John Waggett. John Scott at that time was Secretary of BAPS and had many influential international contacts which included Prof Jannie Louw from Cape Town. Prof Louw was visiting Newcastle in 1975 and John Scott organised with him for a further period of training for Victor Boston in South Africa. In those days the Red Cross Memorial Children's Hospital, Cape Town had training posts which were funded by the South African Government for overseas trainees. This represented a unique opportunity for Victor Boston not only in terms of clinical experience but also in clinical and laboratory research. The volume and extensive case mix of the patients in Red Cross is perhaps unequalled anywhere else in the world.

While he had a general paediatric surgical training in South Africa he was also able to develop special interests in gastroenterology and urology, particularly in Hirschsprung's Disease and hypospadias. The former was the subject of his MD thesis which was presented and accepted in 1982. He returned to Belfast in 1977 where he was appointed as a Consultant Paediatric Surgeon to the RBHSC, UHD and the BCH. During the time from his appointment to his retirement in 2005 he developed close research collaboration with the Department of Surgery, Queen's University Belfast and supervised several postgraduate students during their MD research, an activity which became part of the day-to-day work of the Department of Paediatric Surgery. He had from the beginning an interest in medical politics both locally and nationally. This was initially stimulated by recognition that appropriate funding for the department depended on the level of influence of the contacts which could be developed within the funding establishment. Apart from chairing several Hospital and Department of Health Committees locally in Belfast, he went on play a active role in national and international affairs in Paediatric Surgery. This culminated shortly before he retired in him being elected to the Presidency of the BAPS, of being a member of the European Board in Paediatric Surgery, the councils of both the Royal College of Surgeons in London and Edinburgh and of the Senate of Surgery for Great Britain and Ireland.

Bill Cochran left his post in Belfast when he was appointed as a Consultant Paediatric Surgeon in Glasgow in 1978. His successor was Stephen Brown who was appointed in the same year as a Consultant Paediatric Surgeon to the RBHSC and the UHD. Stephen's training was initially as a General Surgeon where he was a senior registrar in the RVH until he decided that he wished to follow a career in Paediatric Surgery. In 1975 he secured a training position as a senior registrar in paediatric surgery in Manchester with the Ambrose Jollies and Joe Cohen followed in 1976 as a senior registrar in Great Ormond Street, London with Andrew Wilkinson and Harold Nixon amongst others. All of these personalities were influential figures in the international family of paediatric surgery and were presidents of the BAPS in there time. This exposure, particularly in Great Ormond Street, enabled Stephen when he was appointed to RBHSC and the UHD in 1978 to bring experience which further facilitated the development of the spectrum of paediatric surgery in Belfast, particularly in urology.

With the reorganisation of the National Health Service in the late 1980's and early 1990's Stephen became involved in medical administration. He undertook postgraduate studies in medical management and was involved in the local administration of the Hospital being the first Clinical Director for RBHSC. During the latter years of his career he developed the paediatric urology service for Northern Ireland particularly through his involvement in urodynamic assessment of spina bifida patients. He retired in 2004.

When Brian Smyth retired in 1986 his post was replaced by the appointment of Stephen Randal Potts. Stephen had been a registrar in RBHSC rotating through the general surgical training programme. Following that experience, he decided that he wanted a career in paediatric surgery. Most of his postgraduate training was undertaken in Belfast following his appointment as a senior registrar in paediatric surgery in 1982. Stephen Brown, through his previous contacts was able to secure for Stephen Potts, a similar training position in Manchester where he was appointed as a senior registrar in paediatric surgery in 1985. Following completion of his certified training he was appointed to the RBHSC and UHD as a Consultant Paediatric Surgeon to replace Brian Smyth in 1986. While Stephen was a trained general paediatric surgeon he was the first in Belfast to develop the newly emerging field of endoscopic surgery and was a founder and executive member of the British Association of Paediatric Endoscopic Surgeons. Initially during the 1990's, there were considerable difficulties in funding the appropriate hardware to undertake this new surgical discipline. Stephen through a great deal of hard work, almost single-handedly, managed to get the service off the ground. This is now established as a routine method for undertaking an increasing number of surgical procedures in RBHSC and UHD. As a spin-off from this experience of fund raising he became the secretary to the new Helping Hand RBHSC Charity for which he was a tireless worker. Stephen retired in 2005.

During the late 1970's and early 1980's it was apparent to those working in the Paediatric Surgical Service that there was unnecessary duplication of services in the three hospitals providing this service. While initially, there was pressure from the various hospitals to provide a full spectrum of paediatric surgical care in each unit, increasingly, the RBHSC was becoming the centre for provision of the specialist services such as major trauma, neonatal surgery and oncology. The difficulty which was faced was that any rationalisation within the three units would require additional beds in the remaining hospital/s. The logical solution to this problem would have been to concentrate all specialist Paediatric Surgical Services for Northern Ireland in one unit, the RBHSC. Following much debate with the Department of Health and the Eastern Health and Social Services Board (the local health authority for Belfast), a decision was taken to withdraw from the BCH, but to continue services in RBHSC and UHD.

This occurred in 1989 with the surgery previously undertaken in BCH being divided between RBHSC and the UHD where, unusually, at the time there happened to be some spare bed capacity. This resulted in the development of Day Care Surgical facilities in both the RBHSC and UHD. Because of the additional capacity in the UHD compared to the RBHSC, the bulk of this type of surgery was undertaken there. Increasingly, many of these patients were from outside Belfast because many of the province's DGH's were having difficulties in conforming to published standards of surgical care for children. This demographic shift of patients towards the specialist units in Belfast meant an increasing work load, mostly of the generality of paediatric surgical problems. This change in case mix has created difficulties in how to deliver the service most appropriately.

In 1992, the increase in work load in RBHSC and UHD lead to a general recognition of the need for an additional Consultant Paediatric Surgeon. At that time Bill McCallion a rotating general surgical trainee, had expressed an interest. Bill spent 1995 in Red

Cross Memorial Children's Hospital in Capetown with Prof Syd Cywes, then the President of the World Federation of Pediatric Surgeons. This was the position which Victor Boston occupied 20 years previously and gave Bill the same invaluable clinical experience particularly in Gastroenterology. Additional funding was secured from the commissioning authority in Northern Ireland and he was appointed as a Consultant Paediatric Surgeon to RBHSC and UHD in 1996. Since then he has continued to develop the surgical gastroenterology service in RBHSC and UHD particularly with regard to inflammatory bowel disease.

In line with the increasing workload, RBHSC clearly required additional resourses. In 1998 the phase one development of the hospital has given an upgraded A&E department, a new intensive care unit and operating theatres and new out patient facilities. These have greatly improved the services which are provided by the hospital. However, like many developments, by the time planning and building are complete the original expectations for the new build at RBHSC were overtaken by the increased workload once again. Further phase 2 development is anticipated by 2015. Interestingly, this will combine the maternity and paediatric specialist services in the same building.

During the late 1990's and the early part of the new century the case load being transferred to Belfast from the periphery of the province has continued to increase. This has been confounded by the European Woking Time Directive which will reduce the hours worked by staff in the health service. Flowing from this is a recognition that further additional staff are required and to date the Paediatric Surgical Service for Northern Ireland has six Consultants with the prospect of an additional appointment 2009–2010.

A great deal has happened since 1959. While the special needs of children (as compared to adults) are now recognised both in terms of staff and facilities. Children in Northern Ireland paradoxically still have difficulty in competing with other clinical services for money to secure the appropriate standards of care expected by an increasingly demanding general public.

References

1. Fleetwood JF. *History of Medicine in Ireland*, 2nd ed., 1983; pp. 222–224.
2. Fitzgerald J. In: Walker A (ed.) *The Children's Hospital, Temple Street: The Post-Centenary Years (1972–2000)*. Blackwater Press, Dublin, 2000; pp. 64–66.
3. Guiney EJ, O'Donnell B. Personal communication.
4. Clarke AT, Matthews TG. In: Brown A (ed.) *Masters, Midwives and Ladies-in-Waiting*, A & A Farmar, Dublin, 1995, p. 132–133.
5. The Children's Research Centre, https://www.cmrf.org/Background.html

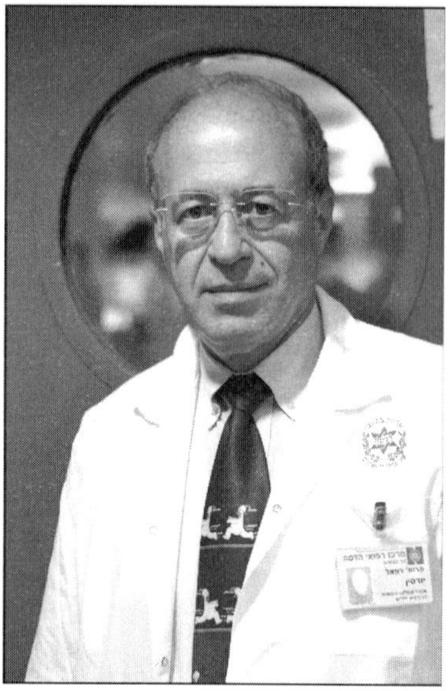

Raphael Udassin

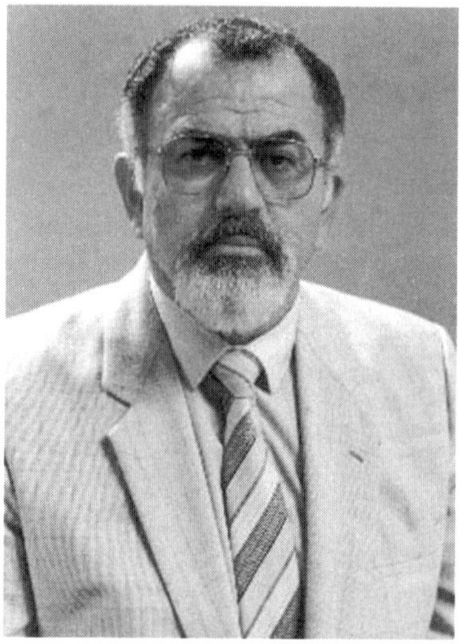

Abraham J. Mares

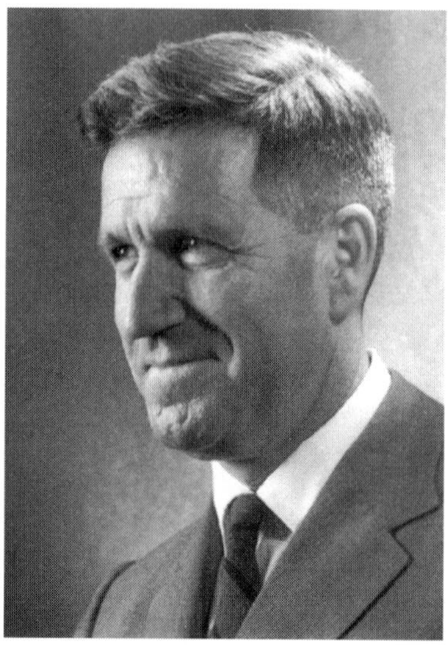

Shemuel Nissan

ISRAEL

Raphael Udassin
Abraham J. Mares
Shemuel Nissan

Introduction

From the second half of the twentieth century, pediatric surgery in Israel developed from the total absence of pediatric surgeons to departments of pediatric surgery that are accredited by the Scientific Council of the Israeli Medical Association to train Pediatric surgeons.

The first pediatric surgeon in the Holy Land and the Near East as a whole was Dr Max Sandrezky, a German physician who established the first Children's Hospital, in Jerusalem in 1872. A chapter describing his pioneer work is included in Section 5 of this book written by Dr Shemuel Nissan. Until the 1950's, pediatric surgery was practiced in Israel almost exclusively by general surgeons, and children were admitted either to pediatric departments or to adult general surgery departments. After the creation of the state of Israel (1948), medical services were formalized and modernized. The need for surgeons that are dedicated to pediatric patients became obvious with the mass immigration of Jews to the state, many of them with large numbers of children per family, as well as a high rate of birth and consanguineous marriages.

The first generation of Israeli surgeons who acquired some knowledge and interest in pediatric surgery were sent to children's hospitals in the United Kingdom and the United States in order that, upon their return to Israel, they would also practice pediatric surgery within the framework of general surgery departments. Two surgeons from the Tel Aviv area, Drs Moshe Soloveichik and Dr M. Dintsman, were trained by Professor Andrew Wilkinson at Great Ormond Street. Dr Avraham Laufer was a surgeon who served in World War II in the British Royal Army Medical Corps in Ethiopia under Colonel Orde Wingate. After the war, Dr Laufer spent some time in Philadelphia under Dr C. E. Koop and was appointed Head of Pediatric Surgery at Hadassah.

Other general surgeons who treated children were Dr Ami-Zakai J. Abrahamson, in Haifa, who was a registrar on Professor A. Wilkinson's service at Great Ormond Street,[1] Dr Antonin Motovic who was trained at the Prague Children's Hospital and worked in Kfar-Saba, Dr M. Dintsman (previously mentioned) at the Beilinson Hospital in Petach Tikva, Dr Erwin Jacob and Dr Mordechai at Asaf-Harofeh Hospital in Zrifin, Dr Isidor Wollfstein at Tel Hashomer Hospital in Ramat Gan and Dr Moshe Soloveichik in Ichilov Hospital in Tel-Aviv. All the above mentioned doctors worked as part of a general surgery service.

The first named pediatric surgical department, with a pediatric surgeon as chief of the service, was established at the newly opened Hadassah University Hospital in Ein-Karem, in September of 1961. Dr Laufer passed away before the inauguration of the new hospital in Ein Karem, and the position of the chief pediatric surgeon of the service was offered to Dr Shemuel Nissan, who spent eight years at the Barnes and Children's hospital in St. Louis Missouri. After passing the board examinations in general Surgery and Thoracic surgery, in preparation for assuming the appointment in Jerusalem, Dr Nissan joined Dr W. Potts at the Children's Memorial Hospital in Chicago. The first step he had taken after assuming the assignment was to appoint two head nurses that were trained and qualified abroad. One was born in the USA and trained at the Boston Children's Hospital, the other born in England and trained at the Hospital for Sick Children at Great Ormond Street. They were to train additional nurses in the care of children. This shows Nissan's concept, later adopted elsewhere, that care for children needs to be comprehensive and does not end with surgery. This concept was later expanded to specialized "child-friendly" wards, playrooms and in-hospital schools. In 1963 Dr S. Nissan was offered the position of the chief of the department of surgery and pediatric surgery, at the Central Emek Hospital in Afula, where a fair-sized building was dedicated to pediatric surgery. It served general and thoracic pediatric surgery as well as urology, orthopedics, E.N.T, neonatal and burn units. The nursing staff was trained specifically to take care of children.

As part of Nissan's comprehensive child care, a research laboratory was established with a biochemist, Dr Edna Rosen on the staff to specifically research surgically related childhood diseases. The studies in the laboratory were on the metabolism of sodium transport *in vitro* and in intact animals during several forms of dehydration.[2,3] Prof Shemuel Nissan has established myectomy for treating the mild form of Hirschsprung's disease (mistakenly termed "short segment").[4,5] He established a very productive neurophysiology laboratory with specific interest on intestinal motility.[6,7] He was the first one to perform colonic intersposition for esophageal replacement in Israel[8] and the first to perform a Swenson operation for Hirschsprung's disease in 1961 in Hadassah later to turn to Duhamel's operation in 1965. Nissan was the first to describe endoesophageal resection for benign strictures of the esophagus[9] and the first to perform Nissen fundoplication in a familial dysautonomia patient.[10,11]

Dr Nissan's place in Hadassah was taken by Dr Moshe M. Feuchtwanger (1963–1968) who later assumed the appointment of head of department of general surgery and Chairman of the Division of Surgery at the Ben-Gurion University (a rotating appointment) — Soroka Medical Center (then the Negev Central Hospital). As of 1968 he began to organize a pediatric surgical service within his general surgery department. This was later taken over by Dr A. J. Mares upon his arrival, as described later. Dr Feuchtwanger introduced the "side-to-side" duodenoduodenostomy,[12] as well as the Pidzerl's gracilis muscle transposition for the correction of anal incontinence.[13]

Following the unification of Jerusalem in 1967, the Hadassah University Hospital on Mt. Scopus was renovated. Dr S. Nissan was

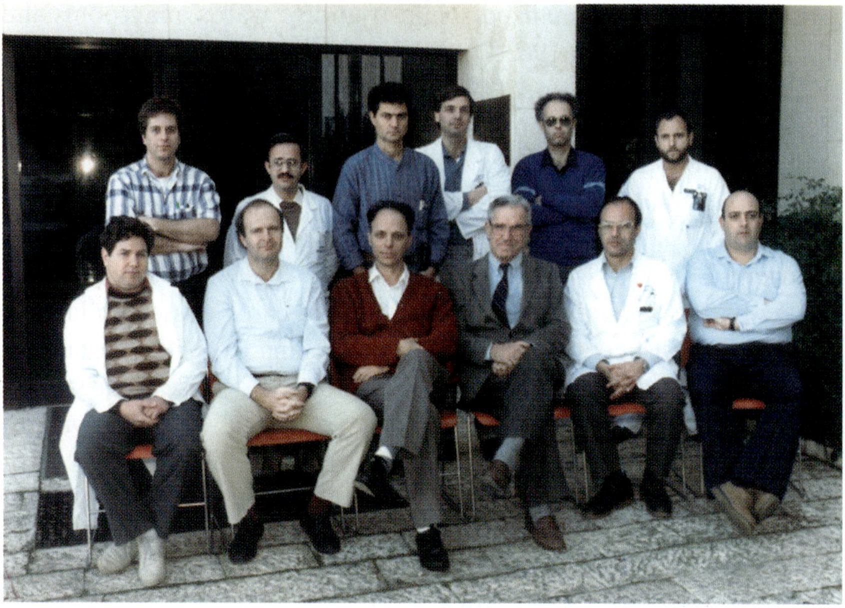

Fig. 1. Prof Shemuel Nissan at 20 years celebration of the Department of Pediatric Surgery at Hadassah Mount Scopus, Jerusalem with Prof Omri Lernau on his right and Prof Raphael Udassin on his left (1987).

appointed the chairman of the department of surgery that included a separate wing of pediatric surgery with facilities for rooming in for parents (Fig. 1). The nursing staffs were trained to care for children. A neonatal intensive care unit was also available.

The second generation of pediatric surgeons consisted of two surgeons that have been trained in both general surgery and pediatric surgery but were willing to dedicate themselves solely to the practice of pediatric surgery, concomitant with the rise of Pediatric Surgery as a distinct profession.

The first of the two was Dr Abraham J. Mares, who obtained board certification in the United States, followed by Dr Medad Schiller. Dr Abraham J. Mares was trained in general surgery at the Beilinson Medical Center in Israel (1963–1965) and at the Beth–Israel Hospital in Boston (1965–1968) and was US Board Certified in general surgery (1969). He then continued his training in

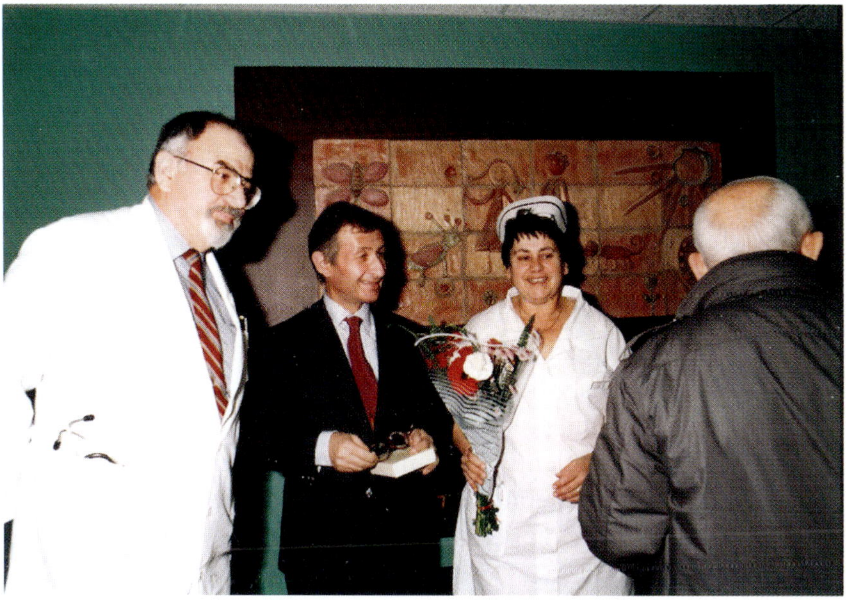

Fig. 2. Prof Abraham J. Mares at the inauguration of the new wing of Pediatric Surgery, Soroka Medical Center, January 1992, at the foyer-entrance to the new Pediatric Surgery Department, with the senior representative of the donors," RASHI foundation" and Mrs Ofra Mares.

pediatric surgery and was chief resident at the Children's Hospital of Los Angeles (1968–1969). Dr Mares returned to Israel in 1970 and was appointed head of a pediatric surgery unit, later to become a separate Department, at the Soroka Medical Center in Be'er-Sheva, covering the whole southern part of Israel (Negev) (Fig. 2). Among others, it serves the largest Bedouin population in Israel with high marriage consanguinity and has the largest number of obstetric deliveries in Israel in a single hospital.

Dr Abraham Mares was the first to perform upper thoracic sympathectomy for palmar hyperhydrosis in children in Israel since 1974,[14,15] the first to introduce the Dartos pouch approach for orchiopexy since 1970 and the only one in Israel who continued for more than 25 years to use successfully the Swenson operation for Hirschsprung's disease.[16] Dr Mares was also asked by the Israeli authorities to train two Arab surgeons from the Gaza strip for a year in pediatric surgery, in the 1980's. Among his other duties, he served as Chairman of the Department of Surgery (all surgical specialties) from 1986–1990 (a rotating appointment) and as Vice Dean of the Faculty of Health Sciences at the Ben Gurion University of the Negev in Be'er-Sheva (1984–1986).

Dr Medad Schiller was trained at the Children's Hospital of Columbus, Ohio (1969–1971). He returned to Israel in 1971 and assumed the position of head of pediatric surgery department at the Hadassah University Hospital Ein-Karem (Fig. 3), the same department previously headed already by Drs Laufer, Nissan and Feuchtwanger. Dr Schiller had a large series of patients operated upon for biliary atresia,[17] patients with familial total colonic Hirschsprung's disease[18] and patients operated upon for hyperinsulinism.[19] He became a worldwide authority on pediatric biliary operations. As part of his

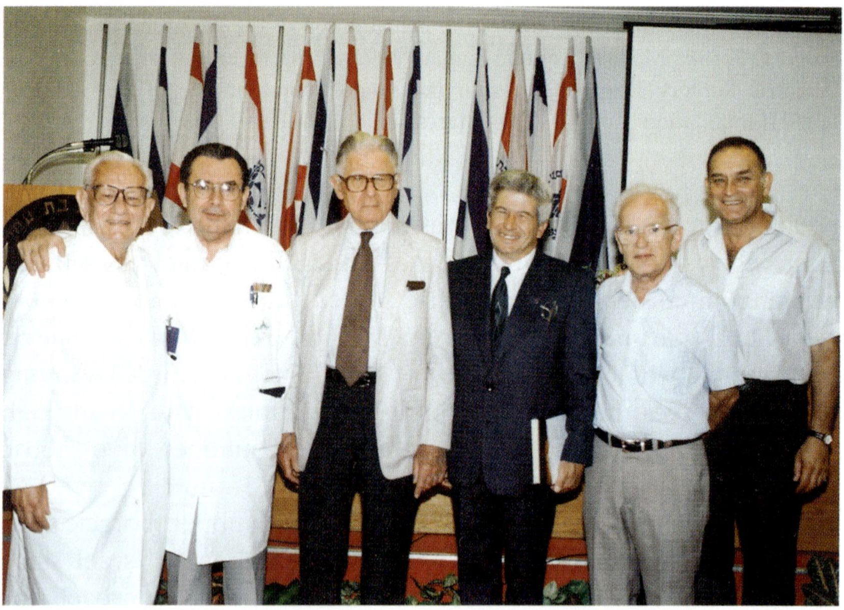

Fig. 3. Prof Medad Schiller at 25 years celebration of the Department of Pediatric Surgery at Hadassah Ein-Karem, Jerusalem (1996). From left to right: Profs Emeric Lax, Medad Schiller, Nathan Saltz, Halil Abu-Dalo, Zvi Eyal, Shemuel Katz.

work, together with his colleagues from other hospitals, he established a system in which sick Palestinian children received regular surgical care in Israel, a system that still exists today.

The "offsprings" of the second generation of pediatric surgeons in Israel expanded the horizons of the profession. Following the training that most of them received already in Israel, they obtained further clinical fellowships in the United States, in Europe, in Australia and South Africa, some with innovations of their own.

Prof Nissan's trainees that became head of services include Dr Bar–Maor at Rambam hospital in Haifa (Fig. 4), Dr Lernau at Shaare–Zedek hospital in Jerusalem (Fig. 1), Dr Vinograd at Dana Children's Hospital in Tel-Aviv and Dr Udassin at Hadassah University Hospital in Jerusalem. Dr Udassin serves presently as the chairman of the Israel Association of Pediatric Surgery (Fig. 4). Dr Mares'

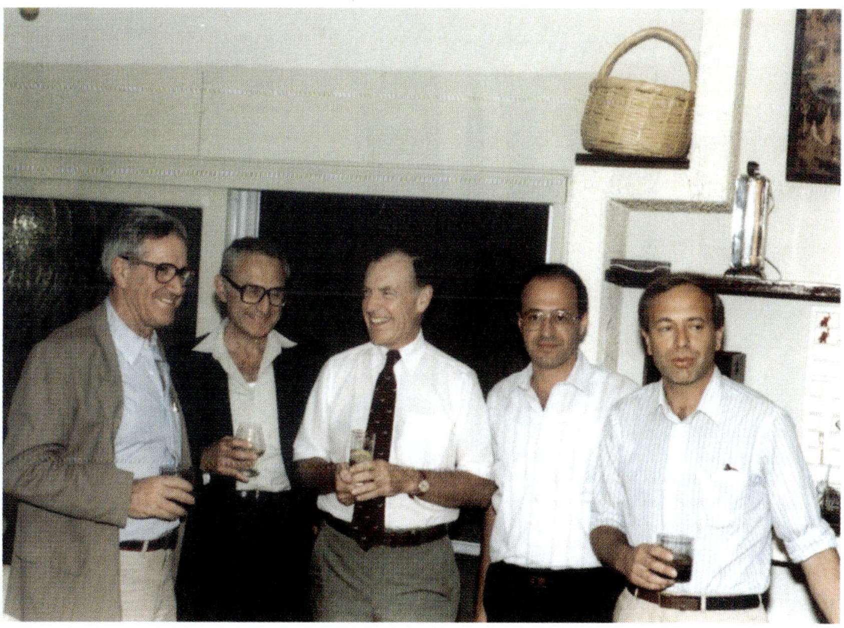

Fig. 4. Prof Shemuel Nissan with Prof James A. O'Neill with Nissan's "off springs" (1985). From left to right: Professors Nissan, Bar-Maor, O'Niell, Udassin, Vinograd.

trainees who became head of services include Dr Siplovich at Central Emek Hospital in Afula, Dr Steiner at Hillel-Yaffe Hospital in Hadera, Dr Freud at Schnieder Children's Hospital at the Rabin medical center in Petach-Tikva, Dr Kurzbart at Barzilai Hospital in Ashkelon and Dr Cohen at the Soroka Medical center in Be'er-Sheva, following Dr Mares upon his retirement in July 2000 (Fig. 5).

Dr Schiller's trainees who became head of services include the late Dr Shemuel Katz, who headed the pediatric surgery department at Sapir hospital in Kfar-Sabba (Fig. 3), and Dr Gorenstein at Wolfson hospital in Holon.

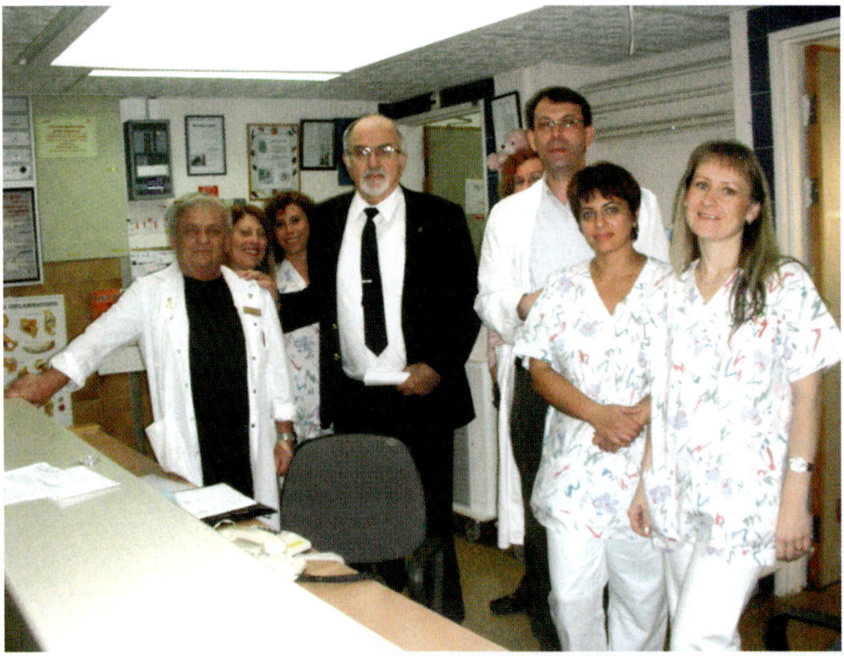

Fig. 5. Prof Abraham J. Mares visiting his former Department of Pediatric Surgery, Soroka Medical Center, on November, 2007 with some of the staff. From left to right: Prof Zahavi Cohen, present head of the Department, Mrs Orit Behar, Secretary, Mrs Ra'ia Madar, Head nurse, Prof Abraham J. Mares, Dr Nitza Neuman–Heiman, Dr Oleg Kleiner and two nurses.

Official Accreditation of Pediatric Surgery and the Formation of the Israel Association of Pediatric Surgery

The main driving force behind the official accreditation of pediatric surgery as a separate profession in Israel was Dr Mares. Upon his return to Israel in 1970 Dr Mares initiated the long process, with the active support of Dr Feuchtwanger, who served at the time as president of the Israel Surgical society. This long process finally ended up with the official declaration of pediatric surgery as a separate profession in 1985, with a separate syllabus, board examinations, and criteria for training program accreditation, a process that took some ten years, the crucial steps being:

1. The general assembly of the Israel General Surgery Association's decision of accepting the separation of pediatric surgery from general surgery (a separate society within the Israel Surgical Association) — November 1975.
2. Founding meeting of the Israel Association of Pediatric Surgery — June 1976 with Dr Mares as the first chairman serving up to 1990.
3. The formation of a syllabus for pediatric surgery training.
4. The acceptance of the syllabus by the Scientific Council of the Israel Medical Council — January 1982.
5. Naming of pediatric surgery founders ("forefathers") and the issuing of the first pediatric surgery specialty diplomas by Prof Baruch Modan, the General Director of the Israel Ministry of Health — 1983.
6. The formation criteria for training program accreditation and its approval by the Israel Medical council — 1985.
7. Official declaration of the new profession by the Israel Ministry of Health — 1985.

The Israel Association of Pediatric Surgery has applied for membership to the World Federation of Pediatric Surgery Associations while Dr Mares was serving as its chairman. Dr Mares was invited to their council meeting in Belgrade (1983) where the Association was formally admitted; the same meeting the Russian Association was also admitted.

Syllabus. The initial approved syllabus for pediatric surgery was of six and a half years of "straight residency", including general surgery and rotations. It was changed in the mid-1990's, somewhat according to the American example, namely, a basic requirement of six years training and board certification in general surgery and then two and a half years in pediatric surgery and in an intensive neonatal unit.

Present status of pediatric surgery in Israel. The population of Israel is 7 million with 2.3 million children and the population of the West-Bank and Gaza strip are over 3 millions. There are 55 active pediatric surgeons and five residents (Fig. 6). These professionals are serving in 17 departments and units all over Israel. Six

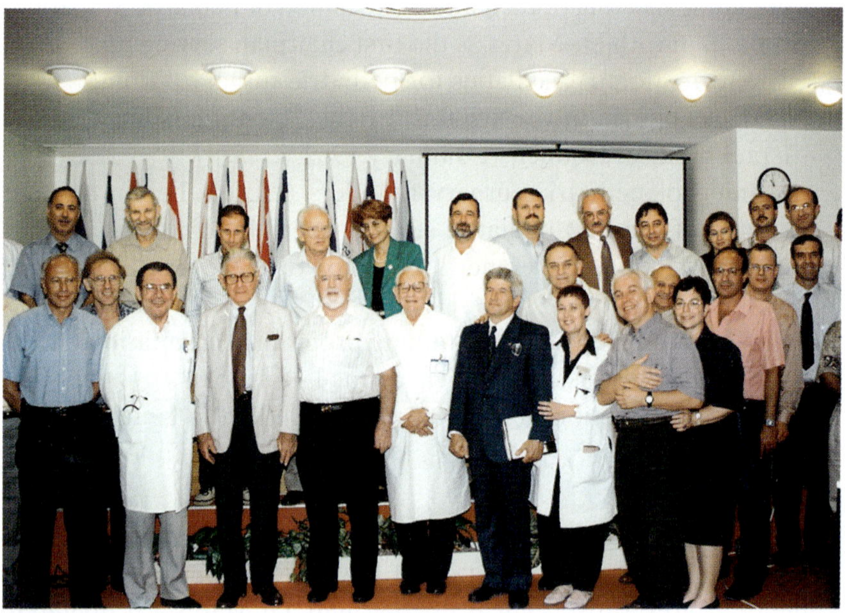

Fig. 6. Members of the Israel Association of Pediatric Surgery, 1996.

of them offer full residency programs; each one of these six services operate on over 1500 children each year. All hospitals in Israel are getting pediatric surgery services from a board certified pediatric surgeon and it will be uncommon for a general surgeon to perform an operation on a child, though the Israeli law permits it. This shows that the concepts by the founding fathers of our profession have been well-ingrained into our system. Today, all pediatric surgical wards are set apart from the adult population and have a staff (doctors and nurses) completely dedicated to child health and welfare.

The fact that abortion is not an option for a large portion of the population for religious reasons (orthodox Jews and part of the Arab population) and the still abundant consanguineous marriages, cause a unique situation in which major congenital anomalies are still frequent. The birth rates in the Palestinian territories as well as in certain parts of Israel (most notably Jerusalem and the Negev) are more similar to less developed countries than to European or North American standards. The relationships with physicians of the West Bank have evolved from willingly admitting complicated surgical patients from the West Bank to Israeli hospitals to extensive fellowships that enabled the establishment of pediatric surgery services in Hebron, East Jerusalem and Gaza strip. Although most pediatric surgical procedures on Palestinian children are performed by Palestinian surgeons, complex cases are still referred to Israeli tertiary centers and are performed free of personal surgeon charge. These fellowship programs lead to close personal and professional relationships between the trainees and the pediatric surgeons in Israel. In the present political atmosphere, these connections define the maxim that medicine and politics do not intermingle.

The **Israel Association of Pediatric Surgery** is very active. There are two annual academic meetings and the required number of pediatric surgeons in Israel is continuously monitored. It promotes additional clinical fellowships in major pediatric surgery services throughout the world and modestly finances some of them.

References

1. Abrahamson J, Shandling B. Esophageal atresia in the underweight baby: a challenge. *J Pediatr Surg* 1972;7(5):608–613.
2. Moyer CA, Nissan S. Alterations in the basal oxygen consumptions of rats attendant upon three types of dehydration. *Ann Surg* 1961;154(6, Suppl):51–64.
3. Nissan S, Aviram A, Czaczkes JW, Ullmann L, Ullmann TD. Increased O-2 consumption of the rat diaphragm by elevated NaCl concentrations. *Am J Physiol* 1966;210(6):1222–1224.
4. Nissan S, Bar-Maor JA, *et al.* Anorectal myomectomy in the treatment of short segment Hirschsprung's disease. *Ann Surg* 1969;170(6):969–977.
5. Udassin Nissan RS, *et al.* The mild form of Hirschsprung's disease (short segment): fourteen-years experience in diagnosis and treatment. *Ann Surg* 1981;194(6):767–770.
6. Nissan Vinograd SY, *et al.* Physiological and pharmacological studies of the internal anal sphincter in the rat. *J Pediatr Surg* 1984;19(1):12–14.
7. Hanani M, Lernau OZ, *et al.* Nerve mediated responses to drugs and electrical stimulation in aganglionic muscle segments in Hirschsprung's disease. *J Pediatr Surg* 1986;21(10):848–851.
8. Bar–Maor JA, Nissan S. Improved vascularization of transplanted colon for esophageal replacement. *Surg Gynecol Obstet* 1970; 131(4):755–756.
9. Nissan S, Bar–Maor JA, *et al.* Endesophageal resection of short benign strictures of the esophagus. *J Pediatr Surg* 1978;13(4):377–379.
10. Vinograd I, Lernau OZ, *et al.* Fundoplication and pyloroplasty — a surgical treatment for intractable "cyclic vomiting" in familial dysautonomia. *J Pediatr Surg* 1982;17(1):80–81.
11. Udassin R, Seror D, *et al.* Nissen fundoplication in the treatment of children with familial dysautonomia. *Am J Surg* 1992;164(4):332–336.
12. Feuchtwanger MM, Weiss Y. Side-to-side duodenoduodenostomy for obstructing annular pancreas in the newborn. *J Pediatr Surg* 1968; 3(3):398–401.
13. Feuchtwanger MM, Ben–Hur N. The surgical correction of anal incontinence by complete perineoplasty: case report. *Plast Reconstr Surg* 1968;41(3):268–272.

14. Mares AJ, Steiner Z, *et al.* Transaxillary upper thoracic sympathectomy for primary palmar hyperhidrosis in children and adolescents. *J Pediatr Surg* 1994;29(3):382–386.
15. Cohen Z, Shinar D, *et al.* Thoracoscopic upper thoracic sympathectomy for primary palmar hyperhidrosis in children and adolescents. *J Pediatr Surg* 1995;30(3):471–473.
16. Halevy H, Mares A, Cohen Z, Finaly R, *et al.* [Hirschprung's disease in the Negev]. *Harefuah* 1994;127(5–6):148–154, 216.
17. Katz S, Freund H, *et al.* [Hepatic portoenterostomy for biliary atresia]. *Harefuah* 1976;91(12):429–434.
18. Schiller M, Levy P, *et al.* Familial Hirschsprung's disease — a report of 22 affected siblings in four families. *J Pediatr Surg* 1990;25(3):322–325.
19. Schiller M, Krausz M, *et al.* Neonatal hyperinsulinism — surgical and pathologic considerations. *J Pediatr Surg* 1980;15(1):16–20.

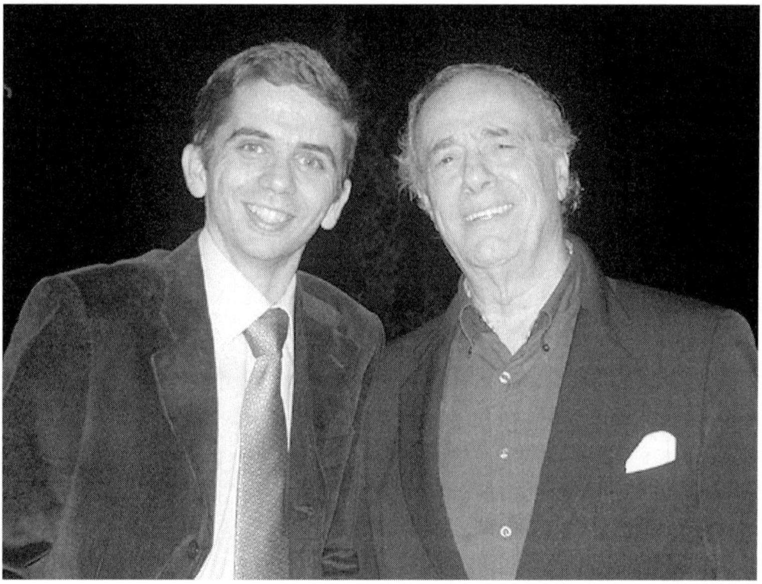

Simone Frediani and Francesco Cozzi

ITALY

Francesco Cozzi
Simone Frediani

In Italy, the "*Spedale degli Innocenti*" or "*Hospital of the Innocents*" is considered the place of birth of the Italian pediatrics. The *Spedale degli Innocenti* was established at Florence in 1419 to give refuge, proper care, and education to abandoned children. The architecture of the *Spedale degli Innocenti* was the work of **Brunelleschi** (1377–1446), the famous designer of the dome of the cathedral of Florence. The structural concept and the porticoes facade (Fig. 1) were new to the civil architecture of the time and embodied the prototype of the Renaissance dwelling. The loggia is adorned with a series of medallions by Della Robbia depicting infants in the swaddling clothes of the medieval period (Fig. 2), portraits which have became the symbol of pediatrics.[1]

The date of birth of the Italian pediatrics is sometimes considered to be March 15, 1780, when **Lorenzo Nannoni** started in the *Spedale degli Innocenti* a course of surgical practice for medical students on the corpse of foundlings. A more appropriate date seems April 8, 1802 when the first teaching of pediatrics was established in the *Spedale degli Innocenti*, and was held be March 16, 1805. At the end of 19th century, in some rooms given by the *Spedale degli Innocenti* to the "*Arcispedale di S. Maria Nuova*", the University of Florence established one of the first Italian official chair of pediatrics and then the first teaching of pediatric surgery. The professorial units of pediatrics and pediatric surgery were subsequently transferred to the new children's hospital which had been opened on February 15, 1891 and called "*Spedalino Meyer*", from the name of the benefactor the marquis

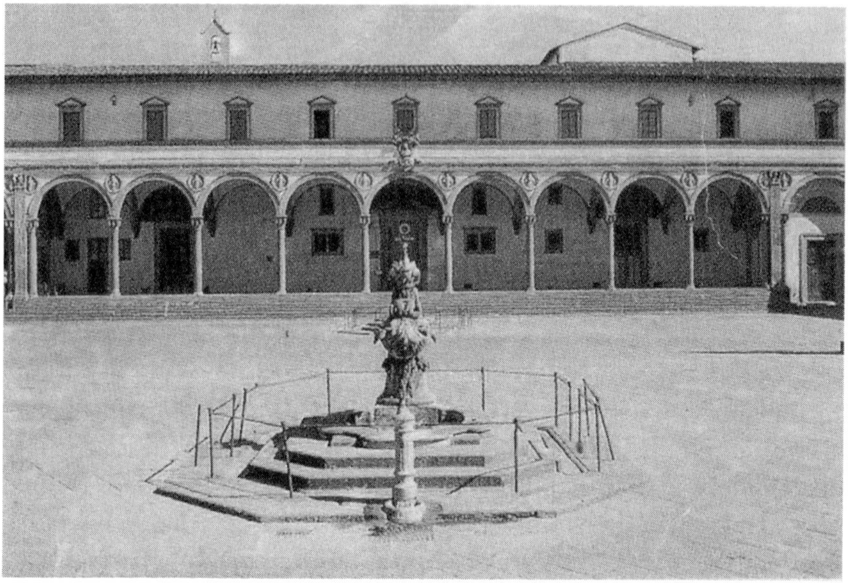

Fig. 1. Portico facade of the Hospital of the Innocents (Florence, 1419).

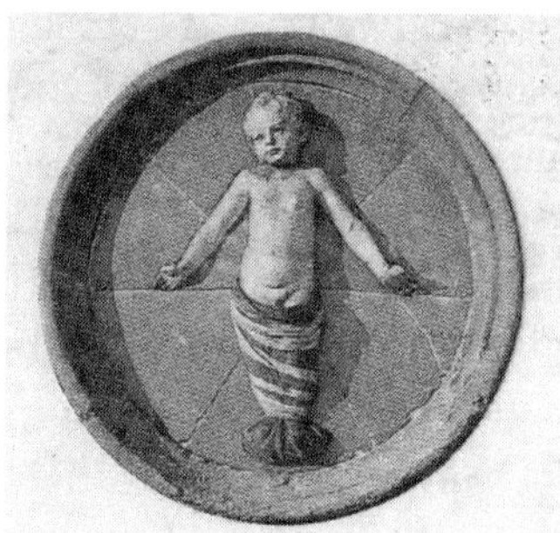

Fig. 2. One of the medallions adorning the loggia of the Hospital of the Innocents depicting infants in swaddling-clothes (Florence, 1419).

Giovanni Meyer, who founded "a hospital to cure sick children, especially those affected by congenital malformations."[2] It is worthy of notice that, in 1891, the professor of pediatrics **Giuseppe Mya** first used the original name "megacolon congenitum" and gave an accurate descriptions of enterocolitis associated with Hirschprung's disease.[3]

The first of present Italian institutions that limited themselves to the care of sick children was probably the "*Ospedale Infantile di Trieste*", which was established November 18, 1856. The institution, which for many years was called "*Ospedaletto*", had 24 beds for "children of both sexes, definitively poor, of any religion, and with curable disease". In 1907 the *Ospedaletto* received a bequest of money by the baroness **Maria di Burlo Garofalo** and since then it was called "*Ospedale Infantile Burlo Garofalo*".

The first mention of a Unit for admission of children with surgical disease is found in the historical archives of the "*Ospedale Bambino Gesù*" of Rome, which was established March 19, 1869;[4] subsequently, in April 1870, it was decided to open also a surgical unit; the chief surgeon was **Alessandro Ceccarelli**. However, the children's hospital exclusively dedicated to pediatric surgery was the "*Ospedale Lina Fieschi Ravaschieri*", which was opened in Naples November 4, 1880. This surgical children's hospital (Fig. 3) was

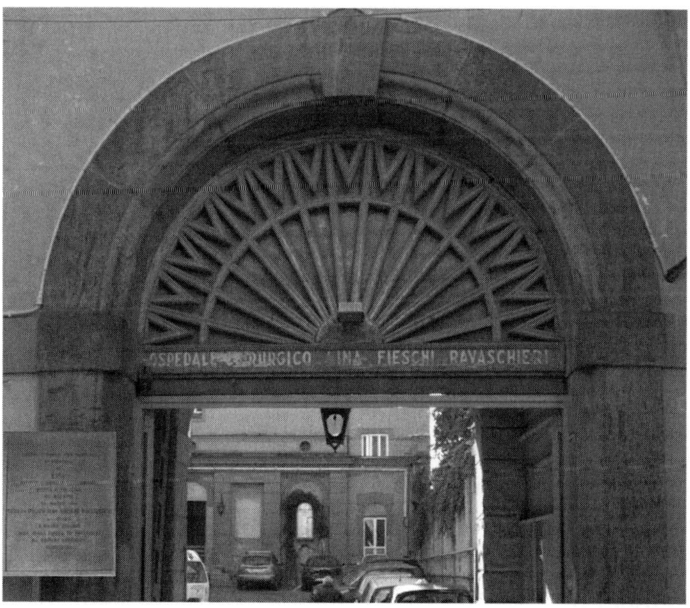

Fig. 3. Main entrance of the *Hospital Lina Ravaschieri* for children with surgical disease (Naples, 1880).

founded by the **Duchess Teresa Filangeri Fieschi Ravaschieri**, and dedicated to her daughter Lina. The girl died at the age of 12 years following an operation for acute appendicitis complicated by peritonitis. The hospital had at the beginning 30 beds for admission of "poor children between three and ten yrs of age affected by disease curable by means of surgical art."[5] The surgeon was **Carlo Gallozzi**, professor of general surgery at the Naples University and senator in the "*Camera Vitalizia*" when the Italian Kingdom was first established. At the present the building of the "*Hospital Lina Ravaschieri*" is used as administrative offices of the Naples Children's hospital Santobono–Pausillipon.

Before the end of the 19th century, the following other institutions, that limited themselves to the care of sick children, were established. In Turin, the "*Ospedaletto Infantile*" (1883), subsequently called "*Ospedale Infantile Regina Margherita*;" in this institution the presence of a surgical unit was first mentioned in the minutes of the meeting of the hospital memberships (1901). In Cremona, the "*Ospedale dei Bambini*" (1887); had 32 beds for children with medical or surgical disease.[6] In Genoa, the "*Ospedale infantile di S. Filippo*" (1888) had 24 beds for pediatrics, and 12 for pediatric surgery; subsequently the hospital was called "*Galliera*." Since 1888, in this institution had admitted children with severe malformations, as indicated by the photos in an atlas (Figs. 4 and 5). In Alessandria, the "*Uspidalet Infantile*" (1890) was established for children between two and seven years of age without infection, therefore mainly with surgical problems. In Milan, the "*Ospedale dei Bambini*" (1897), subsequently called "*V. Buzzi*;" admitted during the first year of activity 110 children in the surgical pediatric unit. The total number of surgical procedures was 187 including operation for inguinal hernia, hydrocele, abscesses, cyst, empyema, sinusitis, cleft lip, congenital dislocation of the hip, club feet, abdominal tumors, angioma and adenitis.[7] The surgeon of the hospital V. Buzzi was **Benedetto Formiggini**, who founded in 1934 the first Italian *journal of Pediatric Surgery* (Fig. 6). The journal had a brief life due to a shortage of papers to publish.

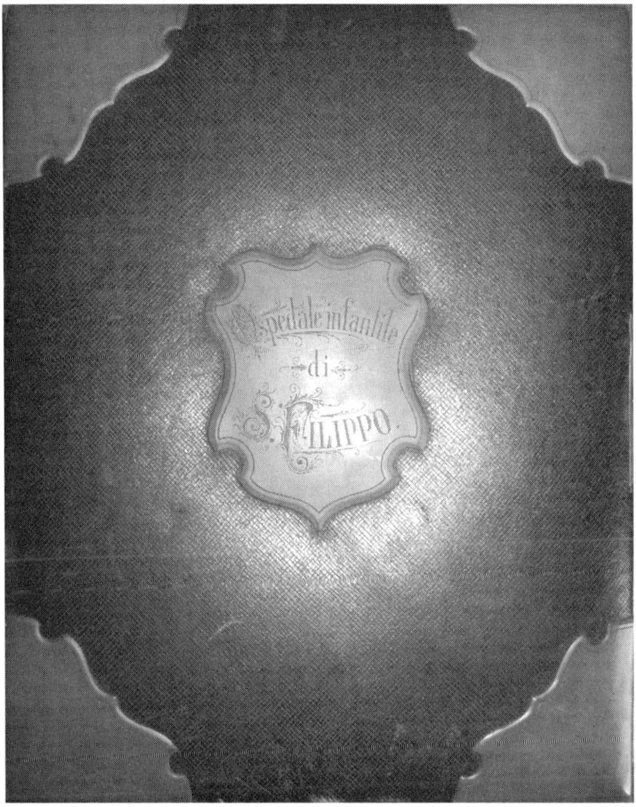

Fig. 4. Atlas containing the photographs of children with rare disease admitted since 1888 at the *Children Hospital S. Filippo* of Genoa (courtesy of Prof G. Romagnoli).

In Ancona, the "*Ospedaletto dei Bambini*" was established April 6, 1900; during this year of activity, the surgeon dott. **G. Branzanti** performed the first 32 operations; subsequently the hospital was called "*Ospedale dei bambini G. Salesi*" from the name of the benefactor who bought the building, which was subsequently transformed in a children hospital.[8] In Brescia, the "*Ospedale dei bambini Umberto I*" was opened on June 1, 1902 with 40 beds for children with medical or surgical problems.[6] During the period between July 1902 and December 1906, 1609 children were admitted; of these 850 were admitted to the surgical pediatric unit. The chief surgeon was

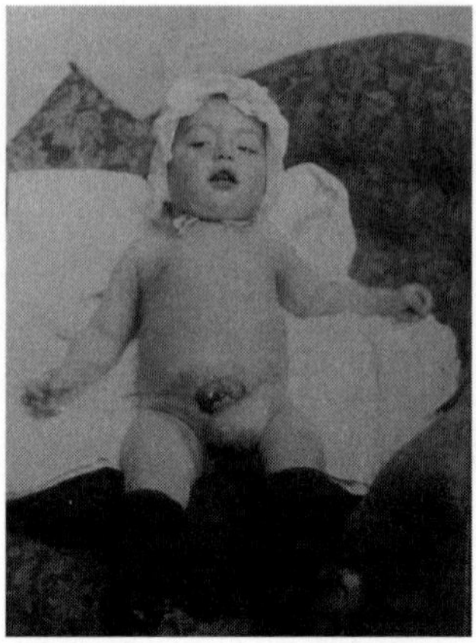

Fig. 5. Clinical photograph of a child with bladder estrophy admitted to the *Hospital S. Filippo* in Genoa (1888) (courtesy of Prof G. Romagnoli).

Artemio Magrassi (Fig. 7). In Parma, the "*Ospedale dei Bambini*" was established December 9, 1900; the surgeon in charge of the pediatric surgical unit was Vittorio Caprara.

In Palermo the "*Ospedale dei Bambini*" was established in 1904, and subsequently entitled to Giovanni Di Cristina, professor of pediatrics. In this hospital, the surgical activity was started by Agostino Giardina.[9] Inside the "*Hospital Vittorio Emanuele*" of Catania, the pavilion "*Costanza Gravina*", was established April 28, 1922. The surgical pediatric unit and the temporary teaching of pediatrics surgery were given to **Giovanni Zurria**.

In 1937, a new pavilion with a unit of pediatric surgery was added to the Department of Pediatrics of the "*Policlinico Umberto I*" of Rome. In this institution, the first surgeon was **Sovena,** who, in 1939, performed 203 operations, including a neonate with duodenal atresia, who died during the post-operative period, and a neonate with a renal tumour who was one of the first neonates to survive after a nephro-ureterectomy; this patient died at the age of 64 years for a malignant tumor on the contralateral kidney (Fig. 8). In 1938, it was established in Genoa the "Children Hospital Giannina Gaslini", after a little girl who died of peritonitis. Her father, **Senator Gaslini**, decided to give to the Children Hospital his considerable heritage.

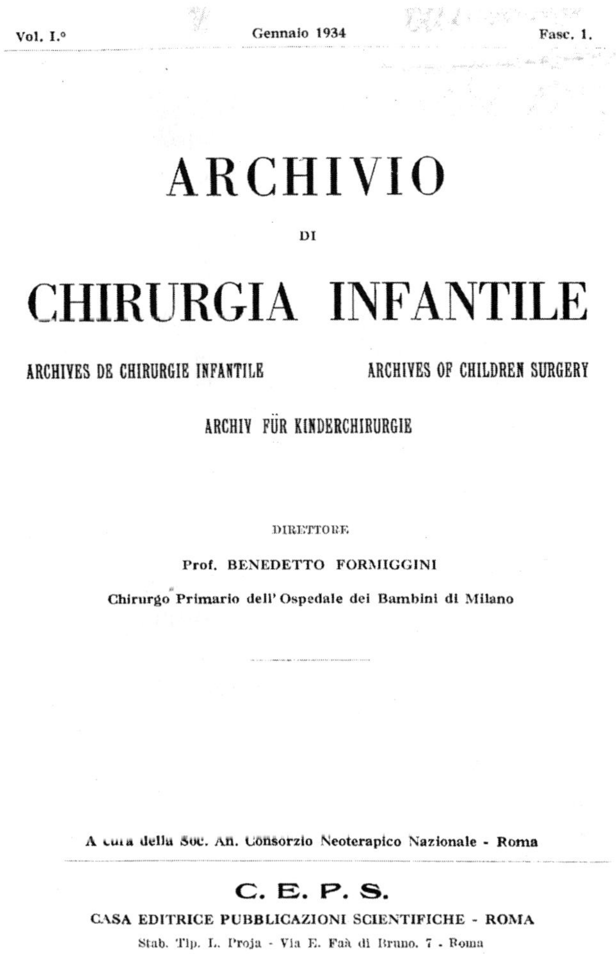

Vol. I.° Gennaio 1934 Fasc. 1.

ARCHIVIO

DI

CHIRURGIA INFANTILE

ARCHIVES DE CHIRURGIE INFANTILE ARCHIVES OF CHILDREN SURGERY

ARCHIV FÜR KINDERCHIRURGIE

DIRETTORE

Prof. BENEDETTO FORMIGGINI

Chirurgo Primario dell' Ospedale dei Bambini di Milano

A cura della Soc. An. Consorzio Neoterapico Nazionale - Roma

C. E. P. S.

CASA EDITRICE PUBBLICAZIONI SCIENTIFICHE - ROMA

Stab. Tip. L. Proja - Via E. Faà di Bruno, 7 - Roma

Fig. 6. The first Italian journal publishing only papers dealing with pediatric surgery (1934).

Furthermore, before the Second World War, other children's hospitals were established in Bologna, Livorno, Novara and Pavia. These institutions had beds for children with surgical problems.

In Italy, the second half of 20th century has seen dramatic progress in pediatric surgery, particularly in neonatal surgery. New procedures have been developed for conditions previously regarded

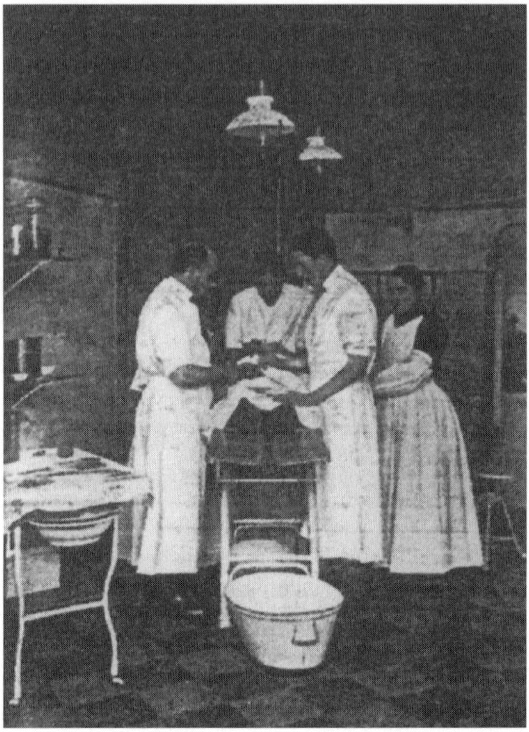

Fig. 7. Operation in progress, at the *Childrens Hospital Umberto I*; on the right the surgeon Artemio Magrassi (Brescia, 1900).

as inoperable. One of the best examples is esophageal atresia, which was considered the epitome of neonatal surgery. In our country, the first successful esophageal anastomosis in a neonate with esophageal atresia[10] was performed ten years after the first report by Cameron Haight. The surgeon was **Raffaele Paolucci**, professor of general surgery at the University of Rome *Policlinico Umberto I*. He was an excellent surgeon and was well known because he had been decorated during the First World War with a gold medal for sinking of the battleship "Viribus Unitis", flagship of Hapsbury Navy.

Many factors contributed to the development of pediatric surgery as a specialty on its own right. Several units of pediatric surgery were re-organized and other new units were established in many

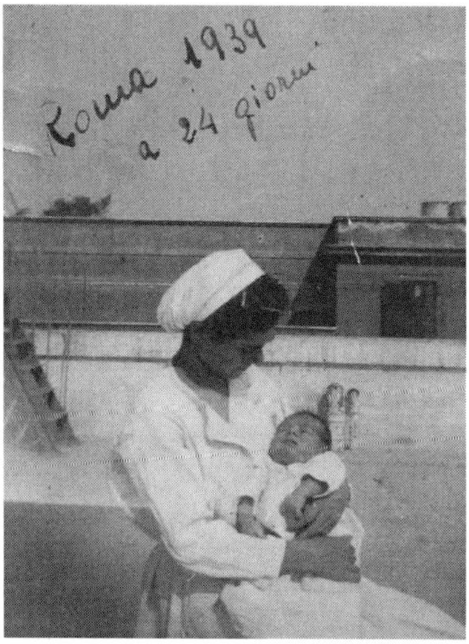

Fig. 8. Post-operative clinical photograph of the first neonate (23 days old) surviving a nephrectomy for renal neoplasia performed at the age of 16 days in 1939 at *Policlinico Umberto I* of Rome (courtesy of Mrs Anna Carluccio Pallotta).

cities throughout all the country, attesting an increasing awareness of the special problems in this field. In addition, the new generation of surgeons started to confine their work to paediatrics surgery. Their training included experience in qualified centers of pediatric surgery in Italy and abroad. A great help for trainees was the translation in Italian by **Carlo Alberto Montagnani** (Fig. 9) of the clinical book *The Surgery of Infancy and Childhood*, masterfully written by R. Gross, a super teacher. The excellent iconography of this book, the good results obtained in the large series of infants and children, induced many surgeons to believe that pediatric surgery had the dignity of a specialty.

Carlo was born in 1916 and studied medicine at the University of Modena. He graduated *cum laudae* in 1940. He trained in Capri and was then appointed an Associate Professor in the University of Florence. After 18 months as a Research Fellow at Harvard he returned to Florence in 1950 to the Department of Surgery, becoming an Assistant Professor in General Surgery and in Paediatric

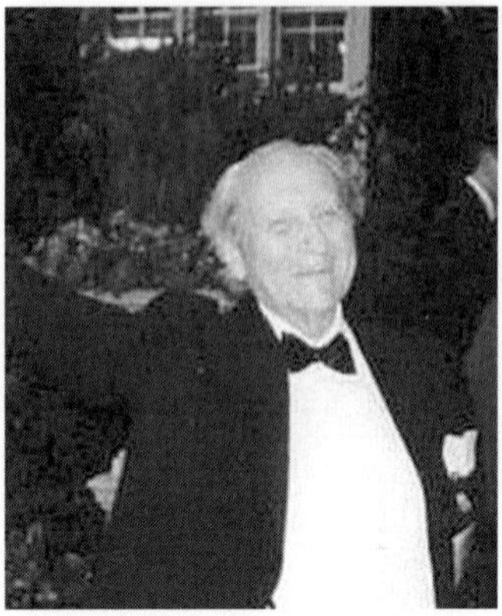

Fig. 9. Carlo Alberto Montagnani (1916–2006).

Surgery. In 1954 as a Senior Lecturer in Paediatric Surgery he was appointed as Chief of the Department of Paediatric Surgery at the Children's Hospital a. Meyer in Florence and appointed as Professor of Paediatric Surgery in the University Medical School.

During his 10 year period teaching he devoted himself entirely to paediatric surgery. Apart from his translation work, he also wrote extensively including on blood transfusion and published 65 papers in various medical journals (Italian, French and English). He also published monographs.[11]

In 1973 Carlo was appointed Head of the Department of Pediatric Surgery at the *Ospendale Nuovo Regina Margherita* in Rome where he worked until his retirement in 1980. He was the Overseas member of the Council of BAPS and Foreign Member of the German Asssociation of Pediatric Surgery. He attended and lectured in many national and international meetings and was a member of the Advisory Board of the *Journal of Pediatric Surgery* and was the President of the Italian Society of Paediatric Surgery. In 1977 he visited the Health Institutions of the States of Bahrain and Kuwait and delivered lectures. He was an offical visitor and gave advice on establishing a Department of Paediatric Surgery in Kuwait.

In 1955, for the first time in Italy Pediatric Surgery was included in those specialities recognized as a field for free teaching

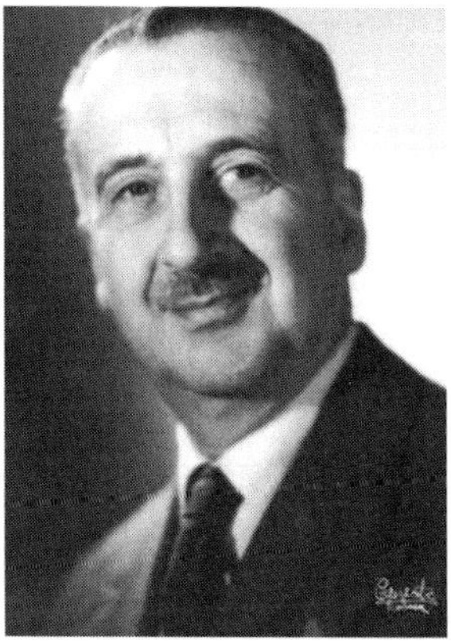

Fig. 10. Pasquale Romualdi (1899–1987).

("*Libera docenza*"), a title which was abolished in 1972. Another important step in the development of pediatric surgery was the foundation in 1959, by **Pasquale Romualdi** of the *Rivista Italiana di Chirurgia Pediatrica* which published paper regarding various topics of pediatric surgery (Fig. 10). A great contribution in the development of pediatric surgery was the foundation of the **Italian Society of Pediatric Surgery (SICP)** in Livorno on February 24, 1963. The aim was: "to promote the progress of the surgical art and science in the pediatric field, to make easier the exchange of ideas among pediatric surgeons, to defend the prestige and the interests of pediatric surgery lowers." The first President of SICP was **Pasquale Romualdi**. In the same year the first Italian SICP congress was organized by **Prof C. A. Montagnani** in Florence.

Born in Notaresco in 1899 Romualdi was a medical student in Rome when he was drafted into the First World war as and assistant surgeon in the military hospital. He was decorated for his work before returning to his studies and graduating in 1923. In 1938 he was appointed consultant paediatric surgeon and Chief at the Hospital "Bambino Gesù in Rome where he worked for more than 30 years, before retiring in 1970.

In 1959 he founded the journal *Rivista Italianaa di Chifurgia Pediatrica* which published papers on a range of pediatric surgical

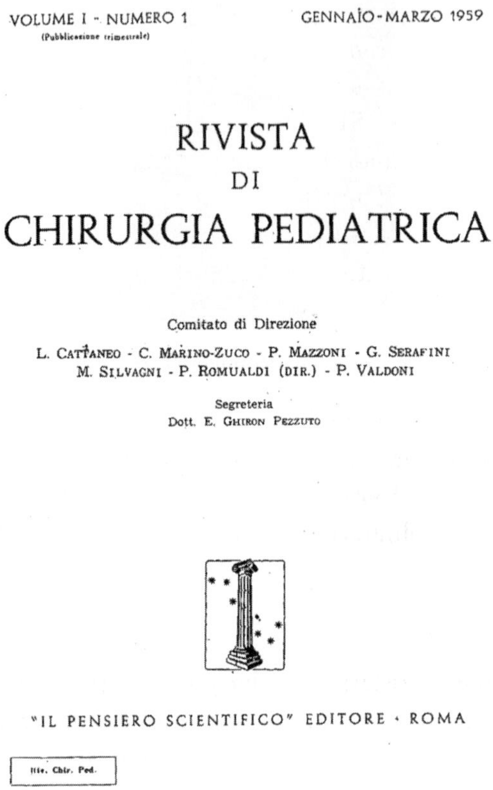

VOLUME I - NUMERO 1 GENNAIO-MARZO 1959
(Pubblicazione trimestrale)

RIVISTA
DI
CHIRURGIA PEDIATRICA

Comitato di Direzione
L. CATTANEO - C. MARINO-ZUCO - P. MAZZONI - G. SERAFINI
M. SILVAGNI - P. ROMUALDI (DIR.) - P. VALDONI

Segreteria
Dott. E. GHIRON PEZZUTO

"IL PENSIERO SCIENTIFICO" EDITORE - ROMA

Riv. Chir. Ped.

Fig. 11. The *Italian Journal of Pediatric Surgery* founded and edited by Pasquale Romualdi (1959).

topics. Romualdi was the first President of the Italian Society of Paediatric Surgery (1965–1967), and was an Honorary Member of National Societies of Spain, France, Germany and Argentina. He died in 1987.

In 1966 the establishment of the first Italian chair of pediatric surgery at Bologna University was a breakthrough in teaching and research. **Remigio Domini**, the inaugural professor brought a sense of excitement and enthusiasm through those areas. In 1992, the SICP decided to stop the publication of the *Italian Journal of Pediatric Surgery*. The *European Journal of Pediatric Surgery*, published in the English language, became the official journal of SICP.

At the present, the SICP has 241 members; the president is **Prof Aurelio Di Benedetto**, who organized in 2008 the 39th congress of the SICP. The venue of the congress was Catania. At the end of the 20th century, the Italian population was around 57,000,000 abitants. In Italy, at the present, there are 61 units of pediatric surgery.

Among the pioneers of Italian pediatric surgery, space permits mention of only a few: **Pasquale Romualdi** (Rome), **Franco Soave** (Genova), **Antonio Righini** (Livorno), **Carlo Alberto Montagnani** (Firenze), **Walter Galluzzi** (Trieste), **Lucio Parenzan** (Trieste, Bergamo), **Giovanni Verga** (Pavia), **Manlio Caucci** (Ancona) and **Remigio Domini** (Bologna).

Acknowledgments

We are very much grateful for the great help and precious information regarding the history of their institution to the following distinguished colleagues: Baraldini V., Canavese F., Corsello G., Di Benedetto A., Domini R., Martino A., La Grutta A., Parigi G.B., Romagnoli G., Schleef J., Seymandi P., Zamparini M. and Verga G.

References

1. Redbill SX. A history of Children's Hospitals. *Am J Dis Child* 1955; 90:411–416.
2. La storia del Meyer in 10 pagine. Vallechi grafiche. Firenze (e-mail: redazioneweb@meyer.it).
3. Mya G. Due osservazioni di dilatazione ed ipertrofia congenita del colon (megacolon congenito). *Lo sperimentale* 1894;48:215–231.
4. Martinelli V. *Dal Tevere al Gianicolo: l'Ospedale Bambino Gesù tra cronaca e storia*. Edizioni dell'Obelisco, Roma, 1980.

5. Jacobacci V. *Io Teresa Filangeri.* Marions Edizioni, Pompei, 2002.
6. Semprini A. *Origini e storia di un ospedale pediatrico. L'Ospedale dei bambini Umberto I di Brescia.* Editcom sas, Brescia, 2002.
7. Sironi AV, Taccone F. *I bambini e la cura. Storia dell'Ospedale dei bambini di Milano.* Editore La Terza, 2006.
8. Mazzoni Ascoli F, Coricelli S, Cardinali F. *Cent'anni d'amore. Le Patronesse del Salesi e L'Ospedaletto dei Bambini raccontati dai protagonisti.* Tecnostampa, Loreto, 2000.
9. La Grutta A, Corsello G. *Celebrazione del centenario della istruzione della Clinica pediatrica nell'Università di Palermo.* Tipografia Alba, Palermo, 2004.
10. Paolucci di VR, Bendondi G. Su due casi di atresia dell'esofago con fistola esofago-tracheale. *Rivista Clinica Pediatrica* 1952;50:509–528.
11. Montagani CA. The prognosis of oesophageal atresia, up to date results of surgical therapy. *Rivista Clinica Pediatr* 1956;58,157–189.

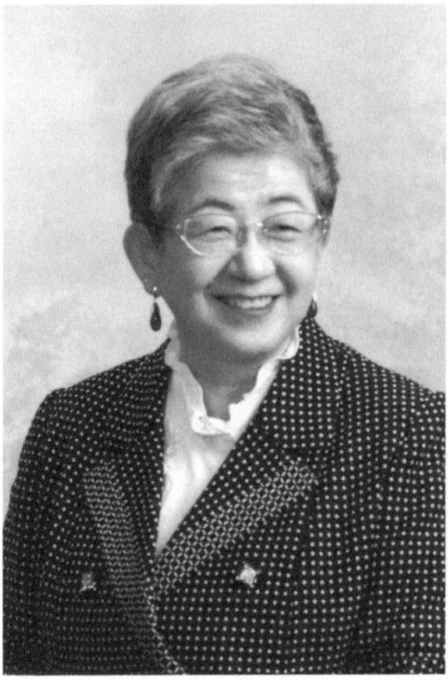

Sachiyo Suita

JAPAN

Sachiyo Suita

Before the Modern Era

Although the start of modern pediatric surgery in Japan was behind by nearly 50 years as compared to USA and European countries, interestingly, there has been several reports about congenital anomalies in Japan since the Edo era (Tokugawa Showgunate 1600–1867). Prof Teruho Kajimoto reported several collections about surgical treatment of congenital anomalies in the President lecture at the 34th Annual meeting of Japanese Association of Pediatric Surgery. For example:

1) Conjoined twins. In Japan, in 1825, as shown in Fig. 1, a conjoined twin body was found floating in the river, which was the first written case of conjoined twin in Japan. In 1926, the first successful separation of conjoined twin was performed for 36 day-old boys, however, one of them died of adhesive ileus later on.
2) Omphalocele and gastroschisis. The earliest report of a description for omphalocele was by Paré in 1634, and the earliest documentation of gastroschisis was by Calder in 1733. In 1887, a baby with exposed stomach and intestine was operated but died after operation, which was reported in the *Journal of Juntendo University Medical School.*
3) Anorectal malformations. Paulus Aegineta wrote that treatment was the rupture of an obstructing membrane with fingers or the point of a knife and the dilation of the track until healing was complete. This approach was used for many years and remained in vogue until the last century. In 1840, this operation

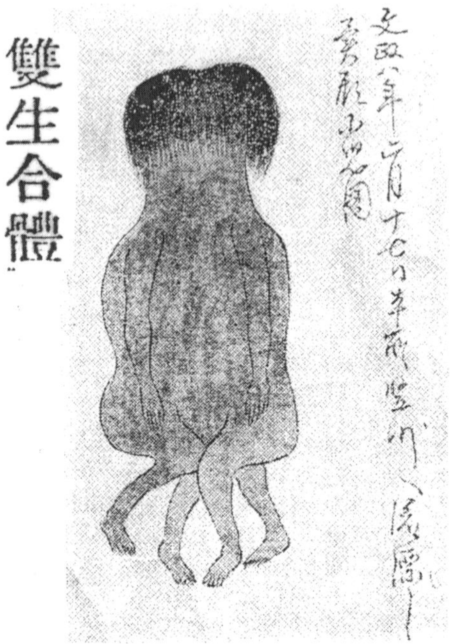

Fig. 1. The First Reported Case of Conjoined Twins.

was described in literature for surgery in Japan, as shown in Fig. 2, it shows the passage of meconium after surgery. Surprisingly, they called this type of disease as *Sako*, which means anal atresia in Japanese.

Then came the 20th century. In 1903, Akira Uno first used the term "pediatric surgery" in Japan and he emphasized that there were many kind of surgical disease during childhood and pediatric surgery was as necessary as adult surgery. Then in 1931, Fumito Honna described in the *Japanese Medical Journal* why there was neither pediatric surgeons nor a Department of Pediatric Surgery in Japan. He also said that there should be research work done in pediatric surgery. However, since then no account of pediatric surgery was mentioned in the Japanese journal, because Japan had rushed into war. The country and people needed only strong soldiers, and

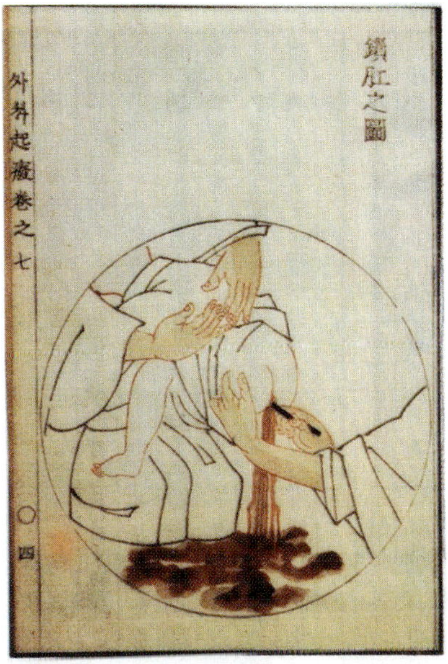

『外科起癈図譜』

Fig. 2. Operation for Anal Atresia.

there was no room for paying consideration for babies with congenital anomalies.

We, the pediatric surgeons in Japan, never forgot the year of 1941; that was the year of the beginning of World War II and also the year when Dr C. Haight in USA succeeded with the first primary anastomosis for a newborn baby with congenital esophageal atresia. Nearly 20 years have passed until the first successful operation of esophageal atresia for newborn baby was done in Japan by Prof Wakabayashi (Fig. 3) and Dr Ueda (Fig. 4).

Pediatric Surgery in Japan in the Early Days After World War II

Around 1950, almost all Japanese medical doctors did not know about pediatric surgery, particularly neonatal surgery, and the

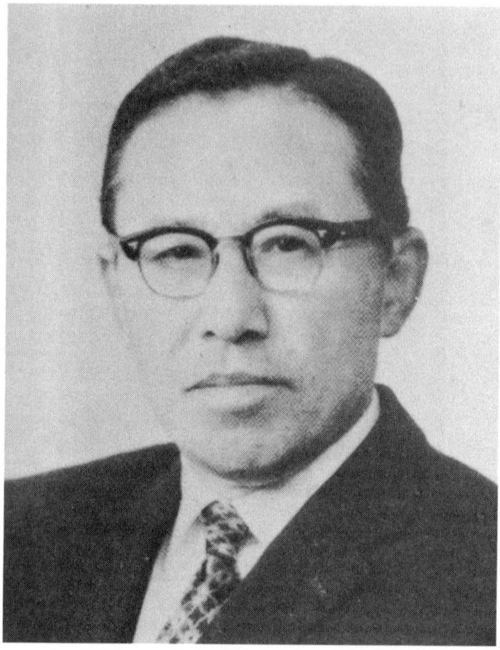

Fig. 3. Prof Wakabayashi.

leaders of Japanese medical society did not understand the importance of pediatric surgery. Many leaders of Japanese medical society thought that it would be better for them not to treat babies with congenital anomalies at all. Therefore, non-medical people, of course with far less understanding about pediatric surgery, and most parents, asked obstetricians or nurses to kill their children if their child was born with congenital anomalies. For example, when a baby was born with an omphalocele or gastroschisis, the obstetrician, at the request of the parents, would not give milk to the baby and leave the baby alone without putting the infant in the incubator, so that the baby would die due to low temperature and malnutrition.

However, several young surgeons could not tolerate or ignore such a miserable situation and they thought there should be some way to save such kind of babies. Fortunately after the World War II, which produced a tremendous variety of surgical specialties, an explosion of pediatric surgery occurred in many advanced countries,

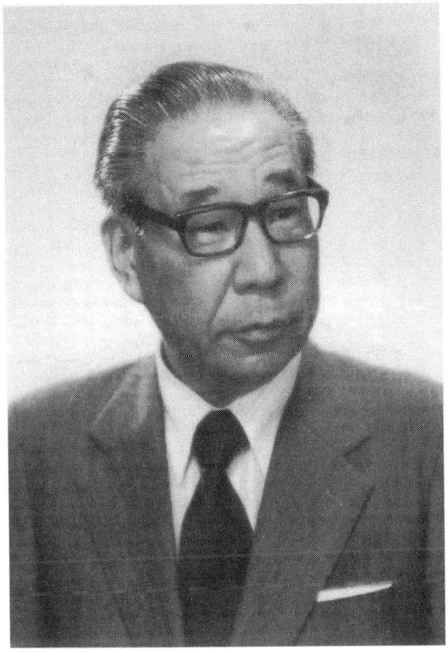

Fig. 4. Dr Ueda.

particularly in USA and European countries. At that time, Japan was under the occupation from USA and much new medical knowledge and techniques were imported from USA and it stimulated Japanese doctors very much.

Under these situations, there were several eminent persons who recognized the need of special area of surgery for children and made it possible to improve pediatric surgery in Japan. All of them were Professors of General Surgery; Prof Hiroshi Miyake of Kyushu University, Prof Komei Nakayama of Chiba University, Prof Tamotu Fukuda of Juntendo University and Prof Seiji Kimoto of Tokyo University. They encouraged their junior surgeons and gave them an opportunity to study about pediatric surgery.

Dr Keijiro Suruga (Fig. 5), who is well-known surgeon and a pioneer of Pediatric Surgery in Japan, was one of such junior surgeons. He operated on a newborn baby with intestinal atresia in 1953, which was the first case in Japan. In 1958, it was the first time a session

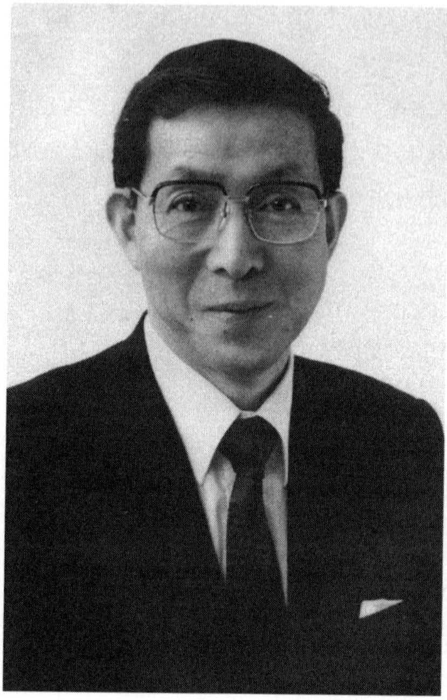

Fig. 5. Prof Suruga.

named Pediatric Surgery was held during the Annual Meeting of Japan Surgical Society under the presidency of Prof Miyake, Kyushu University at Fukuoka city. Then, as I have mentioned previously, in 1959 on almost the same day, the first two cases of successful operation of neonate with oesophageal atresia and tracheo-oesophageal fistula were reported by Dr Wakabayashi and his group at Nihon University and Dr Ueda and his group at Osaka University. This was sensational news and encouraged the doctors who had strong ambition for pediatric surgery.

In the fall in 1960, several doctors interested in pediatric surgery had a meeting to exchange information about pediatric surgery at Tokyo. Among them were not only surgeons who would be pediatric surgeons, but also pediatricians, obstetricians and anesthesiologists who know the importance of pediatric surgery. This meeting played a very important role in improving techniques and knowledge for surgical operations and/or post-operative management for children.

The pre-foundation meeting of the Japanese Society of Pediatric Surgeons (JSPS) was held in December 1963, and at last, in January 1964 the JSPS was founded. Prof Wakabayashi of Nihon University was elected as the first president of this society. In June 1964, the first annual meeting of JSPS was held at Tokyo and since then this meeting has been held annually. The number of members of the JSPS at the beginning were 1041 including surgeons, pediatricians, obstetricians, urologists and orthopedic surgeons who all had interest in pediatric surgery. For the first meeting, 161 papers were accepted and the Presidential address and 6 teaching lectures, 2 symposiums and 4 small group discussions were presented. Also in that year, the *Journal of Pediatric Surgery* in Japanese was published; initially the frequency was four times a year but has since increased to seven times a year. Since then pediatric surgery in Japan has developed with extraordinary speed. There have been many difficulties and obstructions, but these have been speedily overcome with tremendous passion.

Pediatric Surgery in Japan in the Growing Era

In 1965, the first national Children's Hospital was opened in Tokyo as a symbol of congratulations for the marriage of Crown Prince Akihito and Princess Michiko, who are now Emperor and Empress of Japan. There is an epoch making story for opening of this hospital. In 1963, Prof Kimoto of Tokyo University and Dr Suruga of San-Ikukai hospital at that time, invited Prof Sulamaa from Finland to operate a baby with short arms, which was recognized as a side-effect of medical drug thalidomaide. This became very sensational news in Japan and also made a very big impact for many people, including the Japanese government, in realizing the importance of pediatric surgery and necessity of a independent hospital for children. Then, the Committee to found the children's hospital was made by the Japanese Government and at last the National Children's Hospital was opened in 1965.

This Children's Hospital had many departments including pediatric surgery and this was indeed a red-letter day in the history of pediatric surgery in Japan. This hospital played a very important role for progress of pediatric surgery in Japan. In 1969 in Osaka, and in 1970 in Kanagawa prefecture, children's hospitals were opened. Since then a total of 18 children's hospitals were opened in Japan, which made good progress in pediatric surgery. Along with this, in 1968 the first independent Department of Pediatric Surgery was opened at Juntendo University, but it took nearly ten more years to open the independent Department of Pediatric Surgery in National University, first opened at Kyushu University in 1979 by the strong efforts of many people including Prof Kiyoshi Inokuchi and Dr Keiichi Ikeda. Since then pediatric surgery had recognition and several universities, both National and Private Universities opened independent departments of pediatric surgery. An enormous amount of excellent research and clinical work has been done.

It is impossible here to mention all the names of the outstanding men who have been responsible for this remarkable development. I shall talk about three of them, not only because they are my long-standing mentors, but because I believe that they have taken a major part in developing Japanese pediatric surgery: **Prof Keijiro Suruga, Prof Morio Kasai** and **Dr Takashi Ueda**.

Prof Suruga graduated from Tokyo University in 1944. As I have mentioned previously, he is the one of young surgeons who realized the importance of pediatric surgery while he was working at San-Ikukai Hospital, which was located in the down town in Tokyo. After the World War II many babies were born at that hospital. Among them there were lots of anomalies needing the care of pediatric surgery. He worked very hard not only for medical side to improve knowledge and techniques of pediatric surgery, but also he worked very hard to have friendship in the world. He attended many meetings all over the world and carried the message of advancement of pediatric surgery to many colleagues in all parts of the world. He contributed to make the independent department of pediatric surgery in many Universities in Japan and also contributed to open Children's Hospital in Zambia collaborated with JICA. He also played very important role to establish JAPS, PAPS (Pacific Association of Pediatric Surgeons),

AAPS (Asian Association of Pediatric Surgeons) and WoFAPS (World Federation of Associations of Pediatric Surgery). A long-time member of editorial board of *Journal of Pediatric Surgery*, he is still a Consultant Editor of that journal. As a pioneer and father of pediatric surgery in Japan, it is hoped that his explosive energy and vast experience will continue to be used for the benefit of his patients and young surgeons.

Prof Morio Kasai (Fig. 6) graduated from Tohoku University in 1947. Although he stayed as a professor of general surgery during his academic life he studied pediatric surgery at Philadelphia Children's Hospital and he worked very hard to establish the identity of pediatric surgery in Japan. He trained many young pediatric surgeons not only in Japan but he also accepted many young surgeons from overseas. His work on biliary atresia has been one of the great advances in the last century. He went to many countries to teach his operative procedure (Kasai Operation) for biliary atresia. Also he

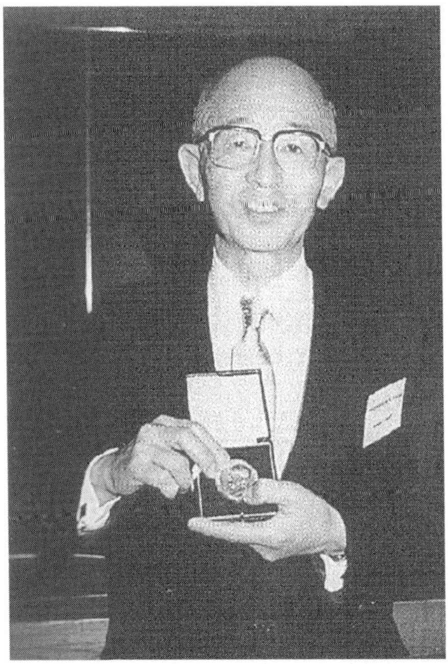

Fig. 6. Prof Kasai with Ladd Medal.

worked hard to develop pediatric oncology in Japan. He and his colleagues made a useful pathological classification of hepatoblastoma. His contribution for pediatric surgery was rewarded through his receipt of the Ladd Medal from APSA, Denis Browne Medal from BAPS and Coe medal from PAPS.

Takashi Ueda (1916–1995) graduated from Osaka University in 1941 and he gradually became interested in pediatric surgery when he met a baby with omphalocele, left on the table without any medical care or newborn care until the end of baby's life. His enthusiasm to learn pediatric surgery brought him to Chicago to work for Dr Orvar Swenson in 1962. After his return to Osaka, he worked energetically to develop pediatric surgery in Japan along with other pioneers Profs Morio Kasai and Keijiro Suruga. He trained many students to become excellent pediatric surgeons in Japan. One of them is Dr Eizo Okamoto. They studied the histology of the embryonic alimentary tract, and described the embryonic intramural ganglion migration theory that brought light to the etiology of Hirschsprung's disease.

The progress of Pediatric Surgery in Japan has been contributed to by overseas pediatric surgeons. Particularly we would like to thank two surgeons: Prof E. C. Koop (USA) and the late Mr P. P. Rickham (UK), who made tremendous efforts for the development of pediatric surgery in Japan. **Prof Koop** visited Japan as the first overseas pediatric surgeon in 1961 and travelled several places lecturing about neonatal surgery in USA. This encouraged and stimulated many young Japanese surgeons. Since then he has visited Japan several times and whenever he came to Japan, he delivered many new messages to us.

Mr Rickham was invited as the guest to the 4th Annual meeting of JSPS held in Hiroshima in 1967. He lectured on "Massive small intestinal resection in the newborn infants," showing the long-term survival with using an intravenous feeding including lipid emulsions. His lecture gave a tremendous culture shock to Japanese Pediatric Surgeons who all had trouble with babies with short bowel syndrome after massive small intestinal resection. He also trained young

Japanese surgeons at his hospital: Drs Suita, Ikeda and Miyano, who all contributed later on to pediatric surgery in Japan.

Also many world famous pediatric surgeons from USA and European countries came as guest speakers at the Annual Congress in Japan, as shown in Table 1. Scientific exchanges made us aware of the backward gap from the world level and encourage us in many different fields of pediatric surgery. We tried all hard to catch up. Many young surgeons went to overseas to learn pediatric surgery. For example, Los Angels Children's Hospital, Philadelphia Children's Hospital, Chicago Children's Hospital in USA, Bremen in Germany, Paris in France, Liverpool and Glasgow in UK and Dublin in Ireland were the main places which gave many young Japanese pediatric surgeons the opportunity both in clinical work and research.

We also recognized that without the development of pediatric anesthesiology, pediatric surgery would never have gotten off the ground. As a pioneer of pediatric anesthesia, we can name Prof Seizou Iwai of Kobe University and Prof Mitsuko Satoyoshi of Juntendo University; both were trained at Los Angeles Children's Hospital, USA and established independent specialty later who worked with Prof Keijiro Suruga for long time (Fig. 7).

The Role and Contribution of JSPS to Other Countries and Associations

The aims of JSPS are to set a standard medical care for children and to popularize them to all surgeons. Included were:

1) National survey of neonatal surgery every five years, which helped to improve neonatal surgery in Japan. At the beginning in 1964 the mortality rate of main neonatal surgery, such as omphalocele, etc. was over 70%, which gradually decreased, and the latest rate in 2003 was 12% on average.
2) Training five-day seminars once a year to educate pediatric surgeons. Both senior and junior pediatric surgeons at least 7 years after graduation were allowed to attend, where the discussions

Table 1. List of president and guests of Annual meeting of JSPS.

No.	Year	President	Oversea Guest Speaker	Title
1	1964	Osamu Wakabayashi		
2	1965	Tamotsu Fukuda		
3	1966	Jiro Mikami	W.H. Snyder, Jr.	The Embryology and Pathology of the Intestinal Tract
4	1967	Ryouichi Uemura	PP. Rickham	Massive small bowel resection for neonate
			LI. Mark	Alterations in pulse rate during anesthesia in children
5	1968	Takeo Hayashida	AH. Bill, Jr.	Studies of the mechanism of regression of human neuroblastoma
6	1969	Eisuke Hamaguchi	von W. Hasse	Diagnostik und Therapie der kindlichen Zwerchfell und Hiatushernia
7	1970	Morio Kasai	DG. Young	Congenital diaphragmatic hernia in the newborn
8	1971	Takashi Ueda	JH. Fisher	Pediatric surgery in the United States
				Pitfalls in the management of Hirschsprung's disease
9	1972	Kiyoto Shibata		
10	1973	Kiyoshi Inokuchi	ED. Smith	Anorectal anomalies
			DM. Hays	Surgery in the management of lymphoma in childhood
11	1974	Masanobu Ishida	JH. Louw	The pathogenesis and management of intestinal atresia
12	1975	Keijiro Suruga	NA. Myers	Unusual problems in the surgery of the oesophagus in childhood
			WH. Hung	Experience in the treatment for Hirschsprung's disease
13	1976	Kenji Honda	SL. Gans	Pediatric endoscopy

(*Continued*)

Table 1. (*Continued*)

No.	Year	President	Oversea Guest Speaker	Title
14	1977	Sakae Asada	AW. Conn	Unknown
			RM. Filler	Unknown
15	1978	Hisao Manabe	J. Lister	The surgeon, the child and the welfare state
			AR. Castaneda	Corrective open heart surgery in infancy
16	1979	Kiichi Muto	MM. Woolley	Management of infant which ambiguous external genitalia
			ET. Bole	Wilms' tumor — 1979
17	1980	Hiroshi Akiyama	JJ. Dowes	Techniques of airway management for upper airway obstruction in infants and children
			EW. Fonkalsrud	New approaches to the management of gastroesophageal reflux in childhood: Experience with 175 children
18	1981	Yoichi Kasai	S. Gans	Methods and application of laparoscopy in infants and children
			L. Helson	Basic chemotherapy for neuroblastoma and maturation in tumor cell
			DM. Hays	Recent results of the treatment on neuroblastoma in USA

(*Continued*)

Table 1. (*Continued*)

No.	Year	President	Oversea Guest Speaker	Title
19	1982	Ken Morita	C-c. Cheng	An antireflux spur valve in Roux-Y anastomosis
			AG. Coran	Preoperative and postoperative care of premature infant
			JG. Raffensperger	Anorecral anomalies in the female
20	1983	Keiichi Ikeda	WG. Williams	Cardiovascular surgery in neonates and infants
20	1983	Keiichi Ikeda	TG. Chisholm	Extrophy of the urinary bladder
			JL. Grosfeld	Management of solid tumors in infancy and childhood, The Indiana experience
21	1984	Sumio Saito	JB. Beckwith	Recent results from National Wilms Tumor Study
			JJ. Corkery	The surgical treatment of congenital anomalies vesicoureteral junction
22	1985	Keizo Katsumata	WH. Hendren	Management of cloacal malformation
			PK. Donahoe	The contributions of Japanese surgeons to the understanding of Mullerian inhibiting substance, its role in intersex abnormalities and development as an antitumor agent
23	1986	Hiromichi Yano	JC. Molenaar	Etiology and diagnosis of innervationrelated motility disorders of the gut
			AJ. Haller	Pediatric trauma — The most lethal disease of childhood
			WK. Kim	A short history of pediatric surgery in Korea

(*Continued*)

Table 1. (*Continued*)

No.	Year	President	Oversea Guest Speaker	Title
24	1987	Eizo Okamoto	LW. Martin	Aganglionosis involving more than total colon
			A. Pena	Management of anorectal malformation
25	1988	Akio Tsunoda	DG. Johnson	Excellence in search of recognition: The struggle for pediatric surgery subspeciality certification in North America
			WI. Norwood	Reconstructive surgical management of hypoplastic left heart syndrome
26	1989	Hideyo Takahashi	EK. Motoyama	Pathophysiology of congenital diaphragmatic hernia
27	1990	Shigeru Kimura	DM. Behrendt	Pediatric heart transplantation
			JB. Otte	Liver transplantation in children
			RJ. Andrassy	Protecting the Gut and enhancing immune response
			DG.Young	Necrotizing enterocolitis
28	1991	Takahiro Ito	D. Kluth	Applied embryology for pediatric surgeons
			MZ. Schwartz	Small intestine transplantation; past, present and future
			MR. Harrison	Prenatal diagnosis and treatment
29	1992	Junichi Uchino	K. Kimura	米国から見た日本の小児外科の現状と将来
			AH. Bill	The unique aspects of pediatric surgery
			Y. Iwaki	組織適合性抗原よりみた移植の手術適応
			AJ. Demetris	Pathology of non-rejection complications of liver allografts

(*Continued*)

Table 1. (*Continued*)

No.	Year	President	Oversea Guest Speaker	Title
			S. Todo	小腸移植ー実験から臨床へ
			J. Valayer	Liver transplantation for treatment of biliary atresia
			JC. Emond	Living related liver transplantation
			L. Helson	Childhood cancer update
			JL. Grosfeld	Role of surgery in pediatric cancer
			JE. Haas	Clinicopathological progress in hepatic tumors of children
30	1993	Yasuaki Naito	TL. Spray	Pediatric lung transplantation: Indication, techniques and early results
			JA. O'Neill, Jr.	Studies on pathophysiology of necrotizing enterocolitis (NEC) and related clinical implications
			SG. Haworth	Pulmonary vascular disease: Evolution, clinical problem and resolution
31	1994	Takuji Totani	FM. Guttman	New challenges in the treatment of inflammatory bowel disease in pediatric surgery
			SW. Beasley	Oesophageal atresia the melbourne experience
32	1995	Yoshiaki Tsuchida	H. Nikaidoh	Neonatal heart surgery in the era of ECMO
			GM. Haase	Recent progress in pediatric solid tumors: A surgical perspective from the children's cancer group
			A. Pena	Advances in the management of anorectal malformation

(*Continued*)

Table 1. (*Continued*)

No.	Year	President	Oversea Guest Speaker	Title
33	1996	Akira Okada	J. Dent	Oesophageal motor function in children
			DA. Lloyd	Energy expenditure in the surgical newborn infant
			AG. Coran	The surgical management of ulcerative colitis, familial polyposis and total colonic aganglionosis in infants and children
			GL. Klein	Parenteral nutrition-associated metabolic bone disease: Old problems and new considerations
34	1997	Makoto Iwabuchi	TE. Lobe	Endoscopic surgery and children
			RM. Filler	Congenital tracheal anomalies
			JB. Atkinson	Current concepts in surgical treatment of neuroblastoma
35	1998	Teruho Kajimoto	SH. von Kap-herr	Personal results and comments based on experiences in anorectal anomalies
			RW. Strong	The many facets of partial liver transplantation
36	1999	Ryuji Ohi	MR. Harrison	The development of minimally invasive fetoscopic surgery: FETENDO
			TR. Karl	Surgery for transposition of the great arteries
			KE. Georgeson	The influence of laparoscopy on the management of pediatric colorectal disorders
37	2000	Sachiyo Suita	AF. Scharli	Further experience with intestinal innervation disorders
			J. Boix-Ochoa	Gastro-oesophageal reflux in pediatrics: State of art

(*Continued*)

Table 1. (*Continued*)

No.	Year	President	Oversea Guest Speaker	Title
			S. Stylianos	Current issues and controversies in pediatric abdominal trauma: The need for evidence-based guidelines
			JD. Goldberg	Perinatal management of women undergoing fetal surgery
38	2001	Morihiro Saeki	FD. Stephens	The embryogenesis of A-R (ano-rectal), VATER and OEIS deformations
			AG. Tzakis	Evolution of gastrointestinal transplantation at the University of Miami
			E-H. Hwang	The 25 years experience of pediatric surgery in a single institute in Korea
39	2002	Takeshi Miyano	AG. Coran	Vaginal reconstruction for ambiguous genitalia and congenital absence of the vagina: A twenty-seven year experience
			P. Puri	Pulmonary vasculature in congenital diaphragmatic hernia
			K. Kimura	Operations I have developed
			JL. Grosfeld	The impact of genetic and biological alterations in the management of pediatric solid tumors
40	2003	Naomi Iwai	AM. Holschneider	Complications following posterior sagittal approach — PSARP

(*Continued*)

Table 1. (*Continued*)

No.	Year	President	Oversea Guest Speaker	Title
			A. Kaminski	Esophageal substitution with interposed intestinal segment
			T. Wester	Notable postnatal alterations in the myenteric plexus of normal human bowel
			SH. Choi	Proper treatment of megacolon after various anoplasties for anorectal malformation
			BM. Ure	Impact of minimally invasive techniques on pediatric surgery
			SNC. Buyukunal	Do MAVIS and dorsal dartos patch procedure improves the complication rates and side effects of mathieu procedure?
			PD. Losty	Recent advances in congenital diaphragmatic hernia
			MD. Stringer	Minimizing surgical morbidity in pediatric cadaveric liver transplantation
			Y. Gac	Minimally invasive repair of pectus excavatum. a single institution's experience
41	2004	Yoji Imamura	R. Lange	Reconstruction of the right ventricular outflow tract with allografts and xenografts
			P. Puri	Altered distribution of interstitial cells of Cajal in motility disorders

(*Continued*)

Table 1. *(Continued)*

No.	Year	President	Oversea Guest Speaker	Title
			KP. Lally	Modern outcomes for infants with congenital diaphragmatic hernia
			TE. Lobe	The use of robotics in clinical pediatric surgery
			DL. Sigalet	Novel hormonal therapy for pediatric short bowel syndrome
			J. Reyes	Rabbit anti-thymocyte (rATG) preconditioning and induction for pediatric intestinal transplantation
42	2005	Naomi Ohnuma	J. Plaschkes	The changing but continued role of surgery in the management of liver tumours hepatoblastoma (HB) and hepatocellular carcinoma (HCC) in children and adolescents in the light of new results from the SIOPEL studies — past experience and future perspectives
			G. Martucciello	Hirschsprung's disease and intestinal neuronal dysplasia
			J-Y. Lai	Bladder auto-augmentation using biodegradable polymer seeded with autologous smooth muscle cells in a rabbit model
			J-N. Lin	From minimal, limited, to maximal posterior sagittal anorectoplasty

(Continued)

Table 1. (*Continued*)

No.	Year	President	Oversea Guest Speaker	Title
			D. Arsic	Evidence for the role of sonic hedgehog in foregut and hindgut development
			C-LS. Lin	The role of macrophage migration inhibitory factor (MIF) in necrotizing enterocolitis and neuroblastoma
42	2005	Naomi Ohnuma	SM. Ahn	The clinical relevance of the survivin expression and the loss of heterozygosity in neuroblastoma
43	2006	Tetsuo Kato		
44	2007	Yasuhide Morikawa	PK. Donahoe	Research in clinical care in pediatric surgery
			HM. Young	Pathophysiology and treatment of hirschsprung's disease — neural crest stem cell biology and its therapeutic potential
			KH. Tam	Hirschsprung's disease: New insights in pathophysiology and therapy
			HB. Kim	The 2005 report from the international STEP data registry: Indications, efficacy and complications — a good first step
			T. Kato	Current issues on pediatric intestinal and multivisceral transplantation
			AT. Hadidi	Surgery for ambiguous genitalia

(*Continued*)

Table 1. (*Continued*)

No.	Year	President	Oversea Guest Speaker	Title
			C-L. Chen	Pediatric living donor liver transplantation
			D. Fauza	Fetal tissue engineering from amniotic fluid progenitor cells
			DK. Gupta	Surgical management of children with advanced neuroblastoma
			DC. Aronson	Recurrence of chest wall tumors
45	2008	Michio Kaneko	M. Yanagisawa	Endothelin and hirschsprung's disease — its discovery and the expansion of successive research-

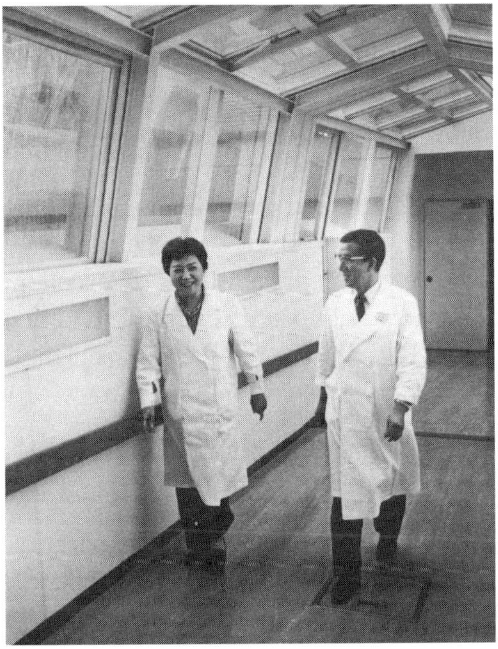

Fig. 7. Prof Mituko Satoyoshi with Prof Suruga.

revolve around pediatric surgery. It started in 1967 and lasted until 1985 when it was thought to finish the purpose of the beginning and subsequently changed to two-day course for junior surgeons who take the Board examination for Specialist of Pediatric Surgery.

3) Autumn symposium. Once a year we gathered to discuss one subject in depth.
4) In 1972, JSPS was allowed to be a member of Japanese Association of Medicine, and in 1978 all pediatric surgeons were allowed to be named Pediatric Surgeons independently from General Surgery.
5) In 1979, specialist systems were started in all medical areas. We are considered board certified pediatric surgeons after having passed the examination.
6) International activation. As I have mentioned previously, we have invited world famous pediatric surgeons to the annual

meeting of JSPS. Now we also invite several young pediatric surgeons from Asian countries who can attend the meeting and exchange ideas to promote knowledge on all pediatric surgical problems and/or techniques.

We, Japanese pediatric surgeons are actively working for International meetings of PAPS, BAPS, APSA, AAPS and WOFAPS not only for attending and presenting our excellent research and clinical works, but also we hosted several times for these meetings with great success (Fig. 8); We have organized the PAPS meeting five times, AAPS three times and one meeting with WOFAPS.

Generation Changes and the Future

Nearly 50 years have passed since pediatric surgery was started in Japan. Many of the first generation of pediatric surgeons have passed away and pediatric surgeons belonging to second and third

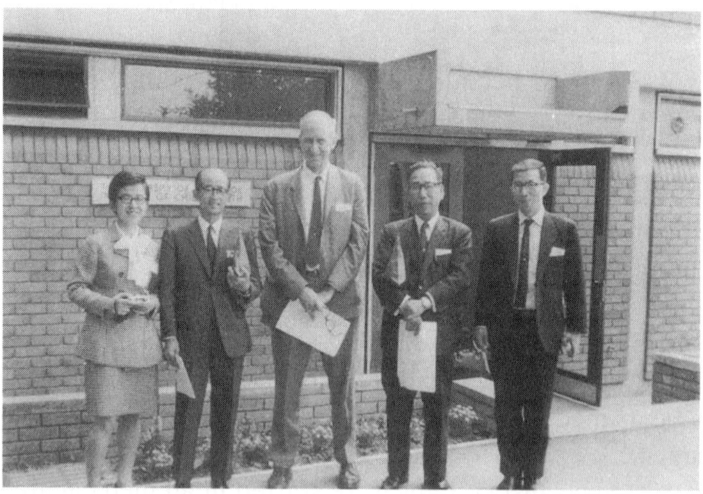

Fig. 8. Dr Suita, Prof Kasai, Prof Bill, Dr Ueda and Prof Suruga at the Institute of Child Health, Liverpool in 1968 during the 15th BAPS Meeting. (Suita was an SHO with Mr Rickham at that time).

generation are retired, or almost so, from active clinical work. We all miss Prof Yoshiaki Tsuchida (1936–2005) and Prof Akira Okada (1938–2007). Prof Tsuchida contributed research works on pediatric oncology, particularly neuroblastoma. He was a leader of nationwide Japanese study of advanced neuroblastoma. Prof Okada devoted his life to nutritional management and research, particularly intravenous nutrition, and without this method we can not save newborn babies with multiple anomalies. Now in Japan the 4th generation of pediatric surgeon is coming up. Also new subjects are emerging such as high technology in molecular medicine and genetic levels are developing. The rapid development of the organ specialties has increased and minimal access approach is becoming a standard method in surgery.

Manpower is decreasing. We have to keep a eye carefully on what direction that may go and will give advice when it may be necessary.

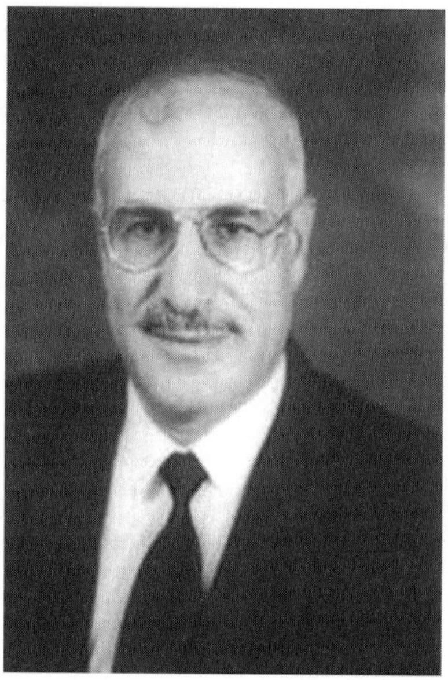

Hayel J. Al-Ejeilat

JORDAN

Hayel J. Al-Ejeilat

Introduction

Jordan health in a glance. Jordan is a small country with a population of 5.6 million, as reported in 2006. The birth rate is 29/1000, the average family size is 5.4 with an infant mortality rate of 22/1000, as published by the Ministry of Health 2006.

The health services are divided between the following sectors:

1) **The Ministry of Health**
   It offers free primary health care for all Jordanians, and its hospitals (4235 beds) offer secondary and tertiary care for about 39.8% of the population through insuring all government employees and their dependants. Its main referral hospital is Al Bashir hospital (650 beds) in Amman, and quite recently Prince Hamza hospital (450 beds).
2) **The Royal Medical Services (RMS)**
   It is the medical service of the Jordan Armed Forces. It offers health care for about 25.5% of the population (1.43 million). It provides secondary and tertiary care services through many hospitals (2119 beds), the main hospital of which being **King Hussein Medical Center (KHMC)**. It caters for the armed forces' personnel and their dependants, police and intelligence forces and their dependants, MPs, ministers, and foreign diplomats. It also provides insurance for certain groups like the Royal Jordanian Airline personnel and their dependants. KHMC serves as a referral hospital in all sub-specialties for all local as well as foreign patients.

3) **The private sector of medical services**
It serves a good percentage of the population (26.9%) and it caters for the privately insured and non-insured personnel working in the private sector. It also provides insurance for certain categories of government employees. It serves a good number of patients coming from various neighboring Arab countries seeking medical advice.
4) **Jordan University Medical School** with its hospital (JUH), and the **Jordan University of Science and Technology** with its hospital (KAH). They both serve about 7.8% of the population through insuring all university staff and their dependants, and providing secondary and tertiary care for the referred patients from the government and private sector.

Health Sector	No. of Hospitals	Number of beds	%
Ministry of Health	20	4235	38.3
Jordan University Hospital (JUH)	1	531	4.8
King Abduallah Hospital (KAH)	1	457	4.1
Royal Medical Services (RMS)	11	2119	19.2
Private Sector	58	3707	33.6

Source: Ministry of Health Website (www.moh.gov.jo).

Care for children. Each of the above-mentioned services has its own pediatric department. Jordan had its first children hospital in the 1960's when it was part of the Ministry of Health. It served for a few years before it was shifted to the central government hospital (Al Bashir) as a pediatric department. In 1995, a 110-bed children hospital was built by the Ministry of Health in the north of Jordan-Irbid (Princess Rahmah Hospital). In 2006, the Royal Medical Services (RMS) started building a 200-bed children hospital at the KHMC premises and is due to open in 2008. Pediatric medicine is well-established in these departments since the early 1960's, but pediatric surgery was not a recognized specialty in those days. Surgery on babies and children was an individual interest under the different surgical sub-specialties until the 1970's. There were no trained pediatric surgeons or surgical baby units. Well-trained adult thoracic surgeons offered reasonable expertise in handling cases like TEF and diaphragmatic hernias with limited successes and high mortality. Trained plastic surgeons offered reasonable help to babies within their domain.

Development of Pediatric Surgery

It was not until 1979 that pediatric surgery as a distinct specialty was known in Jordan, and that was in the KHMC. Before, two hesitant attempts were seen but could not develop properly:

1) The first was **Dr A. Haddadin**, a senior surgeon in the Ministry of Health, who developed a genuine interest in pediatric surgery, and spent a year training in Sheffield, UK, 1970–1971. Upon his return to Jordan, he worked in Al-Bashir hospital, but found great difficulty in establishing a unit there, so he moved to Jordan University Hospital (then Amman Hospital) and stayed for about six months. Again he had to leave from frustration to the private sector (1973) where the medical services at the time where very primitive, and he settled down doing mainly general surgery.
2) The second attempt was by **Dr N. Ajlouni**, a member of the RMS who was sent on a scholarship to Great Ormond Street (G.O.S) hospital (UK) in 1972 to do pediatric surgery for one year. A few months after his return to Jordan, he was satisfied to join the plastic surgery team as, according to him, he found it very difficult to get any cooperation from the various surgical sub-specialties in the RMS to refer cases to him.

Pediatric Surgery at RMS, the Difficult Birth

I feel it is worth going through the details of the painful process of birth of pediatric surgery as I experienced it in the Royal Medical

Services and in Jordan, since it is now almost 27 years since its inception and the new generations of pediatric surgeons are entitled to know the various facts of that birth.

I developed my interest in pediatric surgery through my work as a specialist surgeon in Zarka Military Hospital (1973–1974). In September 1974, I was sent on a scholarship to the United Kingdom. I spent the period until September 1976 between Edinburgh Children Hospital and Glasgow Children Hospital, with two very short periods in Manchester and Great Ormond Street (G.O.S) children hospitals. I came back by the end of September 1976 and was assigned to do pediatric surgery at KHMC. The director of the RMS at that time, General Dawood Hanania, asked me to write a full report on how to implement pediatric surgery, as he was very interested and encouraging. Soon after, the head of Surgery department at KHMC called for a meeting that gathered all heads of surgical sub-specialties and myself. In that meeting, I was asked to define pediatric surgery, and how I envisage the implementation should be; I described the status applied in UK children hospitals and the type of cases that a pediatric surgeon should be dealing with, including all congenital malformations of the genito-urinary, thoracic, plastic, and GI tracts, excluding cardiac, orthopedic and neurosurgery. The reaction to this definition was absurd, as all my surgical colleagues in the meeting refused to give way to any case and asked me to do only general pediatric surgery (??). When I asked them to define what general pediatric surgery meant to them, nothing apart from a hernia, an appendix and an occasional thyroid was outside their interest. It was a very heated discussion that ended nowhere. I finally asked to have a clinic tagged as Pediatric Surgery Clinic, but even this was denied, as it meant to them referring all surgical cases below 13 years of age to this clinic. The meeting ended without any decision. The following day, I was told that I had been transferred to a district hospital, Marka Military Hospital. I insisted on seeing the director of the RMS, who told me that all the surgeons came to him after the meeting and asked that I should do my pediatric surgery somewhere else. He had to see for their demands and transfer me; that was a military order that I had to obey.

I stayed between October 1976 till October 1977 in Marka Military Hospital as a general and pediatric surgeon. I was on my own and could establish a small two-bed baby unit. I was able to solve a good deal of the major pediatric surgical problems. I even started getting referred problems from KHMC. By the time I felt things were going well, I was astonished that another military order of transferring me to a very far district hospital in the south of Jordan, Aqaba Military Hospital, was issued. It came to me like a shock, but I had no choice; I even had to take a six-month old baby with an esophagostomy and gastrostomy, whose parents had left in the unit, refusing to take "a handicapped child" home. I took him with me to Aqaba hospital where, two months later, I gave him a colon conduit; that was when the family came asking for their boy and named him after me. I stayed in Aqaba Hospital until July 1978. I did the same as in Marka Military Hospital until another military order was issued to transfer me back to KHMC. I was very furious until I met the head of surgery there, who told me that the director of the RMS wanted me to establish a pediatric surgery unit, and this had to be at KHMC. Having sensed the support of the directorate, I insisted on having a pediatric surgery clinic and a surgical baby unit. This was granted to me, but I was asked to give up the surgery on spina bifida and its sequels, and cleft lip and palate surgery. I had to compromise, and that was when things started heading up in the right direction. I elected to cover calls for all babies below two years of age on my own and share calls with my general surgical colleagues for children above two years of age. I had to cover general and pediatric surgery at the beginning, as the load was not enough.

The start was relatively slow, and it took until October 1979 (more than one year) until the patient load became big enough to force me to abandon general surgery, with an O/R waiting list of two months.

This achievement could not have been reached without the extra effort that I had to do trying to convince colleagues around me that I can offer a better care and better results:

1) I worked all the time in the baby unit as a doctor and a nurse, teaching nurses and supervising work very closely. This reflected itself on the marked improvement of survival of those surgical newborns. This attitude no doubt had taken too much of my social life, but then those babies were the challenge of my present and future.
2) As always, a few incidents happened in the management of some babies and children by other colleagues (complications) that triggered the change and the referral of all those babies to pediatric surgery. I never hesitated in accepting to take over the management of those complications and the case as a whole. This finally phased out the surgery on those babies and children completely to be in the hands of pediatric surgery.

By October 1979, the great change in the quality of care and results of surgery was quite evident. The head of surgery, then, **Dr G. Shubailat**, called me and informed me that the directorate had decided to establish a separate sub-specialty in surgery named Pediatric Surgery, and that I was assigned head of this sub-specialty. This was a great step forward, as it marked the beginning of the development of pediatric surgery as a specialty, not only in the Royal Medical Services but in the whole of Jordan. It gave me the chance to:

- have separate equipment order;
- have fellows to train and assist in the department;
- have more beds in the baby unit and the pediatric ward; and
- send nurses to get training outside Jordan.

The first fellow to join the newly-formed specialty was **Dr M. Omari** (an American Board graduate in general surgery) from June 1980 to July 1982, after which he was sent to Texas

Children Hospital for 18 months. He was followed by **Dr N. Hamati** (F.R.C.S General Surgery from UK) from 1983 till 1985, after which he was sent to Glasgow Children Hospital for one year. He was followed by **Dr B. Samawi**, who is currently the chairman of the pediatric surgery section at KHMC after the three of us had retired.

Development of Pediatric Surgery in Jordan

The pediatric surgery department at KHMC was the nucleus and the only department in Jordan until 1985. By February 1982, the Jordan Medical Council was born, where its main duty was to supervise training and certify medical trainees in various specialties. We could enforce the adoption of pediatric surgery as a recognized sub-specialty in Jordan and set the standard for training and certification in this specialty. A board of pediatric surgery was given to candidates who:

- had spent four years training in general surgery;
- had spent two years training in pediatric surgery, one of which has to be in a center with a neonatal surgical unit, where the qualified center for training has to have two consultant pediatric surgeons as a minimum requirement; and
- Passed a board examination in pediatric surgery.

This encouraged fellows from the government sector to join the pediatric surgery department at KHMC for training and get their board exam. Foreign examiners from various Arab and European countries assisted in these exams and in the evaluation of the training program at KHMC. Until 1991, all pediatric surgeons, whether trained locally or outside Jordan, had to sit for the Jordan Board of Pediatric Surgery exam. After that, the board exam was limited to the locally trained surgeons, and surgeons trained outside Jordan have to satisfy the training requirement as put by the counsel without the need to sit for the exam, provided their certificate was taken following passing an exam in the training country.

By 1986, the Jordan Association of Pediatric Surgeons was established, with twelve members.

The Royal Medical Services. Pediatric surgery at RMS continued to grow both in beds and staff, and in 1996, another unit of pediatric surgery was established at Queen Alia Hospital (Amman), with two full-time consultant pediatric surgeons. In 2006, three more units were established: one in the north of Jordan (Irbid), one in the south (Karak), and one in Zarqa Military Hospitals. These units are covered by part-time pediatric surgeons from KHMC. At present, the number of pediatric surgeons at KHMC is eight consultants and two fellows. The great expansion of the pediatric surgical service at the RMS required the planning of a national children hospital, which is a 200-bed hospital now being built at the KHMC premises and is due to open early 2008.

Jordan University. In 1985, the Jordan University Hospital assigned a colleague pediatric surgeon — Dr M. Haddad, a graduate of Birmingham, UK. He stayed for three years trying hard to establish a unit, but he finally elected to move to Saudia Arabia and later to the UK. This continued until 1998, with pediatric surgeons joining the university and leaving after one to two years, until Dr M. Omari, who had retired from the army and went to Saudia Arabia, came back and joined the university in 1998. He has now established a unit with two consultant pediatric surgeons.

The Jordan University of Science and Technology. The university assigned a full-time Iraqi pediatric surgeon in 1991. Six years later (1997), she was joined by a Jordanian pediatric surgeon trained in Australia, and a small unit was established there. The Iraqi pediatric surgeon left back to Iraq in 2001 and another Jordanian pediatric surgeon, a graduate of Australia, joined the university's newly-built hospital (King Abdulla Hospital) in 2002. The unit continued working with two consultant pediatric surgeons until four year later, when one of them left permanently to Australia, and the unit was run by one full-time pediatric surgeon and two part-time surgeons from the

Jordan University Hospital. By the end of 2006, the unit lost its full-time surgeon to the private sector, and is now run only by the two part-time pediatric surgeons from Jordan University.

The Government Sector (Ministry of Health). The government sector attracted two pediatric surgeons trained in Greece in 1982. One of them was assigned at Al Bashir Hospital (**Dr S. Ayyoub**) and the other in a district hospital in Zarqa (**Dr J. Nimri**). Both worked as general and pediatric surgeons. By 1985, another pediatric surgeon, trained in UK (**Dr H. Jadid**), joined Al Bashir hospital, where a unit was finally established with two consultant pediatric surgeons. A few fellows joined the unit for training and had part of their training at KHMC as well. The unit is still running at Al Bashir Hospital with two consultant pediatric surgeons, and another unit has been recently established in the newly-built Prince Hamza Hospital (2006) with two full-time consultant pediatric surgeons.

In Zarqa Hospital, a small unit was established in 1984 with one consultant pediatric surgeon. By 1987, he moved to the private sector and another colleague, graduate of Spain, joined the unit in 1988 until he also moved to the private sector four years later (1992), leaving the hospital without any pediatric surgical service up till now. Pediatric surgical cases are referred to Al Bashir or Prince Hamza hospitals in Amman.

In the north of Jordan (Irbid), Princess Rahmah Children Hospital (PRCH) was built in 1995 (110 beds) and is being covered by a full-time pediatric surgeon. A good unit has been established there and is quite active in the management of various pediatric surgical cases.

The Private Sector. **Dr A. Haddadin** has been working in the private sector as a general and pediatric surgeon since 1973. In 1978, two more pediatric surgeons joined the sector, one as a full-time surgeon at the Islamic hospital (**Dr S. Hammoudi**) and one resigned from Zarqa government hospital. In 1988, I retired from the army and joined the Jordan University of Science and Technology for a very short period, and later joined the private sector, helping my three colleagues who were working before me in this sector to establish a decent pediatric surgical service. In the 1990s, a good number of well-equipped and staffed hospitals were built in the sector that attracted a good number of pediatric surgeons, most of whom retired from the army and government services, as well as the bypassers who joined the university for short periods. We have now 13 pediatric surgeons in this sector.

Today, in Jordan, we have 30 pediatric surgeons, covering all the health sectors. Ten of those had their basic training outside Jordan.

Number of pediatric surgeons in Jordan (2006)

Royal Medical Services	10
Government:	
Al Bashir Hospital	2
Prince Hamza Hospital	2
Princess Rahmah Hospital	1
Jordan University H	2
Private Sector	13
Total	30

Impact of the Development of Pediatric Surgery on Children's Health in Jordan

Effect on survival of the surgical neonate. Until the late 1970s, the survival of the surgical newborn was very low, and the main survivors were the anorectal anomalies with their high incontinence rate, and the occasional esophageal atresia, who was lucky to fall in the hands of a well-trained thoracic surgeon. The main reason beside the lack of trained pediatric surgeons was the lack of trained anesthesiologists, as well as the lack of trained nurses and baby units who could care for these babies. By 1978, the first trained anesthesiologist in pediatric surgery, **Dr M. Kilani** (a member of the royal medical services), who got a special training in pediatric anesthesia at G.O.S hospital (UK) came back to the KHMC and was able to influence and train a good number of fellow anesthesiologists. He is now retired to the private sector and is a good help there as well. This was reflected markedly on the operative survival of those neonates. The development of well-equipped surgical baby units, supported by well-trained neonatologists and nurses at KHMC, the Jordan University, as well as three units in the private sector (the Islamic, the Specialty and the Jordan Hospitals) has also significantly influenced the survivals of those newborns.

Effect on early diagnosis

1) Hirschsprung's disease: In the 70s and early 80s, we used to see cases of HD presenting quite late in childhood with full classical picture of malnourished, distended belly patients. Since the development of pediatric surgery, the diagnosis of HD is mostly done in the neonatal period and early infancy. Very occasionally, we see patients beyond two years of age.
2) Biliary atresia: the first successful Kasai operation was done in Jordan in May 1980. He is now 27 years old and leading a normal life. Before that, biliary atresia patients were doomed to die, especially because liver transplant was not a feasible option at that time. We do have now a good number of patients with Kasai porto-enterostomy who are now adolescents or in their twenties, leading relatively normal lives. An exception is one patient who started having problems of recurrent cholangitis at the age of 13 and continued to do so in spite of intussusception of his Roux-en-y loop. His liver continued to deteriorate and he finally required liver transplant donated by his mother when he was age 21 (last year), and has been doing well since.
3) Esophageal atresia patients and upper GI atresia, as well as diaphragmatic hernias, are now diagnosed mostly antenatally, and their prompt management has affected markedly their survival. I still recall cases of esophageal atresia that I had to operate upon intants at age 12–14 days, and cases of diaphragmatic hernias presenting as late as one year with recurrent chest infection. They evidently survived, basically because of nature selection.
4) In 1986, the first trained pediatric radiologist came back to Jordan (**Dr Y. Al Khairi**), who had spent one year of special

training at G.O.S hospital (UK) and was able to influence the development of a pediatric radiology section at KHMC. Before that, we used not only to do the conventional radiological procedures ourselves, but also to interpret them. When he retired to the private sector, he was a great help there as well.

5) Laparoscopic surgery is now becoming an established method in the management of various diseases in pediatric surgery, and KHMC is becoming a training center for this.
6) Jordan is now becoming a regional referral center to handle and solve most major pediatric surgical problems, and we do get a good number of cases referred from the neighboring Arab countries.

In Jordan nowadays, we see a good number of congenital malformations (as shown in the following graph) which keeps all those numbers of pediatric surgeons relatively busy.

Number of Congenital Malformations Seen in Jordan (2006)

	Gov. sector			Private			
	ABH	PRCH	RMS	sector	JUH	KAH	Total
TEF	15	3	13	15	12	1	**59**
Diaph. H	5	1	8	19	5	2	**40**
HD	9	4	7	23	13	7	**63**
Exomph.	6	2	4	13	5	1	**31**
Small Bowel Atresia	7	3	11	23	15	3	**62**
Ectopia Vesice	—	1	3	5	2	—	**11**
Anorectal Anomaly	10	7	15	38	11	5	**68**
Biliary Atresia	7	1	3	4	3	1	**19**

Conclusion

In spite of the difficulties encountered at the beginning, the development of pediatric surgery in Jordan took its course and made great achievements in the care of surgical babies, and definitely reduced markedly the neonatal mortality. But being a small country with limited resources, it took us longer than expected to even establish a pediatric hospital. Several attempts to build a pediatric hospital were made, but they stopped at the design phase as there was no financial support to continue. As it appeared, without the support and encouragement of the Royal Medical Services with its main center KHMC, pediatric surgery could have still been stumbling. He is hoped that the building of a new well-equipped and staffed pediatric hospital at KHMC premises will provide solutions for most of the remaining deficiencies that we still have to overcome in pediatric surgery in Jordan:

1) the establishment of an ECMO service;
2) the establishment of an intrauterine surgical service;
3) the establishment of a pediatric transplant service; and
4) the establishment of a research facility.

Acknowledgments

I would like to thank all my pediatric surgical colleagues for their valuable help in sharing information and providing accurate numbers and figures of their work in pediatric surgery during the year 2006.

I would also like to thank all the hospitals and institutions who allowed me to access their record system and get the needed information.

References

1. Jordan Medical Council. Rules and regulations, 1999.
2. Royal Medical Services. Annual statistical report, 2005.
3. Health Insurance Department. Ministry of Health statistical report, 2006.
4. Ministry of Health website. www.moh.gov.jo
5. KHMC operating room record book.
6. Jordan University computer department.

7. King Abdullah Hospital operating room record book.
8. Al Bashir hospital operating room record book.
9. Personal communication with all pediatric surgeons in the private sector.
10. Princess Rahmah Hospital computer department.

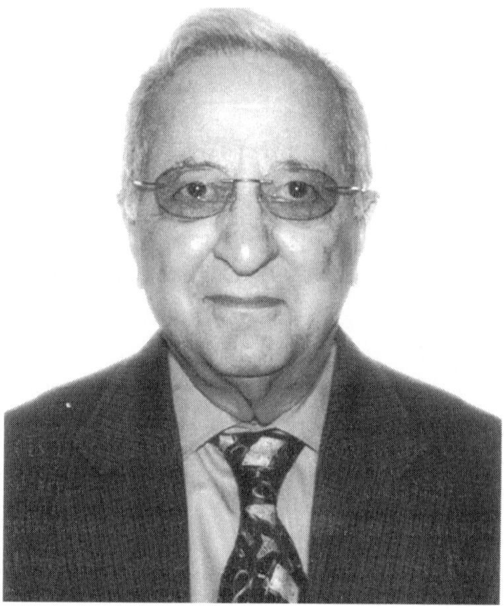

Michel S. Slim

LEBANON

Michel S. Slim

The inception and growth of Surgical Pediatrics (SP) in Lebanon in 1959 are closely related to regional events during the following period: the political turmoil to which Lebanon was repeatedly exposed since its full independence in the mid-forties, and the impetus that the American University of Beirut (AUB) had locally since its creation in 1866. A brief account of these variables would indicate the challenges that the specialty SP had to face during its development.

Lebanon is a relatively small country along the coast of the Mediterranean sea having a surface area of 10,452 square kilometers, with a wonderful ridge of mountains in its background that serve as a summer resort and for sports activities. It has a population of about 3.8 million, of which 90% are literate, and has been a haven for refugees whose number reach about 10% of its natives. Lebanon has been considered as the Switzerland of the Middle East (ME) and, in peaceful times, has been the center of tourism and a bridge between the Western World and the ME Eighteen religious denominations are represented in it. In 1975, it suffered from a civil war that lasted 15 years. Some have referred to this as the "war of others on Lebanese soil". The strife resulted in 170,000 dead and 300,000 wounded. Many people fled abroad, including some of the intelligentsia. The Lebanese diaspora is estimated at present to reach 12 million people. By virtue of the number and proximity of the casualties during the war, the University Hospitals were converted into battle field and front-line units. A total of 270 children were admitted as casualties to the American University of Beirut Medical

Center between 1975 and 1986, of whom 70% had penetrating injuries, with an overall mortality rate of 4.8%.[1] The hospitals witnessed a change in their staffing and a deficiency in their equipment and supplies. The pediatric surgeons had to care for the injured of all ages (whereas the accepted upper age limit is 15 years) when their colleagues in adult medicine were not available. These circumstances led them to introduce innovative techniques to their surgical armamentarium, that included primary repair of splenic and colorectal injuries, successful repair of penetrating cardio-vascular injuries without the use of the heart-lung machine, pancreatic preservation after repair of complex injuries to the retroperitoneal structures, and the exclusive use of non-hemic solutions to prime the heart-lung machine.[2–7] Since the tragic death of Mr Rafic Hariri, the Prime Minister of Lebanon, and some of his staff in February 2005, the country has gone through political and economical instability that has affected the medical community at large and led some pediatric surgeons to leave Lebanon seeking job opportunities elsewhere.

The AUB, founded in 1866 by a protestant missionary from Vermont (US), has become the symbol of American civic values of freedom, tolerance and democracy. The University grants its degrees under the authority of the Regents of the University of New York State. In 1945, Dr J. J. McDonald was recruited from NY as the Chairman of the Department of Surgery and introduced at the AUB the concept of residency training to replace the previous tutorship, a change which was adopted eventually by other local departments and regional universities. During the last three-quarters of a century, five other medical schools came into existence in Lebanon and are listed in chronological order of their establishment: Universite St Joseph, the Lebanese University, the Arab University, the Balamant University, and the Lebanese American University. During the "civil war" the academic performance at the university level was challenged by hospital staff escaping because of security reasons, by assassinations and kidnappings of university administrators and educators and by threats regarding student grades and admissions to Medical Schools.[8] The first full-time pediatric surgeon to start practicing in Lebanon was Dr Henry Mishalany (AUB–MD 1951) in 1959 after he completed his training in Montreal (Canada). For security reasons, he emigrated to the US in 1976.

In January 1963, Dr Michel Slim (AUB–MD 1954), returning from his training in Pittsburgh (USA) with two surgical Specialty Board certificates, joined the Medical Staff at AUB as the Director of a newly created Division of SP and was also appointed as an active member of the Division of Cardio-Thoracic (CT) Surgery. The introduction of SP and pediatric cardiac surgery as new specialties in Lebanon was a time-consuming affair. The operative results confirmed the value of a team approach in the management of complex congenital anomalies,[9,10] thus utilizing the expertise of different specialists. The pediatricians and their colleagues in adult surgery were eventually convinced of the role and need for SP to serve the community. These efforts paved the way for other pediatric surgeons, mainly trained in France, to join forces in Lebanon. They were: Dr George Korkomaz, Dr Sami Kyriakos, Dr Edmond Azzi, and Dr Nicolas Nini. Some of these surgeons included Pediatric Urology in their practices, depending on the type of training they had received. The introduction in 1964 of the program of outpatient inguinal hernia repair on children was a novelty and an oddity to the local practitioners, but proved to be useful to all concerned and strengthened the residency training admirably.[11] This program was implemented because of the increasing number of patients on the waiting list for surgery and the limited space that was available for them on the in-patient service. During the "civil war", Dr Slim was also assigned the directorship of the Division of C T Surgery at AUB and took care of training new perfusionists to run the heart-lung machine, who replaced those that had fled to the USA.

In 1975, Dr Slim organized the first SP Symposium in Lebanon as part of the Middle East Medical Assembly (MEMA), which was an annual event that started in 1951, sponsored by the AUB and its Alumni Association, and that acted as a forum for the exchange of knowledge among the medical scientists. There were guest speakers from the UK, Sweden, Turkey and Lebanon who contributed to the programme, a half-day Symposium.

In 1977, under the leadership of Dr Slim, the Lebanese pediatric surgeons and those associated with SP on a part-time basis agreed to form a Surgical Section as part of the Lebanese Pediatric Society (LPS), comparable to what was founded in 1948 with the American Academy of Pediatrics. The Section then applied for membership to the World Association of Pediatric Surgeons. This move was supported by Prof James Lister, the Secretary-Treasurer of the WOFPSA, and its application was accepted to the three-year old Federation, making Lebanon the first member from the ME In 1992, the Surgical Section was substituted by an independent Lebanese Society of Pediatric Surgeons (LSPS). Initially, the LSPS had 13 full-time members and functioned under the aegis of the Lebanese Order of Physicians. The Presidents of the LSPS are listed here in sequential order: Dr Sami Kyriakos, Dr George Korkomaz, Dr Edmond Azzi, Dr Samir Akel, Dr Paul Daher, Dr Nabil Daoud, and Dr Sleiman Gebran. The Society organized successfully three international Scientific Congresses that were held in Beirut in November 1996, November 1998, and November 2000. These were well attended by regional and international participants.

Special credit goes to the British Association of Pediatric Surgeons (BAPS) that helped to foster friendship and links among pediatric surgeons globally. In July 1985, during the BAPS annual meeting in Vienna, Dr Hayel Ejeilat (Jordan) was delegated by 23 Arab pediatric surgeons attending the Congress to draft the Constitution of a new Arab Association of Pediatric Surgeons (AAPS) and organize the first Congress of the AAPS in Amman. This took place on October 9, 1986 and was very well received internationally. The Surgical Section of the LPS was instrumental in the formation of the AAPS and in the preparation of its Congress. The history of the AAPS is recorded in another chapter of this book.

Dr Slim's connection with the BAPS membership made him an ideal candidate as an overseas member on its Council between 1982 and 1985. In addition, the impact of SP in Lebanon and the

ME had led him to be invited in 1985 as an Honorary Lecturer to the Jordanian Surgical Society, to the Turkish Association of Pediatric Surgeons (TAPS) and to participate in a postgraduate Course in Pediatric Surgery in Lisbon (Portugal).

An Arab Board of Medical Specialists is presently available and requires the SP candidate to train for six years after the MD diploma, and succeed in the written, oral and clinical skills exams before being certified as a pediatric surgeon.

An attrition in the number of the "first generation" of pediatric surgeons practicing in Lebanon occurred during the last 40 years:

1) Dr N. Nini died tragically in a car accident in North Lebanon after having successfully practiced in Tripoli.
2) Dr H. Mishalany emigrated to the US in 1976, and joined the Professorial Staff at the Children's Hospital in Los Angeles. He died in 1991 after a car accident.
3) Dr M. Slim left in the summer of 1986 for a "sabbatical leave", that was extended in NY till he retired in September 2006. He was succeeded at the AUB by Dr S. Akel, who had formal training in SP in the United Kingdom, where he also obtained his FRCS Diploma. During his stay in the US, Dr Slim served as the Director of SP and Pediatric Trauma at New York Medical College/Westchester Medical Center.
4) Dr G. Korkomaz, after having served as the Chief of Pediatric Surgery at Hotel Dieu Hospital (Beirut), passed away in 2006 after a chronic illness.

In summary, in the early fifties, less than one hundred pediatric surgeons existed in the world. At present in Lebanon, 42 pediatric surgeons are registered in the Lebanese Order of Physicians serving a population of over four million with a birth rate of 20/1000 people, with children less than 15 years of age accounting for about 27% of the population. The majority of the Lebanese pediatric surgeons have been trained in Europe, predominately in France.

The concept of establishing a Children's Hospital Medical Center in Lebanon was discussed on several occasions since 1982 with a proposal submitted to different influential and interested Lebanese officials and professionals, but has not received a favorable response. Ideally, such an Institution would collectively be a Center for service, education and research related to health issues in the pediatric population not only in Lebanon but also in the whole Middle East.

It is hoped that Lebanon will soon rise like the historical phoenix so that the Land of Cedars and its Medical Community will shine and excel again.

Acknowledgment

The author thanks Dr S. Akel for his critical review of the manuscript and for the valuable information that he provided regarding the changes in the Lebanese arena since 1986 that affected the course of development of SP in Lebanon. Special thanks are also owed to Ms Julie Slim Nassif for her constructive remarks on the contents and format of the manuscript.

References

1. Slim MS, Her C, Akel SR *et al.* Factors affecting survival of children after abdominal trauma in Lebanese civil war. *Pediatr Surg Internat* 1990;5:188–191.
2. Slim MS. Penetrating injuries of the heart and the great vessels. *Middle East J Anesthesiol* 1978;5:77–84.
3. Slim MS, Najjar NE, Mishalany HG. Preservation of the injured. *Spleen Br J Surg* 1979;66:671–672.
4. Nasser MG, Tahmizian BA, Slim MS. Appraisal of nonhemic prime with hypothermia in open-heart surgery. *Middle East J Anesthesiol* 1979;5:235–247.
5. Slim MS, Makaroun M, Shamma A. Primary repair of colorectal injuries in childhood. *J Pediatr Surg* 1983;16:1008–1011.
6. Slim MS, Srouji MN, Sankari M, Georgio B. A bizarre case of penetrating trauma. *Pediatr Surg Int* 1986;1:252–253.

7. Slim MS, Jaraki KM, Dajani OM. Sphincter-preserving procedure for penetrating pancreato-duodenal-biliary injury in a child. *Ped Cerrahi dergisi* 1989;3:117–121.
8. Slim MS. Cardiac surgery — Challenges and surprises in a country at war. *Middle East J Anesthesiol* 12:37–47.
9. Slim MS. Congenital cardiovascular lesions in childhood (Personal experience with 116 operated cases). *Jordan Med J* 1978;13:6–20.
10. Slim MS, Dajani OM, Hatem J *et al.* Tetralogy of fallot (A report of an experience with total repair of 72 consecutive patients). *Jordan Med J* 1986;21:179–190.
11. Slim MS, Mishalany HG. Outpatient inguinal herniorrhaphy in childhood. *Br J Clin Med* 1971;25:223–225.

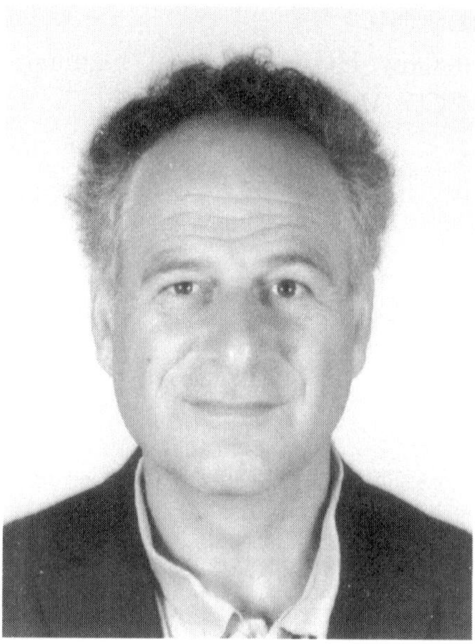

Daniel C. Aronson

NETHERLANDS

Daniel C. Aronson

The Hospitals (1860–1920)

Until well into the 19th century, in most European countries children were treated in the same hospitals and by the same doctors and surgeons, as adults. The first children's hospital in Europe, the *Hôpital des Enfants Malades*, was founded in Paris in 1802, the second in Berlin in 1829, and the third in Leningrad in 1843, but it would take until 1863 for children's hospitals to be opened in The Netherlands.

In the Netherlands, as in all other European countries, the 19th century saw a huge working class that lived under terrible social conditions. Poverty, lack of work and income, poor hygiene, bad housing, and for many a difficult life on the streets. Around 1850, the average life expectancy for a male newborn was 24 years, and for a female infant 30 years. The rich that fell ill were treated at home by visiting physicians, the poor were put in hospitals under sometimes devastating conditions. Children were treated the same way as adults, though sometimes they might be put in an orphanage, or brought to houses in rural areas to be fed and brought into a better physical condition. The aristocracy and the well-to-do bourgeois middle class slowly started to realise that this situation was unacceptable, and some individuals in various cities started initiatives to collect money for a change of care of the poor in general, and more specifically for the care of children.

In 1863, the first Children's Hospital was founded in Rotterdam by Hendrik Willem de Monchy (1830–1905) and Jan van der Hoeven

(1834–1900), two of those individuals who felt that something had to change in the medical care of children of the poor.[1] The Children's Hospital opened on August 12, 1863 in a first floor apartment in the city centre with eight beds in two rooms. Three years later, the children's hospital moved to villa Belvédère which had a large garden, was situated on the outskirts of the city and increased its bed capacity to 16 and later 18. In 1870 it was named after Queen Sophia, the first wife of King Willem III of the Netherlands. The surgeon and co-founder Van der Hoeven, who worked at the Coolsingel Hospital, operated on the children at the Sophia Children's from 1863 to 1890, being succeeded by his son Jan van der Hoeven Jr. who practised as a volunteer surgeon at the children's hospital until 1906. He was further succeeded by C. D. van Rossem who was occasionally substituted by P. Fockens. The latter published the first successful surgical treatment of a child with a small bowel atresia in 1911.[2] In 1913, a second surgeon, H. J. Bouvé was appointed to manage the outpatient clinic, but it would take until 1920, and the appointment of H. A. Jagerink in succession to van Rossem, before both surgeons would start to work together as a team, rather than separately.

In 1865, the second Children's Hospital was founded in Amsterdam by the general practitioner Samuel de Ranitz (1834–1913), who was deeply moved by the terrible social circumstances of the working class.[3] It opened its doors to the first six children on May 1 that year, in the old "English Orphanage" in the city centre, and moved in 1872 to a new location on the edge of the city, overlooking the pastures. In 1899, it was named the Emma Children's Hospital after Queen Emma, the second wife of King Willem III (Figs. 1–4). Prof C. B. Tilanus and his son Prof J. W. R. Tilanus Jr. from the University Hospital "Binnengasthuis", and later Prof J. A. Korteweg and Prof C. L. Wurfbein from that same hospital visited the Children's Hospital to operate on the children as volunteer surgeons. In 1889, Hendrik Timmer was appointed on the basis that he received his surgical training from Prof Korteweg and father and son Tilanus.[4] Timmer proceeded to modernise the surgical unit of the Children's Hospital, introducing chloroform anaesthesia and the disinfection

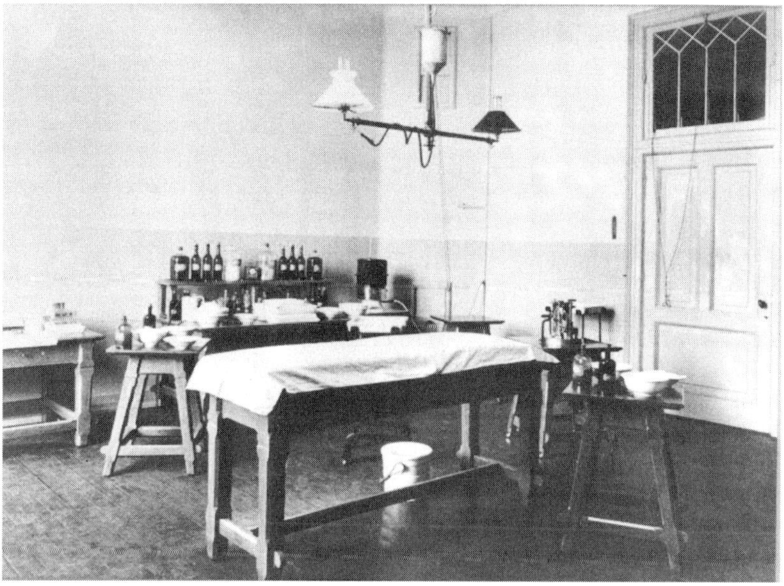

Fig. 1. Emma Children's Operating Room.

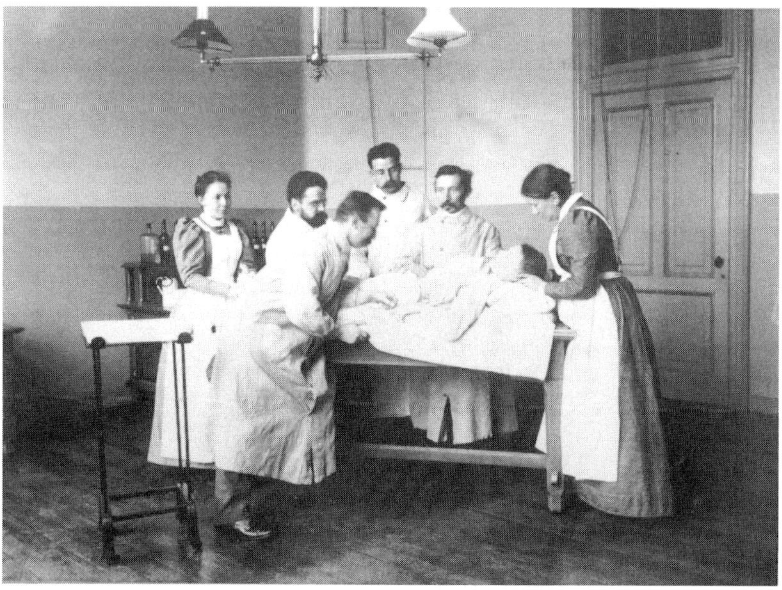

Fig. 2. Emma Children's Operating Room in Action.

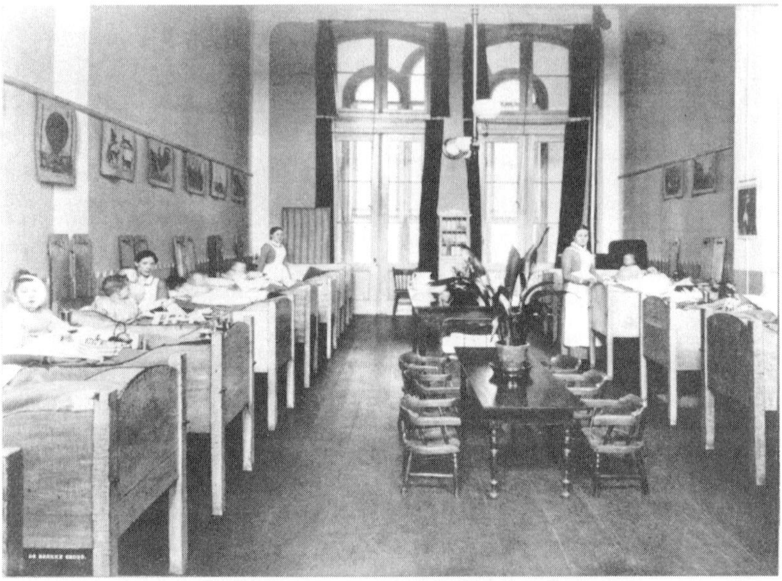

Fig. 3. Emma Children's Surgical Ward.

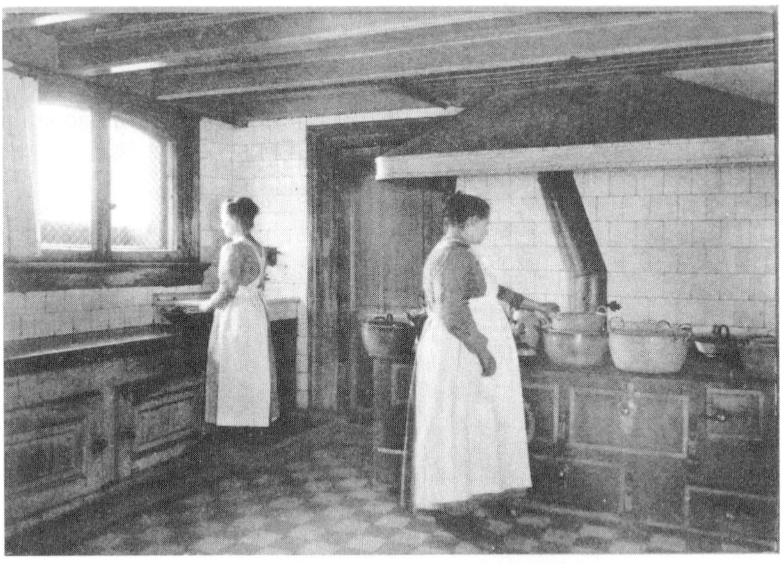

Fig. 4. Emma Chidren's Kitchen.

principles of Pasteur. In 1902, Timmer was one of the co-founders of the Netherlands Association of Surgeons in Amsterdam. He would continue to work at the Emma Children's until 1920.

Within ten years, various Children's Hospitals were founded throughout the country. In Arnhem (1881), The Hague (1885), Dordrecht (1885), Apeldoorn (1887), Utrecht (1888), and Groningen (1890).[5] The children's hospital in The Hague, founded in 1885 as a six beds and one cradle hospital at the Prins Hendrikplein, expanded the following year to 12 beds and four cradles, and moved in 1891 to a modern new building with 62 beds and 20 cradles at the Laan van Meerdervoort where it would remain until 1929.[6] The children's hospital in Utrecht, founded in 1888 with eight beds in two rooms, was located in the city centre at the Oude Kerkstraat. Parents were able to visit their admitted child three days a week, during one hour. In 1898 it moved to its new location at the Nieuwegracht where it remained until 1999. At the opening ceremony in 1898 it was named the Wilhelmina Children's Hospital, after the future Queen Wilhelmina, who was to be crowned that same year.[7]

On June 15, 1892, the directors of these Children's Hospitals founded the Netherlands Association of Paediatricians. The second half of the 19th century saw the development and organisation of paediatrics but it would take until the 1920's for paediatric surgery to emerge. Until then, the surgical care in the Children's Hospitals was usually undertaken by volunteer surgeons who spent most of their time working in general hospitals operating on adult patients. Children also continued to be treated in general hospitals throughout the country, although following the turn of the century attempts were made to concentrate children into separate departments of paediatrics within these general hospitals.

To date, the difference is still visible between those paediatric surgical centres that were naturally stimulated by the existence of a dedicated children's hospital, and centres that developed from the beginning as part of a university hospital where paediatric surgery always remained an integrated part of general surgery.

The Paediatric Surgeons (1920–2008)

Amsterdam. Reinder Johan Harrenstein (1988–1971) is regarded to have been the first full-time appointed paediatric surgeon in The Netherlands.[8] Following his surgical training with van Campen in Amsterdam, he trained with Prof F. Lange in Munich and then with Prof A. Lorenz in Vienna to gain further experience in orthopaedics. He came from an aristocratic family and decided to devote his career to the surgical treatment of children. Harrenstein despised the situation where children were always treated in an inferior manner; they were dispersed amongst adult patients, and were usually placed two in a bed. In 1921, he was appointed successor to H. Timmer at the Emma Children's Hospital in Amsterdam.[3] He called himself a "Paediatric Surgeon", a field of surgery that did not officially exist at that time, and was therefore regarded with scepticism by his contemporaries. He authored many publications, in both paediatric surgery and orthopaedics, and contributed much to the 1920–1940 era when the Emma Children's thrived successfully. As far as we are aware, during this time period until World War II, surgeons working with children did not appear to have organised specific meetings dedicated to paediatric surgery, nor specifically seemed to have collaborated with each other to share clinical problems. Their routine work included fractures, rickets, tuberculosis, orthopaedics, hypertrophic pylorus stenosis, laparotomies, hernia and testicular surgery, bladder stones and the increasing development of urology, cleft lip and palate, haemangiomas, and skin diseases.[3]

In 1948, M. Schoorl joined Harrenstein and was appointed at the Emma Children's in 1950 as a full-time paediatric surgeon. As Harrenstein retired in 1954, Schoorl, joined by W. van Putten from 1965–1974, continued the paediatric surgical practice. Not only did he work with a second paediatric surgeon, but he also established regular contacts with his contemporaries, first ten Kate and later Bom in The Hague, and Vervat in Rotterdam.[9] Until the 1970's, paediatric surgery was mainly located at the children's hospitals of these three cities, although every general surgeon throughout the country would incidentally operate on infants and children.

In 1969, J. C. Molenaar, who had just finished his surgical training at the VU University in Amsterdam decided to become a paediatric surgeon and trained with D. Vervat in Rotterdam. Upon his return to Amsterdam, he started the first academic paediatric surgical department in Amsterdam, at the VU University, and was appointed senior lecturer at that University in 1971. In 1972 he left Amsterdam to succeed D. Vervat in Rotterdam. In the meantime, A. Vos completed his surgical training at the University of Amsterdam, and trained at the paediatric surgical residency program of the Children's Hospital Boston (program director Robert E. Gross and J. Folkman) from 1971 to 1973. Upon his return to Amsterdam, he joined Schoorl at the Emma Children's, and succeeded J. C. Molenaar as head of the paediatric surgical department at the Vrije University.

In 1975 he was joined by Mrs C. G. M. Moorman–Voestermans at the Emma Children's, and when M. Schoorl retired in 1977, E. Krul was appointed as the second full-time paediatric surgeon in 1979. At the VU University, S. Ekkelkamp had been appointed in 1978, the four of them now forming one group of paediatric surgeons, working at two locations and sharing the on-call services. From 1975 to 1982, this group also provided the paediatric surgical care at the Wilhelmina Children's Hospital in Utrecht which did not yet have its own paediatric surgeon at that time.[5] In 1976, A. Vos was appointed senior lecturer at the Vrije University, until the chair was reverted to a full professorship in 1980. In 1988, the Emma Children's merged into the newly built Academic Medical Centre of the University of Amsterdam, to become the Emma Children's Hospital AMC. From this moment, the paediatric surgical department became the Paediatric Surgical Centre of Amsterdam bi-located at the two Academic Hospitals of Amsterdam.

Following the merge of the Emma Children's into Academic Medical Centre, Prof Vos was also appointed Professor of Paediatric Surgery at the University of Amsterdam in 1991. The department focussed on paediatric surgical oncology and gradually the staff members became more active in this field. In the late 1980's and first half of the 1990's, the staff changed and gradually expanded. In 1988,

H. A. Heij joined the staff following his training in paediatric surgery in Rotterdam and Amsterdam. In 1990, E. Borgstein (currently Head of the Department of Paediatric Surgery of the Queen Elisabeth Central Hospital and Postgraduate Dean of the University Malawi) was trained and left for Malawi in 1992. Following the demise of Krul in 1990, D. C. Aronson was appointed in 1991 and became a member of the staff in 1993, followed by Mrs Chr. Sleeboom (1994), Mrs C. F. Kuijper (1995) and Mrs R. van Baren (1996) after their two-year training period. When Prof Vos became emeritus in 1999, Prof Heij became the new chair holder that year. Subsequent to oncological studies, much of the clinical and research activities now focussed on long-term outcome of congenital malformations, including quality of life. In the following years, W. G. van Gemert trained from 1998 to 2000 and left to Maastricht in 2002, M. W. N. Oomen (2005), B. H. Verhoeven (2007) and J. C. H. Wilde (2007) were trained, and the staff were complemented after the retirements of Moorman (2001) and Ekkelkamp (2005), and the departure of Verhoeven to Maastricht in 2007. The current staff consists of H. A. Heij (Head), D. C. Aronson, Mrs Chr. Sleeboom, Mrs C. F. Kuijper, Mrs R. van Baren, M. W. N. Oomen, and J. C. H. Wilde.

Rotterdam. The time period from 1920 until after World War II did not show the thrilling progress of activities seen in Amsterdam during that time period. It would take until the full-time appointment of D. Vervat in 1949 in succession of Bouvé before paediatric surgery started to evolve into a more mature field of surgery. In the early 1950's, the surgical treatment of congenital anomalies like Hirschsprung's disease and pectus excavatum were introduced, and in 1952 Vervat performed his first oesophageal atresia correction.[1] Vervat chose to cooperate with other surgical specialties, a novelty at this time, and with the paediatricians of the Children's Hospital, he often called himself a "surgical paediatrician".[10] He also had regular contacts with Schoorl in Amsterdam, and first with ten Kate and later Bom in The Hague, and made the activities and developments at the Sophia Children's visible at national and international paediatric surgical meetings which slowly started to be organised.[11] His international contacts were also reflected being among the founding members of the British Association of Paediatric Surgeons (BAPS), together with Schoorl and Bom. In 1960, J. A. Noordijk joined the paediatric surgical department as the second paediatric surgeon.

A new development occurred in 1965 with the opening of the medical faculty at the Erasmus University of Rotterdam. In 1969, D. Vervat was appointed senior lecturer at the University, the department becoming the first in the country to acquire an academic status. Eventually in 1971, the Sophia Children's Hospital formally became the academic children's hospital of Rotterdam. That same year professor Vervat was appointed Director of the Sophia Children's Hospital and ceased his surgical activities. In 1972, J. C. Molenaar succeeded Vervat and was also appointed senior lecturer at the Erasmus University until 1976, when the chair changed and Prof Molenaar became the first full Professor of Paediatric Surgery.

Molenaar's vision, to increase the research activities of the department by the appointment of Abram Provoost, a biochemist, as full-time researcher to work in close collaboration with other departments such as developmental biology and genetics, gave rise to an internationally acknowledged and very productive research program.[12] Latterly, a second full-time researcher, R. Rottier joined the laboratory staff. This research program eventually culminated in the foundation of a chair in experimental paediatric surgery, to which D. Tibboel, a paediatrician who had taken the lead of the research program, was appointed in 1993. During this period, the staff increased with the appointment of N. M. A. Bax (1977) who had trained in paediatric surgery with Prof P. P. Rickham in Zürich and Prof J. Louw in Cape Town (1977), and F. Hazebroek (1978) who had trained with Schoorl and Prof Vos in Amsterdam. D. Noordijk retired in 1982, after which Mrs M. Rövekamp (1982) and B. J. Pull ter Gunne (1982) entered the training program. In 1982 Bax left Rotterdam to establish a paediatric surgical department in Utrecht, followed by Rövekamp and Pull ter Gunne in 1983 and 1984 respectively, who joined him at the new department in Utrecht.

J. H. Bergmeijer (1982), R. A. T. Th. M. Langemeijer (1983), G. C. Madern (1984), and E. Heineman (1987) trained in Rotterdam and were appointed to the staff following their two years of training. H.A. Heij trained in Rotterdam in 1986, but left Rotterdam in 1987 to continue his training in Amsterdam with Prof A. Vos. In 1991, Heineman went to Maastricht where he was appointed as the first full-time paediatric surgeon.

From 1986 onwards, a close collaboration between the Sophia Children's Hospital and the Juliana Children's Hospital in the Hague took place under the initiative of J. J. Hamming, and further organised by F. Hazebroek. This lead to a paediatric surgeon from the Sophia Children's working there on a part-time basis in order to increase the quality of care of the general paediatric surgical service.

In the 1990' much attention was drawn to medical-ethical questions in the treatment of severe life threatening congenital malformations. For the first time, fundamental questions were raised as to whether treatment should cease under certain dreadful medical circumstances. Molenaar, Tibboel and Hazebroek were pioneers who reported on their studies regarding the difficult decisions to cease life-prolonging measures and the medical management to be taken once those decisions were taken.[13]

In 1996 Mrs. Th. L. van den Hoonaard was appointed staff member after training at the Sophia Children's, and the following year, in 1997 Prof J. C. Molenaar became emeritus. In 1998 he was succeeded by Prof F. Hazebroek as professor of paediatric surgery and head of the department. C. P. van de Ven was trained (1998–2000) and was appointed a staff member in 2000. In 2002 Bergmeijer retired, and Mrs G. W. Zijp, who trained from 2004 to 2005, left Rotterdam in 2006 to become a paediatric surgeon in the Juliana Children's Hospital in The Hague. In 2005 Prof F. Hazebroek became emeritus and was succeeded in 2006 by Prof N. M. A. Bax. In the period from 2006 to 2008 another young surgeon, Mrs C. Meeussen, was trained in paediatric surgery. Early in 2008 Langemeijer retired. The current staff consists of Prof N. M. A. Bax (Head), Prof D. Tibboel, G. C. Madern, Mrs Th. L. van den Hoonaard, C. P. van de Ven, and Mrs C. Meeussen.

The Hague. Until the Second World War, infants and children at the children's hospital would be operated by general surgeons working in one of the nearby city hospitals. In 1913, J. Exalto (1881–1966), one of the surgeons at the Rode Kruis Hospital, was appointed in 1913 as volunteer surgeon for the children's hospital, and in 1919 A. M. Streef was appointed as the second surgeon.[6]

After moving to its third location in 1929, the newly built Children's Hospital was opened by the Queen-Mother Emma, and named after her grandchild Princess Juliana: the Juliana Children's Hospital.

In 1944, J. ten Kate, former head of the trauma unit of the Municipal Hospital "*De Zuidwal*" was appointed as the third surgeon. He performed the first successful oesophageal atresia reconstruction in an infant who survived. After his early death, ten Kate was succeeded in 1951 by K. Waldeck, a trainee of Exalto at the Rode Kruis Hospital. Exalto retired in 1952 and was succeeded by J. D. Bom, head of one of the two general surgical departments of the Zuidwal Hospital. Streef retired in 1957, and was succeeded by J. K. Bakker of the same department as Bom.

When the Municipal Hospital moved from the old Zuidwal Hospital to the modern newly constructed Leyenburg Hospital in 1971, Bom and Bakker provided the surgical service at the Juliana Children's from the Leyenburg Hospital, and Waldeck from the Rode Kruis Hospital. Bom, together with Schoorl (Amsterdam) and Vervat and Noordijk (Rotterdam), played a pivotal role in the emerging identity of paediatric surgery within the national Surgical Society by forming national and international contacts.[11]

When Waldeck retired in 1974, he was succeeded by J. J. Hamming, general surgeon at the Rode Kruis Hospital. After Bom retired in 1985, a Hammings initiative of 1986 saw close collaboration with the Sophia Children's Hospital in Rotterdam further compounded by Bakkers retirement in 1987. At that time, the paediatric surgical team of Prof Molenaar participated in the surgical patient care at the Juliana Children's, the only children's hospital without an academic status, and this continues to be supported by the Rotterdam team to the present day. In 1993 Hamming retired and was first succeeded by Boutkan the same year and in 1995 by J. H. Allema, both appointed as surgical staff of the Juliana Children's Hospital, having been general surgeons at the Rode Kruis Hospital.

In 1997, The Juliana Children's Hospital and the Rode Kruis Hospital combined into one organisation, and in 2004 the Leyenburg Hospital also merged into this collaboration forming the new Haga Hospital. Nevertheless, the Juliana Children's remained in a separate building. In 2005 Mrs G. W. Zijp, who trained at the Sophia Children's Hospital the two previous years, was appointed as a new member of the paediatric surgical staff. The current staff consists of J. H. Allema, Mrs G. W. Zijp, and Mrs Th. L. van den Hoonaard (Sophia Children's Hospital) in a part-time position.

Nijmegen. In 1923 the Catholic University of Nijmegen was founded, but it would take until 1951 to develop a medical faculty, and in 1956 the Academic Hospital St. Radboud was opened. In the 1950's and 1960's, children were operated upon by various general surgeons, in the latter years more specifically by Prof D. De Moulin.

C. Festen, who had trained in general surgery with Prof Schmidt was asked by him at the end of his training to gain further experience in paediatric surgery. Festen tutored under Prof Vervat (Rotterdam), Prof Rehbein (Bremen), Prof William B. Kiesewetter (Pittsburg), Prof C. Everett Koop (Philadelphia), and Prof Ehrenpreis (Stockholm), and returned to Nijmegen in 1970.[14]

In 1974 a separate Department of Paediatric Surgery was established, and the following year, in 1975, a chair of paediatric surgery was opened and Prof Festen was appointed as senior lecturer. The department had its own paediatrician (F. Kuijper) and its own anaesthesiologist (P. Ponsioen).[15] In 1974, Mrs C. G. M. Moorman–Voestermans started her training in paediatric surgery, after one year she left for the Emma Children's Hospital in Amsterdam. In 1980 the staff would be increased through the addition R. S. V. M. Severijnen and in 1981 a second full-time staff member, F. H. J. M. van der Staak, was appointed, following their training in Nijmegen. The following years saw much research on biliary atresia, short bowel syndrome and congenital diaphragmatic hernia. Experience was gained with extracorporeal membrane oxygenation (ECMO), and the department became one of the two centres in the Netherlands with the exclusive governmental permission to administer ECMO treatment.

As the clinical workload increased, the staff again increased with the appointment of P. N. M. A. Rieu (1989) and R. M. H. Wijnen (2000), both of whom had two years of paediatric surgical training in Nijmegen. During these years, the focus also turned towards ano-rectal malformations and haemangioma's and many international contacts were established in these fields. In 2000, Prof Festen became emeritus, and Severijnen was appointed head of the department until his retirement in 2007.[15] In this period, M. H. W. A. Wijnen (2003) and I. de Blaauw (2004) were appointed new staff members.

The retirement of Severijnen in 2007, saw succession by P. N. M. A. Rieu as head of the department "*ad interim*", who currently leads the staff: F. H. J. M. van der Staak, R. M. H. Wijnen, M. H. W. A. Wijnen, and I. de Blaauw.

Utrecht. Sporadically, only small operations would be performed in the Wilhelmina Children's Hospital, usually by surgeons from the Academic Hospital ("*Stedelijk en Academisch Ziekenhuis*" or SAZU), otherwise, children would be transferred and operated at the Academic Hospital. Throughout the years 1930–1969, the children's hospital was gradually modernised and expanded; the early 1950's saw the first true operating theatre, which was rebuilt with an additional theatre in the early 1970's.[7]

From 1975 to 1982, at the request of Prof J. Stoop, who was appointed Professor of Paediatrics and Medical Director of the Wilhelmina Children's in 1974, M. Schoorl and later the whole group of paediatric surgeons from Amsterdam served as part-time paediatric surgeons for the Wilhelmina Children's Hospital.

In 1982, N. M. A. Bax was appointed as the first full-time paediatric surgeon, joined by Mrs M. Rövekamp in 1983, and B. J. Pull ter Gunne in 1984. D. C. van der Zee, who started his training at the Wilhelmina Children's Hospital in 1988, eventually joined the staff in 1991. In 1990, the forth chair of paediatric surgery, established at the University of Utrecht, saw Prof Bax appointed as Professor of Paediatric Surgery. From 1992 onwards, this group pioneered minimally invasive paediatric surgery, developing and gaining experience in a broad range of laparoscopic and thoracoscopic procedures in children and infants. A stream of scientific publications describing these new endoscopic techniques, and many educational courses in this field resulted from these forerunner activities.

In 1994, Thomas Boemers, a pediatric urologist entered the training program to become a paediatric surgeon, and left for Hamburg in 1997 after he finished and defended his thesis. When Pull ter Gunne and Mrs Rövekamp left in 1996 and in 1997, respectively, W. L. M. Kramer and B. Ure were appointed new members of the staff that same year.

In 1999, the hospital moved to "*De Uithof*" on the outskirts of the city, where the Wilhelmina Children's Hospital was built next to the Academic Hospital, to form the University Medical Center Utrecht together with the Academic Hospital and the Medical Faculty. These developments lead to formation of a centre of excellence in paediatric laparoscopic surgery.

In 2000, B. Ure left for Hannover to be appointed Professor of Paediatric Surgery at the University of Hannover. That same year, Mrs D. Travassos was appointed new staff member. S. H. A. J. Tytgat was trained in the period from 2004 to 2006, and became a staff member in 2007. In the mean time, Prof Bax left Utrecht to succeed Prof Hazebroek as a Prof of Paediatric Surgery at the Sophia Children's Hospital in Rotterdam in 2006. J. R. de Jong was trained from 2005 to 2007, and started as paediatric surgeon in Maastricht in 2008. The current staff consists of D. C. van der Zee (Head *ad interim*), W. L. M. Kramer, Mrs D. Vieira-Travassos, and S. H. A. J. Tytgat.

Groningen. Professor L. D. Eerland (1897–1977), chief of the academic surgical training program, developed a major interest in thoracic surgery and the surgical treatment of infants and children.[16] In the late 1940's he travelled to the United States and learnt from

Swenson in Boston the treatment of oesophageal atresia. His return saw the second successful oesophageal atresia repair in the Netherlands in 1947, just two weeks prior to Schoorl who operated on the third patient in Amsterdam.[17]

Eerland was succeeded in 1966 by Prof P. J. Kuijjer who shared the same interest for the surgical treatment of infants and children, and asked L. J. M. Vos in the late 1960's to establish a paediatric surgical service. Due to the absence of possibilities for an academic career in paediatric surgery, he left and was succeeded by G. Kootstra, who had trained with Kuijjer, and who combined paediatric surgery with transplant surgery.

When Kootstra left for Maastricht in 1980 to establish a transplant unit in that hospital, R. P. Zwierstra, became the first full-time dedicated paediatric surgeon in Groningen. He was joined in 1989 by Z. J. de Langen, who changed from head end neck surgery to paediatric surgery. R. Zijlstra was trained from 1986–1988, but left in 2002. Zwierstra, who was devoted to medical education, decided in 1998 to develop the new curriculum full-time. In 1990, De Langen became the head of the Paediatric Surgical Department. P. M. A. Broens trained in Groningen from 2003 to 2005 and was appointed to the staff in 2005. Mrs R. Rassouli trained with Holschneider in Cologne, Germany until 2005 and was appointed a staff member in 2006, followed by I. Jester (2008) who trained with Professor K.-L. Waag in Mannheim, Germany. Currently the staff consists of Z. J. de Langen (Head), P. M. A. Broens, Mrs R. Rassouli, and I. Jester.

Maastricht. In 1980, G. Kootstra left the university hospital in Groningen to commence a kidney transplant program at the Academic Hospital Maastricht. On his request, Prof Greep the chief of the Surgical Department, allowed him to also start a small paediatric surgical service. With the help of G. Sie and C. Baeten the paediatric surgical activities began to take shape, but it would take until 1991 when E. Heineman, trained by Prof J. C. Molenaar in Rotterdam, and appointed as the first full-time paediatric surgeon in Maastricht that a research program focussed on gut integrity offered a sound basis for national and international collaboration.[17] Further development of paediatric surgical activities saw L. W. E. van Heurn, trained in paediatric surgery in London, Maastricht and Hong Kong, and he became an additional staff member in 1997, following the departure of Heineman for New Zealand where he was appointed Professor of Paediatric Surgery from 1997 to 2001.

Upon his return in 2001, Prof Heineman was appointed Professor of Paediatric Surgery in Maastricht, the fifth chair of paediatric surgery. When Prof Heineman departed in 2007, van Heurn succeeded him as head of the department of paediatric surgery and the staff increased by the appointment of B. H. Verhoeven (2007) who had been trained in Amsterdam and J. R. de Jong (2008) who had been trained in Utrecht. Currently, the staff consists of L. W. E. van Heurn (Head), G. Sie, B. Verhoeven, and J. R. de Jong.

The Organisation of Paediatric Surgery in The Netherlands (1950–2008)

In the late 1940's and 1950's, Dutch paediatric surgeons had increasing contact with each other and started to work together. Schoorl in Amsterdam regularly discussed patients with ten Kate in The Hague and with Vervat in Rotterdam, and in difficult cases they sometimes operated together. Two months after ten Kate had reported on his first successful case of a reconstructed oesophageal atresia in 1947 — his 13th case of oesophageal atresia and the first surviving patient in the Netherlands — ten Kate came to Amsterdam to help Schoorl perform his first oesophago-oesophagostomy. This made Schoorl the third Dutch paediatric surgeon to perform this operation, the second, Prof Eerland in Groningen had performed his first case two weeks previously.[18]

In 1953, the British Association of Paediatric Surgeons (BAPS) was founded, with Vervat, Schoorl, and Bom as founder members, improving emerging and soon intensifying international collaboration. Three years later, in 1956, over three days the first international paediatric surgical meetings took place in Amsterdam, the Hague, and Rotterdam, hosted by Schoorl, Bom and Vervat.[11] Dutch and

Scottish participants discussed whether surgical organ specialists or paediatric surgeons should undertake the surgical care of children. In 1964, Vervat was among the founder members of the *Journal of Pediatric Surgery* (JPS), the first journal dedicated to paediatric surgery. He was one of the early supporters of the concept of having such a journal. A gathering was held in Rotterdam at the 1964 BAPS meeting amongst a few interested people that were positive about the new journal. The JPS started in 1966. Later, Prof Molenaar served as the Editor for Europe for ten years.

While in America and in many other European countries paediatric surgery evolved as a separate speciality with specialised paediatric surgical departments, in 1967 a meeting was organised in Nijmegen to discuss the position of paediatric surgery in the Netherlands.[19] Vervat argued in favour of separate paediatric surgical units within Children's Hospitals, while den Otter, the chief of one of the major academic surgical training programs, made the suggestion for training a few surgical specialists for children, working in paediatric surgical units within some of the general surgical training hospitals. This meeting reflected the first common opinion, that surgical care for children required specific knowledge within the vast field of Surgery, and somehow had to be centralised to gain sufficient experience with rare paediatric surgical diseases and (congenital) anomalies.

In 1973, thoughts that had originally emerged in 1967 culminated in the foundation of the Working Group for Surgery in Children & Neonates by Schoorl, Bom Vervat and Noordijk, that was acknowledged in 1974 as a separate entity within the Netherlands Association of Surgeons.[20] In their statement, the Executive Board of the Association of Surgeons declared Paediatric Surgery should become a speciality within Surgery, rather than a separate specialty, to be centralised in specific paediatric surgical centres as part of academic surgical training, and performed by specifically trained full-time paediatric surgeons. This Working Group would be responsible for education and research within the field, with the due aim to strive for the establishment of a chair for Paediatric Surgery. In 1981, the Netherlands Association of Paediatric Surgeons was founded by the first Executive Board that consisted of Prof C. Festen, President, F. W. J. Hazebroek, Secretary, and S. Ekkelkamp, Treasurer.[21] It was the first sub-Association of the Netherlands Association of Surgeons, followed that same year by sub-Associations of Surgical Oncologist, Vascular Surgeons, and later of Trauma Surgeons (1982), Gastrointestinal Surgeons (1989) and Lung Surgeons (1995).[22]

In 1989, the Public Health Council published their crucial report "Surgery in children. The need for concentration" in response to the Secretary of State of Public Health, who had asked the Council in 1984 for advice regarding the need for concentration of paediatric surgery.[23] This report described the field of paediatric surgery very accurately, distinguishing the so-called "specific" paediatric surgery that required centralisation, from "surgery in children" that could remain under the care of the general surgeons. The remit of a Paediatric Surgical Centre was carefully defined, and the requirement for the country was calculated to be no more than six, but optimally probably four. Following this advisory recommendation in 1993, the Executive Board of the Netherlands Association of Surgeons instructed her members to concentrate on five specifically identified patient categories in centres for paediatric surgery: (1) all at term born infants below the age of one month, and all preterm infants below the age of six months; (2) children with surgical diseases so severe or rare that they belong in a centre; (3) children with surgical diseases with such high risk and increased chance for complications (like poly-trauma) that they belong in a centre; (4) children with oncological diseases; and (5) children with a need for organ transplantation. These services were to be located within the six Paediatric Surgical Centres at the Academic Hospitals in Amsterdam, Groningen, Maastricht, Nijmegen, Rotterdam, and Utrecht. Other additional children could be treated outside these centres in general hospitals.[24]

From 1992 onwards, the paediatric surgeons had representation within the Executive Board of the Netherlands Association of Surgeons. Until the mid-1990's, the Netherlands Association of Paediatric Surgeons devoted much time and energy discussing the possibility of becoming a separate specialty, Paediatric Surgery, with the Netherlands Association of Surgeons, their Council for the Surgical Training and Education (Concilium Chirurgicum), the Council for the Registration of Specialists (Central College), and the Government (Department of Public Health). The discussion to adopt this form of organisation, in parallel to most of the surrounding countries, came to an end in 1996. In that year the Council for the Registration of Specialists concluded that it was undesirable to increase the number of specialties. Following clear recognition of paediatric surgery by the Netherlands Association of Surgeons by the Council's advice to their members to follow the guidelines for concentration of children within the five paediatric surgical categories, the need for further separation ceased. In 1994, the European Board of Paediatric Surgery (EBPS) was established within the "monospecialist section paediatric surgery" of the *Union Européenne des Médecins Spécialistes* (UEMS). In the meantime, the Dutch paediatric surgeons had become certified by the EBPS, who also performed site visits to some Paediatric Surgical Centres that gained EBPS recognition (Amsterdam 2002, Rotterdam 2004). In 1999, the training program requirements for paediatric surgery in the Netherlands were accepted by the membership of both the Netherlands Association of Paediatric Surgeons and the Netherlands Association of Surgeons. In the years thereafter, the first site visits took place in Amsterdam (2002), Rotterdam (2003), Utrecht (2003), Nijmegen (2004), and Groningen (2007) by the Council for the Surgical Training and Education (Concilium Chirurgicum) that approved their two year training programs, necessary for a general surgeon to become a paediatric surgeon.

Currently, the optimal number of paediatric surgical centres is still under debate. Increasingly the attention of the public is drawn to medical activities and also to patient safety and quality of care. It seems inevitable that quality is linked to volume, and to increase volume especially of rare (congenital) anomalies, it will be necessary to combine centres to increase patient numbers per centre. In an era where paediatric surgical centres in the Netherlands increase their cooperation through mutual clinical and research projects, it will be the challenge of the future to unify activities by mutual consent.

The modern paediatric surgeons humbly stand on the shoulders of giants. The achievements of the current generation of paediatric surgeons and their leadership would not have been possible without the hard work of the paediatric surgical pioneers who have shaped the extent and boundaries of the (paediatric) surgical contribution to the benefit of children. It is imperative to realise that there is no present or future, without the past.

Acknowledgements

It has been very difficult to describe the history of Paediatric Surgery in the Netherlands with such little sources available in the literature. I am therefore much indebted to all who have been of help. I have to especially thank Mak Schoorl — the oldest living paediatric surgeon in the Netherlands, who at 94 has been willing to be interviewed for many hours and who gave me all of his tokens left from the past. Throughout the years, Jan Molenaar has always sent me documents regarding Paediatric Surgery in the Netherlands, that all have been of great help. Anton Vos, Jan Molenaar and Kees Festen have critically read the manuscript, and have added and changed what was necessary. All heads of the Paediatric Surgical Departments, Jan-Hein Allema, Frans Hazebroek, Hugo Heij, Erik Heineman, Ernst van Heurn, Ries de Langen, René Severijnen, and David van der Zee have critically read the history of their institution and filled out the blank spots. Without all of their help, this endeavour could not have been accomplished.

References

1. Lieburg MJ. *The History of the Sophia Children's Hospital in Rotterdam* (*De Geschiedenis van het Sophia Kinderziekenhuis te Rotterdam*). Erasmus Publishing, Rotterdam, 2004 [Dutch].
2. Fockens P. Congenital small bowel atresia, a case healed by surgery (Over aangeboren atresie van den darm, met een door operatie genezen geval). *Ned Tijdschr Geneeskd* 1911;54:1658–1665.

3. Wijsenbeek Th. *Sick Darlings. 125 Years of Children's Care in the Emma Children's Hospital* (*Zieke Lievertjes. 125 Jaar Kinderzorg in het Emma Kinderziekenhuis*). Uitgeverij Ploegsma, Amsterdam, 1990 [Dutch].
4. De Wilde PA. The golden jubilee of H. Timmer, surgeon in Amsterdam. (Gouden ambtsjubileum H. Timmer te Amsterdam). *Tijdschr Geneeskd* 1938;82:3389–3390 [Dutch].
5. Bax NMA. The world can only become smaller (De wereld kan alleen maar kleiner worden) Inaugural lecture. Utrecht, 1991 [Dutch].
6. Haeseker B, Lieburg MJ. *The History of the HagaHospital in The Hague, 1823–2007* (*De Geschiedenis van het HagaZiekenhuis, 1823–2007*). Erasmus Publishing, Rotterdam, 2007 [Dutch].
7. 't Hart PD. *The Sick Child in Good Hands. 100 Years of Health Care at the Wilhelmina Children's Hospital* (*Het Zieke Kind in Goede Handen. 100 Jaar Gezondheidszorg in het Wilhelmina Kinderziekenhuis*). Uitgeverij Cathena, Zwolle, 1988 [Dutch].
8. Schoorl M. Dr. R. J. Harrenstein, the first paediatric surgeon in the Netherlands. (Dr. R. J. Harrenstein, de eerste kinderchirurg in Nederland). *Tijdschr Kindergeneeskd* 1987;55:125 [Dutch].
9. Deurloo JA, Aronson DC. Dr. Mak Schoorl, paediatric surgeon: 'If I went hunting I'd put a blue flash light on top of my car' (Dr. Mak Schoorl, kinderchirurg: 'Als ik ging jagen zette ik een blauw zwaailicht op mijn auto'). *Ned Tijdschr Heelkd* 2005; 14:178–179 [Dutch].
10. Molenaar JC, Visser HKA. Obituary D. Vervat (In memoriam D. Vervat). *Ned Tijdschr Geneeskd* 2000;144:2223.
11. Schoorl M, Bom DJ, Vervat D. Paediatrc Surgery (Kinderchirurgie). *Ned Tijdschr Geneeskd* 1956; 100:1886 [Dutch].
12. Provoost AP, Hagoort J. *From Fata Morgana to Reality. Twenty Years of Research in Pediatric Surgery*. Erasmus University School of Medicine and Health Sciences, Sophia Children's Hospital, University Hospital Rotterdam, Rotterdam, 1997.
13. Hazebroek FW, Tibboel D, Mourik M, Bos AP, Molenaar JC. Withholding and withdrawal of life support from surgical neonates with life-threatening congenital anomalies. *J Pediatr Surg* 1993; 28:1093–1097.

14. Festen C. Medicine as teamwork (Geneeskunde in groepsverband). Inaugural lecture. Nijmegen, 1976 [Dutch].
15. Festen C. 25 Years of Paediatric Surgery in Nijmegen (25 jaar Kinderchirurgie in Nijmegen). Farewell lecture. Nijmegen, 2000 [Dutch].
16. Eerland DL. *The Scalpel and the Candle* (*Het Scalpel en de Kaars*). Van Gorcum & Comp. NV, Assen, 1970 [Dutch].
17. Kootstra G. Bye, bye scalpel (Vaarwel scalpel). Farewell lecture. Maastricht, 2000 [Dutch].
18. Deurloo, JA. Oesophageal atresia. History, treatment, and long term results. Doctorate thesis, University of Amsterdam. Febodruk BV, Enschede, 2005.
19. The Surgical Treatment of Children: In *Proceedings of the 19th Congress of the Netherlands Association for the Advancement of Surgical Sciences*. Nijmegen, 1967 [Dutch].
20. Molenaar JC, Hagoort J, Hazebroek FW. One hundred years of the Association of Surgeons in the Netherlands. IX. Pediatric surgery. *Ned Tijdschr Geneeskd* 2002;146(33):1551–1556 [Dutch].
21. Molenaar JC, Hagoort J, Hazebroek FW. Paediatrc Surgery (Kinderchirurgie). In: *Heelkunde op schrift. Hoofdstukken uit de recente geschiedenis van de Nederlandse Vereniging voor Heelkunde 1977–2005*. Van Zuiden Communications BV, Alphen aan de Rijn, 2006, pp. 51–63 [Dutch].
22. Wereldsma JCJ. The sub-Associations (De subverenigingen). In: *Heelkunde op schrift. Hoofdstukken uit de recente geschiedenis van de Nederlandse Vereniging voor Heelkunde 1977–2005*. Van Zuiden Communications BV, Alphen aan de Rijn, 2006, pp. 33–51 [Dutch].
23. Surgery in children. The need for concentration; an advisory by the Public Health Council to the Minister and the Secretary of State of Welfare, Public Health and Culture No. 1989/18 The Hague, 1989.
24. Molenaar JC. Surgery in children. The need for concentration; an advisory by the Public Health Council. *Ned Tijdschr Geneeskd* 1990; 134(3):139 [Dutch].

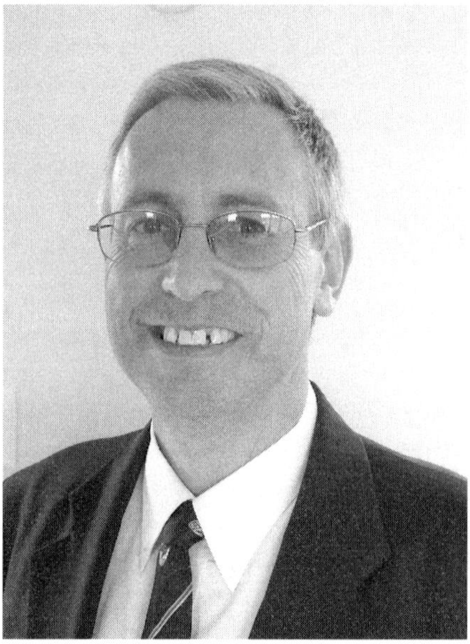

Spencer W. Beasley

NEW ZEALAND AND THE SOUTH PACIFIC

Spencer W. Beasley

Introduction

Although Australia and New Zealand have much in common, including the Royal Australasian College of Surgeons ("Australasian" refers to Australia and New Zealand), and a bi-national training programme in paediatric surgery, the history of the development of paediatric surgery has been quite different. Whereas paediatric surgery in Australia has been well-established and accepted for over half a century, in New Zealand, at least outside Auckland, it has only become recognised as a speciality in its own right in the last decade or so. Indeed, in the mid-nineties there was still some discussion as to whether paediatric surgeons were needed at all outside the tertiary centre in Auckland!

History, Demography and Topography

New Zealand is a young country geologically, thrust upwards as the massive Pacific tectonic plate collides with the Australian plate, producing varied and dramatic topography. The South Island is characterised by a ridge of high mountains running its length (the Southern Alps), with mountain lakes and fiords, and the slightly smaller North Island is volcanic in parts with other areas of rugged mountains and forest.

Its recent formation and isolation account for its unique flora and fauna, and explain why it was not colonised until the 13th century

AD during the period of widespread Polynesian ocean exploration.[1] The origin of the Maori settlers has been controversial,[2] but recent evidence suggests that their migration across the Pacific in various waves may have started on the east coast of Asia, perhaps from Taiwan about 6000 years ago, via the Philippines and Indonesia and acquiring a Melanesian contribution to their genetic make-up, eastwards across the Pacific to East Polynesia and ultimately south to New Zealand.[3,4] If this is correct, it may explain the higher incidence of hepatobiliary conditions such as biliary atresia seen in Maori compared with Europeans.[5]

In December 1642, the Dutch explorer Abel Tasman was the first European to see New Zealand, although the violent reception he received from Maori caused him to turn away without ever stepping foot on the land. Thus New Zealand was not to become a Dutch colony. Instead, 127 years later, James Cook circumnavigated it, and mapped its coastline in great detail. He was followed in the early 1800's by settlers and missionaries, and by 1840 when the Treaty of Waitangi was signed, there were already substantial of pakeha (European) settlers, mostly from the United Kingdom. Since then, there has been substantial immigration from other Pacific Islands, Asia and continental Europe.

Now, the population of New Zealand is over four million, with three million people living in the North Island, and fewer than one million people occupying the whole of the South Island. Apart from the largest city Auckland which has a population of about one million, Christchurch and Wellington each have about 360,000. Four centres have paediatric surgical units (Fig. 1).

The Specialisation of Paediatric Surgery

For many years surgery on children was viewed as part of general surgery, and surgeons would operate on children relying on their general surgical training. Outcomes, particularly for neonatal and other rare congenital conditions reflected this, leading to efforts by a number of paediatricians and surgeons throughout the country to concentrate this surgery into the hands of a few surgeons who had

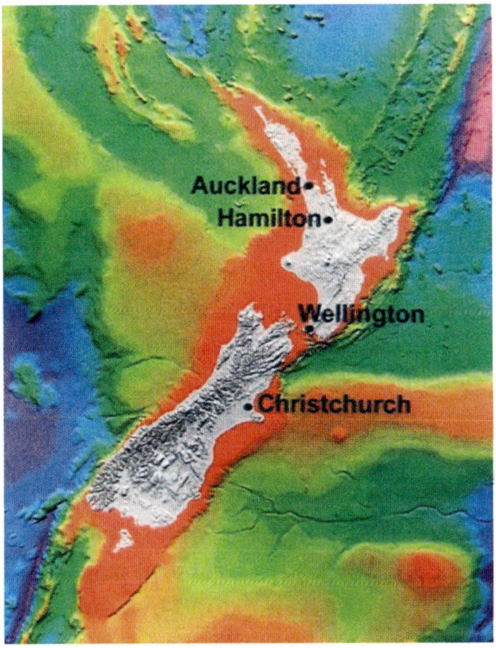

Fig. 1. Map of New Zealand showing the ridge formed by collision of the two tectonic plates, and identifying the location of the four paediatric surgical units; Auckland, Hamilton, Wellington and Christchurch.

demonstrated skills and a particular commitment or interest in the work. This arrangement continued until the 1980's or later in many regions.

General surgeons with an interest or expertise in children's surgery included Sam Burcher and Laurie Smith (Auckland), Graeme Campbell (Hamilton), Alan A. "Joe" Pullar, RT "Dick" Aldridge and John McIlwaine (Wellington), Rob Davidson and Robbie Robertson (Christchurch), Victor Pearse and Mike Shackleton (Dunedin).

On occasions, general surgeons working in a provincial hospital had a significant achievement, despite having limited resources at their disposal. For example, the first survivor of oesophageal atresia in the southern hemisphere was born and treated in New Plymouth in Taranaki by a provincial surgeon, Henry Barrett — much to the consternation of Gordon Bell, the then Professor of Surgery in Dunedin.[6]

Auckland. After World War II, a pre-fabricated American military hospital was turned into Princess Mary Hospital, and this was occupied from about 1946. Initially, a number of general surgeons operated on children there, namely Ted Jeffard, Kevin MacNamara, Cole and a few others. During the late 1940's and early 1950's Pud Lindsay did much of the paediatric surgery, but was a very slow surgeon who confined himself to the simple common general surgical procedures and did no urology or thoracic work. Just before the end of the 1940's Sam Burcher returned to New Zealand having done some paediatric surgery in the UK and he was responsible for setting up a separate paediatric surgical unit in the Princess Mary Hospital. At those times they were only paid two-tenth (equivalent of one day/week) by the public hospital system so he co-opted the help of Campbell McLaren, John Gilman and Keith Ewan. For many years a total of eight of ten of a paediatric surgeon shared the burden. Again, they confined themselves to general paediatric surgical problems, with the urology work being done by adult urologists.

In the early 1970's Laurie Smith was appointed as a part-time paediatric surgeon. Trained as a general surgeon he had a wealth of experience in trauma and had spent three years with Sir Douglas Robb and Sir Brian Barrett–Boyes, so was fully versed in cardiothoracic and thoracic surgery. He was an extremely hard worker and remained involved in paediatric surgery for the next 20 years. He pioneered the conservative management of solid organ trauma in New Zealand. He set up renal transplantation and paediatric renal transplantation in Auckland, and helped set up the thoracic surgical unit.

In 1974, Stuart Ferguson returned to New Zealand (virtually all New Zealanders did a period of post-Fellowship surgical training overseas) to do paediatric surgery, but found he had to continue with some adult general surgery. He was an early advocate of the advantages of day surgery in children. Also, he brought paediatric urology into what he referred to as "its rightful place" under the umbrella of paediatric surgery. For a while, there was a lot of resentment from the adult urologists, but with the backing of Sir Brian Barrett–Boyes and Sir William Manchester, he was successful.

Percy Pease was appointed in the 1970's, and brought with him an interest in paediatric thoracic surgery. Subsequent appointments included Anne Kolbe (interest in trauma), Vipul Upadhyaya (urology), Derek Rothwell (urology), Erik Heinemann (Professor of Paediatric Surgery from 1998 to 2002), Philip Morreau (hepatobiliary), James Hamill (trauma) and Michael Nightingale.

Waikato. Graeme Campbell started up paediatric surgery as a separate entity at Waikato Hospital in Hamilton, and was joined in the 1980's by Stuart Brown. Subsequently, and after the retirement of Graeme Campbell, two further paediatric surgeons were appointed: Margot Allen and Udaya Samarakkody. Margot Allan departed for Tasmania within a year, and was replaced by Russell Blakelock. Russell moved to Christchurch in 2002, and his position was taken up by Askar Kukkady.

Wellington. At the time Alan A. Pullar, or "Joe" Pullar as he was always called, left India to take up a position as the Resident Surgeon at Wellington Hospital surgery on children was being performed by all the general surgeons, albeit reluctantly, as none had any particular interest in it. Joe was an unobtrusively quick and highly competent surgeon with experience in many fields, including children, and soon accepted overall responsibility for their surgical care.

After he retired, first Richard "Dick" Aldridge and then John McIlwaine, both adult surgeons with some paediatric training, continued doing the paediatric surgery in Wellington, the other general surgeons by now having ceased all work in the specialty. Both were technically highly skilled surgeons, although John McIlwaine tended to do the more complicated cases. Dick Aldridge, like so many of the paediatric surgeons in New Zealand, had received his paediatric surgical training at the Royal Children's Hospital in Melbourne: it was while there that he performed the original research that enabled the diagnosis of Hirschsprung's disease to be made by suction rectal biopsy.[7]

In 1987 Kevin Pringle (Melbourne-trained) returned to New Zealand from Iowa as Wellington's first full-time paediatric surgeon, taking over from Dick Aldridge. In addition to his paediatric responsibilities he was appointed Acting Head of the Department of Surgery in 2000, the Head of the Department of Obstetrics and Gynaecology from 2001 and Head of Surgery from 2003 to 2005. When John McIlwaine retired, he was replaced by Brendon Bowkett in 1997, and Toni-Marie Wilson became the unit's third paediatric surgeon in 2004.

Brendon Bowkett has lead a Wellington based surgical team on 5 visits to East timor since 2001. These have proved a crucial bridge to ongoing support for paediatric surgical development in that country particularly given the complete loss of almost all local surgical specialist staff since the violence and turmoil during the late 1990s.

Christchurch. In Christchurch, in the late 1950's and early 1960's, Rob Davidson was the designated general surgeon responsible for paediatric surgery, and subsequently he was joined by Robbie Robertson. For a brief period after Rob Davidson's retirement at the end of 1985 Greg Robertson, a colorectal surgeon, assisted with this work.

It was not until 1996 that Spencer Beasley, a surgeon who had worked at the Royal Children's Hospital in Melbourne for 13 years, was appointed Professor of Paediatric Surgery in Christchurch as the first specialist paediatric surgeon in the South Island. He was joined by Kiki Maoate in 1998 and Russell Blakelock in 2002 and together they have provided a comprehensive service to all the public hospitals of the South Island. The scope of practice of all three surgeons included thoracic surgery and urology, sharing the urological work with Stephen Mark, an adult urologist with paediatric urological training and an interest in the neurogenic bladder.

Christchurch was one of the first centres in Australasia to embrace laparoscopic surgery in adults. This meant that laparoscopy became routine early on, and when Kiki Maoate was appointed to Christchurch in 1998 he was able to expand its applications in children and spearhead the introduction of advanced laparoscopic techniques.

Dunedin. Victor Pearse was an extremely good surgeon technically and had a reputation for being quite a character. He drove a Jaguar and would park it outside the front door of the hospital with a stethoscope draped over the front seat to deter traffic officers from giving him a ticket. In the late 1960's he was joined by Michael Shackleton, with a subsequent contribution by Ross Pettigrew and support from Kevin Pringle in Wellington until 1996.

The limited drainage population of Dunedin (the region, Otago, has a population of 145,000) ensured it would never be able to support it own paediatric surgical unit, so from 1996 the Christchurch paediatric surgeons provided a regular outreach service to Dunedin Hospital, including both clinics and operating.

The First Specialists

As mentioned, the development of paediatric surgery in New Zealand as a speciality in its own right lagged a long way behind Australia, despite their shared a training scheme and examination through the RACS. Unlike Australia, New Zealand did not have the benefit of purpose-built free-standing paediatric hospitals (until Auckland's Starship Children's Hospital was opened in 1990), with the inevitable consequent concentration of expertise.

For many years it was generally considered that outside New Zealand's biggest city, Auckland, it would be impossible for there to be full time paediatric surgeons — the population would be insufficient, and any general surgeon could perform surgery in children for all but a few of the more complex neonatal conditions. Advances in paediatric surgery were slow to take on, and clinical outcomes for children varied enormously as a consequence.

Before 1985 most of the recognised paediatric surgeons had a RACS Fellowship endorsed in (adult) general surgery, and their expertise in paediatric surgery was gained overseas as post-Fellowship training. The first New Zealand surgeons to obtain a RACS Fellowship endorsed in paediatric surgery as well were Stuart Brown and Spencer Beasley in 1985, both of whom were trained at the Royal Children's Hospital in Melbourne. Stuart Brown returned to Hamilton in that year, whereas Spencer Beasley stayed in Melbourne until he moved to Christchurch in 1996.

From about 1995 most trainees went directly into the paediatric surgical training programme, without acquiring a general surgical Fellowship first. As a result of the bi-national training scheme this was done mainly in Australia (Melbourne has been involved in the training of 11 of the 14 current surgeons in New Zealand) but some have received additional training in the United Kingdom and USA. Of course, not all New Zealanders have returned to New Zealand, and there is a sprinkling of them around the world.

Other Paediatric Sub-specialities

A few surgeons from other specialities have subspecialised in paediatrics, but this process has been handicapped by the small population of the country. Thus, by necessity, most have been appointed to Starship Children's Hospital in Auckland, the main tertiary referral hospital for paediatrics in New Zealand.

Cardiac surgery. Greenlane Hospital in Auckland was a leading institution in the 1960's and 1970's as cardiac surgery was being pioneered and techniques of cardiopulmonary perfusion (bypass) were being developed to allow surgery on congenital heart defects. Sir Brian Barrett–Boyes led a team of medical and paramedical experts at Greenlane Hospital when he returned from Birmingham, Alabama, in the early 1960's after working there with Kirklin. In particular, Sir Brian developed a method of cooling babies before stopping the circulation, i.e. circulatory arrest, which allowed repairs to be carried out on small infants and children. At that time bypass methods were only safe in older children and adults and most infants had to have inferior palliative procedures, in the hope that they would survive until old enough to have a definitive repair. Sir Brian's results in infants using this technique represented a major advance for that era and some of the concepts are still used today, albeit with more sophisticated equipment.

Later in the 1970's through to the 1990's coronary artery disease overtook congenital heart disease as the major indication for heart surgery and children suffered as they competed with adults for resources. By 1995 it became clear that paediatric cardiac surgery needed to split from the adult cardiac area and become a speciality in its own right. By then more than 50% of operations were on infants under 1 year and many infants had complex problems involving other organ systems such that they would be advantaged by being looked after in a specialist paediatric centre. Planning for the move to Starship Children's Hospital began in the mid 1990s but did not occur until 2003. Current results are comparable to some of the best institutions world-wide.

Orthopaedic surgery. Colin Hooker (Hamilton), Geoff Lamb (Auckland) and Hugh Stevens (Christchurch) recognised early the importance of paediatric sub-specialisation in orthopaedics, and in their own regions help establish the infrastructure that permitted subsequent development of the speciality.

Graham Smaill (Wellington), had a daughter born with congenital dislocation of the hip. This prompted him to set up a neonatal screening service in Wellington from 1962, and subsequently the service was adopted throughout much of New Zealand: this significantly reduced the morbidity of the condition, as delays in diagnosis and treatment are associated with markedly worse outcomes.

Since then, each major city hospital has identified at least one person with expertise and responsibilities for paediatric orthopaedics. Some of these, such as Alan Panting in Nelson, have had substantial paediatric training, and were they to have been employed in a larger centre would likely have had greater involvement.

A number of events helped establish paediatric orthopaedics: first, the Paediatric Orthopaedic Society of New Zealand was set up in the late 1980's, the first sub-speciality society of the New Zealand Orthopaedic Association. Geoff Lamb was its first President, with Mike Barnes its Secretary.

Secondly, several full-time paediatric orthopaedic appointments were made: the first was Richard Nichol, followed by David Clews (Hamilton) who remained full-time throughout his life.

Thirdly, the opening of Starship Children's Hospital in Auckland allowed concentration of paediatric orthopaedic expertise and provided a referral centre for the rest of the country. Geoff Lamb and Tony Hardy were already part-time paediatric, but were joined by

Richard Nichol in 1988 and it was he who was tasked with setting up the unit. Subsequently, he was joined by Mike Barnes, Stuart Walsh, Sue Stott (Associate Professor, and as such the first senior paediatric orthopaedic academic appointment), Teri Bidwell, and two spinal surgeons: Hamish Crawford and John Ferguson (the son of Stuart Ferguson).

Otorhinolarngology (ORL). Otorhinolaryngology is a speciality that treats large numbers of children, mostly for minor operative procedures. There would be few ENT surgeons in New Zealand who do not manage at least some children. The more complex and difficult surgery is now referred to Starship Hospital. Gavin S. Douglas, affectionately known as "Ru", was joined there by Colin Barber, the first dedicated paediatric otolarnyngologist. In more recent years a number of other appointments have been made: Colin Brown, Murali Mahadevan and Lesley Salkeld, with support from a number of others including Brennian Dorman and Michel Neeff.

Ophthalmology. Virtually all ophthalmologists in New Zealand treat children, but some have developed a special interest in paediatrics or made specific research contributions. For example, Richard Clemett, a Christchurch ophthalmologist, and Brian Darlow (neonatologist) developed New Zealand screening guidelines for retinopathy of the premature (Clemett and Darlow, 1990), guidelines that have subsequently been validated and adopted elsewhere in the world. Cryotherapy became available in Christchurch in 1986, markedly reducing the adverse visual outcome of eyes that had reached "threshold disease". Rod Suckling, a Christchurch ophthalmologist, set up a *de facto* national service for retinoblastoma, which for many years concentrated expertise for the treatment of this malignancy. With Auckland's population increase, some of these tumours are now treated in Auckland as well.

Neurosurgery. The first neurosurgical unit in New Zealand was established in Dunedin in 1943, with Auckland, Christchurch, Wellington and Hamilton gaining units subsequently (in that order).

All neurosurgeons undertook to treat children as part of their general workload, and it was not until the opening of Starship Children's Hospital that paediatric neurosurgery acquired particular focus. There remains considerable paediatric expertise in the other centres, particularly in Christchurch.

Plastic surgery. Sub-specialisation has also occurred in plastic surgery which was initially done at Middlemore by Sir William Manchester, and later by John Williams and others. Each of the four plastic surgical units in New Zealand (Middlemore in Auckland, Hamilton, Lower Hutt near Wellington, and Christchurch) have dealt with a broad range of paediatric plastic surgery, including burns and cleft lips and palates.

The Starship Children's Hospital

After World War II, a prefabricated American military base in Auckland was turned into Princess Mary Hospital and this was occupied from about 1946. This was clearly inadequate in many respects but it took much negotiation and time before a replacement facility was constructed. Stuart Ferguson who was on the Auckland Hospital Board for 6 years was one of those who argued strongly for the new hospital. Auckland's Starship Children's Hospital, is now the flagship of tertiary paediatric services in New Zealand (Fig. 2).

Quite apart from the improved facilities that the building of a modern designated paediatric hospital in Auckland provided, it was important because it facilitated the concentration of tertiary child health expertise, and many of these services required specialist paediatric surgical involvement.

New Zealand Society of Paediatric Surgeons

The New Zealand Society of Paediatric Surgery (NZSPS) was set up in 1996 to replace the older New Zealand Society for Paediatric Surgery (established in 1985), an informal group whose membership had included nurses, pathologists and surgeons who shared a common

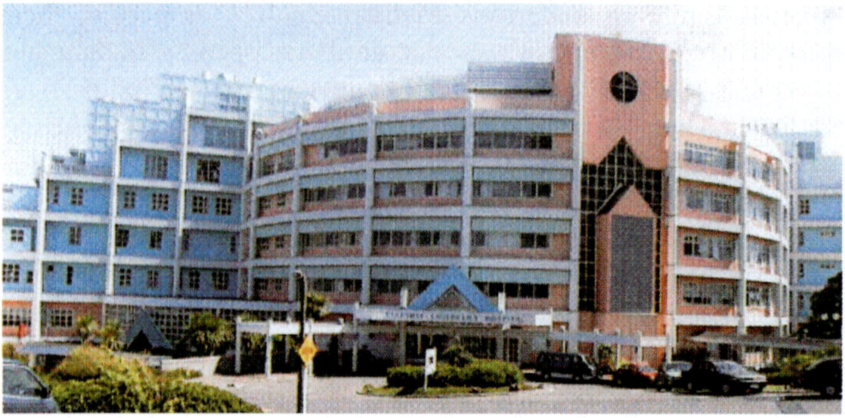

(a)

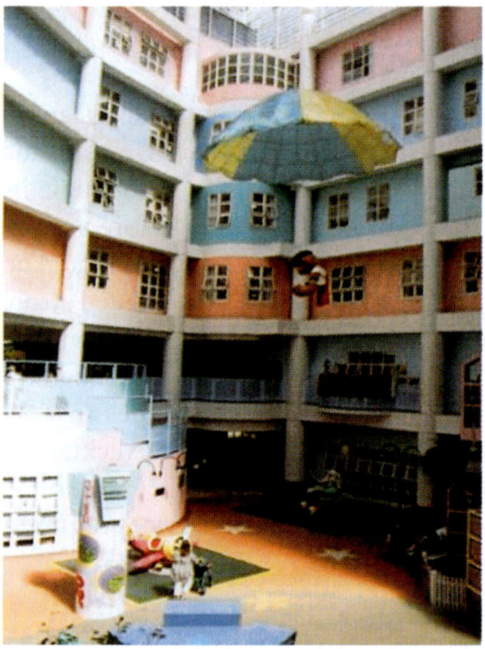

(b)

Fig. 2. The Starship Children's Hospital in Auckland provides tertiary services to the whole country. Recently, it has expanded, but is chronically under-resourced and struggles to meet demand. (a) external view, and (b) The massive entrance foyer.

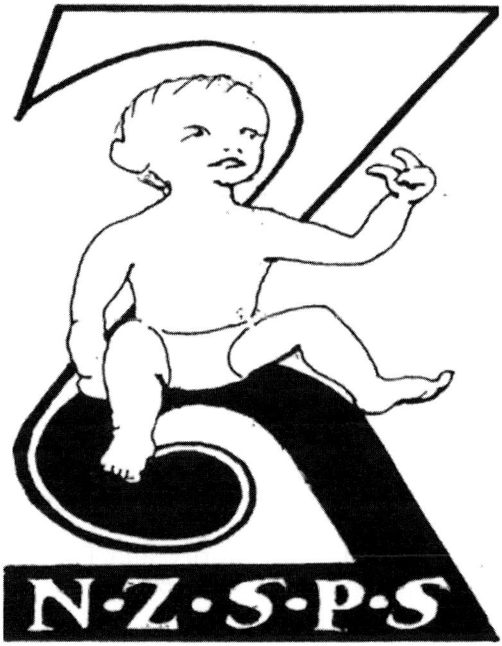

Fig. 3. The logo of the New Zealand Society of Paediatric Surgeons.

interest in children's surgery. The new NZSPS (Fig. 3) remained inclusive to the degree that its membership included surgeons whose practise was predominantly or substantially in children (to involve general surgeons and urologists who still performed surgery on children, but were not specialists), but with time and the recent expansion of workforce numbers (from six paediatric surgeons in 1995 to 14 in 2006) it has become a society of specialist paediatric surgeons.

The NZSPS has provided the political arm of children's surgery in New Zealand and has worked closely with the Paediatric Society of New Zealand on issues of mutual strategic importance. It has been the body that has met with the Minister of Health as required, and with senior ministry officials. In 2004, Brendon Bowkett moved from Secretary to President of the Society, replacing the inaugural President, Spencer Beasley; James Hamill was elected the new Secretary. The society meets annually, sometimes in conjunction with other scientific meetings. It has provided an opportunity for all 14 paediatric surgeons to get together on a regular basis, although there are now additional annual business meetings of the four Clinical Directors (Auckland, Waikato, Wellington and Christchurch). The emphasis has been on provision of a national service, rather than having 4 units working completely independently.

The NZSPS has identified a number of extremely rare but potentially difficult conditions, e.g. long gap oesophageal atresia, biliary atresia, major hepatic surgery, bladder exstrophy, DSDs (ambiguous genitalia) and advanced laparoscopic surgery, where between one and three surgeons in the country have been designated as "experts" and at least one of these experts is involved in each new case.

HFA/PSNZ Review of Tertiary Paediatric Services

In 1998, the Health Funding Authority and Paediatric Society of New Zealand, in conjunction with the NZSPS undertook a comprehensive review of tertiary paediatric services, including paediatric surgery and paediatric urology.

This was symbolic of the recognition of paediatric surgery in New Zealand, and provided the template that was used from which the specialty could develop and expand its service to all parts of New Zealand. It forced consideration of a number of contentious issues that related to the configuration of paediatric surgical services in New Zealand. It recognised the importance of providing a service that was accessible to all children, even in the more remote areas, and the requirement for the highest standards of care.

In many ways, it represented the "coming of age" of paediatric surgery as a specialty in New Zealand, and gave credibility to the concept of outreach services to the smaller centres. Amongst other things, it encouraged application of the South Island model of care to outreach services in the North Island.

Outreach Services

Many aspects of the health services in New Zealand are compromised by the country's small and sparse population, and difficult

Table. Configuration of paediatric surgical services in New Zealand, December 2007.

Hospital	Staff	RACS Training Posts	Oncology	PICU	Cardiac
Starship Children's Hospital, **Auckland**	Phil Morreau (CD) Stuart Ferguson Vipul Upadhyay James Hamill Michael Nightingale	2*	✓	✓	✓
Waikato Hospital, **Hamilton**	Udaya Samarakkody (CD) Stuart Brown Askar Kukkaday	1*			
Wellington Hospital, **Wellington**	Kevin Pringle (CD) Brendon Bowkett Toni-Marie Wilson				
Christchurch Hospital, **Christchurch**	Spencer Beasley (CD) Kiki Maoate Russell Blakelock	1	✓		

topography. In both islands, but particularly in the larger and more mountainous South Island, substantial communities are more than 4 hours by car from the nearest hospital, and in winter poor weather and high mountain ranges can make emergency air retrieval and transport difficult. The additional inconvenience and disruption caused to families who have to travel long distances to receive quality specialist opinion and treatment is also recognised. For these reasons, regular and comprehensive paediatric surgical outreach services have been developed to most of the smaller centres and more remote regions. Many of these involve paediatric surgeons travelling from the tertiary centres to perform outpatient clinics and day surgery, although sometimes more substantial surgery is also performed in the larger hospitals (e.g. in Dunedin). As necessary, a specialist paediatric anaesthetist accompanies the surgeon, expanding the range of conditions that can receive surgery locally without compromising safety. For example, the Christchurch surgeons provide regular clinics and surgery to all the public hospitals of the

South Island, with only the more complex conditions that require the additional facilities that Christchurch can provide as the tertiary centre. Auckland provides outreach services to Whangarei, New Plymouth and Gisborne; the Hamilton-based surgeons are responsible for the Bay of Plenty and Waikato; and Wellington covers the area south of Wanganui to Hawkes Bay.

The Pacific

New Zealand has long felt an obligation to its neighbouring countries in the South Pacific (Fig. 4). This has certainly been true of paediatric surgery.

Tonga and Samoa. Percy Pease (Auckland) visited Tonga and Samoa for about 20 years. He ran clinics and performed many procedures locally, organising the transfer of complex cases to New Zealand. Since his retirement efforts have been made to formalise the organisational and logistical arrangements, primarily with

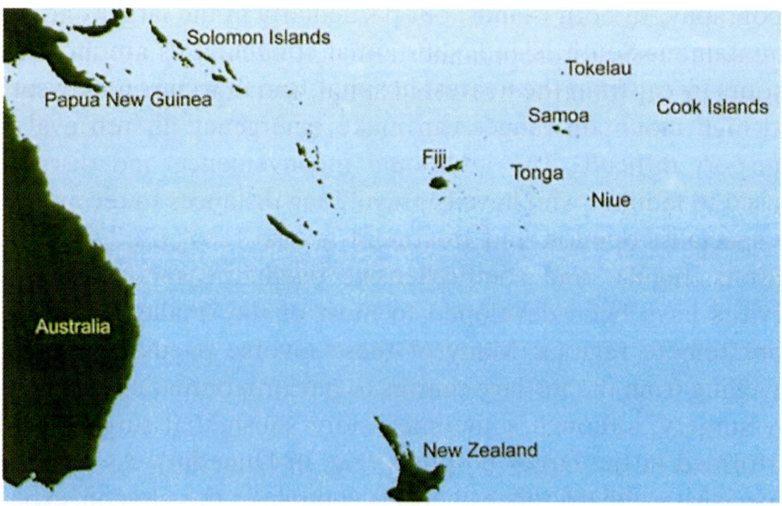

Fig. 4. Map of the main islands of the South Pacific: Europe would fit easily within this area. Apart from Fiji, each country has a small and widely dispersed population.

Starship Children's Hospital. Tonga is fortunate in having Viliami Tangi, a surgeon who received some paediatric surgical training in Auckland and Newcastle (NSW), as its Minister of Health. He has a Fellowship of the RACS endorsed in general surgery, but also has the distinction of being responsible for Tonga's first oesophageal atresia survivor. It is hoped that in the future other surgeons from Tonga and Samoa may obtain paediatric surgical training in New Zealand as part of their overseas training.

Cook Islands, Niue, Tokelau Islands. Citizens of these sparsely populated countries, whose islands are so widely dispersed, are also citizens of New Zealand. This means that major cases can be transferred to New Zealand, subject to financial constraints. These islands have major problems with retrieval: many of the islands have no airport or landing strip, such that patients have to be transferred to larger islands first by boat — and often by small boat — and it may take days for them to receive definitive care. Trauma and infections predominate.

Kiki Maoate, himself originally from the Cook Islands, has been involved in initiatives matching workforce training with local needs, organising training programmes relevant to their communities, and improving health infrastructure. He has been instrumental in setting up a National Research Framework in conjunction with the Health Research Council of New Zealand.

Fiji. Fiji is by far the most populous of the nations of the South Pacific, with almost 800,000 people, mostly of indigenous Fijian or Indian ethnicity.[8]

The Royal Australasian College of Surgeons Pacific Island Project (RACS PIP) has been running there for 13 years. The project is funded by AUSAID, and the RACS administers it. It has predominantly involved outreach visits by surgeons of all specialties, both from Australia and New Zealand. Fiji, by virtue of its population, is the only island in the South Pacific that has justified RACS PIP involvement by paediatric surgeons, and many Australian and

New Zealand paediatric surgeons have participated in this project. However, that so many different surgeons have been involved, in itself has led to lack of continuity and limited its usefulness in some respects. Apart from Kevin Pringle (Wellington) and Russell Blakelock (Christchurch, and himself part-Fijian), most surgeons have visited only once. Another problem related to the difficulties organising a paediatric anaesthetist to be permitted to join the visits — for this Kiki Maoate argued long and hard. The visits have continued annually (with additional visits as required), predominantly by Russell Blakelock, with an emphasis on continuity, teaching and identification of students who may be suitable for further training.

It was always recognised that the RACS PIP programme represented an interim solution only, until Fiji had its own surgeons and infrastructure in place. In 2001, Jitoko Cama, a quiet unassuming but talented surgeon, was identified as a potential paediatric surgeon. He received paediatric surgical training in Christchurch, Auckland and Melbourne and is about to return as Fiji's first fully-trained specialist paediatric surgeon.

The Fiji School of Medicine was set up in 1885 after a measles epidemic wiped out a third of the population. Its medical school is highly regarded, and over the years a number of New Zealand paediatric surgeons have contributed to defining the paediatric surgical component of its curriculum.

Papua New Guinea (PNG) and Solomon Islands. Paediatric surgical input in PNG has largely been under the auspices of Australia, although Kiki Maoate has been involved in providing surgical support to the adjacent Solomon Islands. Now, some of that work has been taken over from PNG by McLee Mathew who received training in Melbourne organised by Paddy Dewan. Douglas Pikacha, a general surgeon with an interest in paediatrics, received his training from the teams visiting the Solomon Islands and Fiji, and has now returned to the Solomon Islands. He has used modern technology with great success there, making use of email and internet communication with colleagues overseas to overcome some of the problems of isolation.

Support to the Pacific from other specialities. Over the years a number of surgeons have contributed to improving the plight of children with surgical conditions in the Pacific region.

For example, in 1967, through the Red Cross, a Wellington orthopaedic surgeon, Wyn Beasley, studied the incidence and causes of crippled children in Western Samoa. Polio was identified as being a major cause (ironically, epidemics of polio occurred in the 1930's and 1950's, in part attributable to an earlier programme to inoculate against yaws). This research led to a return visit with a cask of Sabin vaccine! The other cause of significant morbidity was clubbed feet; the incidence in this community being many times higher than in New Zealand.

A paediatric cardiac surgery outreach service is well developed in Tahiti and is now being extended to Samoa and Tonga. Infants with correctable forms of congenital heart disease such as transposition of the great arteries are being diagnosed and transferred to New Zealand earlier instead of dying, as happened only three or four years ago. Some infants are sent home if the lesions are too complex to repair with one operation.

Rheumatic valvular repair surgery remains a challenge, as the insertion of mechanical valves leads to major issues with adequate monitoring and supervision of Warfarin levels. The development of registers in each country to administer penicillin regularly to those who have been diagnosed may prove to be an important public health initiative.

Royal Australasian College of Surgeons and Its Training Programmes

New Zealand paediatric surgeons have had a high profile in College activities. Anne Kolbe, formerly at Auckland Starship Children's Hospital, became the first female President of the RACS, having previously been an examiner in paediatric surgery and Censor-in-Chief. Spencer Beasley was Chairman of the Board of Paediatric Surgery for 6 years before becoming the New Zealand Censor, senior examiner in paediatric surgery, member of the Education Board and Councillor RACS. Phil Morreau is a current member of the Board of Paediatric Surgery and on the committee responsible for the running of the Basic Surgical Training.

Many, if not most of the New Zealand paediatric surgeons, are or have been instructors for the EMST, APLS or Surgical Teachers Courses run by the RACS. For about 10 years Christchurch has run the pre-Fellowship examination course for paediatric surgery, in recent years these were organised by Kiki Maoate. Percy Pease, Kiki Maoate and Spencer Beasley have represented paediatric surgery on the NZ National Board RACS.

Roles in International Organisations

In 1990, the AAPS changed its name from Australian to Australasian Association of Paediatric Surgeons to allow it to include New Zealand paediatric surgeons. This occurred when Spencer Beasley, then working in Melbourne, was the Secretary/Treasurer (1989–1993). It was felt that the development of paediatric surgery in New Zealand would be helped by support from Australia, and that the relationship between the Board of Paediatric Surgery (then also the Training, Education and Accreditation Committee of the AAPS) would be simpler if both nations were on an equal footing and both had representation. Since then, New Zealanders have always had representation on the executive committee of AAPS, Spencer Beasley was elected President 2005–2007, and Philip Morreau was Secretary/Treasurer from 2004.

New Zealand has provided two Presidents of the Pacific Association of Paediatric Surgeons: Stuart Ferguson (1985) and Kevin Pringle (2006). It has also had representation on the publication committee for the PAPS issue of the Journal of Paediatric Surgery: Kevin Pringle (1995–2001) and Spencer Beasley (1994–2001). Kevin Pringle was a founding member of the International Fetal Medicine and Surgery Society in 1987, to become its President from 1989–1990.

Academic and Research

All four centres (Auckland, Hamilton, Wellington and Christchurch) have had active involvement in clinical research, and published widely. Several studies have been collaborative, including data from all centres. Prevention of childhood accidents has been a frequent theme, particularly driveway accidents (which are very common in New Zealand, especially in Auckland, in part due to the design of state housing), and handlebar injuries.

In Wellington, Kevin Pringle has led a group initially studying lung development, and subsequently renal development in obstructive uropathy: These experiments have used a fetal lamb model, and represent continuation of his previous work in Iowa. He has been assisted by four Japanese Fellows: Marc Matsumura, Hiro Kitagawa, Atsuyuki Yamataka and Yasuji Seki. Part of their research involves ongoing collaboration with Keio University in Tokyo.

In Christchurch, research has used the Adriamycin and ETU rat models of the VATER association to study oesophageal atresia and anorectal malformations (Qi Bao Quan, Parkash Mandhan and Andrew Williams), and — following the formation of the Child Cancer and Developmental Genetics Research Unit — the role of Sonic Hedgehog in embryogenesis and oncogenesis (Dejan Arsic and Michael Sullivan). This work received recognition and support by the RACS with the award of the John Mitchell Crouch Fellowship to Spencer Beasley in 2001.

The focus of research being undertaken by the cardiac surgical unit at Starship Hospital is shifting towards improved brain protection during cardiac surgery. A major study of infants who had heart surgery in the first two months of life is occurring currently in collaboration with Melbourne.

New Zealand has had three professors of paediatric surgery: Erik Heinemann (Auckland School of Medicine, University of Auckland, 1998–2002), Spencer Beasley (Christchurch School of medicine and Health Science, University of Otago, 1997–present) and Kevin Pringle (Wellington School of Medicine and Health Science, University of

Otago, 2001–present). Erik Heinemann has subsequently returned to Maastricht, the Netherlands.

The Future

Rural general surgeons in New Zealand are becoming increasingly reluctant to treat children, partly because their specialty training now includes little (if any) exposure to paediatric surgery, and partly for reasons of credentialling and a perception of medicolegal vulnerability. Yet the majority of acute cases (outside the neonatal period) seen in paediatric surgical practice affect older children and involve conditions with which general surgeons are already familiar, such as appendicitis, testicular torsion and abscesses. Therefore, it should not be difficult for rural surgeons to remain competent in dealing with these conditions, with support from their regional paediatric surgical service for the less common or more complex cases. The challenge for the paediatric surgeon is to ensure that rural surgeons are adequately equipped to deal with these acute cases, and provide a sufficiently comprehensive outreach service to the smaller centres so that the highest standards of care are available for the elective cases, such as herniotomies and orchidopexies. Indeed, the HFA/PSNZ review of surgical services recognised that this was where a paediatric surgical service could make the greatest contribution to improving outcomes in children (HFA/PSNZ review 1998).

Agreement amongst the paediatric surgeons themselves is likely to result in increasing specialisation for the extremely rare or complex index cases, such that for many conditions there would be only one or two surgeons in the country with primary responsibility for their management; and for some patients it may even be that transfer to Australia (or bringing an Australian surgeon to New Zealand) is the most appropriate action — this has already occurred on a number of occasions. Guidelines are being developed for infants born with an intersex abnormality (now called Disorders of Sexual Development).

Workforce numbers could be affected by safe hours of practice legislation, lifestyle and gender issues (already a majority of surgical trainees in paediatric surgery are female), and outreach requirements to the provincial hospitals. The small population of the country and relatively poor incomes in New Zealand compared with Australia and beyond, mean that a proportion of New Zealand trainees will always be attracted elsewhere: the so-called "kiwi brain-drain".

It is likely that New Zealand's role in training the future paediatric surgeons of the Pacific region will increase. Trips to the Pacific Islands to perform surgery will gradually be replaced by initiatives that will decrease the reliance of the various nations of the Pacific on overseas support, although their small populations are such that for some cases transfer to New Zealand or Australia will still be necessary.

But irrespective to any changes in the environment in which paediatric surgeons have to work, their objectives and goals will remain unchanged: to continue to improve the quality of the surgical care that can be provided to the children of New Zealand and the South Pacific.

Acknowledgements

I am grateful for the information and assistance provided by Stuart Ferguson, Philip Morreau, Kirsten Finucane, Richard Nichol, Brennian Dorman, John McIlwaine, Kevin Pringle, Wyn Beasley, Kiki Maoate and Russell Blakelock in the preparation of this manuscript.

References

1. King M. *The Penguin History of New Zealand.* Viking Books, 2004, pp. 48.
2. Hurles ME, Irven C, Nicholson J, Taylor PG, *et al.* European Y-chromosome lineages in Polynesians: a contrast to the population structure revealed by mtDNA. *Am J Hum Genet* 1998;63:1793–1806.
3. Horstman M. Maori men and women from different homelands. ABC Science Online: http://www.abc.net.au/science/news/ancient/Ancient Republish_817069.

4. Carpinter B. Where did the Maori come from? Part of the answer is falling into place thanks to new techniques for analysing human DNA. http://nzsm.webcentre.co.nz/article1834.htm
5. Yu T, Morreau P, Beasley SW, Brown S, *et al.* Long-term outcome of biliary atresia in New Zealand. *Aust NZ J Surg* 2007;77(Suppl):A57.
6. Myers NA. Oesophageal atresia: the first survival in the Southern Hemisphere. *Aust NZ J Surg* 1992;62:973–974.
7. Aldridge RT, Campbell PE. Ganglion cell distribution in the normal rectum and anal canal. A basis for the diagnosis of Hirschsprung's disease by anorectal biopsy. *J Pediatr Surg* 1968;3:475.
8. Penington AH. The Fiji School of medicine — a brief history. *Hawaii Med J* 1984;43(9):314–318.

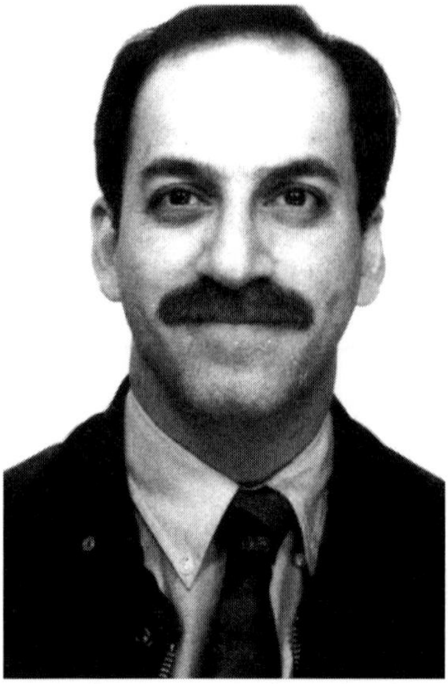

Basith Amjad

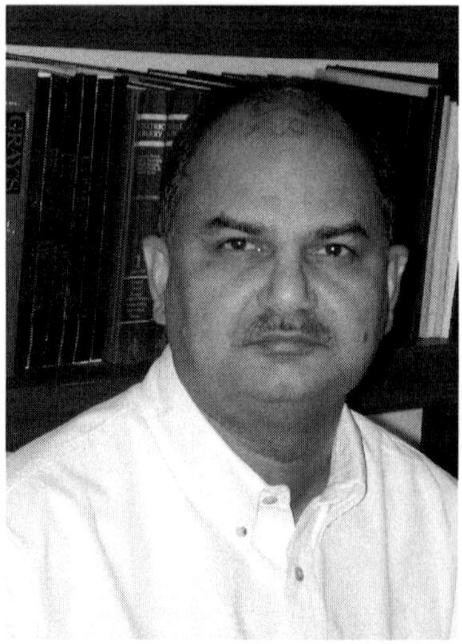

Zafar Nazir

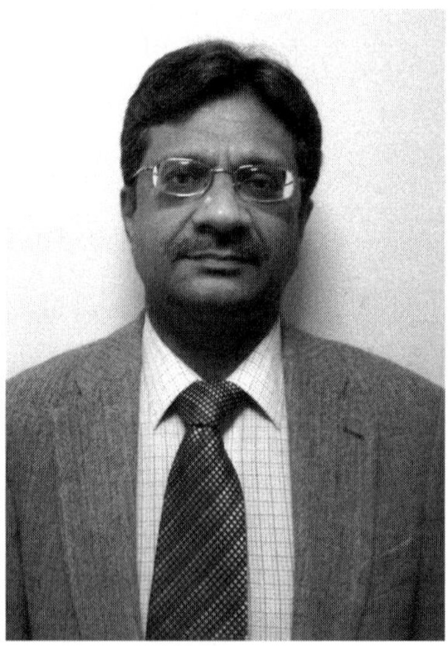

Khalid Rasheed

PAKISTAN

Basith Amjad
Zafar Nazir
Khalid Rasheed

The division of British India in the year 1947 led to the creation of Pakistan. When the new nation came into being, the regions of the Indian subcontinent it encompassed were far from the centre of governance and population masses, and thus the medical services were poorly developed. The few hospitals were confined to the big cities and a few were associated with military institutions established during the Second World War. There was one solitary medical school in the whole country, the King Edward Medical College, at Lahore, in the Punjab. Considering this history and the time and effort it took to set up basic health services in the country, paediatric surgery took its roots just thirty years after its recognition as a separate speciality in the West.

Birth of Paediatric Surgery in Pakistan

The Government of Pakistan with the collaboration of the World Health Organisation (WHO) and UNICEF set up the first Children's Hospital in the country in Karachi, then the capital, in 1958. Dr **Hamid Ali Khan,** a renowned paediatrician, was appointed as the head of the institution and Dr **Amanullah Khan** (Fig. 1), a general surgeon at the Dow Medical College in Karachi, was appointed as the first paediatric surgeon to this hospital. After his appointment Dr Khan proceeded to the **Karolinska Institute** in Stockholm Sweden

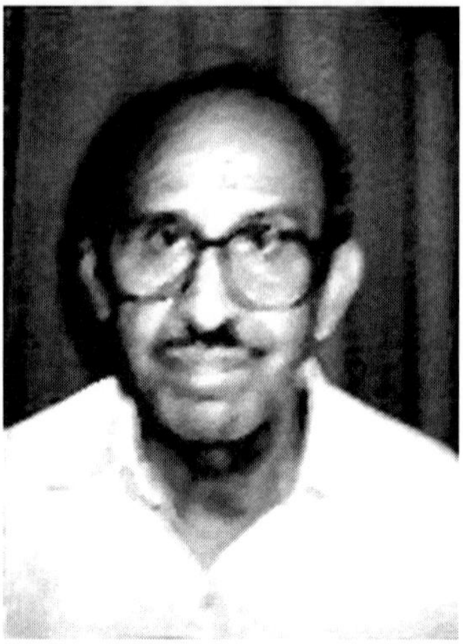

Fig. 1. Prof Amanullah Khan — The First Pediatric Surgeon of Pakistan.

for training in paediatric surgery. This was for a period of one year on a WHO scholarship.

In the spring of 1959 after his return Dr Amanullah Khan set up the department (20 beds) at the old casualty block of the Jinnah Central Hospital (now the Jinnah Postgraduate Medical Centre JPMC). He continued his interest in adult general surgery as well and shared on call commitments for paediatrics with the general surgeons.

In 1963, after the formation of the **Jinnah Postgraduate Medical Centre** (JPMC) Dr Amanullah Khan was appointed the country's first Professor of Paediatric Surgery. In the same year Dr **Nizam ul Hasan** (Fig. 2) trained in the United Kingdom, was appointed as honorary paediatric surgeon at the hospital. Dr Nizam ul Hasan confined his practice solely to children and thus was the first full-time paediatric surgeon in the country.

Initially anaesthetic and critical care was provided by cross cover from the department of anaesthesiology at the JPMC by Prof **A. M. Attar** but in 1964 a separate department was set up when Dr **Muniruddin** was appointed as Assistant Professor of Paediatric Anaesthesiology. Over the course of the next five years a new

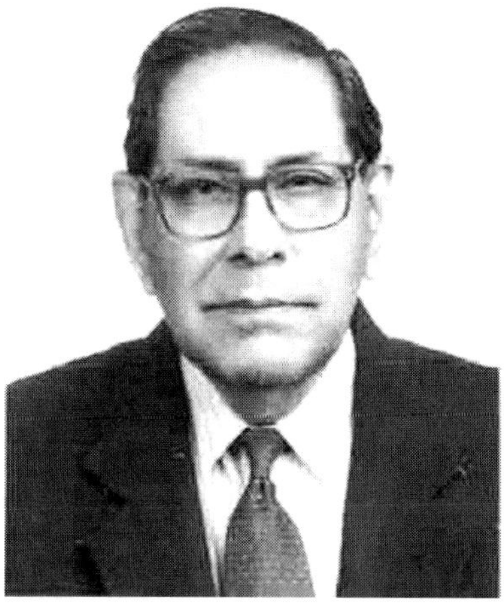

Fig. 2. Prof Nizam ul Hassan — The First Full-Time Pediatric Surgeon and Ex-President of Asian Association of Pediatric Surgeon.

purpose-built children's hospital was set up under the leadership of Dr Amanullah Khan.

In 1972, the department was shifted to its new premises within the confines of the Jinnah Postgraduate Medical Centre. This unit consisted of 300 beds and had two wards of 80 surgical beds, a surgical intensive care unit with a separate surgical nursery, a 10-bed burns unit, three suites of modern operation theatres, an emergency operation theatre, and a separate out-patient department.

With the development of different paediatric medical and surgical services, including a separate paediatric pathology department and ancillary services, this unit was declared by a charter as the **National Institute of Child Health** in 1979. This institute became the first centre for the training of paediatric surgeons in Pakistan.

Dr Khan retired in 1976 due to ill health and Dr Nizamul Hasan took over as the new head. Prof Hasan was one of the early pioneers who steered the formative years of paediatric surgery both on the national and international forums, eventually retiring in 1991. Currently he runs an NGO, a child aid foundation and has helped to establish a paediatric oncology unit at the National Institute of Child Health.

Development of other Centres

Over the decades, with the establishment of further medical schools, more units of paediatric surgery were opened. The second department of paediatric surgery was established at the **Nishter Medical College** in Multan. This was the work of Prof **Abdul Hamid** (Fig. 3) who was appointed as Assistant Professor of Paediatric Surgery in 1967. Prof Hamid had trained in **Dublin**, **Belfast** and **Great Ormond Street Hospital**. Over a period of six years, with hard work and perseverance he had established a full-fledged unit with a well trained staff. He went on to become the second professor of paediatric surgery in Pakistan in 1974. Professor **Nasim Raza** joined him in 1976 as assistant professor.

In 1980 Prof Abdul Hamid moved to **King Edward Medical College** Lahore to set up the third paediatric surgical unit in the country. In 1982 this unit moved to a new purpose built building with 107 beds including an intensive care unit and modern operation theatre facilities. Prof Abdul Hamid has to his credit the training of about 40 paediatric surgeons who occupy responsible positions across the country. He retired in 1993 and was succeeded

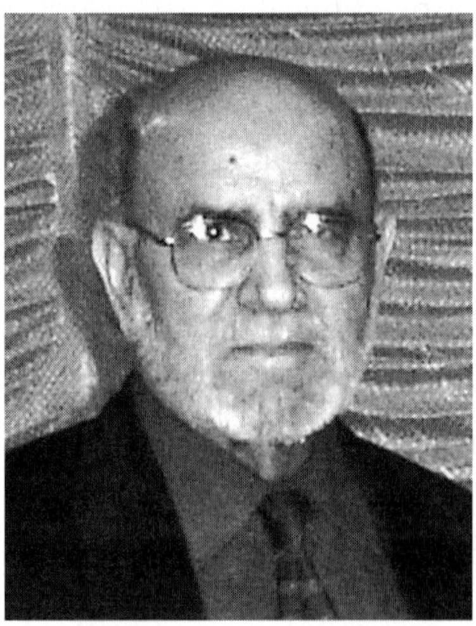

Fig. 3. Prof Abdul Hamid.

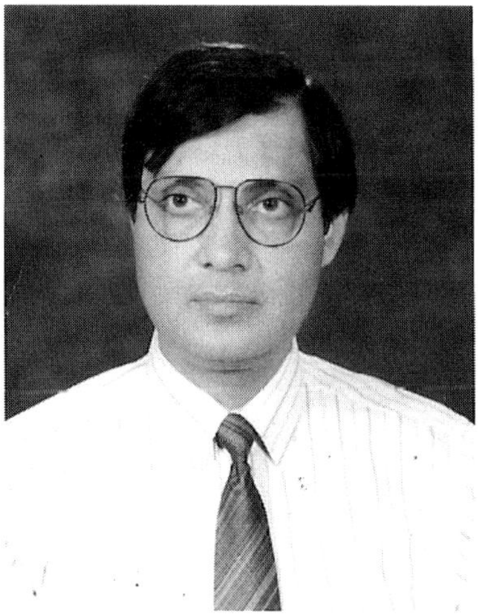

Fig. 4. Prof Moshin Ali.

by Prof Nasim Raza. He continues his interest in paediatric surgery apart from being an avid golfer and terrific story teller. Prof Nasim Raza during his tenure at Nishtar Medical College also trained at Great Ormond Street Hospital London on a one-year scholarship.

Two new paediatric surgical centres were established in 1985. The first was by Prof **Mohsin Azhar Ali** (Fig. 4), current Dean of Ziauddin Hospital and Medical School at the **Dow Medical College** and **Civil Hospital Karachi**. Trained initially under Nizam ul Hasan and later in the UK, Prof Ali has also inspired a generation of paediatric surgeons.

His book "*Notes on Paediatric Surgery*" has benefited not just paediatric surgeons but also general surgeons and all others who have been involved in the care of children in Pakistan.

The year 1985 also saw the appointment of Prof **Farhat Moazam** (Fig. 5), an eminent paediatric surgeon trained in the USA as the chairperson Department of Paediatric Surgery at the newly established **Aga Khan University Hospital** in Karachi. A very reputable and structured surgical residency programme was established under her leadership, the first of its kind in the country. She was later

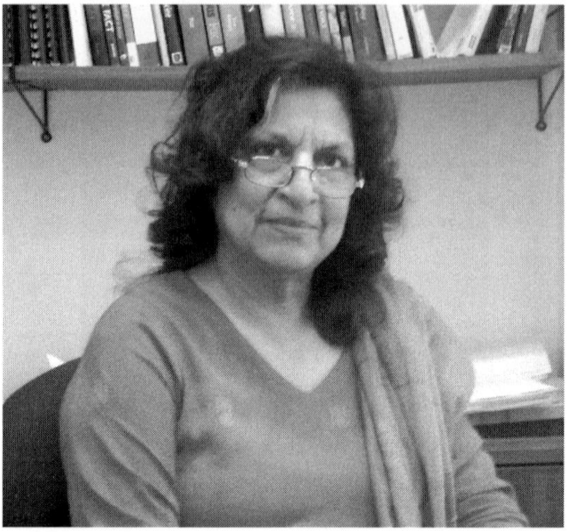

Fig. 5. Prof Farhat Moazam — Pediatric Surgeon, Teacher and Ethicist.

joined by **Khalid Rasheed** in 1991 and **Zafar Nazir** in 1994. AKUH was the first medical school to have paediatric surgery as part of its undergraduate curriculum. Prof Moazam, has since left to establish the Centre of Bioethics at the Sind Institute of Transplantation and Urology, Dow Medical University.

Prof **Naeem uz Zafar Khan** (Fig. 6) also trained at the Great Ormond Street Hospital, set up the first paediatric surgical centre in Islamabad. The **Children's Hospital Islamabad** was established with the help of the Government of Japan in June 1986. He was later appointed as the Professor of Paediatric Surgery at the Quaid-e-Azam University in Islamabad. He is the author of "*Paediatric Surgery Problems*", "*Ectopia Vesicae*" and "*An Atlas of Paediatric Surgery*". Prof Naeem Khan's unit was the first to successfully separate conjoined twins (1992) in Pakistan (Fig. 7). He was later joined by Dr **Zaheer Abbasi** and Dr Iftikhar Jan. Dr Abbasi, who currently heads the department trained in Glasgow in 1982.

In 1987 the Pakistan Army established a paediatric surgical unit at the **Armed Forces Medical College and Military Hospital** in Rawalpindi. This unit has two consultants and a 40-bed paediatric

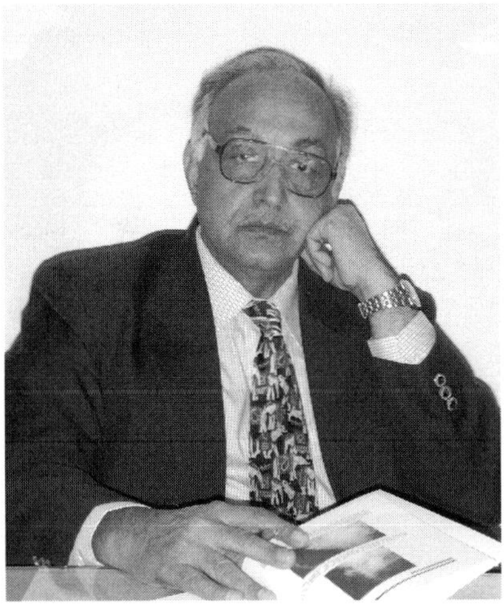

Fig. 6. Prof Naeem Zafar Khan.

surgical unit. The research arm of this unit has produced important clinical and basic research papers. The unit was established by Col **Arshad Hashmi**.

A new unit of paediatric surgery was also established at the Khyber Medical College and Lady Reading Hospital Peshawar in 1988 under Dr **Fazal Rehman**. Since the 1990's further units were established at Bolan Medical College, Quetta, under Dr Iqbal Lashari, the Abbasi Shaheed Hospital, Karachi, under Dr Zeba Attar, the Chandka Medical College, Larkana under Dr Sikander Mughal and at the Punjab Medical College Faisalabad, under Dr Younus Awan.

In 1995 a new children's hospital was established in Lahore called the **Children's Hospital**. It was established by the hard work of **Irfan Mirza** and **Mahmood Shaukat**. It has a close working relationship with the Royal Hospital for Sick Children Glasgow, and is twinned with it. There is an exchange programme in place and personnel have visited either centre to establish liaison and training.

(a)

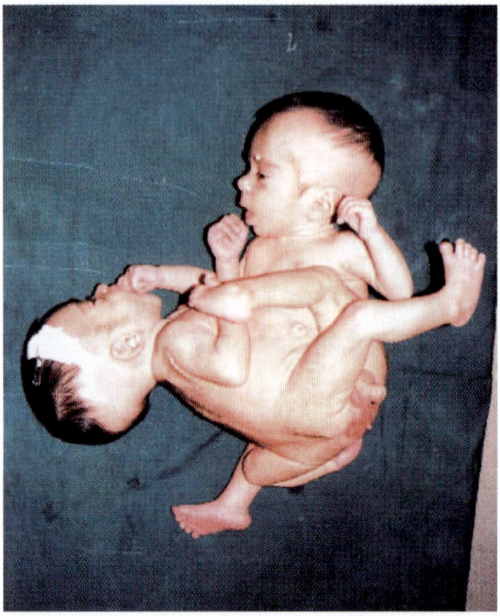

(b)

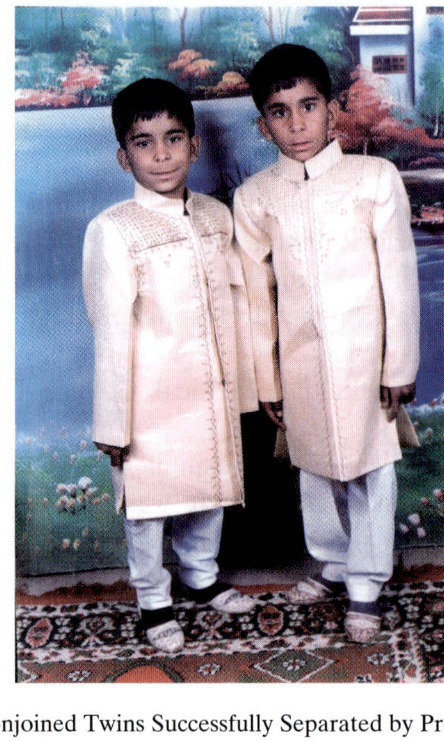

Fig. 7. Conjoined Twins Successfully Separated by Prof Naeem.

Training in Paediatric Surgery

With the development of paediatric surgery as a separate surgical discipline, need for training of paediatric surgeons was soon realised. An exchange programme was set up between the Royal Children's Hospital in Melbourne with the late Prof **Nate Myers** and the National institute of Child Health. Dr **Abdul Aziz**, who later headed the NICH was sent as a trainee to Melbourne for one year. Similarly Dr **Zeba Attar** was sent for a year to work at Kobe Children's Hospital Japan under Dr **Chikara Tsugawa**.

The University of Karachi established a Masters Degree in Paediatric Surgery in 1985. This higher degree did not receive much enthusiasm in the surgical community. Eventually the College of Physicians and Surgeons of Pakistan also established a Paediatric Surgery faculty at the college in 1985 and established an exit examination in the speciality leading to a fellowship in Paediatric Surgery. The first fellowship examination was held in October of 1990 and Prof Amanullah Khan was the first convenor. Over the years about 94 candidates have received this fellowship in Paediatric Surgery.

At present seven institutions are recognized by the College of Physicians and Surgeons of Pakistan (CPSP) for paediatric surgery training (two years general surgery and four years of paediatric surgery). Paediatric surgeons have played a significant role in the governing and academic affairs of CPSP. Prof Aziz Ahmed and Prof Saghir Ahmed have served as Vice President and Secretary of the college respectively. At present the college is accepted by the paediatric surgical community as the sole authority to prepare the curriculum, inspect the training institutions, conduct the examinations and grant the diploma of fellowship in Paediatric Surgery.

Academic Paediatric Surgery

In 1977 the paediatric surgeons in Pakistan were offered an opportunity to join the World Federation of Association of Paediatric Surgeons in Spain. The provision was that a national association must have at least ten members. As there were only six qualified paediatric surgeons in the country, an associate membership was offered to those surgeons whose work involved treating children. Thus a meeting was held in 1977 and an **Association of Paediatric Surgeons in Pakistan (APSP)** was founded in the presence of Prof Amanulah Khan and Prof Nizam ul Hasan. It was formally accepted as a member of the world body in July 1977.

In December 1980, the Association of paediatric Surgeons in Pakistan hosted the Vth Congress of Asian Association of Paediatric Surgeons. Thirty paediatric surgeons from around the world attended the conference and it coincided with the first national congress of APSP. Prof Nizamul Hasan was elected president and Dr Abdul Majid as secretary of the association.

The association with overseas paediatric surgery has continued as both Prof Abdul Hameed and Prof Farhat Moazam have been on the overseas committee of the British Association of Paediatric Surgeons and both Prof Nizam ul Hasan and Prof Mohsin Azhar Ali, on the executive committee of the Asian Association of Paediatric Surgeons.

Future of Paediatric Surgery in Pakistan

At the advent of the new millennium the surgical care of children in Pakistan is still far from satisfactory. Pakistan is a country of 165 million people with an annual growth of 2.03%. Seventy percent of the population lives in rural areas and children below 14 years comprises 40% of the population. Current infant mortality is around 75/1000 live birth. Poverty, illiteracy, poorly developed health infrastructure and difficulties in transportation of sick children has made it difficult for the approximately hundred full-time paediatric surgeons (who are concentrated mainly in large cities) to deliver appropriate paediatric surgical care. Many paediatric patients are still treated by general surgeons. There is a projected need for about 300 paediatric surgeons. Due to poor living conditions surgical emergences are challenges. These include accidental trauma, burns, pyogenic infections and acute abdomen secondary to worm infestation, typhoid and perforated appendices. The elective workload is phenomenal especially in government hospitals. The support facilities such as pathology, anaesthesiology, radiology and intensive care are less than optimal. Late presentation is common and it is not unusual to see exstrophy of the bladder presenting in a patient in his mid-twenties. As a result mortality and morbidity in children undergoing a surgical procedure is high compared to regional and international standards. Due to overwhelming clinical work, poor working environment, few available paediatric surgical positions in government and private sector, poor compensation and desire for better quality of life has made an increasing number of young qualified paediatric surgeons to switch to other specialities. As a result academics and research in paediatric surgery lags behind the current international standards. In spite of these difficulties a few paediatric surgeons are pursuing basic research relating to paediatric surgery and embracing modern technology such as laparoscopy and developing subspecialties such as paediatric urology and oncology.

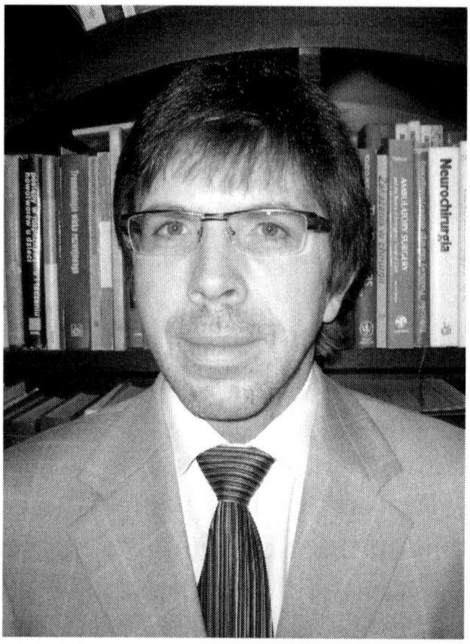

Maciej Baglaj

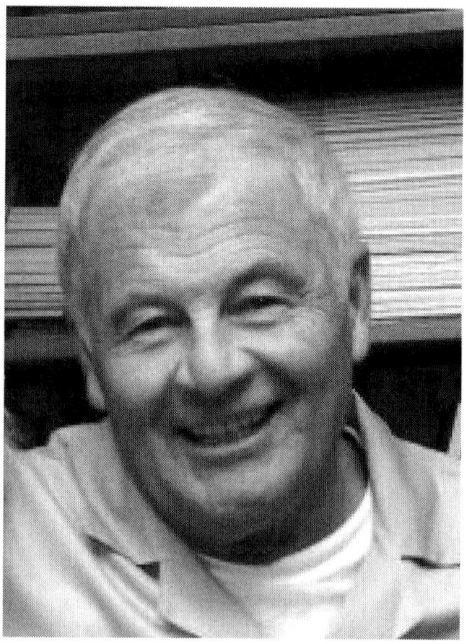

Jerzy Czernik

POLAND

Maciej Baglaj
Jerzy Czernik

Background

The first Polish trace of interest in paediatric diseases which, at present, are univocally considered as indication for surgical treatment has been found in the work from 1583 "*De orbis puerorum tractatem locupletissim*" the author of which was Jan Chróściejewski, a lecturer of Medical University of Venice but native of Poznań. In his treatise, he included a number of descriptions concerning paediatric surgical diseases such as inguinal hernias, rachischises, palatal clefts and even anal atresia.

The beginnings of paediatric surgical treatment in Polish territories dates back to 19th century. The preserved literature reveals the incidental attempts of surgical treatment of both acquired and congenital deformities even in the first decades of the century. In 1810, the first manual in Polish language was published. Its title was "*Paediatric Diseases*" and the author, Jakub Szymkiewicz, gave a detailed description of diagnosis and treatment concerning many acquired childhood diseases such as skin haematomas and abscesses, bone inflammations, fractures and dislocations, head injuries or phimosis. Also, he discussed developmental anomalies like myelomeningoceles, inguinal and umbilical hernias, cleft lip, anal atresia and limbs deformities.

19th Century

Only with the rise of first infirmaries and children's hospitals was paediatrics distinguished as an individual medical discipline. The first children's hospital was founded in 1845 in Lwow (St. Sophie's Children's Hospital) and the next hospitals dealing only with paediatric patients were raised in Warsaw in 1869 (Children's Hospital at Solna Street), in Kraków in 1876 (St. Lewis' Hospital), in Poznań (St. Joseph's Hospital) and the second hospital in Warsaw (Berson's Hospital). On the basis of St. Lewis' Hospital in Kraków, the first in Poland and the third in the world, the University Department of Paediatrics was founded and its first Head was Maciej Leon Jakubowski, the professor of Jagiellonian University. However, in the second half of the 19th century, the number of paediatric hospitals was still too small and majority of ill children were referred to hospitals specialising in treatment of adults.

The development of paediatric surgery in Poland in 19th century was initiated both by surgeons and paediatricians. At that time, children were treated surgically either by surgeons additionally employed in paediatric hospitals or in hospitals for adults. The range of surgical procedures was limited so, for those reasons, mainly children with traumatic injuries, osteoarticular tuberculosis, foreign bodies and superficial tumours were operated on. However, in some centres, children with skeletal deformities, hernias or facial clefts were treated as well. The literature evidencing the condition of medicine of those days includes reports concerning the attempts of treating anal atresia, intussusception, urolithiasis, hydrocephalus, myelocele, torticollis and haemangiomas. The fact that, apart from their regular job in general hospitals, the surgeons were additionally involved in medical practice in children's hospitals did not prevent them from significant achievements in the field of paediatric surgical treatment. Some of those achievements undoubtedly largely contributed towards the development of surgery. Tomasz Drobnik was the first to carry out successful subperiosteal translocations of tendons in children with cerebral palsy. He also described original method of osteotomy with Achilles tendon elongation in rachitic deformation as well as in talipes varus. In years 1890 to 1899, he was the Head of Children's Hospital in Poznań. In 1899 in Kraków, Maksymilian Rutkowski, a head physician of St. Lewis' Hospital Surgical Department, performed a pioneer reconstruction of bladder extrophy with the use of ileal segment.

An outstanding and highly estimated contribution towards the development of medicine is that of Jan Mikulicz–Radecki's whose pioneer work gave absolutely new basis and prospects for world surgery. In his professional activity, he mainly concentrated on adult patients. However, his significant role in laying paediatric surgery foundation has always been widely recognised. Mikulicz–Radecki was a pupil of Prof T. Billroth, and early during his activity in Vienna, in cooperation with J. Leiter he invented the first oesophagoscope and gastroscope initiating a new era in endoscopy which gave him the title "father of endoscopy" in medical literature. In 1882, he became the Head of Surgical Department of Jagiellonian University in Kraków and in years 1882 to 1887 he was in charge of the first paediatric surgery department in Polish territories in St. Lewis Hospital. In 1887, he described the technique of pyloroplasty known as Heineke–Mikulicz operation. (The procedure was performed by Heineke in 1886). In 1890, Jan Mikulicz–Radecki took on the post of the Head of the Surgical Department in Wrocław and it was a culminant period in his surgical activity. His pioneer permanent ventricular drainage was performed for the first time in 1895 in a hydrocephalic child. It was ventriculo-subgaleal system with gold-plated metal tubes as its main element. In 1893, for the first time, Mikulicz performed staged resection of the large intestine due to carcinoma. The technique of intestinal double-barrel fistula described by Mikulicz was subsequently adapted by paediatric surgeons in treating intestinal deformities and acquired diseases. His most outstanding achievements were clinical and experimental studies carried out with his pupil — F. Sauerbruch — which resulted in foundations of thoracic surgery. Wrocław was the centre where the first open thoracotomies were carried on.

The pupils of Mikulicz took over his work which resulted in significant improvement of medical care of children who required surgical treatment. One should not forget about Hilary Schramm who was the author of the first Polish manual "*Paediatric Surgical Diseases*" published in Lwow in 1901. After moving from Krakow to Lwow, in 1886, he expanded the activity of Surgical Department of St. Sophie's Hospital. His clinical as well as organizational achievements were of great importance and in 1887 he included clinical classes in the curriculum of studies for the students of Medical Faculty of Lwow University. His inauguration lecture which was also the thesis qualifying him as assistant professor pointed at the need to recognize paediatric surgery as an individual clinical specialty.

Assistant professor Bossowski, who took after Mikulicz the post of the Head of Surgical Department in St. Lewis' Hospital, largely broadened the range of operative procedures. The new scope of operations included corrections of post traumatic and burn scars, hand recontructive operations, treatment of spina bifida, hepatic and renal neoplasms or treatment of congenital megocolon by ileoanal anastomosis.

20th Century

In the first decades of 20th century, sudden political transformations in Europe inhibited the development of medical science. Only with the independence regain, after 120-year period of the partitions of Poland, did the welfare system reconstruction began. Although the number of paediatric wards was still small, the development of the system included also the medical care of children. Hospitals founded in 19th century in Kraków, Warsaw, Poznań and Lwow were still the leading centres of paediatric treatment. In 1911 a new Children's Hospital in Lublin was opened following the foundation of Anna-Maria's Hospital in Łódź and in 1913, Charles and Mary's Hospital was built in Warsaw. Children were treated also in St. Jacob's General Hospital in Vilnus and all these hospitals had seprate surgical wards.

Warsaw Children's Hospital at Kopernik Street largely contributed towards the development of Polish paediatric surgery. In the inter war period, it was the biggest and the most active paediatric surgical department in Poland. Its heads still had to divide their attention and time for children and adults. In 1931, Dr Jan Kossakowski joined Warsaw Children's Hospital. He was the pioneer and founder of modern paediatric surgery in Poland. Initially he was an assistant of Dr Zaorski who was also the Head of surgical department for adults in St. Elisabeth Sisters Hospital in Warsaw. However, Dr J. Kossakowski devoted himself to paediatrics only and he belonged to the group of a few surgeons interested in development and independence of paediatric surgery. The group also comprised of Alojzy Maciejewski, Edward Drescher, Tadeusz Hroboni from Warsaw Children's Hospital, Matylda Tomaszewska from Łódź and Józefa Dowgiallo–Moszyńska from Vilnus. Dr Kossakowski focussed especially on surgical diseases of newborns and infants giving the basis for surgical care of neonates in Poland. In 1937, Jan Kossakowski (Fig. 1) left the Hospital at M. Kopernik Street and took the post of the Head of Surgery and Orthopaedics Department of University Hospital at Litewska Street.

The Second World War suddenly interrupted the development of paediatric surgery in Poland as not only was the hospital infrastructure completely destroyed but also the group of young talented

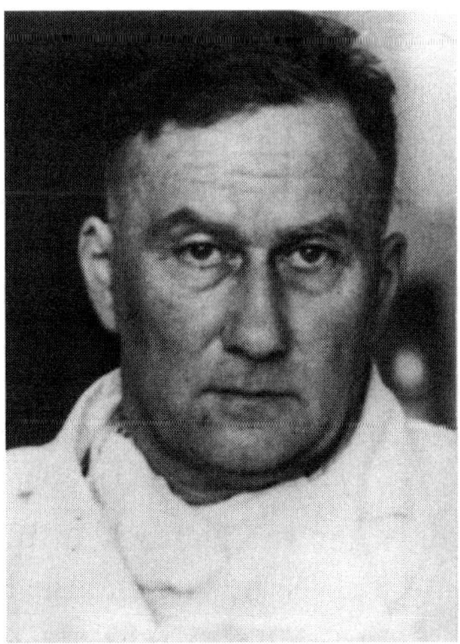

Fig. 1. Prof Jan Kossakowski.

surgeons had to leave the places of their work for a long time. Their extreme effort in coming to the rescue and medical assistance for civilian inhabitants of invaded Warsaw cannot be avoided here, especially during The Warsaw Rising in 1944. Apart from clinical activity, many of them were also involved in secret medical classes. After the Second World War, the surgeons got back to work and start to organise the basis for medical service not only in Warsaw but in the whole country. Paediatric University Hospital at Litewska Street returned to its normal activity under the supervision of Dr J. Kossakowski. Dr Edward Drescher got the post of the Head of Paediatric Surgery Department of Polish Red Cross at Unia Lubelska Street in Szczecin. Dr Alojzy Maciejewski became the Head of Surgery and Orthopaedics Department in Gdańsk and Dr Zbigniew Tabeński organized The Municipal Hospital in Gliwice in which, in 1945, Paediatric Surgery Unit was founded. In January, 1946, Children's Hospital in Poznań resumed its medical activity with Dr Suwalski as the Head and Dr Matylda Tomaszewska again got the same post in Children's Hospital in Łódź. In 1945, Warsaw Children's Hospital at M. Kopernik Street returned to its activity. Also Charles and Mary's Hospital, after total destruction during the war, was opened again in 1947 in a new seat at Działdowska Street under the supervision of Dr Tadeusz Hroboni.

After World War II

After his return to the Paediatric Department of Warsaw University Hospital, Dr Jan Kossakowski became an expert in surgical treatment of children both in Poland and abroad. His incredible committal and passion gave the foundation for modern paediatric surgery in Poland. His great interest in surgical treatment of the youngest patients was reflected in his monograph and habilitation thesis "*Indications for Surgical Treatment of Newborns and Infants*". In 1948, Dr Kossakowski began the lectures at the Medical Faculty of Warsaw University and in 1951 he became the holder of, the first in Poland, Chair of Paediatric Surgery. He got the professor title in

1957. Due to his scientific, clinical and organisational activity, the Chair of Paediatric Surgery acted as the cradle of Polish paediatric surgery. Prof Kossakowski not only initiated development of surgical treatment of newborns and children in Poland but also influenced significantly development of paediatric cardiac surgery and thoracic surgery. In 1955, Prof Kossakowski performed for the first time in Poland Blalock–Taussig procedure, and in 1963, he and his associates, for the first time, repaired ventricular defect in extracorporeal circulation. Apart from his rare surgical skills, Prof Kossakowski was extraordinarily active in the scientific field. He conferred 22 doctors and seven habilitation theses and was the author of six manuals of paediatric surgery and 138 scientific papers. A large group of his pupils included 16 heads of paediatric surgery departments and the circle who carried on with his achievements and largely contributed towards the development of this medical specialty in Poland included: Prof Wanda Poradowska, Prof Kazimierz Łodziński, Prof Irena Gizycka, Prof Krystyna Wysocka, Prof Irena Smólska, Prof Eugenia Zdebska, Prof Jarosław Stodulski, Prof Zygmunt Kaliciński and Dr Andrzej Kamiński.

Prof Kossakowski helped to recognise paediatric surgery as an individual medical discipline and in 1949 he was appointed to the post of state consultant in paediatric surgery. In 1951, in Kielce, the group of leading surgeons: Jan Kossakowski, Wanda Poradowska from Warsaw, Edward Drescher from Szczecin, Zbigniew Tabeński from Gliwice, Alojzy Maciejewski from Łódź, Aleksander Naumik from Lublin, Stefan Kiełkiewicz from Kielce and Tadeusz Hroboni from Warsaw constituted a Team of Regional Specialists in Paediatric Surgery to form the basis for modern surgical care for children. For the first time, the curriculum of specialization in paediatric surgery was elaborated. In the same year, during 2nd Conference of Regional Specialists in Paediatric Surgery, the Paediatric Surgery Section of Polish Association of Surgeons was brought into being.

Prof Kossakowski's services for the development of paediatric surgery in Poland made his pupils create the Chapter of Prof Kossakowski Medal with the motto "*Serere ne dubites*" in 1994. The medal is awarded to Polish surgeons with the recognition of their achievements in paediatric surgery.

The 1950's and 1960's were the period of formation of paediatric surgical departments within the organisational framework of Medical Universities. Not only did it prove the dynamic development of this specialisation but confirmed full acknowledgement of its importance.

Building a fully professional didactic basis both for students and postgraduate teaching was of great importance. In 1954, the Paediatric Surgery Department in Gdańsk came into being followed by opening of Paediatric Surgery Departments in Łódź and Wrocław a year later. In 1957, the Surgical Department of Paediatric Institute in Szczecin was founded and in 1963, the Paediatric Surgery Department of University Hospital in Lublin was opened. In 1966, in Kraków, a modern Paediatric Institute with surgical unit was established which later was transformed into Paediatric Surgery Department.

In 1953, the Paediatric Surgery Department of Mother and Child Research Institute was founded, the first head of which was Prof Wanda Poradowska, one of those most meritorious for paediatric surgery development. She was one of a few post-war surgeons who did the training in centres abroad as in 1948, she was awarded Rockefeller Scholarship and worked in Children's Hospital in Boston. She created a leading centre of paediatric surgery where many specialists from the whole country were trained. Independently from Prof Adam Michejda from Paediatric Surgery Department of Medical University of Wrocław, in 1956 Prof Poradowska successfully performed the first successful repair of oesophageal atresia in Poland. Among her numerous achievements, the most eminent were: modern medical care of burns, treatment of congenital defects in neonates as well as development of paediatric thoracic surgery. Prof Poradowska created the first Polish centre for craniofacial clefts treatment. In the 1970's, her Paediatric Surgery Department started cooperation with American centres focussed on a complex treatment and rehabilitation of neural tube defects resulting in therapeutic management adapted to all sections in the country. In 1972, Prof Poradowska, Prof Kubicz and Dr Reszke published a manual in

English "*Surgical Lung Diseases in Children*". Her initiative resulted in the first intensive paediatric care unit formed in the structures of Mother and Child Research Institute and later transformed into the Department of Intensive Care and Anaesthesiology with Prof Z. Rondio as the Head. It was definitely a "milestone" in the development of paediatric anaesthesiology and intensive care and it largely influenced the progress of paediatric surgery and especially neonatal surgery. From 1960 to 1982, Prof Poradowska (Fig. 2) was the State Specialist in Paediatric Surgery. She was the editor-in-chief of the manual "*Paediatric Surgery. Selected Problems*" published in 1977 and revised in 1992. The successor and the one to continue her eminent work was Prof Kazimierz Łodziński who directed the Paediatric Surgery Department of Mother and Child Research Institute till the year 1992.

In 1962, at the Mother and Child Research Institute in Warsaw, the Oncological Department for Children and Adolescents was formed under the supervision of its founder and the first head, Prof Józef Bożek. It was the first Polish centre offering complex multimodal treatment of paediatric solid tumours and became a very

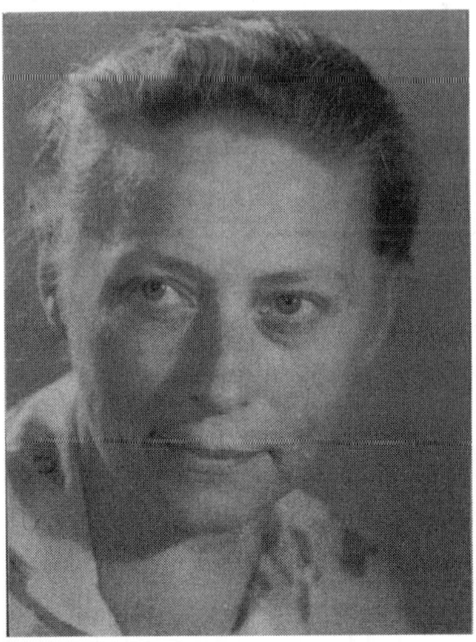

Fig. 2. Prof Poradowska.

active scientific and didactic centre involved in training of many paediatric surgeons interested in paediatric oncology.

In 1965, Paediatric Surgery Section of Polish Association of Surgeons was changed to Polish Association of Paediatric Surgeons, which was a significant event laying emphasis on the advance of this medical discipline in Poland. Its first President was Prof Jan Kossakowski and in 1967, in Warsaw, the first Congress took place. Subsequently, it would be organised once every three years.

In 1974, the first issue of "*Paediatric Surgery Problems*" as Polish Association of Paediatric Surgeons' annual was published. It appeared until 1996 and its editor-in-chief was Prof Kazimierz Łodziński.

The combined Congress of British Association of Paediatric Surgeons and Polish Association of Paediatric Surgeons organized in Sheffield and Warsaw in 1976 was an acknowledgement of distinct achievements of Polish paediatric surgeons. J. Lister was the contemporary President of the British Association and Prof K Łodziński was the President of the Polish one and the Warsaw Congress promoter was Prof Z. Kaliciński. It was the first congress of such a dignity in Central and Eastern Europe of those days.

The 1960's and 1970's were the years of dynamic development of paediatric surgery in Poland. Apart from Warsaw departments, other university paediatric surgical departments played an important role in advances of this specialty. In many of them, significant achievements of international acknowledgement were made. Prof E. Drescher was the author of an original method of conservative treatment of extensive omphalocoele. Prof Jan Słowikowski, the Head of Paediatric Surgery Department in Wrocław, invented his own method of meso-caval anastomosis in portal hypertension. He was also the author of modified procedure for pancreatic cysts. Dr Roman Gross from Paediatric Surgery Department in Gdańsk elaborated inventory techniques of hypospadiasis repair. Prof Marian Koszla from Children's Hospital in Warsaw largely contributed towards the development of paediatric orthopaedics and traumatology in Poland. He was the author of the first manual on paediatric traumatology, "*Koszla's Dilator*" is his most outstanding achievement which is still used in conservative treatment of congenital hip dysplasia and dislocation in neonates and infants. Prof Zygmunt Kaliciński was the promoter and first head of Paediatric Surgery Department of Military University of Medicine in Warsaw. He elaborated original methods of treatment of megaureters, ureteral duplication and posterior urethra valves. The method of ureteral plication known in literature as Kaliciński's method (1977) gained general acceptance in urological practice in the world.

In 1966, in Krakow, a modern children's hospital was founded in the structures of which, Paediatric Surgery Department was formed with Prof Jan Grochowski as its first head. Due to American partners' support, the hospital was transformed into Polish-American Institute of Paediatrics and was one of the best paediatric centres in the country. Apart from paediatric surgery, it included departments of plastic surgery, microsurgery, urology, neurosurgery, orthopaedics, traumatology and cardiosurgery. Conferences and courses organised by Hope Foundation in co-operation with American paediatric surgeons gave excellent training forum for Polish doctors in the eighties.

Another important aspect of Polish paediatric surgery advance was international co-operation and trainings in paediatric centres abroad. They not only enabled learning the most contemporary achievements in paediatric surgery but also gaining new experience, which was transformed and adapted to Polish reality. Under the initiative of the Association led for many years by President Prof Zygmunt Kaliciński (Fig. 3), this resulted in the rise of four foundations which enabled education of Polish surgeons in medical centres in the United States, Great Britain, Japan or France. Among many foundations, the support of the following cannot be avoided here: Children's Medical Care Foundation from Los Angeles started by Richard Fine and Stefan Wilk, MD, Dr Stefan Glowacki's foundation from Detroit, Polish Children's Foundation from New York set up by Maria Niemirska, and Prof Hagiwara's foundation from Kyoto. Brunehilde Mai and Prof R. Pilchmeyer played an important role in organization of trainings for Polish surgeons in Hannover.

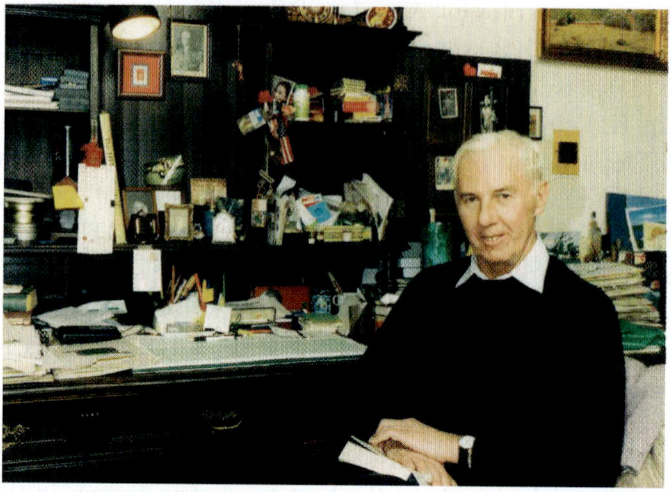

Fig. 3. Professor Zygmunt Kaliciński

In 1993 Prof Łodziński (the editor-in-chief) published the first issue of the periodical "*Surgery in Childhood International*". The Editorial Board included the most outstanding paediatric surgeons from many countries and at that time, it was one out of four international journals devoted to paediatric surgery only.

In 1980, in Warsaw, a new hospital was opened, Children's Memorial Health Centre which also included departments of surgery, urology, neurosurgery and cardiosurgery. From the very beginning, it became a leading centre of paediatric treatment in Poland. The the first Head of Surgical Department was Prof Z. Kaliciński and from 1981, the post was taken over by Dr Wojciech Kamiński. The latter one constituted the team specialising in the paediatric treatment of abnormalities of gastrointestinal system, liver, bile duct, pancreas as well as metabolic diseases and endocrine glands disturbances.

The Paediatric Urology Department headed by Prof Czesław Szymkiewicz was the first unit in Poland of this profile. Its outstanding achievements were elaboration of original diagnostic and therapeutic procedures in children with abnormal sexual differentation, in children with neurogenic dysfunction of the lower urinary tract as well as introduction of original complex surgical treatment of bladder extrophy.

In the Paediatric Surgery Department of Children's Memorial Health Centre, in 1984 the solid organ transplantation programme for children was initiated. Being the first paediatric transplantology centre, it has made new prospects for treating children with renal or liver diseases. The first successful kidney transplantation in a child was made in 1984 and since 1990, liver transplantations have been made as well. Transplantation programme has been realized until nowadays thanks to incredible committment of the whole team headed by Prof Piotr Kaliciński. Organ transplantation has become one of main goals of the Department activity and in 2002 the Department was transformed into the Department of Paediatric Surgery and Transplantology. In this centre, for the first time in Poland, successful transplantation of liver from family donor was made. Also the pioneer combined transplants of liver, intestines and pancreas were made there. At present, the Warsaw centre is one of leaders in paediatric transplantology in Europe which is proved not only by mere statistics but through the excellence of results as well.

In the 1990's, Paediatric Surgery Department of Medical University of Wrocław became an important neonatal surgery centre headed by Prof Słowikowski's pupil, Prof Jerzy Czernik. A modern system of neonatal care has been created which has improved the results of congenital diseases surgical treatment in Lower Silesia Region. Since 1993, Prof Czernik has been the State Consultant in Paediatric Surgery. His efforts have resulted in recognition of Paediatric surgery as an individual clinical specialty.

In 1997, a modern hospital complex in Łódź was opened — Polish Mother's Memorial Research Institute in the structures of which, modern departments of paediatric surgery, neurosurgery, and cardiac surgery started their activity. The organiser of the Surgical Department was Prof A. Chilarski, who has been its Head up to the present moment. Polish Mother's Memorial Research Institute was the first clinical centre in Poland in which the system of a complex prenatal care of mother and her child was established. There, first surgical prenatal interventions were made in foetuses affected by hydrocephalus and urinary tract anomalies.

In 2000, Upper Silesia Mother and Child Research Institute opened and it included modern paediatric surgery and urology department headed by Prof Bohosiewicz. Special achievement of the department team was introduction of prenatal management of myelomeningocoele. However, the first surgical procedure in a foetus with myelomeningocoele in Poland was performed in 2003 by Prof Stoba, the Head of Paediatric Surgery Department in Gdańsk.

Since 1995, in Poland, a dynamic development of minimally invasive surgery has been noted. The first centres to introduce modern endoscopic techniques in routine clinical practice were the Paediatric Surgery Department of Wrocław Medical University headed by Prof Jerzy Czernik as well as the Department of Paediatric Surgery and Traumatology from Zabrze headed by Prof J. Dzielicki. At present, minimally invasive techniques are widely used in many departments of paediatric surgery.

In 2005, in Gdańsk VII EUPSA Congress was held and the Presidents of Organizing Committee were Prof Czesław Stoba and Prof P. Czauderna — the former and present heads of Paediatric Surgery Dept. of Medical University of Gdańsk.

Nowadays, in Poland, paediatric surgery is fully recognised medical sepciality. There are over 80 paediatric surgery departments or units and over 80% of children requiring surgical care are treated by paediatric surgeons.

The long period of over 200 years of surgical treatment of children shows how important proper medical assistance for children has always been in Polish territories. Paediatric surgery development in Poland has been interrupted by many dramatical events which inhibited or totally interrupted its progress. However, Polish surgeons' steadfastness and determination helped to maintain medical care for the youngest patients. Dynamic development of this discipline is still continued. Prof Kossakowski and his followers began a new era in the advance of this specialty and Polish paediatric surgeons have always been opened to new achievements of world paediatrics and declared cooperation with other countries surgeons to implement new experience into their everyday clinical practice in order to improve treatment results. Today, Polish paediatric surgery can positively be considered a stable pillar of modern paediatric surgery in united Europe.

References

1. Aschoff A, Kunze A. The first permanent shunt implantation in the history by Mikulicz 1893 in Wrocław/Breslau. *Neur Neurochir Pol* 1996;30 (Suppl 4):298–301.
2. Bogusz J, Kudowski W. *Sylwetki chirurgów polskich*. Wroclaw, 1982.
3. Drescher E. Observations on the conservative treatment of exopmpholos. *Arch Dis Child* 1963;38:135–137.
4. Drobnik T. O przenoszeniu czynności mieśni przy porażeniach dziecięcych. *Gaz Lek* 1893;5:120–125.
5. Gorecki P, Gorecki W. Jan Mikulicz–Radecki (1850–1905) The creator of modern European surgery. *Dig Surg* 2002;19:313–320.
6. Gross R. Subcutaneous continous pullout sutures in hypospadiasis repair. *Z Kinderchir* 1979;28:67–76.
7. Karcz D. Jan Mikulicz — twórca ezofagoskopii i gastroskopii. *Arch Hist Med* 1997;40:327–331.
8. Kossakowski J. *Wskazania do zabiegow chirurgicznych u noworodków i niemowlat*. Lek Inst Nauk Wyd, Warszawa, 1949.
9. Kossakowski J. *Chirurgia wieku dziecięcego*. Czesc ogolna. PZWL, Warszawa, 1952.
10. Łodziński K. Rozwój chirurgii dziecięcej w Polsce. In Jerzy Czernik (ed.) *Chirurgia Dziecięca* PZWL, Warszawa, 2005, pp. 5–13.
11. Kalicinski ZH, Kansy J, Kotarbińska B, *et al.* Surgery of megaureters — modification of Hendren's operation. *J Pediatr Surg* 1977;12:183–187.
12. Kalicinski ZH, Joszt W, Perdzynski W, *et al.* Completely duplicated ureters. A new concept of reimplantation. *J Pediatr Surg* 1992;27:70–73.
13. Łodziński K. Krajowy Zespół. Specjalistyczny w dziedzinie Chirurgii Dziecięcej. *Probl Chir Dziec* 1993;20:17–19.
14. Łodziński K. 35-lat działalności Kliniki Chirurgii Dzieci i Młodzieży Instytutu Matki i Dziecka. *Prob Chir Dziec* 1990;16:10–21.

15. Poradowska W. Stan chirurgii dziecięcej w Polsce. *Probl Chir Dziec* 1973;5:5–10.
16. Rejmanowski T. Chirurgiczne leczenie dzieci w Polsce w XIX w. *Arch Hist Fil Med* 1988;51:213–219.
17. Schramm H. O potrzebie nauki chirurgii pediatrycznej. *Przegl Lek* 1897;36:605–606, 619–620.
18. Smólska I, Dziak A. Historia chirurgii dziecięcej w Polsce. *Arch Hist Fil Med* 1989;52:293–307.
19. Smólska I, Kaliciński ZH, Kamiński A, Lodziński Kamieński. *Historia chirurgii dziecięcej w Polsce.* Invest-Druk, Warszawa, 1999.
20. Smólska I, Łodziński K, Cedro A. *Historia chirurgii dziecięcej w Polsce. Wydawnictwo Diecezji Pelplińskiej, Bernardinum*", Pelplin Warszawa, 2003.
21. Słowikowski J. Własne modyfikacje operacji Mariona w leczeniu nadciśnienia wrotnego u dzieci. *Pol Tyg Lek* 1964;19:728–731.
22. Słowikowski J. Modyfikacja operacyjnego leczenia torbieli trzustki. *Pol Przegl Chir* 1966;38:783–785.
23. Woźniewski Z, Wieczorek J. Drogi rozwoju chirurgii dziecięcej w Polsce. Pamiętnik I Zjazdu Polskiego Towarzystwa Chirurgów Dziecięcych, Warszawa, 1967, p. 3–8.
24. Wronecki K. Jan Mikulicz Radecki — wielki chirurg wrocławski. *Probl Chir Dziec* 1993;20:136–142.

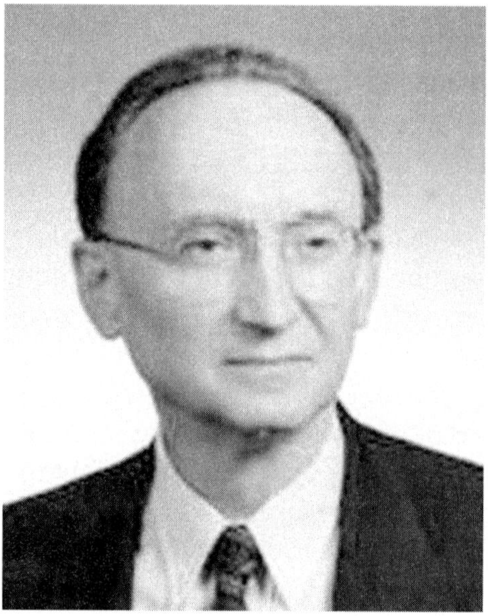

António Gentil Martins

PORTUGAL

António Gentil Martins

Paediatric surgery started in Portugal, as in the rest of the world, with a strong element of children's orthopedics. The first journal, published in 1921, was called "*Archives of Paediatrics and Orthopedics*". Jaime Ernesto Salazar d'Eça e Sousa, Chair Professor of the Surgical Sector of Lisbon's Medical School since 1910, was invited, in 1911, to chair the teaching of Paediatrics and Orthopedics, having previously obtained his Diploma in both areas, in the USA, in 1897 (Fig. 1).

In 1914, Francisco Gentil, as the Head of Lisbon's Civil Hospitals, which included the *Hospital D. Estefânia* (Lisboa's main Children's Hospital and one of the oldest in Europe, opened on the 17th July 1877, under King Peter the IVth, and according to the wishes of his prematurely deceased wife, Queen D. Estefânia), decided to create separate wards, one for Medical diseases of children and another for Orthopedic and Surgical patients.

Jaime Salazar de Sousa became responsible for both, what was officially consecrated by Law 4.563 of the July 9th, 1918. He became internationally known by identifying the hypersplenism syndrome and treating Kalazar by splenectomy, as well as through the use of placental blood for measles immunisation. His Doctoral Theses, in 1899, was on "*Bone Surgery in Infancy*" and the first surgical operation in children, performed at the Hospital D. Estefânia, was the removal of an osteocondroma in 1910. The designation of Medical Paediatrics and Surgical Paediatrics was only officially referred to, on the January 25th, 1929, through

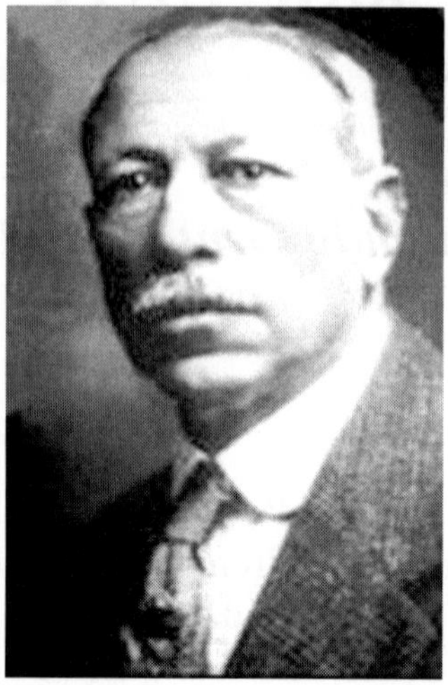

Fig. 1. Jaime Salazar de Sousa.

Law 16.419. Later, Jaime Salazar de Sousa, became Chair Professor of Paediatrics, at Lisbon's Medical School.

As had happened with him, some of his medical and surgical disciple, namely his son, Carlos Salazar de Sousa and Leonardo Castro Freire, also became Chair Professors of Paediatrics at the same Medical School.

Only in 1940, after his death, was a full separation between the two branches of Paediatrics completed, when a full-time Surgeon, Abel Pereira da Cunha, took full care of the surgical ward, having performed the first correction of an intestinal atresia.

After Abel da Cunha's death, in 1959, Eduardo Rosado Pinto e Luciano and José de Carvalho, divided between them the responsability for two surgical departments that resulted from the reorganisation of the Hospital D. Estefânia, confirming the clear separation of Paediatric Surgery and Orthopedics from Medical Paediatrics. In the following years at the *Hospital D. Estefânia*, the very first units, for Neo-Natal Surgery and for Childrens' Burns, were developed by Luciano de Carvalho, the first one being substituted later by a multi-disciplinary Medico-Surgical Intensive Care Neo-Natal, as it stands today.

In the 1960's, paediatric orthopedics was so essential (in the tradition of Ombredanne and Denis Browne), that, for the only Medical Career in Paediatric Surgery and Training Program that then existed in Portugal, the admission examination for a position of Consultant at Lisbon's city hospitals, one of the two patients, to be examined and discussed, had always to be an orthopedic one, the other being of any other surgical pathology. Nevertheless, now, children's orthopedics is no longer a must, having become optional.

Fernando Afonso followed Rosado Pinto and divided his department in General and Neo-Natal Surgery, Urology, Plastic Surgery and Orthopaedics. On the other end, Gentil Martins considering the need for postgraduate teaching and also the need for multidisciplinary emergency work preferred a formal rotation through all the sectors of pathology.

When Fernando Afonso retired in 1996, orthopedics separated completely from paediatric Surgery, and later became directed by an adult orthopedic Surgeon (with a special interest in children's work). In Porto and Coimbra, orthopedics was always out of the scope of paediatric surgery, although include in the Program of Training, as defined by the Ordem dos Médicos (Portuguese Medical Association and Council), until it became optional.

António Gentil Martins author started his work at the *Hospital D. Estefânia*, in 1960, as the first Portuguese Paediatric Surgeon to be fully trained abroad. Before, he had been a British Council Scholar for Paediatric Surgery, training in London, mainly with Sir Denis Browne and David Innes Williams, and in Liverpool, with Isabella Forshall, Peter Rickham and Herbert Johnson, from 1956 to 1959. From there he brought the ideas of a Neo-Natal Surgical Unit and of a Burns Unit, later implemented at the *Hospital D. Estefânia*, by Luciano de Carvalho, his Chief. In 1960 he created the World's first multi-disciplinary (Medico-Surgical) Unit for Paediatric Cancer, at the *Instituto Português de Oncologia Francisco Gentil*, Lisboa, with a totally independent ward since 1966.

He had not only national but also important international activity, having been the Portuguese representative in the Founding of EUPSA (European Union of Paediatric Surgical Associations,

1973) and of WOFAPS (World Federation of Associations of Paediatric Surgeons, 1974), of which he was a Member of the Executive. He was also, for two years, President of the World Medical Association, and was Founder and Honorary Member of the International Societies of Paediatric Oncology (SIOP) and Pediatric Surgical Oncology (IPSO), having been Member of the Scientific Committee of the first and Member of the Board of the second.

Apart from having been for ten years President of the *Ordem dos Médicos*, and Member Emeritus of the Portuguese Academy of Medicine, he was also the leader for the creation of the Portuguese Association of Pediatric Surgeons in 1964, (of which, he was the first President), more formally organised after a General Assembly held at the *Hospital D. Estefânia* on the June 29, 1974. He was also leader for the recognition of paediatric surgery, by the *Ordem dos Médicos*, as an autonomous speciality, in 1964, and also became the first Portuguese Professor of Paediatric Surgery, in 1986, at the same time the *Hospital D. Estefânia* became affiliated to the Lisbon´s Faculty of Medical Sciences (*Faculdade de Ciências Médicas de Lisboa*).

A further paediatric surgeon became a Professor, affiliated also to the Lisbon's Faculty of Medical Sciences: Fernando Mena Martins (having also worked in Uppsala, with Gunnar Grotte).

After the *Ordem dos Médicos* recognised paediatric surgery as a medical speciality of its own right in 1964 and created the College Board of Paediatric Surgery (a consultative body (initially appointed by the Executive of the *Ordem dos Médicos* and now elected within its membership), the state hospitals implemented Training Program in Paediatric Surgery. José Augusto Antunes (who later became the Head of the Paediatric Orthopaedic Department), in Lisboa, and José Manuel Lemos Pavão (who later became Head of Surgery at the Hospital Maria Pia), in Porto, were the first to apply for this formal training.

In Lisboa, at the Lisbon's city hospitals, the emergency treatment of Paediatric Surgical Patients was, till 1985, performed by paediatric surgeons, but working at the main City Emergency

Department, at the *Hospital de São José*. That changed when, in the eighties, in the *Hospital D. Estefânia*, a PNNICU and a PICU were opened. At the Hospital Santa Maria, paediatric surgeons are kept on call.

In 1950 a Paediatric Surgical and Orthopaedic Ward for Children was opened at the *Hospital de Montemor o Novo*, a charity facility (run by the Monks of the Order of *São João de Deus*), directed by Eduardo Rosado Pinto and later by Fernando Afonso).

In 1957, at the Teaching Hospital of Santa Maria, a Paediatric Surgical Unit was created within the Paediatric Department. Jorge Rosa de Oliveira, a general surgeon who had trained in paediatric surgery for a year, in the USA (with Ladd and Gross), became the Surgeon-in-charge. Now a busy paediatric surgical department exists, run by paediatric surgeons, but still included in the general Department of Paediatrics.

In the north of Portugal, on the February 4, 1945 opened, at the Children's Hospital Maria Pia, in Porto, a surgical ward, directed by Armando Tavares (a Paediatrician performing occasionally surgery in children) until his death. Initially, for surgery in children, some general surgeons worked there, like José Barbeitos de Sousa (whom later dedicated himself primarily to children's surgery.) followed, in 1954, by Cardoso da Rocha, who replaced Armando Tavares after his death, in 1965. Historically, Cardoso da Rocha can be quoted as the main Paediatric Surgeon in the North of Portugal.

At the Hospital de Santo António, Babo de Magalhães, Ferreira de Abreu, José Mendo and António Canedo (General Surgeons, with an interest in children's surgery), started working in Paediatric Surgery. A surgical ward was officially opened on the February 18, 1961 and Cardoso da Rocha was appointed its Head. (Apart from being responsible for Neo-Natal Surgery at the *Maternity Hospital Júlio Diniz*, also in Porto, Cardoso da Rocha (Fig. 2) remained Head of Paediatric Surgery at the Hospital Maria Pia until retirement. He organised several National and International Meetings of Paediatric Surgery, and developed a personal technique for pharyngoplasty, in cleft palate.

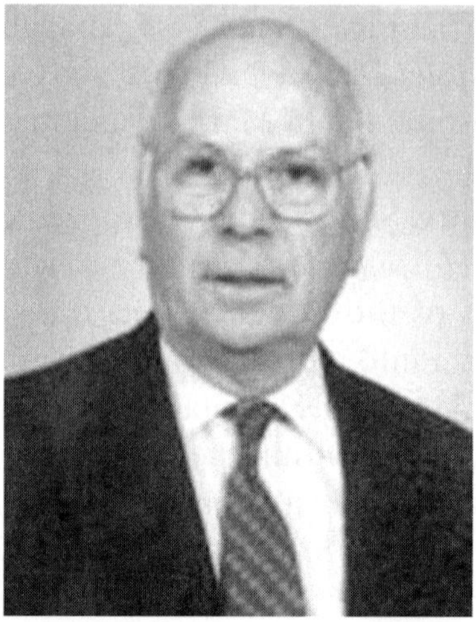

Fig. 2. José Cardoso da Rocha.

In 1963, at the *University Hospital de S. João* (similarly to what had happened in Lisboa, at the University Hospital of Santa Maria) a surgical ward in the Paediatric Department was set up. However, it was, not under the responsibility of the Chair Professor of Paediatrics, but under the Chair Professor of Surgery. Barbeitos de Sousa become the paediatric surgeon-in-charge (until retirement, when Cardoso da Rocha took over). Another Professorship was later created, in the Paediatric Department of the Faculty of Medicine of Porto University, with Estêvão Costa, but another paediatric surgeon, Bessa Monteiro, remained Head of the Unit. Another paediatric surgeon, Jorge Correia Pinto, also became Professor of Physiology, at the new School of Health Sciences, in Braga.

Now, there are three paediatric surgery departments in the north of Portugal, one at the University Hospital of S. João (the only one officially accredited by the European Board), another at the Hospital Maria Pia and the third in the Vila Nova de Gaia City Hospital.

In the Center of Portugal, in Coimbra (site of one of the oldest European Universities), at the Children's Hospital, a surgical ward was opened in 1977, and Carlos Pereira da Silva (a general surgeon with an interest in children, who had spent some time in England) was appointed as its Head. He was replaced in 1978, by Antonio Matos Coimbra, a paediatric surgeon trained at the *Hospital D. Estefânia* and in the UK (Liverpool and Sheffield). António Matos Coimbra was in fact the real first full-time paediatric surgeon, in the center of Portugal, where a full and active department was developed. A paediatric surgeon has now also obtained a professorship: Maria Francelina Lopes. More than 50% of the Portuguese paediatric surgeons had their training at the *Hospital D. Estefânia*. From that hospital, paediatric surgery progressed almost to the whole Country.

Units were later opened in the *Hospital do Espírito Santo*, Évora, with Rui Rosado, in the *Hospital de S. Bernardo*, Setúbal, with Luciana Cunha, in the Hospital de S. Teotónio, Vizeu, with Conceição Salgado), in the *Hospital Garcia de Orta*, Almada, with Orlando Cordeiro, in the *Hospital Fernando Fonseca, Amadora*, with Paolo Casella in the *Hospital do Funchal*, Madeira, with Filomeno Paulo Gomes, and in the *Hospital S. Francisco Xavier*, Lisboa, with Fernando Mena Martins. A further Unit, in the North (with paediatric surgeons trained at the *Hospital de São João*) was opened in Vila Nova de Gaia.

For a time, there was a split within paediatric surgery, and two Paediatric Surgical Societies existed. Finally an agreement was reached, and now only one Society remains: the *Sociedade Portuguesa de Cirurgia Pediátrica* (Fig. 3). During the time when two Societies existed, *José Manuel Pavão*, President of one of them, edited a short-lived "*Portuguese Paediatric Surgical Journal*".

The scope of paediatric surgery in Portugal is defined by the College of Paediatric Surgery of the *Ordem dos Médicos* and training lasts six years, including six months of compulsory paediatrics, one year of general surgery, three years of paediatric surgery (general and including neo-natal surgery), with optional three four-month periods (totaling a year), chosen between orthopaedics, urology, plastic surgery, intensive care, neurosurgery and oncology.

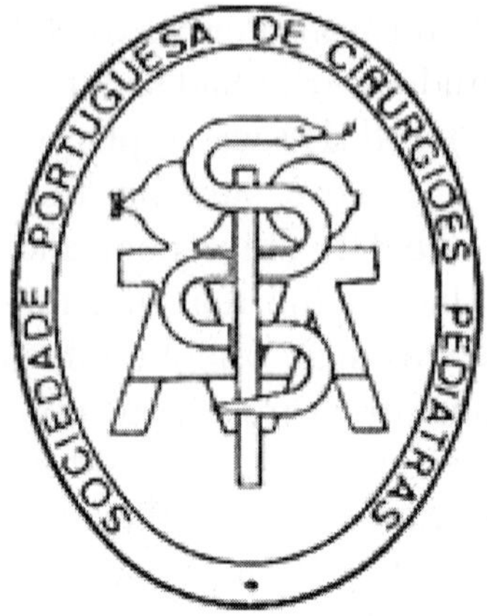

Fig. 3. *Sociedade de Cirurgia Pediátrica* crest.

State of the Art of Paediatric Surgery at the Main Portuguese Centers

Hospital D. Estefânia, Lisboa. One Paediatric Surgical Department with the Sections: General and Neo-Natal Surgery, Urology, Plastic surgery (with a burns unit), Neurosurgery (with paediatric neurosurgeons), and Ambulatory Surgery, and one Paediatric Orthopedic Department (headed by an orthopaedic surgeon, dedicated to Children's Orthopaedics). Malignant tumours are generally cared for (by specialised oncological paediatric surgeons) at the multi-disciplinary Paediatric Department of the **Portuguese Cancer Institute of Francisco Gentil**, although some, requiring post-operative intensive care, are operated by the same surgeons, at the ***Hospital D. Estefânia*** (under a specific Institutional agreement). This hospital is affiliated to the Lisbon's Faculty of Medical Sciences. Some pre-graduate paediatric teaching is done; Margarida Espana being in charge.

Hospital Santa Maria, Lisboa. There is a unit, within the Department of Paediatrics dedicated to general and neo-natal Surgery. Orthopaedics and plastic surgery are dealt mainly by adult specialists, although burns are usually transferred to the burns unit at the *Hospital D. Estefânia.*

This hospital is a University Hospital, linked to Lisbon's Medical Faculty. Some pre-graduate Paediatric Surgery teaching is done; Miroslava Gonçalves being in charge.

Hospital Pediátrico, Coimbra. The hospital has a Paediatric Surgical Department, with separate Sections of General and Neo-Natal Surgery, Urology and Plastic Surgery. Orthopaedics is performed by adult Orthopaedics Specialists.

Hospital de S. João, Porto. There is a Department of Paediatric Surgery (within the Department of Paediatrics), dedicated to General and Neo-Natal Surgery, Urology and Plastic Surgery. Orthopaedics is performed by Adult Orthopaedic Specialists. This department is particularly motivated for research, and it is so far the only one officially accredited by the Paediatric Surgical Board of the UEMS (European Union of Medical Specialists). This hospital is a University Hospital, linked to the Porto's Medical Faculty. Some pre-graduate teaching of paediatric surgery is done, and Estêvão Costa being in charge.

Hospital Maria Pia, Porto. There is a Department of Paediatric Surgery, dedicated to General and Neo-Natal Surgery, however, urology, plastic surgery and orthopedics cases are performed by adult surgeons.

Some teaching of paediatric surgery, at pre-graduate level, is also done at the University Institute of Health Sciences, in Braga, where Jorge Correia Pinto is in charge.

Author's background: Prof Dr António Gentil Martins

António Gentil Martins organised several international Meetings, namely the 1st Luso-Brasilian (1971) and the first Luso-Spanish (1972), Meetings of Paediatric Surgery, the XIth SIOP International Congress (1979) as well as several postgraduate Courses. He was the first to implant a valve for the treatment of hydrocephalus, to perform a colonic transposition for long gap oesophageal atresia, to cure oesophageal atresia associated with a ano-rectal malformation, to perform a total neo-natal bladder exstrophy reconstruction, having also developed innovations (e.g. pre-operative polychemotherapy for nephroblastomas and also partial nephrectomy for unilateral tumours), and original techniques (e.g. for vaginal reconstruction, the treatment of plagiocephaly, funnel chest, jaw and long bones tumours, rectal incontinence, etc.). He was the first to perform pulmonary assisted ventilation, in the post-operative period in surgical neonates and he was the only portuguese surgeon that successfully separated Siamese twins (with nine survivors in seven pairs, certainly one of the world's best results for any individual surgeon). In 2002, after retirement, he was allowed to start a Project of Telemedicine at the *Hospital D. Estefânia* (ended in 2006).

He was awarded the Knighthood of the Infant D. Henrique, the gold Medal of the Portuguese Ministry of Health and the Medal of Honour of the Ordem dos Médicos. He presided the Portuguese League Against Cancer., CAVITOP (Portuguese Center for support of Victims of Torture), and OP (Portuguese Olympic Athletes Association). He is also Specialist in Plastic, Reconstructive and Aesthetic Surgery and was founder of the Portuguese Society of Plastic Surgery and also founder of the so-called "Inside Meetings" (dedicated to a Data Bank on Complications in Paediatric Surgery and Telemedicine), an idea of Prof Gunther Willital (1996). He has the sub-specialization in Paediatric Oncology and is one of the Vice-Presidents of the International College of Surgeons, after having been President of its Portuguese Section.

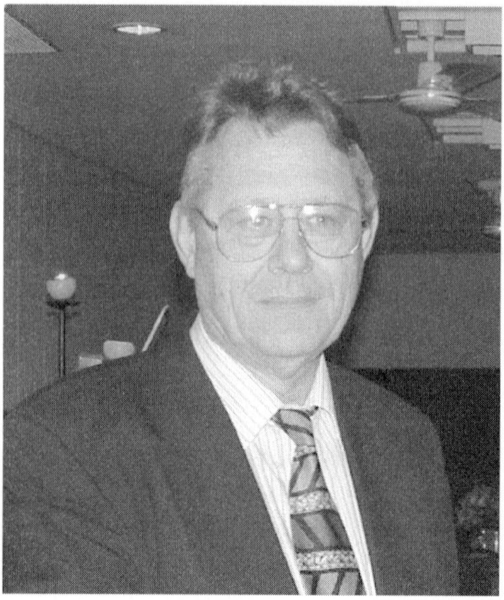

Heinz Rode

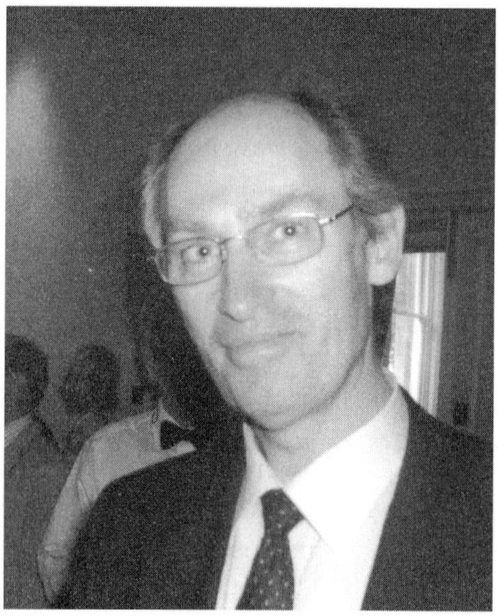

Alastair J. W. Millar

SOUTH AFRICA

Heinz Rode
Alastair J. W. Millar

***"Die erfenis van die verlede is die saad waaruit die vrug van die toekoms spruit."* ("The heritage of the past is the seed from which the future grows.")**

Introduction

Surgery in some shape or form has been has been practiced in Africa since the dawn of time. This craft of primitive man, from as early as the Paleolithic period, included skull trepanations, finger amputations, circumcisions, the treatment of flesh wounds with herbs and the setting of fractures with mud pacts and bark splints. Elective surgery took the form mainly of traditional rites some of which required considerable surgical skill as in the practice of left orchidectomy in boys as recorded by early Dutch settlers in some tribes in and around the Cape of Good Hope. The testis was removed, the vas and vessels ligated and the scrotal sac filled with sheeps fat prior to skin closure with suture with a bone needle and sinew thread. The whole procedure lasted but a few minutes and it seems most survived the experience.

Western medicine was introduced into South Africa by mostly uneducated "barber surgeons" and "apothecary-surgeons" with the arrival of Dutch settlers at what is now Cape Town, in 1652.[1] They were rated in the fourth class, being grouped with constables and tree-watchers. Their surgery was no more than an empirical art limited to anatomy, the technique of opening a skull, tending of wounds and setting fractures, blood letting, draining of abscesses, lithotomies, amputations, removal of musket balls and assegai (spear) tips with crude surgical instruments.[2]

Until the mid-19th century there were only a few European trained doctors and unqualified medical practitioners in South Africa.[3] Training of local surgeons (usually a candidate enlisted from itinerant soldiers and sailors) was by apprenticeship to a European trained barber-surgeon. They were uneducated and not all surgeons were of good repute and the practice of surgery has less attraction for most surgeons than had commerce or exploration. There were a few notable exceptions however. The most famous of these was James Barry, who spent a lifetime as a physician/surgeon to the British Army and achieved the rank of Surgeon General, but was found to have been a normal female at her death in London in 1865. During a secondment to the Cape not only did she rapidly gain a wide reputation for excellence but became the first surgeon in the English speaking world to perform a Caesarean section (in 1826) where both mother and child survived.[4]

However, as from the latter half of the 19th century, practitioners were required to be trained in Europe, initially in Holland and later in the United Kingdom. They were educated and respected and brought surgery on par with that of Europe. In the country districts medical practitioners were mainly retired regimental surgeons and immigrant surgeons from Europe. Qualified surgeons from especially Edinburgh, London, Leyden and the Durham-University in Newcastle-upon-Tyne, England, had a profound influence on the subsequent training and practice of surgery and indirectly paediatric surgery. The first civilian hospital was established in 1818 in Cape Town. Dr Henry Bickersteth was the first surgeon with a degree (M.R.C.S., L.R.C.P.) to practice the art of surgery in this country.[2]

Hospitals exclusively designed for children were built during the 19th century in most West-European countries: Canada, Australia and the United States. Paediatric surgery as a functional discipline is considered to have been introduced as an entity separate from paediatrics, in 1802 in the *Hospital Enfant-Jesus* in Paris.[5] However, recognition of the special nature of children's diseases and their management was slow to develop in South Africa and lagged behind developments elsewhere in the world.

It was only just prior to the World War I that public awareness in South Africa was awakened regarding the special requirements of children and the potential role that hospitals dedicated to the needs of children, could play .The human tragedy and suffering that followed in the wake of World War I, the social-economic problems of that time and the fact that there was no separate provision for children in the various Government Hospitals, were the driving forces behind these developments. These early pioneers, mainly socially conscious women, had to overcome much prejudice and resistance from provincial authorities and from those accustomed only to the needs of adults. By succeeding in these efforts they also underscored the rightful place of pediatrics and subsequently of pediatric surgery as a major discipline.

Paediatric Surgery as a Discipline

The scope and practice of surgery has undergone considerable changes over the past century and can be divided into four phases;

The birth and infancy period. From the 1920's to the early 1950's paediatric surgery was in the hands of paediatricians and part-time surgeons. The prevailing attitude was that a surgically ill child could not be entrusted to a surgeon and senior general surgeons were scathing about a young enthusiast wanting to treat conditions such as intussusception and pyloric stenosis, which they felt were far better, managed in their own capable hands.[6] During this period many children died prior to diagnosis or were moribund on admission. The disease spectrum was dominated by sepsis, peritonitis, tuberculosis of bone and joints, bowel obstruction, empyema, burns, lymph adenopathy, urologic conditions and ear, nose and throat diseases. Only a few congenital abnormalities were reported with a generally dismal outcome.

The second period. From the early 1950's to the middle of the 1960's significant progress in medical sciences was made. The development of new surgical techniques and the increasing interest of surgeons who chose to specialise in paediatric surgery were responsible for the survival of children with conditions that previously were universally fatal The surgical staff was selected from amongst those whose interest was children's surgery.[7] Another important addition has been the introduction of experimental surgery, which changed surgical practice and yielded excellent results. The reductions in the mortality for intestinal atresia from 90% to 58% within four years after a change in technique resulting from experimental work carried out in Cape Town by Christiaan Barnard and Jan H. Louw is a classical example.[8] This period also heralded in the development of subspeciality services, the latter remaining under the auspices of adult surgeons for many years to come.

The third period. The era of recognition of paediatric surgery as an entity, from the early 1960's to 2005:[6,9] Substantial and rapid advances were made during this period in diagnosis, investigations, management, prognosis and understanding the causation of diseases. The emphasis has been on the overall care of the surgically sick child, in particular newborn infants and patients undergoing major surgical procedures. Disease patterns also changed and the volume of work rapidly increased particularly with the development of the neonatal ICU. In recognition of the importance of this new emerging speciality, Chairs in Paediatrtic Surgery were established in 1975 in Cape Town and Johannesburg and in 1984 in Durban. Paediatric surgery was recognized as a sub-speciality with certification by the South African Medical and Dental Council (SAMDC) in 1983 and paediatric surgery was included from the beginning in the curriculum of undergraduate medical students. An ever increasing number of well-trained paediatric surgeons has attested to the need and value of paediatric surgery during these years.

The fourth period was when paediatric surgery became a full speciality in its own right. It was always a sub-speciality of general surgery with certification by the South African Medical Council and became a full speciality only in 2007. The speciality now requires a six year training period in an accredited paediatric surgical academic department with an exit examination and dissertation. Paediatric surgery however, despite all modern developments, continues to be a challenge judging by the large number of sick children, disease patterns specific to this region, late presentations, advanced pathology and financial constraints.[7] At present there are 37 registered paediatric surgeons of whom 24 are either in university/provincial service, six in private practice, four living outside South Africa. Three have retired from active practice. Paediatric training facilities are inspected on a regular five-yearly basis by the Health Professions Council, examining facilities, interviews with staff and trainees to ensure that standards are maintained.

Facilities for Paediatric Surgery

The development of paediatric surgery in South Africa was greatly influenced by the establishment of children's hospitals. Surgery was predominantly practiced within Provincial Hospitals under the auspices of university departments, where the majority of children were treated. With the rapid expansion of private hospital facilities in the 1980's, paediatric surgery outside academic institutions developed. Initially surgery on children was performed by general surgeons with an interest and experience in paediatric surgery and later on by qualified paediatric surgeons, the majority of whom maintained an active affiliation with academic institutions.

In South Africa four children's hospitals were built as freestanding and independent centers and one was recently promulgated as a children's pavilion within an adult hospital. These hospitals were the Transvaal Memorial Hospital for Children (1923–1978), The Children's Memorial Hospital, Durban (1931–1990), the Red Cross War Memorial Children's Hospital (1956–present) and the Pretoria Children's Hospital (1947–1987). These facilities were committed to provide active, quality, cost effective, primary, preventative and specialised care to children in need. Facilities such as these also served as regional centers and engaged in cutting-edge research in children's health.

Sadly, three of these children's hospitals, which became centers of innovation and excellence in child health, were closed as large academic hospitals with paediatric surgical facilities were built and maintaining a stand-alone Children's Hospital was deemed too costly. This happened due predominantly to a lack of understanding of the specific role that a children's hospital can play in child health as well as financial considerations.[10] However there is no doubt that these hospitals played a most important role in the surgical management and care of sick children over the past century.

Paediatric Surgery and Apartheid

The social separation of races had been present in varying degrees since early European settlement but formal separation of races was promulgated and legalised in 1948 with significant consequences for the underprivileged black communities of South Africa. Medical and Hospital services were segregated and hospitals were especially built to accommodate non-white patients, including Baragwanath Hospital in Johannesburg, King Edward VII in Durban, Kalafong and Medical University of South Africa (MEDUNSA) Hospitals in Pretoria and Pelanomi in Bloemfontein, while in others duplicated facilities were built in the same building. This system of segregation prevailed across the cities and rural areas of South Africa. As the political climate in South Africa changed in the late 1980's some of these hospitals unofficially changed their segregation policies and progressively became integrated. The Red Cross Hospital, as an example, had segregated wards but a multiracial cardiac surgical intensive care unit under the supervision of Christiaan Barnard was present in the 1960's and the rest of the hospital increasingly became integrated during the 1970's and was fully integrated by the middle 1980's. Country-wide full integration was only established in 1994.

The policy of racial segregation created moral and ethical dilemmas, which resulted in the emigration of many health professionals including paediatric surgeons. A notable number became prominent members of the international paediatric surgical community, especially in the United States, Canada, Australia, New Zealand, Israel and the United Kingdom. Others however remained in South Africa often under difficult circumstances. They felt the need to continue serving the children of this country and engaged in teaching and researching the unique surgical problems of Southern Africa and the developing world. Over the last seven decades they have rendered exceptional services to this country and its children and in this process laid the basic and solid foundations on which pediatric surgery in South Africa exists today.

Transvaal Memorial Hospital for Children and Paediatric Surgery

Paediatrics as an independent speciality was established in Southern Africa during the early 1920's when the **Transvaal Memorial Hospital for Children (TMHC)** was formally opened in 1923 (Fig. 1). This facility over the subsequent years rendered exceptional services to the children of this country and set the foundations of what was to come. At the same time the first Faculty of Medicine was established in Cape Town with the Professor of Medicine responsible for Paediatrics until 1927 when Dr Louis Leipoldt was appointed the first honorary lecturer in Paediatrics. These were pioneering

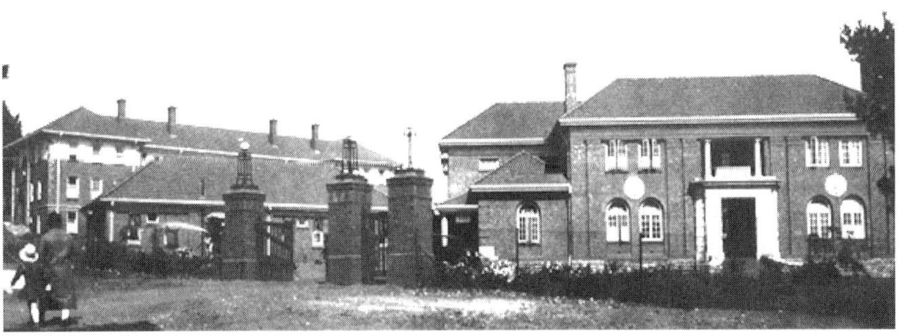

Fig. 1. The Transvaal Memorial Children's Hospital (circa 1930's).

days. At both these hospitals medical and surgical cases were the responsibilities of senior paediatricians with no separate surgical departments.

At the TMHC, Dr B. G. Melle was appointed in the dual post of part-time honorary medical and surgical registrar. The importance of the unique role of surgery in the care of sick children was recognized soon afterwards and Mr R. A. Ross was appointed to the senior post with Mr J. A. Douglas as his assistant surgeon both having marked ability for clinical teaching and surgical practice.[11] Shortly after the opening of the hospital the first group of medical students attended lectures in "Diseases of Children and Children's Surgery". Other surgeons followed in their wake over the years including Mr A. Lee McGregor renowned for his textbook "*A Synopsis of Surgical Anatomy*" first published in 1932 with continuing editions being published well into the 1980's where congenital malformations and embryology were emphasised.[12] These surgeons and paediatricians were the first to start the long and sustained battle for the rightful place of paediatrics, and subsequently paediatric surgery, as a major discipline in practice and teaching in South Africa.

These early pioneers had the vision to recognise the importance of expanding the discipline of paediatric surgery and part-time surgeons were appointed to undertake care of ophthalmic, otorhinolaryngology, orthopaedic, plastic surgery and burns patients. To accommodate the growing need of surgical patients, new operating theatres were opened in 1938 and adolescents were also accommodated as well as facilities for mothers.

From a modest beginning, sufficient to render basic surgical services in 1923, the Institution evolved into a modern and progressive facility able to provide adequate medical and surgical care to the children of Johannesburg and beyond. Fiscal restraints during and after the Second World War resulted in the curtailment of much needed development. For many years surgery remained the responsibility of general surgeons at these facilities. Dr S. Trubshaw was the first and was followed by J. Douglas, A. Wolfowitz and M. Dinner. Dr Michael Dinner joined the staff in 1956 and was appointed full-time paediatric surgeon in 1966. In recognition of the ever increasing importance and need for paediatric surgical services, a sub-department of paediatric surgery was established with facilities in all three major hospitals in Johannesburg. In 1969 Dr Dinner was appointed as the first full-time head, a significant milestone for paediatric surgery. Surgeons who contributed significantly to the establishment and development of a vibrant and dynamic department included Jack Wolpowitz, Jos Lannon, John Beck, Lewis Spitz, P. Perdikus and John Chappel. They had to be expert in general paediatric surgery, urology, thoracic and neurosurgery and were masters in embryology, anatomy, surgical technique and patient care. From the onset part-time surgeons also played an essential role in clinical and academic activities — M. Katzen, "Buzzy"Gampel, F. Kalk, S. Skapinker, W. Saunders, and E. Kessler. Dr Dinner retired in 1978 and his chair was subsequently filled by J. Chappell.[13]

The national policies of segregation created a very difficult situation and to accommodate all the sick children, additional hospitals were built or others converted. For many years paediatric surgery remained the responsibility of junior consulting surgeons at the **TMHC**, **Baragwanath** and the **Coronation hospitals**. The Baragwanath Hospital, initially a British military hospital during World War II and subsequently tuberculoses facility, opened to black patients in 1948. Coronation Hospital was designated for Indian and Coloured patients (mixed race). Integration of patients in these hospitals was finally achieved after 1994.

With the opening of the new **Johannesburg Hospital** situated in Parktown the clinical facilities at TMHC were run-down and closed. Paediatrics were one of the first group of patients to be transferred into this hospital, into a new block, the yellow coded section exclusively designated for paediatric cases. Within the X-ray and operating theatre sections, custom design facilities for these patients were provided for. From 1978 white and, in special instances, patients of colour were admitted to surgical wards at this hospital. ICU beds were shared with paediatrics. Paediatric surgical cases at Coronation Hospital were managed by the Johannesburg Hospital staff where an outpatient's clinic and weekly minor case surgical lists were performed.

The paediatric surgical services at the Baragwanath Hospital and Johannesburg Hospitals functioned as entirely separate units offering equal patient care except for organ transplantation which was done only at the latter hospital. This situation subsequent to full racial integration during the 1990's has remained unaltered. Prof M. R. Q. Davies succeeded John Chappell in 1983. Consultant staff during his tenure were Peter Beale, Graham Pitcher, P. Erpicum; at the Johannesburg Hospital and J. de Fonseca, B. Saunders, F. Kalk, A. Mohamed, M. Selebe, and B. Banieghbal at the Baragwanath Hospital. K. Lakhoo functioned in a similar fashion for a short period of time as did Leonie Schoeman. By virtue of the national and international standing these units both have drawn postgraduate fellows on secondment from many centres across the world. Training at Baragwanath and the General Hospital was sought after by especially trainees from Israel; Uri Kovacs, Bassem Kawar, Asher Pressmen, Meier Goldberg, Tommy Oksenberg, George Mogilner, Leo Siplovitch and others — M. Barrett, A. Kiss, D. Prusniefsky.[14]

The King Edward VIII Hospital and Paediatric Surgery

Another centre in South Africa where paediatric surgery developed as an independent discipline was in Durban at the general teaching hospitals affiliated to the University of Natal.[15,16] **The King Edward VII Teaching Hospital** was established in 1936 and the Natal Medical School in 1951. Ten years later a children's surgical service was introduced under the directorship of Prof David Chapman, a general surgeon. The children's ward was on the top floor of a four-storey building .The open-plan ward was subdivided into four sections: one for neonates, for older children, for burns and for orthopedics (mostly osteitis and fractures). Prof Chapman performed all the neonatal surgery at that time. Dr R. Mickel returned after four years at the Royal Hospital for Sick Children in Edinburgh and was appointed as senior registrar in the professorial unit, partly responsible for children. Although facilities, surgical techniques, anesthesia, pre- and post-operative care were still in their infancy, they had to deal with every pathology from cleft lip, spina bifida, fractured femurs, oesophageal atresia, tumours, snake bites and the rest of the paediatric surgical spectrum. Dr Mickel was a very innovative surgeon and amongst many other contributions, designed special warming methods during surgery and a unique operating table, transparent to X-ray. When Prof Chapman left to become a missionary, the paediatric work load was shared with adult surgeons notably Profs L. Baker, Leslie Linder, Bunny Angorn and others who managed children while on call.

However at the beginning of the 1970's the work load became excessive and, Dr Mickel still had to manage adult patients and the support from pediatricians remained limited. It was only after future pediatricians served as surgical registrars that the prevailing attitudes changed. As part of amalgamating all surgical departments into a division of surgery, paediatric surgery was established as a separate sub-department on the February 1, 1975 in the Division of Surgery and as a separate and independent department in March 1984. In 1974 an additional full-time paediatric surgical post was created and Dr Donald Nuss was appointed from 1975 to 1977 and was subsequently succeeded by Dr David Lloyd, who brought research and clinical excellence to the department. This tradition of service delivery and searching for answers to surgical diseases of Africa was further expanded and developed with the appointments of Larry Hadley in 1983 and Rinus Wiersma in 1986. Additional staff included E. Simpson, Jose Carvalho D. Constantinides, H. Grant, Amadeo Zanotti, Samad Shaik and Mohammed Sheik–Gafoor. As in other parts of South Africa, part-time consultants rendered excellent services to the department. Mike McCormick, Anvir Goga, Dileza Mji, Craig Campbell and R. Mickel on retirement. During the 1980's and onwards a number of trainees from across the world were educated in the principles and practice of paediatric surgery; Jose Carvalho, Amadeo Zanotti, Erroll Simpson, Vivienne Breckon, Samad Shaik and Mohammed Sheik–Gafoor.

The third Chair in Paediatric Surgery was established at this University in 1982 with Prof Robert Mickel as the first incumbent was followed by Larry Hadley in 1989.

From 1974 to 1975 a metropolitan pediatric surgical service was established which included beds at the Addington and RK Kahn Hospitals. These facilities were for white, Indian and Coloured patients. Black patients were treated at the King Edward VII Hospital. Although separate the same surgical staff rendered the services at these hospitals. Building of an ultra modern hospital, the **Nkosi Albert Luthuli Central Hospital** was completed in 2002 where all tertiary paediatric surgical services are now been concentrated.

The history will not be complete without reference to the **Children's Memorial Hospital** in Durban (Fig. 2). It was a beautifully constructed child-friendly hospital on the beach front, serving the need of sick children with great efficiency and pride. Women's guilds created the memorial and commemorative wards and decorated them with stainless glass window, nursery rhymes and other architectural features — a home from home for sick children. The hospital was predominatly for white and coloured children from 1977 onwards and black children were treated at the King Edward VIII Hospital. The types of illnesses encountered have changed over the years with medical science and immunisation have gained control over many diseases which used to fill the wards — polio, TB, measles and rheumatic fever to mention a few. The infrastructure

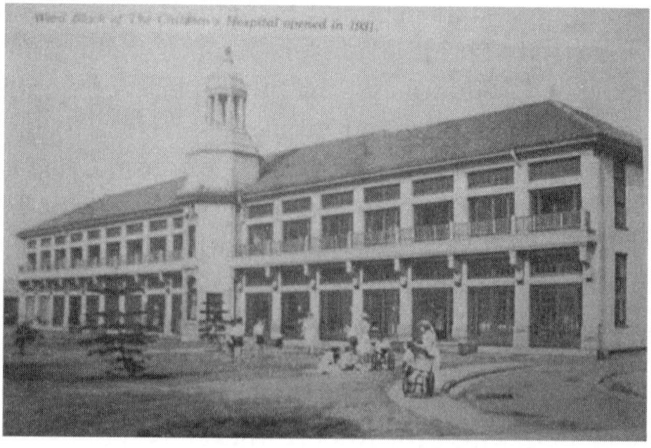

Fig. 2. The Children's Memorial Hospital, Durban (circa 1935).

and old-fashioned operating theaters could not accommodate the increasing demands for services and the hospital was allowed to deteriorate slowly. The doors were closed in the 1990's.[15]

The red cross war memorial children's hospital and paediatric surgery. Although the Cape Hospital Board was considering establishing a children's hospital from 1918 the first 22-bed children's hospital in Cape Town, the **Dennis Buxton Memorial Hospital for Children,** was only erected in 1920 .Thereafter nothing further was done apart from providing children's units in the various Peninsula hospitals. However, paediatric surgery was of little interest to general surgeons and the children's general wards in the Groote Schuur Hospital were occupied mostly by patients suffering from burns, chronic osteitis and empyema. Neonatal emergencies were almost universally fatal. The advantages made in surgery during the Second World War and the return of medical ex-serviceman left a lasting influence on surgical practice. Operative techniques had become gentler, operative mortality less and results vastly improved. It was only in 1948 that Dr J. H. Louw, (Nuffield Dominion Traveling Fellow 1951) whose interest in paediatric surgery was awakened by Mr David Waterston from the Great Ormond Street Hospital for Sick Children, whom he met while on active service in North Africa during WWII and the birth of his first son with intestinal atresia, was put in charge of all 28 general surgery beds for children in the adult Groote Schuur Hospital. These beds were eventually consolidated into a proper paediatric surgical department in 1952.

Children's wards were under the care of paediatricians and surgeons were mostly regarded as technicians with the senior pediatricians firmly in control of the diagnosis and the pre- and post-operative care. Under Dr Louw's care paediatric surgery flourished and he set an example in patient care that few could emulate. Professor Louw is regarded as the Father of Paediatric Surgery in South Africa. When the Red Cross War Memorial Children's Hospital opened in 1956, 50% of the allocated beds were for surgical patients, an indication of the new philosophy and urgent need for facilities (Fig. 3). Sid Cywes (1961) was the first surgeon in South Africa to restrict his

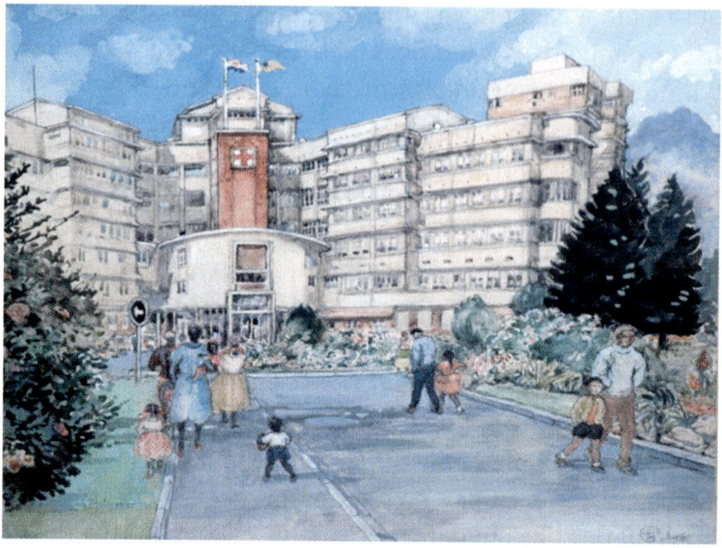

Fig. 3. Red Cross War Memorial Children's Hospital (circa 1987). The artist depicted the right profile of the future development of the hospital.

practice entirely to the surgical care of children and in 1975 succeeded Prof J. H. Louw as Head of Paediatric Surgery when he was appointed to the newly established Charles FM Saint Chair of Paediatric Surgery at the University of Cape Town. Mr Arnold Katz, a general surgeon who had spent time at the Hospital for Sick Children, Great Ormond Street was appointed in 1961 as part-time surgeon in charge of a general ward as well as the children with osteitis, and Dr R. van der Riet (1966) assisted with overall management of the burns ward although the surgical management of the burn wound was done by part time plastic surgeons.

Significant developments and expansion occurred during the 1970–1990 period with the establishment of a neonatal surgical unit with neonatal intensive care (1976), a general intensive care unit (1985), a trauma unit (1984), liver transplantation (1987) and on-site renal transplantation (2000). The Burns unit developed under the headship of H. Rode to one of the largest and most successful in the world treating up to 900 burned children a year. The Child Accident

Prevention Foundation of Southern Africa (1978) was established to try and raise awareness and focus attention on the devastating effect of the trauma epidemic in children. A day case surgical unit was opened in the 1960's and effectively run by three surgically trained general practitioners; A. Bass, J. Levitt and I. Gordon. Further appointments were made in 1974 with Drs M. Davies, H. Rode 1975, A. J. W. Millar 1984, D. Bass (Trauma) 1987, R. A. Brown 1988, S. W. Moore 1990, A. Van As (Trauma) 1999, A. Numanoglu 2001, S. Cox 2005, J. Karpelowsky 2006 and A. Alexander, 2007. Sub-speciality services were also developed as adult specialists began to focus more on their paediatric practice. Foremost amongst these was Ian Aaronson who was appointed as a urologist in 1978 to be followed by Larry Jee in 1987.

Paediatric surgeons recognised from the beginning that they were confronted not only by common diseases but also by surgical pathologies predominantly seen amongst children from the developing world.[17] Much of their scientific and research efforts were directed towards finding solutions for these. The first major contribution dealt with the clinical and experimental work on intestinal atresia, which was internationally acclaimed and paved the way for intra-uterine foetal surgery.[8] Other interests have been in the fields of trauma, congenital abnormalities, Hirschsprung's disease oncology, caustic injuries, ano-rectal abnormalities, conjoined twins, thermal injuries, and diseases unique to the developing world such as parasitic infections and surgical infections of soft tissues and bone.[18] A high incidence of conjoined twins has been noted in Southern Africa resulting in the Red Cross Children's Hospital having one of the largest single centre experiences, with 47 sets seen since 1964.[18] Prof Louw was awarded the coveted Denis Browne Gold Medal from the British Association of Paediartric Surgeons in recognition for outstanding contributions to paediatric surgery.

The hospital's exceptional value to paediatric surgery is underscored by the training of 84 surgical fellows over five decades, many who have filled chairs or became heads of departments in their respective countries; South Africa, Canada, Argentina, Brazil, Paraguay, the USA, England, Australia, Iran, Taiwan, Israel and several countries in Europe. Since 1994, 13 postgraduate fellows from Sub-Saharan countries particularly from Cote d' Ivoire, Cameroon, Gabon, Nigeria, Kenya, Malawi, Tanzania have been trained and have returned to their individual countries.

Pretoria Academic Hospital and Kalafong

There is very little information regarding the management of children in the Province of Northern Transvaal during the 19th and early part of the 20th century. The foundation stone for a general hospital in Pretoria was laid in 1927 and children were accommodated in this new hospital. In 1947 some paediatric patients were moved to pre-fabricated wards that were converted into a medical facility for children. These wards were originally for World War II convalescent soldiers. However, both black and white surgical children were managed in the general hospital in separate but equal facilities. The Andrew McColm Hospital was earmarked as a potential racially integrated children's hospital, but because of administrative indifference and national segregation policies, the hospital never materialised and paediatric surgical services remained spread out through the main hospital complex.[19]

C. H. Derksen, a professor of general surgery, was the first surgeon to practise some paediatric surgery and establish a subdepartment of paediatric surgery in Pretoria.[20] He spent time at the Alder Hey Children's Hospital, Liverpool and the Hospital for Sick Children, Great Ormond Street in 1963. He was succeeded by Dr J. J. Jacobs who took a great interest in surgical conditions of childhood. Dr Jacobs received postgraduate training in Paediatric Surgery at the Great Ormond Street and Red Cross Children's Hospitals and returned in 1961 to be appointed as part-time head of the paediatric surgical unit in Pretoria. Dr Jacobs, with his enthusiasm and dedication had a profound influence on young surgeons and no fewer than nine of his prodigies pursued a lifelong career interest in paediatric surgery, namely J. B. Fichardt, M. R. Q. Davies, H. Rode, C. J. C. Nel, J. H. R. Becker, P. Beale, M. van Niekerk, C. Schoeman and A. Jacobs.[21]

Dr Jacobs was succeeded by Prof Becker who trained with Prof Dan Young at the Yorkhill Children's Hospital in Glasgow in 1980. Paediatric surgical services were also expanded into the Kalafong hospital complex in 1973 and was designated for black children. With minimum technology, hard work and dedication, even to the extent of ventilating children by hand for up to 72 hours and good nursing care, results were acceptable. Professor G. O. Ionescu became head of the department in 1993 and he was followed by Dr C. Schoeman and Dr E. Muller. Prof Becker published a handbook on paediatric surgery in Afrikaans entitled "*Kinderchirurgie — 'n werksboek*" ("*A Handbook of Paediatric Surgery*") in 1992.

Paediatric surgery in the private sector was performed by general surgeons at the Zuid Afrikaanse Hospitaal. Dr C. A. R. Schullenburg was the driving force behind this development in 1976. At that stage there was little cooperation between surgeons and paediatricians. Surgery was after this period predominantly performed by Dr I. Venter, N. Grobbelaar and subsequently by Dr M. L. van Niekerk, although general surgeons continued to manage the non-complicated paediatric surgical conditions.

Karl Bremer and Tygerberg Hospitals

The establishment and clinical practice of paediatric surgery at the University of Stellenbosch Medical School began in 1965 with the appointment of R. Van Der Riet, a general surgeon in private practice with a particular interest in thermal injuries.[22] As he bagan his work he found himself challenged by the management of children with thermal injuries and it became a lifelong interst. In 1972 the 70-bed unit was moved from **Karl Bremer Hospital** to the new **Tygerberg Hospital**, and served as the referral hospital for major pathology from the North-Western part of the country and Namibia.

The department remained within the main structure of the adult hospital, although several attempts were made to establish a children's hospital during the 1970's. All children's services were eventually consolidated in 2005 into a children's pavilion with 300 beds.

The first head was J. J. Heydenrych, who was a general surgeon/ engineer and received post graduate training in Liverpool, Sheffield, Bristol and London from 1970 to 1971. Upon his return in 1971 paediatric surgery was consolidated as a separate discipline within the department of general surgery. He was an early investigator into organ transplantation especially liver and pancreatic transplantation. He was innovative and resolved many technical problems pertaining to the surgical management of children. Prof S. W. Moore was appointed in 1991 as the second head of the department D. Sidler, M. McCormack, B. van Vuuren and K. Saczek trained under his tutelage. Paediatric surgery had undergone significant developments as a speciality particularly in terms of technical achievements expanding academic programmes and the development of new services. In 2007 the department attained the status of a full division within the University of Stellenbosch.

Bloemfontein and Paediatric Surgery

In Bloemfontein paediatric surgery was performed by general surgeons in private practice on part-time bases at provincial level before the medical school was established in 1968.[23] Major cases and congenital abnormalities were referred to larger centres. Dr J. B. Fichardt, a general surgeon in private practice, was appointed on a sessional basis in 1973 at **Pelanomie Hospital** to attend to paediatric surgical cases. All paediatric surgery was performed except anorectal malfomations which were referred to the Witwatersrand, Pretoria or Cape Town for specialised care. In 1975 Dr C. J. C. Nel, who was a full-time consultant in the department of surgery, continued this service after his appointment as Professor and Head of the department of Surgery. From 1982, Dr R. Barry assisted with the paediatric surgery. He was followed by Dr S. Smit for two years. Dr Alic Jacobz, a general surgeon was appointed part-time Head of the department of paediatric surgery. He reorganised and upgraded the Department and attended to paediatric surgical patients, both at Pelanomie and the Universitas hospitals. In 1995, he left for the Middle East. During his tenure, he was responsible for postgraduate surgical training in paediatric surgery. Following his departure, Dr Andre Loubscher attended to the paediatric surgical patients. In January 2003, Dr Esme Le Grange, who trained at the Red Cross Hospital, was appointed full-time Head of the department of paediatric surgery. She was in fact the very first fully trained paediatric surgeon appointed at Bloemfontein and is currently responsible for training general surgical registrars.

Paediatric Surgery in the Eastern Cape

The Eastern Cape developed slightly different medical traditions from the Western Cape. The majority Xhosa population had healing practices of their own while white medical practice had become more remote from modern western medicine. Missionary medicine was relatively under developed at this period in this frontier territory. The advent of the British Settlers after 1820 placed a strong British stamp on the practice of Eastern Cape medicine. British military doctors also encouraged scientific societies, and in the absence of other medical men, treated civilians both black and white.[24]

As in other parts of South Africa paediatric surgery was initially practiced by general surgeons some of whom worked as general practitioners although they had FRCS qualifications.[25] By the 1930's surgery was done in East London at the **Frere Hospital** by a group of GP surgeons including Drs Andrew Pollock, Philip Ziervogel, George Smyth and Dr Alabster and in the post-war years by Tom Baker, Ken Goldstein and Jack Watt. The first specialist surgeon was Dr Jan Hofmeyer in the 1950's.

East London functioned as the main referral centre for a vast rural area. Surgery was also practiced at many of the mission hospitals scattered throughout these areas. Dedicated and committed ex-patriot doctors worked in these hospitals and maintained at least a rudimentary paediatric service. Unfortunately patients presented late, special investigations were limited and transport rudimentary. Surgical practice consisted of corrections of anorectal malformations, exomphalos, myelomeningocele, cleft lip and palate, appendicitis, intestinal obstruction and burns.

By the 1960's a number of qualified surgeons and other specialists migrated to this area including Peter Comfort and Arthur Webster, who added their experience to those of the GP surgeons. The status quo remained with general surgeons both in the public and private sectors treating neonates and the surgical conditions of children. Children with cancer and major congenital anomalies were referred to Cape Town for management.

In 1995 at the invitation of the MEC for health, Dr Colin Lazarus, a general surgeon with addition training in Paediatric Surgery was invited to establish the **Eastern Cape Paediatric Surgical Service in East London**, with the aim of being a main referral and training centre for the Eastern Cape. Under trying circumstances the department developed into an excellent service platform covering the full range of general paediatric surgery, neonatal surgery, paediatric urology, and oncology. The department now have three consultants, registrars in training and medical officers. Since 2003 the department was recognised as one of seven accredited training centre for paediatric surgery in South Africa.

Paediatric Surgery in Port Elizabeth began in the **Livingstone Hospital** in 1964 as a sub department of general surgery. Mr D. Procter, a general surgeon was responsible for paediatric surgery and he was replaced in 1969 by Mr M. Wynne. After some years Dr C. S. Hoffman was appointed. In 1994 Mr Procter returned with responsibilities to manage children with surgical diseases, an important development at that time. In 1996 Dr Ricardo Gonzales Vergara, a Cuban paediatric surgeon came to South Africa under the government to government agreement and joined the department of paediatric surgery in 1998. He has maintained and expanded a comprehensive paediatric surgical service for that region.

Introduction of specialist paediatric surgery was delayed in the rural areas of the Eastern Cape. Prior to 1988 all general paediatric emergencies were performed by general surgeons attached to the Umtata General Hospital. Neonatal surgery and surgery on infants was only occasionally done at the hospital when expertise from general surgeons was present. All the remainder were referred to the King Edward Hospital in KwaZulu Natal. Dr Charles Tackie, a Ghanaian Paediatric Surgeon commenced work at the Umtata Hospital in May 1988. Great difficulties were initially experienced in areas such as Paediatric Anaesthesia, Paediatric Intensive Care and the availability of trained paediatric nurses. He educated, trained and developed a functional 47-bed unit which was reallocated in 2004 to the **Nelson Mandela Academic Hospital** in Umtata.

South African Association of Paediatric Surgeons

In 1970 the *South African Journal of Surgery* devoted a special issue exclusively to paediatric surgery. Prof Sid Cywes proposed the formation of an Association for Paediatric Surgeons in 1974 which was enthusiastically endorsed by Profs M. Dinner and J. H. Louw. During the golden Jubilee Congress of the South African Medical Association, the South African Association of Paediatric Surgeons was established on the July 16, 1975 (SAAPS) (Fig. 4). This was indeed a red letter day in the annals of Paediatric Surgery in South

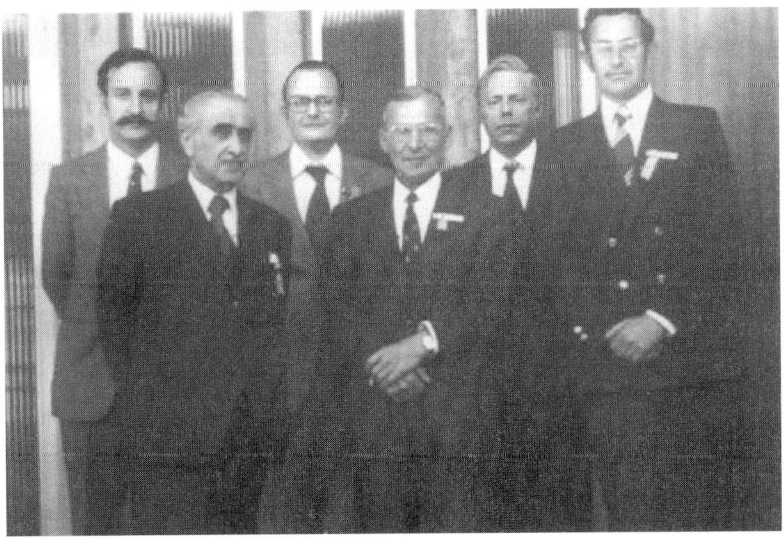

Fig. 4. The first Committee of the S. A. Association of Paediatric Surgeons 1975: Left to right: F. Kalk, M. Dinner, M. Davies, J. H. Louw President, R. Mickel and S. Cywes.

Africa. Prof J. H. Louw was elected the first President and Prof Peter Rickham as the first honorary member. Biennial multidisciplinary conferences with the South African Paediatric Association (SAPA) have been held since 1975 and is the showcase for academia and research. Subsequently honorary membership has been bestowed on 43 eminent surgeons from across the world and this association has been most beneficial to South African Paediatric Surgery over the years (Fig. 5). Eponymous J. H. Louw Lectures addressing new frontiers in Paediatric Surgery have been delivered on 12 occasions. The Association has 107 members and 43 honorary members.

Colleges of Medicine of South Africa

The Colleges of Medicine was founded in 1954 and functions as an independent national postgraduate examining body for registration. All paediatric surgeons in South Africa have qualified either through universities or through College examinations. An exit examination was introduced in 2002 and 17 surgeons have since qualified as paediatric surgeons. The College has since 1990 conferred Honorary Fellowships on five eminent paediatric surgeons; E. Durham Smith (Australia), S. Cywes (South Africa), B. O'Donnell, (Ireland); L. Spitz (United Kingdom); J. Boix–Ochoa (Spain).

What about the Future?

Much of the history of paediatric surgery in South Africa is reflected in the writings of its paediatric surgeons, J. H. Louw, Sid Cywes, B. Mickel, Mike Davies, Larry Hadley, Sam Moore, Alastair Millar, Heinz Rode, Rinus Wiersma, Peter Beale, Rob Brown, Colin Lazarus and Graham Pitcher. Many others following in their tracks have contributed their services, research and teaching with equal ability and devotion.

For more than a century many idealistic men and women have fought for the interest of children and treated the sick with great

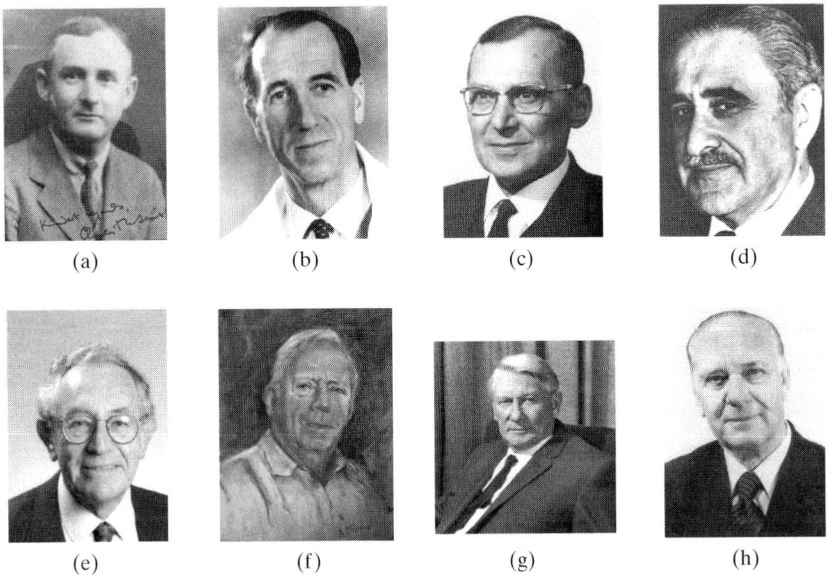

Fig. 5. Pioneers of paediatric surery in South Africa. (a) Prof Charles F. M. Saint, First Professor of Surgery, University of Cape Town 1920–1946: (b) Prof David Chapman, Professor of Surgery, University of Natal, 1961–1967: Prof JH Louw, The Father of Paediatric Surgery in South Africa, Second Professor of Surgery, University of Cape Town, 1955–1981: Prof Michael Dinner, First Professor of Paediatric Surgery, University of the Witwatersrand, 1975–1977: Prof Sid Cywes, First Charles F. M. Saint, Professor of Paediatric Surgery, University of Cape Town, 1975–1996: Prof R.E. Mickel, First Professor of Paediatric Surgery, University of Natal, 1982–1991: Prof C. H. Derksen, Professor of Surgery, University of Pretoria, 1956–1971: Dr J. J. D. Jacobs, General and Paediatric Surgeon, University of Pretoria, 1962–1980.

loving and dedicated care. They deserve our gratitude, admiration and acknowledgement. We are celebrating their traditions, their philosophy and their teachings. It is incumbent upon the current and future generations to continue to build on the solid foundations that have been laid by our ancestors. Working and living in Africa calls for a particular dedication to serve the children of this Continent, a commitment, which they desperately need and so richly deserve.

References

1. Laidler PW, Gelfand M. *South Africa: Its Medical History 1652–1898.* C. Struik, Cape Town, 1971.
2. Louw JH. *In the Shadow of Table Mountain.* C. Struik, Cape Town, 1969.
3. Bornman PC, *et al.* Surgery in South Africa. *Arch Surg* 1996;131(1): 6–12; discussion 13.
4. Du Preez H, Dr James Barry: The early years revealed. *S AFr Med J* 2008;98(1):52–58.
5. Ehrenpreis T. 100 years of pediatric surgery in Stockholm, with personal memories from the last 50 years. *Prog Pediatr Surg* 1986;20:17–33.
6. Cywes S, Millar A, Rode H. From a 'louw' beginning ... paediatric surgery in South Africa. *J Pediatr Surg* 2003;38(7 Suppl):44–47.
7. Editorial: Paediatric Surgery — has it arrived. *S Afr Med J* 1967; pp. 1047–1050.
8. Louw JH, Barnard CN. Congenital intestinal atresia; observations on its origin. *Lancet* 1955;269(6899):1065–1067.
9. Bickler SW, Kyambi J, Rode H. Pediatric surgery in sub-Saharan Africa. *Pediatr Surg Int* 2001;17(5–6):442–447.
10. Rode H, Davies MR, Berg A. The rise and fall of children's hospitals in South Africa. *S Afr Med J* 2006;96(9 Pt 2):849–853.
11. Heymann S. The Transvaal Memorial Hospital for Children, 1923–1973. *S Afr Med J* 1973;47(40):1827–1833.
12. Lee McGregor A, Du Plessis D, J. *Synopsis of Surgical Anatomy*, first edition 1932.
13. Davies MR, Chappel J, Kotzen M, Kessler E. Personal Communication, 2006.
14. Veller M. Department of Surgery, University of the Witwatersrand — a brief history. *S Afr J Surg* 2006;44(2):44–51.
15. Mickel R, Winship B, Hadley GP, Personal Communication, 2006.
16. Robbs JV. History of the Department of Surgery, Nelson R. Mandela School of Medicine, University of KwaZulu-Natal. *S Afr J Surg* 2005; 43(4):154–157.
17. Louw JH. The first two decades of the Red Cross War Memorial Children's Hospital. *S Afr Med J* 1976;50(27):1037–1047.

18. Rode H, *et al.* Four decades of conjoined twins at Red Cross Children's Hospital–lessons learned. *S Afr Med J* 2006;96(9 Pt 2):931–940.
19. Becker J, H, Haasbroek A. Personal Communication, 2006.
20. Mieny CJ. *The History of the Faculty of Medicine of the University of Pretoria 1943–1992.* Chirurgie, UP Geneeskunde, 1993; p. 55–64.
21. Franz RC, Mieny CJ, Becker JH. The Department of Surgery: University of Pretoria. *S Afr J Surg* 2005;43(1):6, 8–12.
22. Moore S, W, Heydenrych JJ. Personal Communication, 2006.
23. Theron E, Personal Communication, 2006.
24. van Heyningen E. Medical practice in the Eastern Cape. *Clio Med* 2004; 74:169–194.
25. Lazarus C. Personal Communication, 2006.

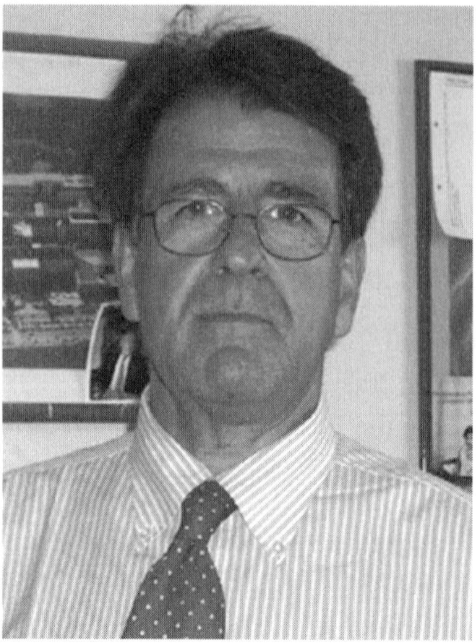

Juan A. Tovar

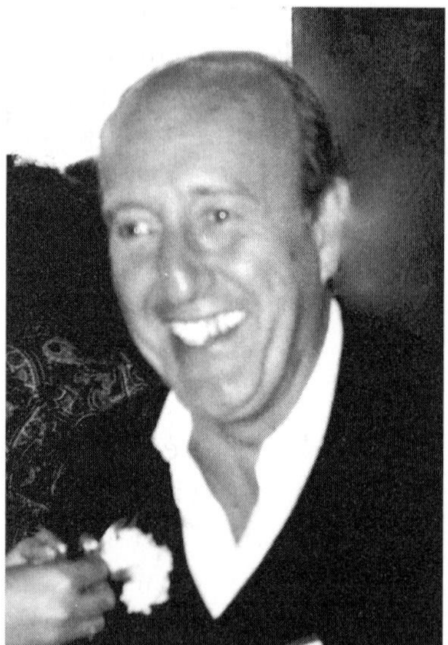

Alfredo Marques–Gubern

SPAIN

Juan A. Tovar
Alfredo Marques–Gubern

Like in other countries, pediatric surgery existed long ago but until the second half of the 20th century it was only embryonally developed due to the rudimentary knowledge on neonatal physiology, anaesthesia and nutrition in small children. Modern anaesthesia authorized undertaking of more complex pediatric surgical procedures only after the 1940's.

Our specialty existed, of course, well before this time but it was embedded into the field of general surgery. However, not only surgeons, but also some pediatricians undertook operations like circumcisions, herniotomies, pyloromyotomies, or correction of foot deformities in children, as attested by textbooks from that period in which pediatric surgical chapters were included. In 1887 Dr Jose Ribera (Fig. 1), Professor of Surgery and attending surgeon at the Hospital del Niño Jesus (the first children's hospital in the country, founded in 1877) published his treaty "*Cirugia Infantil*" ("*Pediatric Surgery*"), and Dr Sebastian Recasens published his two-volume- "*Tratado de Cirugía Infantil*" ("*Treaty on Infantile Surgery*") in 1901.

Modern pediatric surgery originated mainly in Barcelona in the late 1940's and early 1950's. Dr Roviralta (Fig. 2) opened in 1940 a surgical service in the children's' clinic "*Camitas Blancas*" and Dr L. Gubern did so in the Maternidad Provincial at about the same time. They were followed in Madrid by Dr J. Monereo [Fig. 1(d)] at the Maternidad Provincial in 1956, Dr B. Agra (Fig. 3) at the *Hospital de la Cruz Roja* in 1959 and Dr J. Garrido–Lestache,

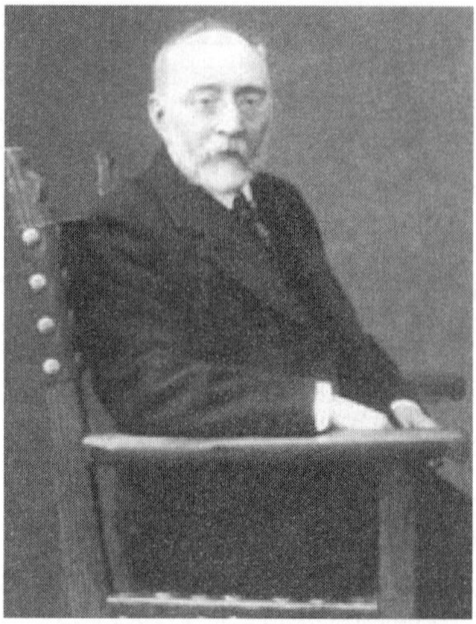

Fig. 1. Dr J. Riberia.

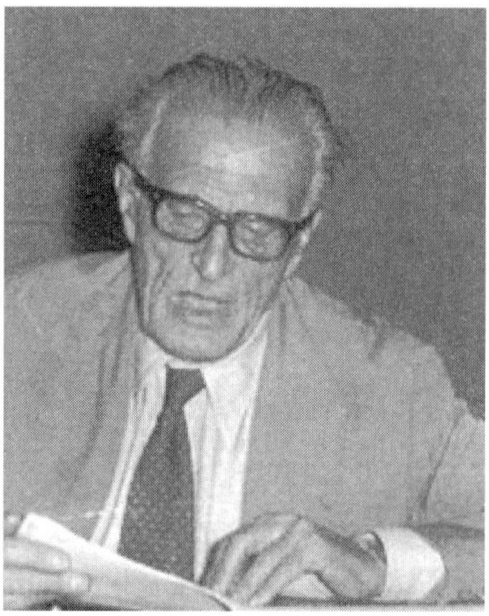

Fig. 2. Dr E. Roviralta.

at the *Hospital del Niño Jesús* in 1963. Other regional hospitals located in various cities followed.

The first survivor to neonatal treatment of Esophageal Atresia was operated upon in three steps with ultimately esophageal

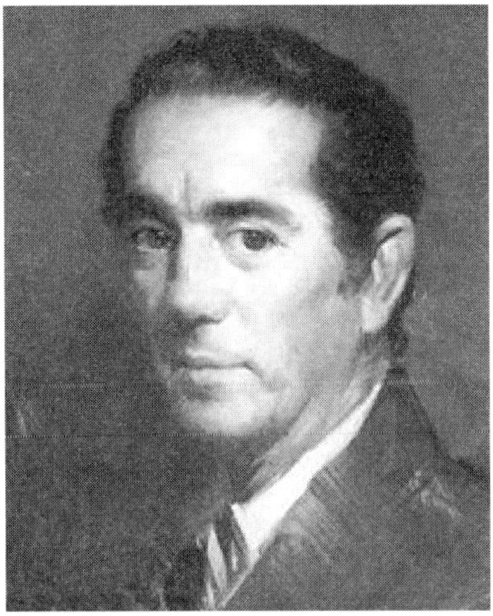

Fig. 3. Dr B. Agra.

replacement by a relevant Professor of General Surgery from Madrid (Dr P. Gonzalez–Duarte). However, the first successful primary anastomosis was reported by Dr I. Claret from Barcelona in 1957.

When the hospital network of the National Health Service attained fully modern standards in the early 1960's pediatric surgery developed very rapidly. The pioneer institution at that time was the Children's' Clinic of Hospital Universitario La Paz founded in 1964 by a relevant pediatrician, Prof E. Jaso who invited in 1965 Dr J. Monereo (Fig. 4) to join him as the first Head of the Pediatric Surgical Department. Monereo had general and pediatric surgical training in the UK and the US and transposed to his new institution what he had already seen. He first attracted a large group of surgical specialists coming from the adult specialties to devote themselves to pediatric urology, ENT, ophtalmology, orthopedics, cardiosurgery and neurosurgery and, at the same time brought into his team his former associates as well as some surgeons who trained abroad. The hospital setting and equipment were modern and the parallel development of pediatric specialties in the hospital brought about large

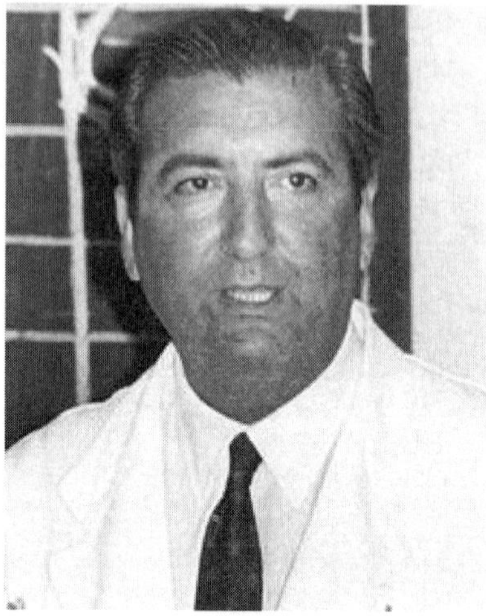

Fig. 4. Dr J. Monereo.

series and rapid progress in the results. The surgical NICU (first in the hospital and in the country) opened in 1969.

Almost simultaneously, the *Hospital del Vall d'Hebron* in Barcelona was build and organized in a very similar way. The founder pediatrician was Prof A. Ballabriga and he, in turn, invited Dr J. Boix Ochoa, who trained with Prof Rehbein in Bremen, to join him taking approximately the same functions that Monereo had in Madrid. The size and organiztion of the Hospital were very similar and it immediately knew a similar explosive development of specialties, series and results.

But these were not the only institutions that benefited of the progressive economic and technical development of the country: The Hospital of San Juan de Dios in Barcelona, in association with the Clinic University Hospital became a large-size facility directed by the very active Dr I. Claret and sub-specialized in the same way. Other institutions in Valencia, Santiago, Zaragoza and Granada followed.

The remarkably good facilities for training residents in these pioneer hospitals created in a few years a critical mass of specialists (enriched by some more coming from other countries) that scattered to the new regional and provincial centres created by the public health system in a way that, at the end of the 1970s, there were major regional pediatric surgical services in Sevilla (Dr A. Martinez Caro), Valencia, (Dr S. Ruiz Company), Zaragoza (Dr J. Alba) and Bilbao (Dr U. Ruiz) and three new ones: two in Madrid (Hospital Provincial, Dr L. Martin Sanz and 12th of October University Hospital, Dr Berchi) and one in Badalona (*Hospital Germans* Trías, Dr Martinez Mora). The network was soon expanded to other provincial capitals like Oviedo (Dr J. Teixidor), Santander (Dr F. Sandoval), San Sebastian (Dr J. A. Tovar), Alicante (Dr A. Gambarini), Mallorca (Dr C. Borras), Murcia (Dr M. A. Gutierrez-Cantó), Granada (Dr C. S. Lopez–Tello), Córdoba (Dr J. M. Pcaña), Malaga (Dr G. Lopez), Tenerife (Dr V. Sancho), Badajoz (Dr E. Blesa), Burgos (Dr J. Dominguez) and Orense (Dr J. Cuadros). Later on, another wave of new and smaller services completed the coverage of the country.

Pediatric surgeons joined to found the first scientific and professional association, the Surgical Section of the Spanish Pediatric Association in 1961 and celebrated their first Congress the same year. The first President was Dr J. Picañol, from Barcelona and the first Secretary, Dr J. Monereo, from Madrid. This association met every year in different cities ever since and became independent of the Asociacion Española de Pediatría in 1984 as the Spanish Pediatric Surgical Association.

A constant collaboration was established with fellow associations from Europe and common meetings with the Portuguese (1970, 2002 and 2005), Scandinavian (1972), French (1973) and Italian (1976) associations were organized. Animated by Drs Z. Kalicinski and G. Lopez–Perez, the Polish and the Spanish Associations of Pediatric Surgeons organized several bilateral visits and meetings along the years (Fig. 5).

The close cultural and linguistic links of Spain with Central and South American countries favoured a constant participation of surgeons from both sides of the Atlantic in the meetings of their

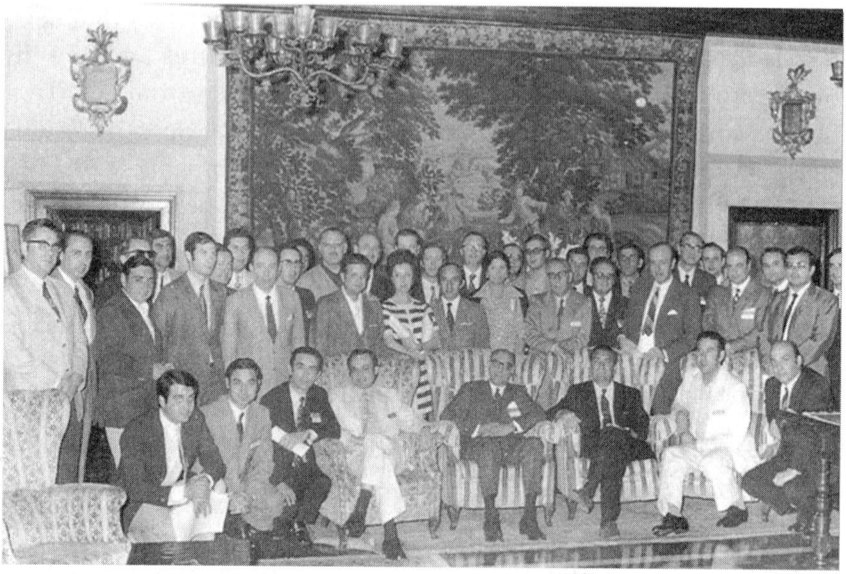

Fig. 5. Spanish Association of Paediatric Surgeons Meeting in 1972.

respective countries and particularly in those of the Southern Cone (CIPESUR) and Panamerican Associations. A Latin-American Congress was organized in Bilbao in 1985.

Participation of Spanish pediatric surgeons in other European and world professional and scientific organizations increased progressively. The first International Symposium of Pediatric Surgery (an embryo of the future WOFAPS Congress) was organized in Barcelona in 1977 by Dr J. Boix–Ochoa and the Spanish Association had its congress together with the BAPS in Madrid in 1982 organized by Dr J. Garrido–Lestache. Dr J. Tovar took in charge the organiztion of the 2nd Congress of the European Union of Pediatric Surgical Associations in Madrid in 1997 and of the 14th International Symposium on Pediatric Surgical Research in 2003. Dr V. Martinez–Ibañez organized in 2006 the VIth Congress of the Mediterranean Association of Pediatric Surgeons in Barcelona.

Pediatric surgery was officially recognized by the *Consejo Nacional de Especialidades* as an independent specialty in 1979 and the training programs ever since had to be accredited by the corresponding section of this government body entirely formed by pediatric surgeons. The vast majority of pediatric surgeons working in Spain were trained in our country although many of them took some additional training abroad.

The quality of care and results reached soon the standards of the surrounding western countries. The success of the training programs is illustrated by the early and successful development of solid organ transplantation in children performed exclusively by pediatric surgeons in our country. The first pediatric kidney transplant was carried out in the 1970s in Valencia and the first liver transplant in 1985 in Barcelona soon followed by Madrid in 1986. Pediatric small bowel transplantation was introduced by *Hospital Universitario La Paz* in 2001 and lung transplantation by *Hospital del Vall d'Hebron* at about the same time.

Although hospital acknowledgement of our specialty was obtained right from the beginning (pediatric surgical services are autonomous and independent of either Pediatric or Surgical Departments), academic acknowledgement has been much slower in the universities. All pre-graduate teaching is carried out within the frame of Pediatric or, less often, of Surgical programs and the majority of pediatric surgeons are involved in University teaching at Associate Professor level. Only a few (Drs Claret, Varela, Morales, Blesa, Moran and Tovar) became Full Professors and still fight to enlarge the space of the specialty within the academic arena.

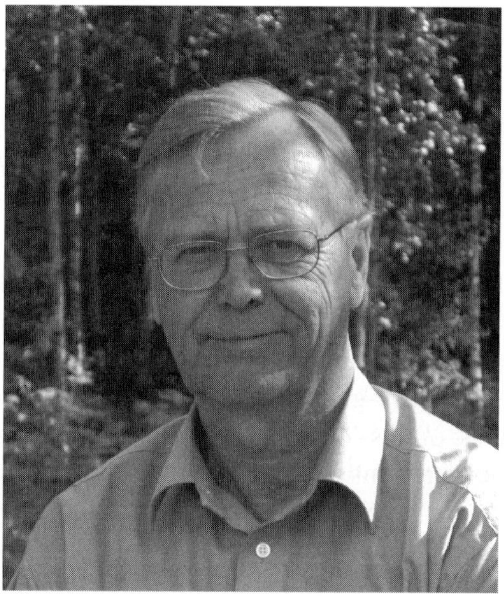

Leif Olsen

SWEDEN

Leif Olsen

The Beginning

The year 1885 is usually stated as the year of birth of the Swedish paediatric surgery. It started in **Stockholm** where **Crown Princess Lovisa's Hospital for Children (CLH)** had been founded in 1854. In 1885 a surgical unit was added to the medical unit, thus constituting the first target-oriented surgery in paediatric patients. The professor of general surgery was responsible for the unit, serving as consultant surgeon. Seven years later an independent chief was appointed. The hospital was small, but the surgical ward contained about 75 beds, as many as the medical. It took a rather long time until the first autonomous paediatric surgical department in Sweden was started at the Karolinska Hospital in 1952.

In 1970 CLH, and with it the paediatric surgical activity, was transferred to St Göran's Hospital. In 1982 the surgical department at Karolinska Hospital also moved to St Göran's Hospital, merging into one department. But in 1998 all paediatric surgery in Stockholm was concentrated to the Karolinska Hospital with its new Astrid Lindgren Hospital for Children, where they still are. The name was a very good choice, because Astrid Lindgren was a world famous writer of children's books, loved by children all over the world. The most famous of Astrid Lindgren's characters is of course Pippi Longstocking, a rebellious young girl with enormous strength and a golden heart. So the children coming to the hospital were expected to love the hospital as well!

In **Gothenburg** a Children's Hospital had been founded in 1859, and in 1912 a self independent surgical ward was established.

In 1999 they named their hospital the **Queen Silvia Children's Hospital** after our much loved and popular Queen.

In **Uppsala** paediatric surgery started in 1960 and in 1979 it became part of the new **University Children's Hospital**. It might have been a better idea to name the hospital Carl von Linné Hospital after the internationally known Swedish scientist, Carl Linnaeus, who lived and worked in Uppsala during the 18th century and who was raised to the peerage.

In **Lund,** finally, paediatric surgery started in 1969 and since 2001 it is part of the new **Children's Hospital**.

The Pioneers

The Swedish paediatric surgical pioneers very early realized the importance of recognition by the medical society, and in 1947 paediatric surgery was declared an independent speciality by the Swedish Medical Association. In 1952, only four years after the AAP, the Swedish Paediatric Surgical Association was established. As a comparison the BAPS was founded in 1953, the Scandinavian Association in 1964, the APSA in 1970, and the EUPSA in 1973.

In Stockholm there were some important surgical profiles at CLH during the early 20th century; Floderus, Perman and Hindmarsch, but not until the end of the world war in 1945 did the era of modern paediatric surgery start. **Philip Sandblom** (Fig. 1), chief surgeon at CLH from 1945 to 1950, lead one of the most dynamic and stimulating periods in the history of paediatric surgery in Sweden. As a general surgeon, he went to USA to learn from the leading centres. He was introduced to surgery of congenital anomalies and to intrathoracic surgery among other things. Unfortunately he left CLH and paediatric surgery, having been offered the Chair of General Surgery in Lund in 1950.

He was succeeded by **Theodor Ehrenpreis** (Fig. 2), known by all as "Prisse", who had an important international impact, well known for his extensive work on Hirschsprung's disease. He was a very elegant surgeon as well as author and speaker. He was awarded the BAPS gold medal in 1974. Ehrenpreis had been appointed head of

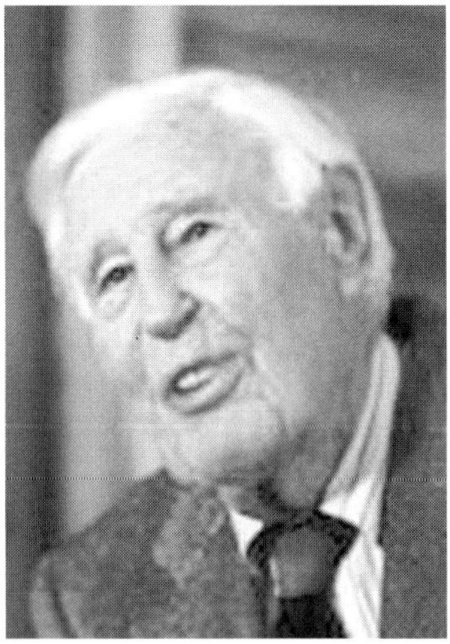

Fig. 1. Philip Sandblom.

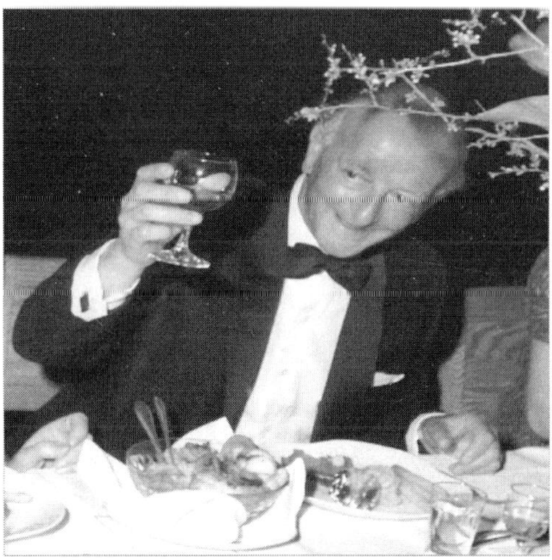

Fig. 2. Theodor Ehrenpreis.

the new surgical department of the Children's clinic at the Karolinska Hospital in 1952, where he stayed till his retirement in 1974. He was succeeded at CLH by Gunnar Ekström (Fig. 3) who served till 1974. N. O. Ericsson (Fig. 4) brought paediatric urology to

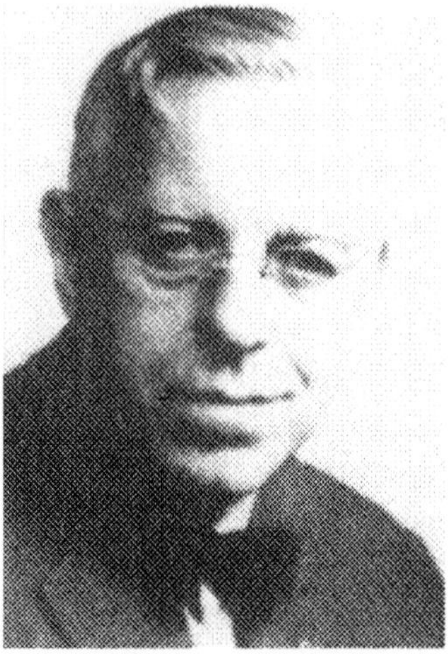

Fig. 3. Gunnar Ekström.

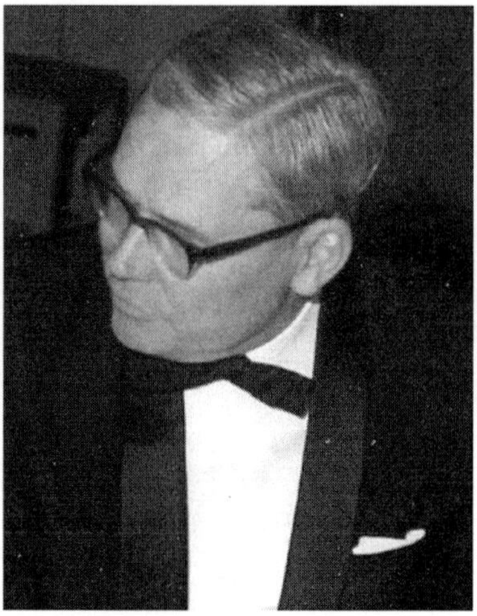

Fig. 4. N. O. Ericsson.

the highest international standards. He was co-author of the textbook "*The Lower Urinary Tract in Childhood*". His contribution is one cause of the strong position of urology in Swedish paediatric surgery today.

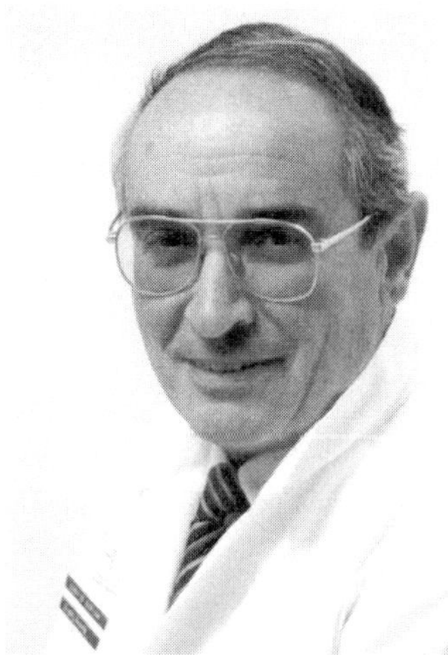

Fig. 5. Ludvig Okmian.

Ludvig Okmian (Fig. 5), later head of the department in Lund, improved respiratory treatment in neonates by adapting the Engström respirator after extensive experimental, clinical and laboratory studies. Among other things he started studies of oesophageal atresia, especially the problem with long gap, where he initiated the circular myotomy. Although not a paediatric surgeon, Clarence Crafoord in 1944 successfully performed the first operation in the world on an 11-year old boy with coarctation of the aorta.

In Gothenburg Gustav Pettersson (Fig. 6) was chief surgeon from 1942 to 1968. He was a brilliant surgeon with special interest in cardiac surgery and plastic surgery. In 1959 he also performed the first successful colonic interposition in the world for long gap oesophageal atresia in a premature boy, two days old. Sture Hagberg (Fig. 7) who continued till 1988, had an extensive knowledge of post-operative fluid therapy. He also had an interest in thoracic surgery and surgery of the urinary tract. He was succeeded by Kelm Hjälmås (Fig. 8), who was a well-known paediatric urologist specialising in micturition studies and urinary incontinence.

Paediatric surgery in Uppsala started in 1960 with Gunnar Grotte, internationally one of the most well-known Swedish paediatric

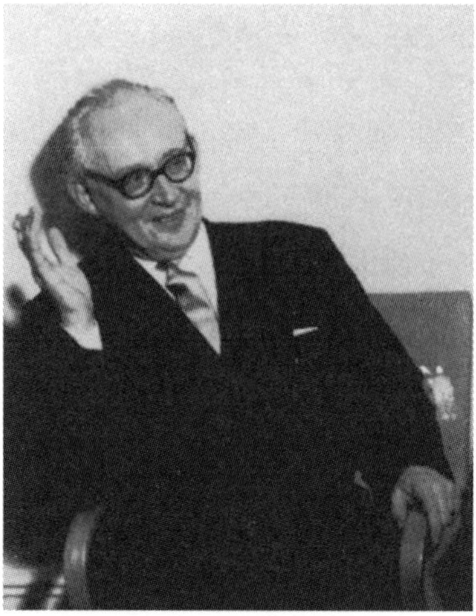

Fig. 6. Gustav Pettersson.

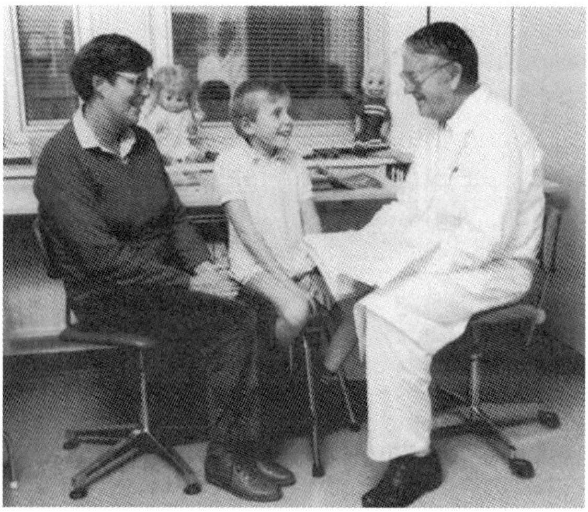

Fig. 7. Sture Hagberg.

surgeons ever. He has friends in the paediatric surgical family all over the world. He has always emphasised the importance of national and international contacts and exchange (Fig. 9). He was one of the first Swedes to join the BAPS and the SPUS. In his dissertation he was first to clarify the passage of Dextran® across

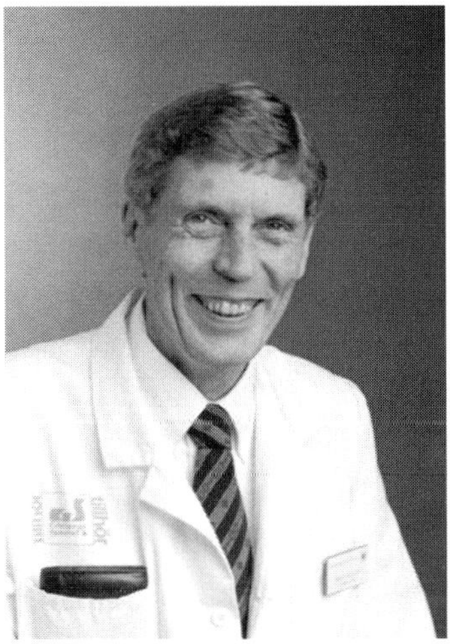

Fig. 8. Kelm Hjälmås.

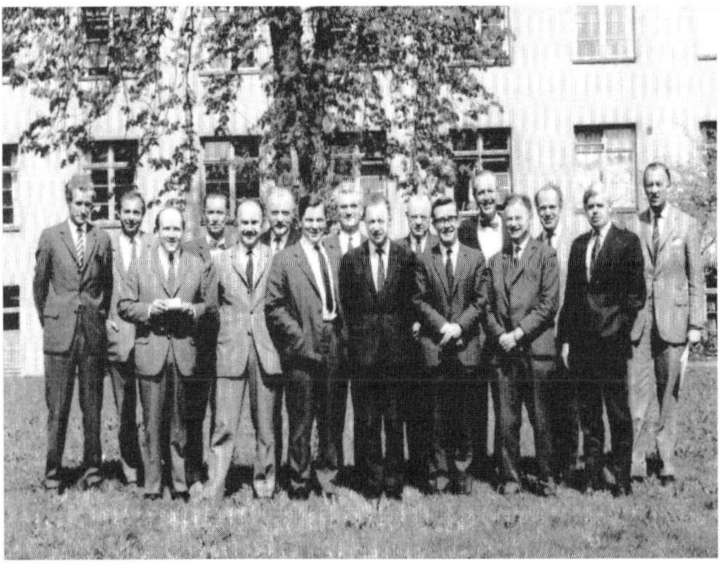

Fig. 9. SPUS 1969, Gunnar Grotte on the Right.

capillary membranes from plasma to lymph, a work that for a long time was one of the most cited Swedish papers in medicine.

In Lund, Okmian, already mentioned, became the first paediatric surgeon-in-chief in 1969.

The Successors

The development of Swedish paediatric surgery has been continued by many people. Among them are a number of persons who have served at different associations. Chairmen of the Swedish Association of Paediatric surgeons in recent years have been Jan Gierup, Leif Olsen, Lars Torsten Larsson, Gunnar Göthberg, Swedish representatives in the Scandinavian Association of Paediatric Surgeons have been Gunnar Grotte, Björn Thomasson, Leif Olsen. Swedish representatives in the EUPSA have been Björn Thomasson, Leif Olsen, Tomas Wester. Wester is the present Secretary in the UEMS.

Most of the Swedish paediatric surgeons are involved in research. For some of them this leads to a doctor's degree, which is more or less a prerequisite of getting a leading position at the centres. It is not possible to mention all researchers, but examples of some of the research performed will give a conception of the breadth of this research.

In *Stockholm* urological research has traditionally been very strong including hydronephrosis, bladder physiology, hypospadias, cryptorchidism. In gastroenterology Hirschsprung's disease and anal function have been thoroughly studied as well as oesophageal atresia with the invention of circular myotomy. Very interesting fields are genetics in paediatric urology and Hirschsprung's disease, and tissue engeneering. Experimental and clinical studies of diaphragmatic hernia and of ECMO are also performed.

In *Gothenburg* also, urology has been dominating with clinical and experimental studies of normal and pathological urinary bladder function, posterior urethral valves, vesicoureteral reflux, myelomeningocele, hypospadias, renal transplantation, self-catheterisation of the bladder, renography. Colonic and rectal motility have been studied, as well as childhood accidents and fractures. In cardiac surgery especially coarctation of the aorta has been investigated.

In *Uppsala* the main field of research has for a long time been paediatric urology including hydronephrosis, vesicoureteral reflux with the invention and use of Deflux®, enuresis and cryptorchidism. Furthermore a strong line has been on malignant tumours especially on neuroblastoma and on angiogenesis. Metabolism, intravenous nutrition and liver research, Hirschsprung's diease and development of the human enteric system are others. Hydrocephalus is a subject of longstanding interest.

In *Lund* there is a strong gastrointestinal research line. Hirschsprung's disease and other dysmotilities, bowel innervation and neurontransplantation as well as oesophageal atresia have been studied in detail in a number of dissertations. Urology, with bladder exstrophy and vesico-ureteric reflux, has been an important field, as well artificial ventilation in children. In 2006 robot surgery was introduced with clinical and experimental applications.

The Situation Today

Today there are still four paediatric surgical centres in Sweden: in Stockholm, Gothenburg, Uppsala and Lund. Sweden has just above nine million inhabitants. The population density is very sparse, about 22 inhabitants per square kilometre. As Sweden is a rather elongated country, 1572 kilometres from north to south, it is obvious that those living in the northern part have to make a long journey to reach the nearest paediatric surgical centre.

The four centres are all part of complete Children's Hospitals with expertise in the care of children with, for instance paediatrics, paediatric radiology, neonatology, anaesthesia, intensive care, physiotherapy, pathology, clinical physiology, dietetics, play therapy school system, etc.

In Stockholm there is an important ECMO-activity. Depending on local tradition some centres also do neurosurgery like hydrocephalus and myelomeningocele, some do orthopedics, others do some thoracic surgery. But common to all, besides the "essential paediatric surgery" is a heavy load of general paediatric surgery with 24 hour primary and secondary duty.

All four centres do paediatric urology, which has always belonged to and been an important part of paediatric surgery. Today it constitutes more than 30% of the total workload. The reason for this paediatric surgical affiliation is not obvious. But as the paediatric surgical pioneers in Sweden all had an interest in urology, and as adult urology was not as strong and developed as it is today, it might be natural that paediatric urology should belong to paediatric surgery and be performed by the paediatric surgeons.

So, within paediatric surgery there has always been a genuine and strong interest in developing the urological part, and during the years a lot of scientific research has been performed, among other things displayed in several doctoral theses. During the last 30 years, 22 paediatric surgeons have taken a doctor's degree in paediatric urology. Probably, most of the paediatric urology in Sweden will continue to be performed within paediatric surgery by specialised paediatric urologists. However, there have been discussions in the European Society for Paediatric Urology (ESPU) and also in Sweden to further strengthen the urology and make it self-independent as an own specialty beside the paediatric surgical specialty.

Beside research, teaching students in medicine and nursing among others is especially important. There is a tight cooperation with EUPSA and other European organizations, especially concerning educational issues.

All centres are working in accordance with the Nordic Association for the need of sick children (NOBAB) and the European Association for children in hospital (EACH) whose charter is a common norm, emanating from the UN Convention on the rights of the child.

Females in Paediatric Surgery

The first Swedish female chief surgeon was Sigrid Söderlund (Fig. 10) at CLH in 1974. There has been only one after her, Christina Clementson Kockum, who is the present chief in Lund. However, the total number of certified female paediatric surgeons is 38% out of a total number of 126, which is the highest percentage of all operating disciplines in Sweden. As a comparison hand surgery has 24%, plastic surgery 23%, general surgery 14%, thoracic surgery and urology 11%, neurosurgery and orthopaedics 9%. But we still have a distance to go to reach the 45% of paediatrics! There are only

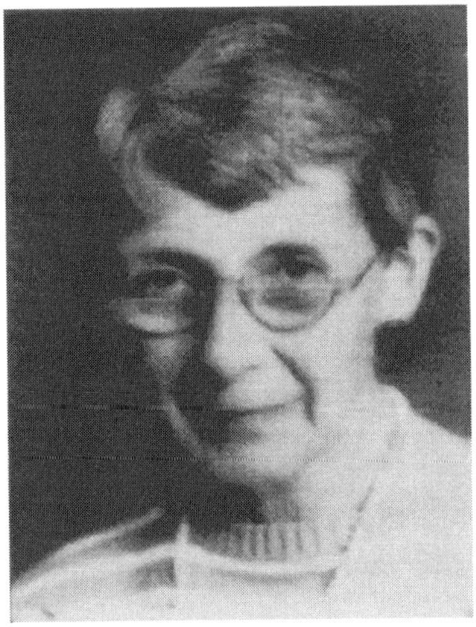

Fig. 10. Sigrid Söderlund.

two female Professors in paediatric surgery, Ulla Sillén in Gothenburg and Agneta Nordenskjöld in Stockholm.

The Future

At the present there are a lot of enthusiastic, promising young doctors wanting to specialize in paediatric surgery. One problem, however, is that there are not enough index cases, or rather, there are already too many specialists! But the heavy 24-hour duty, often with a lot of "non-specialist" general surgical cases due to an ambition that children have a right to be treated by specialists, has lead to this "overproduction" of specialists.

According to the European Union of Monospecialists, there should be one paediatric surgeon per 500,000 inhabitants, and one paediatric surgical centre per 2,5 million inhabitants. In Sweden, the total number of certified paediatric surgeons in the four centres is 62. This implies one surgeon per 145,200 people.

Within the speciality there are now discussions to distribute some of the uncommon diseases with small numbers of patients to one or two of the four centres. This might increase the individual

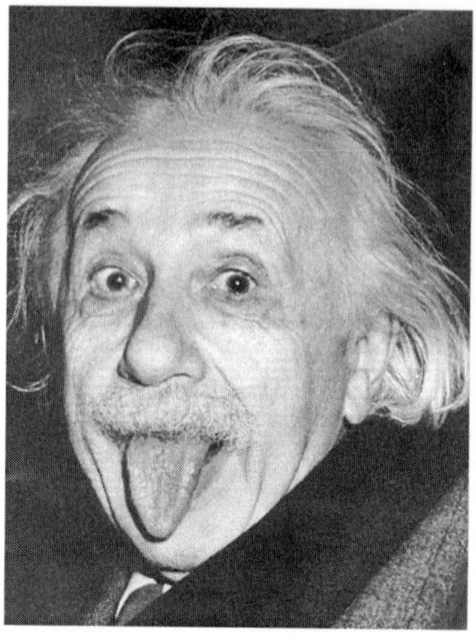

Fig. 11. A genius.

experience in the centres in question. A reduction to three centres is another option, however a very hard task to accomplish.

Swedish paediatric surgery has a long tradition of international contacts and cooperation, a tradition that has to continue in order to keep the activity on a high level. Participation in the European and other international legislative bodies is preferential.

With many young doctors interested in our speciality, the future still looks promising. We try to support their interest by "quoting" a well known scientist (Fig. 11): "You don't have to be a genius to realize that Paediatric Surgery is the best (surgical) speciality in the world!!"

Acknowledgement

I appreciate the valuable information given by Christina Clementson Kockum, Joar Crafoord, Björn Frenckner, Lars-Göran Friberg, Jan Gierup, Gunnar Göthberg, Björn Henrikson, Lars-Torsten Larsson, Gösta Löhr, Johan Nathorst-Westfelt, Arne Stenberg, Johan Wallander, Tomas Wester.

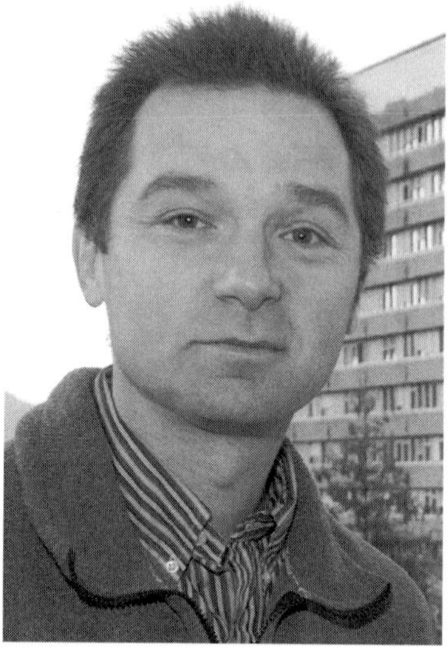

Nicolas Lutz

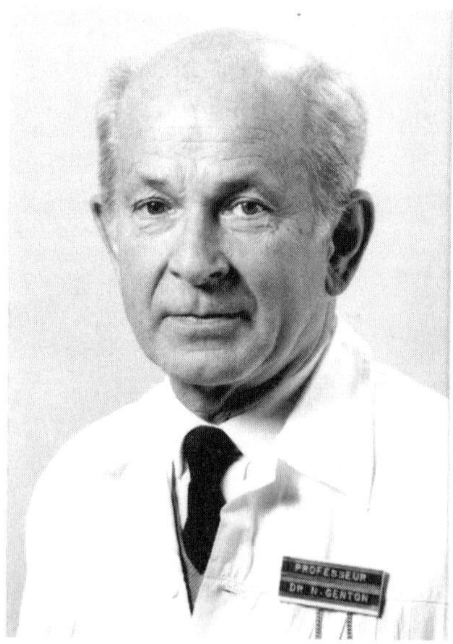

Noël Genton

SWITZERLAND

Nicolas Lutz
Noël Genton

The Beginning

On 24 November, 1689, Elizabeth and Catherine Meyerin were born as conjoined twins in Basel, Switzerland. **Johannes Fatio** (1649–1691), renowned master barber surgeon successfully proceeded to separate the xypho-omphalopagus twin with a silken cord in front of an audience of many medical men and lord mayors. Although published by E. König one year later, this case illustrates the dawn of paediatric surgery in Switzerland, with J. Fatio being its first remarkable representative. In the fourth section of his only printed book "*Helvetic Reasonable Midwife*", more than 17 greatly detailed chapters describe the diseases of neonates and infants, together with their treatment. He describes mouth to mouth respiration as the most efficient method of resuscitation, warns of the danger of bleeding from cutting the lingual frenulum, writes about a peno-scrotal hypospadias operation using a trocar from the glans along the shaft of the penis and passing a leaden tube along the newly made channel into the bladder. He clearly distinguishes between umbilical hernia (which rarely needed any treatment) and exomphalos (to be closed with continuous strapping over the often ruptured membranes).[1]

Until the late 19th century, Switzerland was still a poor and underdeveloped country with significant emigration. Compared to France, the slightly later opening of paediatric hospitals was also due to the relatively small size of our country as well as to the very low

Table 1. Origin of hospitals for children in Switzerland.

Year	Place	Name	Funding
1811	Neuchatel	Pourtalès	Jacques-Louis de Pourtalès
1846	Basel	Kinderspitäli	Frau Burckhardt
1861	Lausanne	Hospice de l'enfance	Aimé and Caroline Steinlen
1862	Bern	Kinderspital	Frau Von Jenner
1866	Aarau	Kinderspital	Sandra Cagnazzo
1871	Zürich	Kinderspital	Dr Conrad Cramer (Eleonoren-Stiftung)
1872	Geneva	Maison des enfants malades	Mr and Mrs Duval-Rillet
1903	Biel	Wildermeth	Johanna and Sigmund Wildermeth
1909	St Gallen	Säuglingsheim	City of Sankt Gallen

income of its inhabitants. As in many parts of Europe, sick Swiss children lucky enough to have access to medical treatment stayed at home or were treated in adult hospitals.

Under the influence of the *Hôpital des Enfants Malades*, founded in 1802 in Paris, Swiss doctors actively participated in the opening of hospitals specially dedicated to the care of children (Table 1). The first was in Neuchatel (1811) followed by Basel (1846), Lausanne (1861), Berne (1862), Aarau (1866), Zurich (1871), Genève (1872), Bienne (1903) and finally Sankt Gallen (1909).[2,3]

Most of these new hospitals were privately funded and were commonly run by general surgeons who had an interest in paediatrics. For example, the ***Kinderspitäli* in Basel** was opened by **Frau Burckhardt** in part of her own house. A housekeeper looked after the patients who were treated by Dr Carl Streckeisen (1811–1868), "for the love of God".[2] Contrary to orphanages and homes for lost children, these hospitals were directed by doctors eager to apply and improve their scientific knowledge. In the 1840s, influenced by the Viennese school, doctors were starting to do auscultation, percussion, to measure temperature and introduce microscopic analysis in their daily practice. Surgery was becoming slightly more reliable, thanks in part to the advent of anaesthesia with ether and chloroform. The 1840 book on paediatric surgery by Gersant was translated from French into English and became an international reference.

Highly symbolic of the success of modern surgery, ironically appendectomy only slowly became popular among the medical societies in Switzerland. Doctors, surgeons and the population in general were not convinced that removing the inflamed appendix was an adequate solution. Over a period of two decades (1880–1900) the American surgical elite was working hard to scientifically study and justify appendectomy. In 1888, Cesar Roux, an influential Swiss general surgeon asked one of his interns at the *Hôpital Cantonal de Lausanne* to study appendectomy for his thesis. Once convinced of the adequacy of the procedure, he quickly performed enough appendectomies to be able to present more than 100 specimens of appendix at the National Exhibition in Vevey in 1901.[4] This had a significant impact on both the population and the local medical community, allowing further generalisation of the procedure.

At the beginning of the 20th century, most of the surgeons operating on children were mainly treating adults, including Prof Monnier in Zurich, Dr Vuillet in Lausanne, Dr Lauterburg in Bern and Dr Nicole in Basel.

Max Grob* (1901–1976)

Born in Zurich in 1901, this man was certainly the most influential Swiss paediatric surgeon, not only for being the first Swiss surgeon to devote his entire work to children, but also because of his many "firsts" in Swiss paediatric surgery and his central role as teacher of many future Swiss paediatric surgeons. Margrit Stockmann (1915–2008, Clinic Santa Anna, Luzern), Marcel Bettex (1920–1997, Bern), Noel Genton (1925–, Lausanne) all trained in Zurich.

The first appointment of Max Grob (Fig. 1) was as a first-year resident at the cantonal infants hospital of his native town in 1928. He then worked with Prof Monnier in the surgical department of the

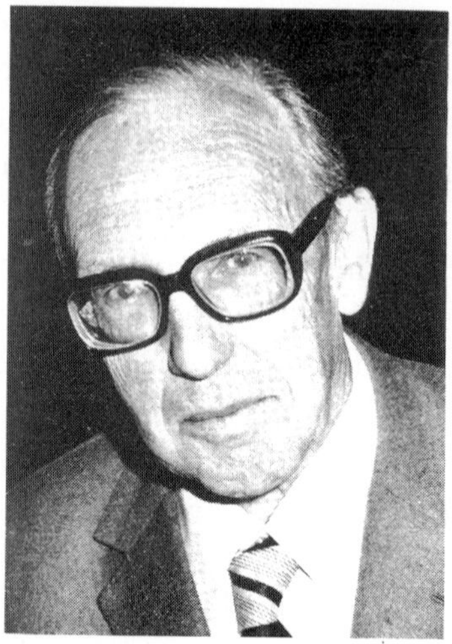

Fig. 1. Max Grob.

same hospital and was so fascinated by his task that he decided to devote himself exclusively to paediatric surgery. He completed his training with P. Clairmont at the University Hospital of Zurich in 1936. This was followed by a six months course in the surgical department directed by L. Ombrédanne at the *Hôpital des Enfants Malades* in Paris. With Professor Veau, he familiarised himself with the treatment of cleft lip, jaw and palate. Back in Zurich, he opened a private practice as a specialist in paediatrics and surgery. The title of specialist in paediatric surgery was neither recognised nor allowed at that time. Two years later, he was elected to be the successor to Monnier at the children's hospital. It was wartime, and there was no exchange of experience on an international level. His main interests were in the surgical correction of congenital malformations and cardiac surgery. He carried out the first successful heart operation in a child in Europe in 1947, performing a Blalock–Taussig operation for Fallot's teralogy. He operated on a wide variety of congenital heart defects, introduced artificial hypothermia in 1957 and, two years later, used a heart-lung machine for the first time (Fig. 2). He also did pioneering work in the treatment of cleft lip, jaw and palate

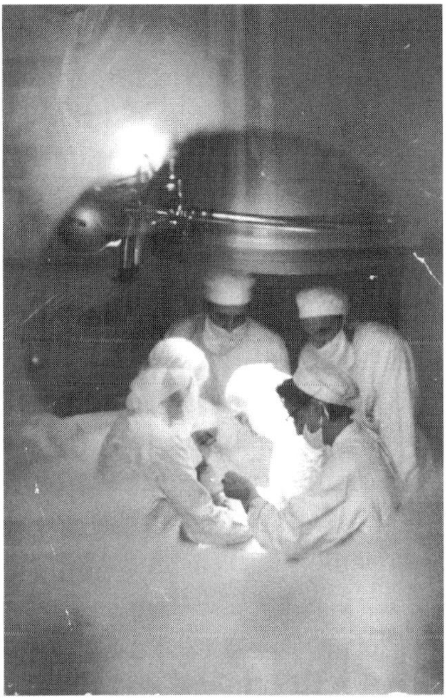

Fig. 2. A Daily Scene in Zürich Kinderspital in 1958: The Operating Room (courtesy of Noël Genton).

surgery. Furthermore, he was the first surgeon in Switzerland to perform a pull-through operation for Hirschsprung's disease and to correct a hiatus hernia. He published a renowned teaching book on paediatric surgery in German, "*Lehrbuch die Kinderchirurgie*", in 1957. In 1982, the second edition of this book edited by M. Bettex, N. Genton and M. Stockmann, involved the vast majority of paediatric surgeons working in Switzerland at that time.

The brilliant career of Max Grob was recognised by many international paediatric surgical associations, from which he received numerous awards and distinctions. In 1969, he was awarded the Dennis Browne Memorial Medal of the British Association of Paediatric Surgeons (BAPS), of which he was a active member from the start in 1953. He was a man of integrity and modesty, with a high sense of criticism and perseverance.[5]

Birth of the Swiss Society for Paediatric Surgery

From 1963 onwards, Swiss paediatric surgeons held yearly meetings to share their knowledge and experiences. The first meeting in 1963 was organized by **Noël Genton** in Lausanne. In the 1960s, many medical specialities led to the foundation of new Swiss societies including a society of Orthopaedics and one of Urology. Even though Max Grob was not very much in favour of a society for paediatric surgery separated from the Swiss Society for General Surgery, he could not stop the movement initiated by his colleagues and pupils. The Swiss Society for Paediatric Surgery was formed in Bern in the Theodor Kocher Institute club room on 20 October, 1969. **Max Grob** became the first president of a society including 18 members from all over Switzerland. Robert Morger from St. Gallen was vice-president and cashier. Marcel Bettex from Bern became general secretary. Fabio Muggiasca and Alois Schärli were appointed to check the accounts.[6] The first society meeting took place the same day in the afternoon. In 1974, the society was officially recognised by the Swiss government official medical council (FMH, *Federatio Medicorum Helveticorum*) implying that its members could then hold the official title "paediatric surgeon FMH". The Swiss Society for Paediatric Surgery became part of the "UNION" in 1978, a joint venture of six surgical societies including General Surgery, Neurosurgery, Urology, Plastic Surgery and Orthopaedics. The aim of the UNION was to achieve quality control without state bureaucracy and to coordinate postgraduate and continuous medical education in the various fields of surgery. A. Schärli from Luzern was general secretary of the UNION for more than 15 years.

The Years 1960 to 1990

In this fast evolving part of the 20th century, several renowned Swiss paediatric surgeons led the way to autonomy from adult surgery in the five university hospitals (Basel, Bern, Geneva, Lausanne, and Zurich) and in three district hospitals (Luzern — A. Schärli, St. Gallen — R. Morger and Biel — J. Ehrensperger).

In Zürich, Peter Paul Rickham (1917–2003), came from Liverpool to succeed Max Grob in 1971. He had just published a book "*Neonatal Surgery*" (1969) and had started a scientific periodical entitled "*Progress in Paediatric Surgery*" (1970). Urs Stauffer worked with him and took over in 1983.[7] In Bern, Marcel Bettex took charge of a few surgical beds in the Children's hospital in 1958. By the time he had retired in 1987, he had created an independent modern department of paediatric surgery. He was appointed president of the World Association of Paediatric Surgeons in 1984, remaining until 1987.[8,9] In Lausanne, Noël Genton obtained an independent paediatric surgical unit in 1961. Antoine Cuendet started a similar unit in Geneva in 1962, Aloïs Schaerli in Luzern in 1971.

A man of endurance with a good sense of humour, **Dr Schärli** (Fig. 3) used to call himself "son of Bettex, grandson of Grob"! With his friends from all five continents, he founded "*Pediatric Surgery International*", a medical journal which contributed greatly to the spread of scientific knowledge in the field of paediatric surgery. He remained editor-in-chief for 18 years. In Basel, Peter Herzog took over responsibility from Prof Nicole in the Kinderspital in 1973.

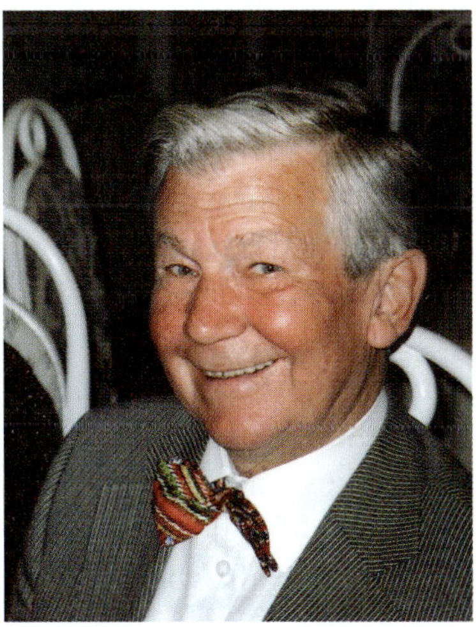

Fig. 3. Alois Schärli.

Over those years, as competition grew amongst centres, their leaders redefined the spectrum of paediatric surgery in Switzerland with the advent of several sub-specialities. They used their friendship with other members of the BAPS to send their pupils for further training to prestigious and renowned paediatric surgical centres both in Europe and the United States.

Today and Tomorrow

With 68 ordinary members, six life members, 48 extraordinary members and 19 corresponding members, the Swiss Society for Paediatric Surgery has steadily grown into an active multi-lingual society supervising sub-specialities such as paediatric neurosurgery, urology, hand, plastic, trauma and neonatal surgery. Recently, our society became a founding member of a new federation of paediatric health care providers, *fPmh* (*Federatio Peditrioca Medica Helveticorum*). Created in 2007 in conjunction with both Swiss Paediatric and Paedo-psychiatric societies, this federation aims to better support child health and medical needs at a national level. With its nearly 8 million inhabitants, Switzerland has 26 cantons with varying health systems and organisations. A national regulation of highly specialised surgery is underway and will require some lobbying from the *fPmh*. A significant link with adult surgery will also be necessary to strengthen the transition in the treatment strategies of our "adult-to-be" patients.

Paediatric surgeons have long performed most visceral and orthopaedic procedures. Over the last decade, orthopaedic surgeons have sub-specialised in paediatric orthopaedics and taken over most orthopaedic procedures, except for fractures, which tend to remain in the hands of general paediatric surgeons. Nowadays, most Swiss paediatric surgeons working in university hospitals have a special field of interest in which they have gained expertise and for which they are renowned nationwide if not further abroad. Some paediatric surgical specialities have also been concentrated in specific university centres such as liver surgery in Geneva, heart transplantation in Zürich and Bern. Paediatric coelioscopic surgery started in

Lausanne and Geneva, following the French influence. It is now well established in most centres.

Following bilateral agreements between the European Union and Switzerland, our society has engaged in a major brainstorming process to "Europeanise" our postgraduate training. The priorities of life today and the legal maximum weekly workload of 50 hours for interns have significantly changed the mentality of the young surgeon. This will require major adjustments in teaching and training.

Our main challenge for the future is to find the best way to train efficiently and work ethically while respecting legally defined working hours and maintaining the high quality level of care established by our predecessors.

References

1. Rickham PP. The Dawn of paediatric surgery: Johannes Fatio. *Prog Pediatr Surgery* 1986;20:94–105.
2. Suter S, *et al.* Ages et Visages de la Pédiatrie: La genèse du Département de pédiatrie. Editions GeorG, Genève, 2001.
3. Rapport annuel. Fondation hôpital d'enfants Wildermeth, Bienne, 2004.
4. Donzé PY. L'ombre de César. Editions BHMS, 2007.
5. Bettex M, Genton N. Nachruf Prof Dr. med. Max Grob. *Zeitschrift für Kinderchirurgie und Grenzgebiete* 1977;20:203–204.
6. Bettex M. *Hat sich das alles gelohnt? Memoiren eines Kinderchirurgen.* Simowa Verlag, Bern, 1999.
7. Lüönd K. *Für Kind und Familie, Der weg des Kinderspitals Zürich ins 21. Jahrhundert.* Rio Verlag, Zürich, 2004.
8. Sommer P. *Das Jenner-Kinderspital in Bern.* Jennerstiftung Verlag, Bern, 1978.
9. Schärli A. Marcel Bettex 1920–1997. *J Pediatr Surg* 1998;33:543–544.

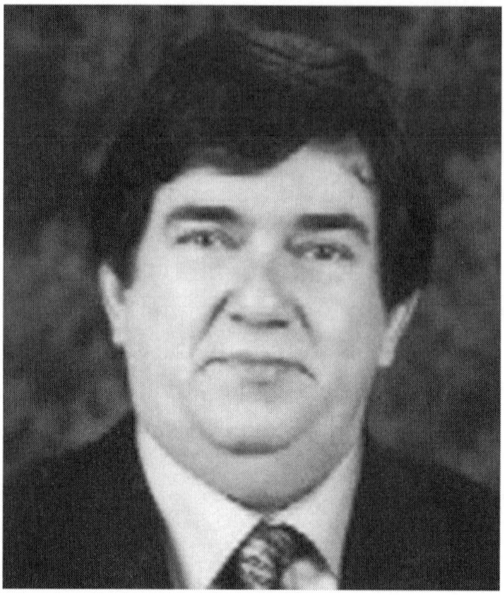

S. N. Cenk Büyükünal

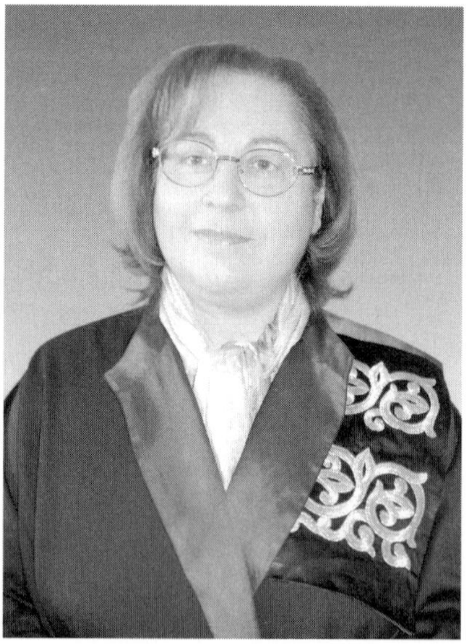

Nil Sari

TURKEY — ANATOLIA

S. N. Cenk Büyükünal
Nil Sari

Anatolia has been one of the main sources for medical discoveries, famous physicians, and developments in medicine. Galen (130–190 AD) born in Pergamon, Aegean cast of Anatolia was the first physician to use the term "hypospadias" for the description of a very well-known genital problem. Besides he described the chordee problem and mentioned the difficulty in ejaculation during sexual intercourse.[1,2]

During the Byzantine period Oribasius (325–403 AD), mentioned the details of the operation for distal type hypospadias: "cutting thc glans a little bit above the coronary sulcus"! By means of this surgical procedure he thought that he was going to be able to bring the meatus to the tip and central part of glans tissue.[3]

In Ottoman period, Şerafettin Sabuncuoğlu was one of the main important corner stones as far as the development of paediatric surgery is concerned. He was from the northern part of central Anatolia and he was the author of the first paediatric surgical textbook and atlas called: "*Cerrahiye-i Ilhaniye*" (Fig. 1). This book was presented to the Ottoman Emperor Mehmet the Second in 1460.[4–7] In this manuscript, the details of surgical treatment of hydrocephalus, short frenulum of tongue, intcrscx-clitorectomy, excision and treatment of superfluous and webbed finger, surgery for inguinal hernia, imperforate anus and hypospadias were described. Besides proper surgical techniques for circumcision, reasons for erroneous circumcision performed by unqualified people practicing surgery were discussed. Surgical instruments such as hypospadias instruments, special lenticular

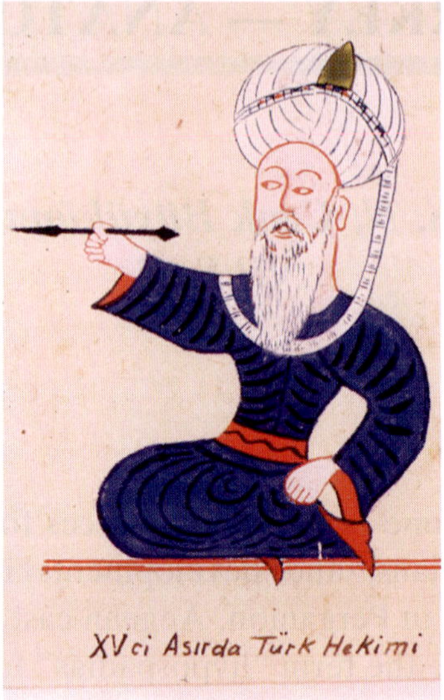

Fig. 1. Sabuncuoğlu Şerafettin, XVth Century (Fatih National Library).

cautery, urinary catheters, designed by himself were presented with colourful pictures. It is observed that the book of Sabuncuoğlu contains many important and major new contributions to surgical and paediatric surgical literature. This historical textbook, as a piece of art, could also be accepted as the first paediatric surgical atlas.

The history of the Ottoman Period was full of positive efforts for the children's health and children rights. There were strong community efforts to save the children's rights and public organizations for the care of pediatric patients. According to Islamic religion, there were special ethical principles in medical practice as far as patient's and surgeon's rights were concerned.[8–11]

For the Patients

a) Ethical rules were basically the same for adult and pediatric patients and this was extremely important in the Ottoman Empire.
b) Community and health organizations were very sensitive about children's rights.

c) Before every operation, a special consent called "*huccet*" was taken from the parent or guardian of the child or from the judge (if there is no parent or relative).

Huccet

Before every operation a special contract of consent "*Huccet*" was signed in order to withold parents or guardians from starting suits for compensation against the surgeon in case of death or complications:

a) This contract of consent was a legal obligation 11–13.
b) In this consent, it was also noted that the surgeon was going to operate the paediatric patient skillfully and going to do his best.
c) If the surgeon treated his patient honestly and used his skill properly, no compensation was to be claimed in case of death, complication or injury.
d) If the surgeon was found to be negligent or faulty, he had to compensate the harm which was given to the child.
e) These contracts were signed by the parents and surgeon with the agreement of witnesses.
f) In some of these contracts, the surgeon's fee and the amounts to be given before and after the operation, was also mentioned.

What were the Responsibilities of a Surgeon?

a) A surgeon was obliged to treat every paediatric patient and was not approved to refuse any of them, unless there was another surgeon in the neigboorhood.
b) There were certain ethical rules for candidates and practitioners of surgery. These special ethical rules were described in major manuscripts of surgery and these were given as advices for the trainees and practitioners. Besides, every main hospital was ruled according to its deed of trust, which described ethical issues expected to be obeyed by the surgeons to be appointed.

c) Every surgeon was expected to acquire the basic medical knowledge of the age. Surgeons were also responsible for the follow-up of the paediatric patients and post operative treatment.
d) Surgeons were not responsible for orthopaedics and ophtalmology. These two branches were considered different fields of practice.

When was the Surgeon Regarded as Responsible in the Case of any Injury and Complication?

a) When a written consent was not taken.
b) When there was an unacceptable surgical or medical failure.
c) When his surgical technique is found to be below or under the standards of that period of time.
d) When ill-will was found in his practice.
e) When the surgeon was scientifically under the standards and unqualified and not skillful and efficient enough.

In Ottoman Hospitals there were some certain rules for the appointed surgeons. Besides, every health personnel or workers were individually responsible for what they did. There were some ethical advices in well-known surgical manuscripts or medical textbooks:

Ethical Advice in Surgical Manuscript Cerrahiyetü'l Haniye of Sabuncuoglu Ş̧erafeddin from Amasya (mid XVth century)[4–7]

a) Every surgeon must be conscious of the potential risks of exstensive bleeding and major infections.
b) Extraction of bladder stones may be dangerous for some paediatric patients. Surgeon has to be meticulous and gentle in these cases.
c) Before the operation, inform the patient's family/parents about the details and potential risks of the operation.
d) Do not operate if there is a certain risk for the patient.
e) Do not operate any patient only for your self-interest. Priority should always be known as patient's interest!

Ethical Advices in Surgical Manuscript Alâim-i Cerrahîn (XVth Century by Ibrahim bin Abdullah)

a) A surgeon should be good-humoured, honest and modest.
b) Should behave respectfully to his masters.
c) Should be quick enough and skillful.
d) Should have enough basic medical knowledge.
e) Should be informed of the methods of preparing ointments, dressings and, coatings.
f) Must prepare drugs suited for children (Fig. 2).
g) His surgical instruments must be gold-plated, silver or at least tin.

Examples of Copies of Contracts Signed by Fathers Giving Consent for Pediatric Urological Procedures

A contract signed by the father of the child and the surgeon

Name of the patient: İbrahim (male)
Name of the father: Son of Kinyas Mahlî

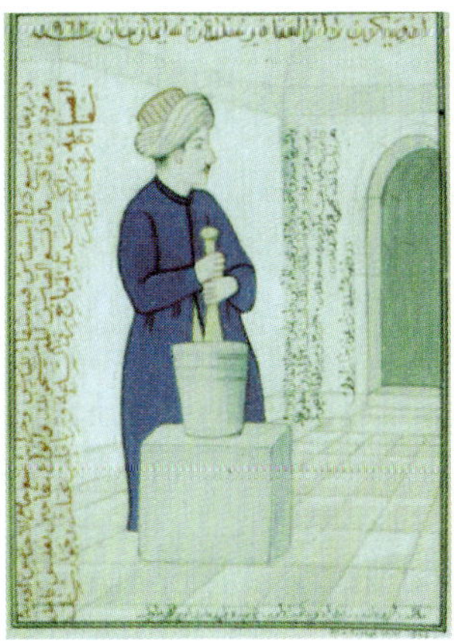

Fig. 2. A Surgeon Preparing Ointments and Creams for Postoperative Wound Care.

Name of the surgeon: Budak bin Nazar
Operation: Removal of a bladder stone "vesicolithotomy"
Surgeon's fee: 4 gold coins
City and year: Gaziantep (Southeast of Turkey, 1539)
Witnesses: Osman oğlu Cakin, Ali Musa Can Cavus
Judicial registration no: 2, p. 282.

Another contract signed by the parents and the surgeon

Name of the child patient: Gullu Bali (female)
Name of the father: Yanli Bali son of Penayedu
Name of the surgeon: Ahmed bin Musa
Surgical procedure: Vesicolithotomy
Year and city: 1652, Isparta (South Anatolia)
Judicial registration number: Unread

In the Ottoman Empire, some of the courts were in charge of cases which were related to surgical problems. The following case is an example for that:

Case, register number 122, p. 73, February 1765, Gaziantep. Omer and his wife from Sehrekustu, a district from Gaziantep, accused the son of Mustafa, Molla Mehmed, the surgeon, who lived in the same neighborhood and claimed, "A mass had developed on our son Mehmed's back (possibly an abscess?) and we took him to the accused surgeon for treatment. The accused incised the mass and as a result, our son died in four days".

The surgeon defended himself saying, "The illness called "*ummussibyan*", known as "*duzumcu*" in our city, was on the back of the child. This illness is treated by incising and than draining the liquid in it called "ma-i cedîd". Later, the wound is treated medically. This treatment modality has been practiced successfully for a long time. I had the plaintiff's conset for incising and treating the swelling." And he also presented a "fatwa" (a decision on legal matter), providing the truth of what he had said in his defense. The plaintiff said that he did not have their consent. So, the accused was asked to prove his defense. The witnesses who were heard, said that the operation was performed on the plaintiff's consent. They also added that Molla Mehmed was an efficient surgeon. "Judgement was given in favor of the surgeon."

In conclusion, in Ottoman Empire, surgical practice and ethical rules exactly the same for adult and pediatric patients. There were no difference for male and female patients. Besides, community, health organizations and hospitals were very careful and sensitive for children's rights and health problems. There were certain ethical rules for major hospitals and their surgeons. Surgeons regarded as responsible for pediatric surgical procedures; preparation of drugs, creams and ointments which are used in the postoperative period. Surgeons were also responsible for pre and post operative treatment and follow-up of the children. This was a major difference between a barber and a modern surgeon.

Surgeons should be up-to-date with modern medical and surgical knowledge. In the Ottoman period, urolithiasis was a well-known surgical disease in pediatric age group and it was possible to treat it with surgical techniques.

In Ottoman Empire, during the reign of Sultan Abdulhamid-II the end of 19th century is extremely important for child health. The first children's hospital with a separate pediatric surgical pavillon was in service in Istanbul, the Hamidiyye-i Etfal Children's Hospital (Figs. 3, 4). There was a separate pavillon with 16 beds, reserved for the care of children of tourists, foreign guests and embassies. All medical care was free of charge.

The Paediatric Surgery Department had two separate wards and Operating Room (O.R.). One of the two operation rooms was reserved for major operations. The other one is used for minor surgical procedures. An X-ray room, a laboratory for the design and production of new surgical instruments, and a laboratory for orthopaedic prostesis made up the other parts of this department. The O.R had whole anesthesiology equipment, steamed hot water, modern surgical instruments and electricity as well. There was a special air circulating system and microbiological analysis for O.R and wards were performed in routine basis.

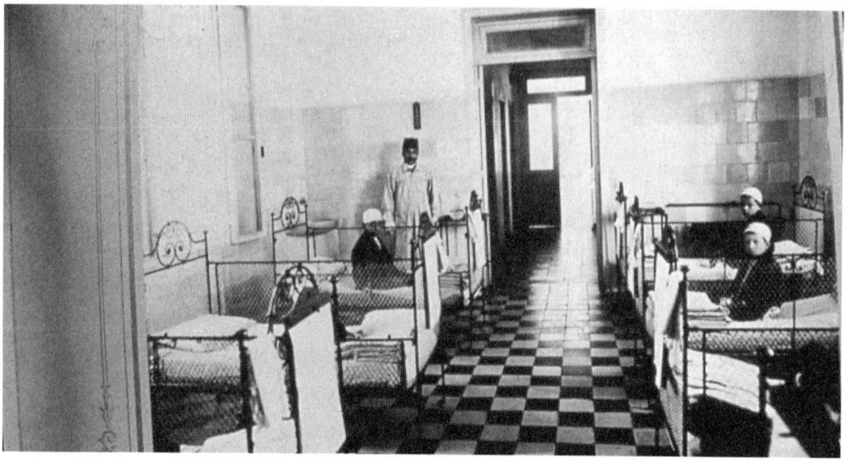

Fig. 3. Paediatric Surgery Ward.

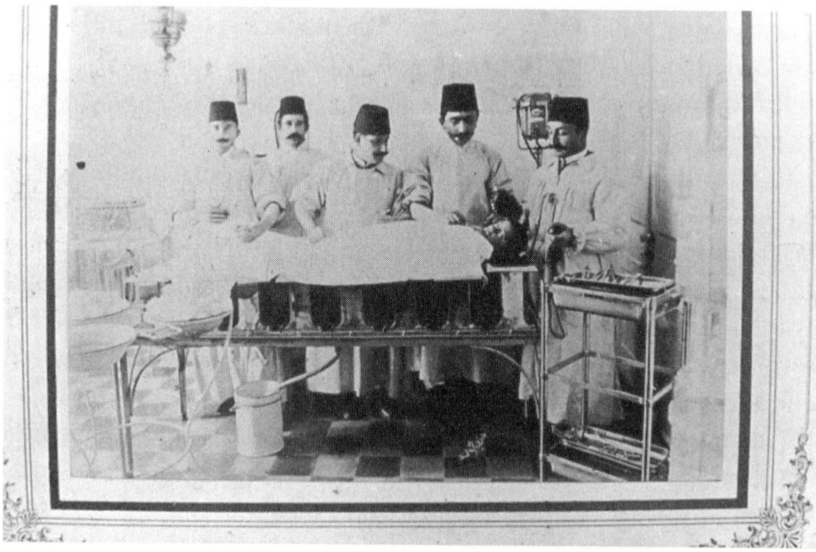

Fig. 4. Operating Room (P. Surgery).

The central heating system, sterilization unit, a mechanical steam-powered dishwasher, and a special steam machine for the sterilization of milk bottles were the new technological developments in this unit. Moreover there was an animal research laboratory with whole

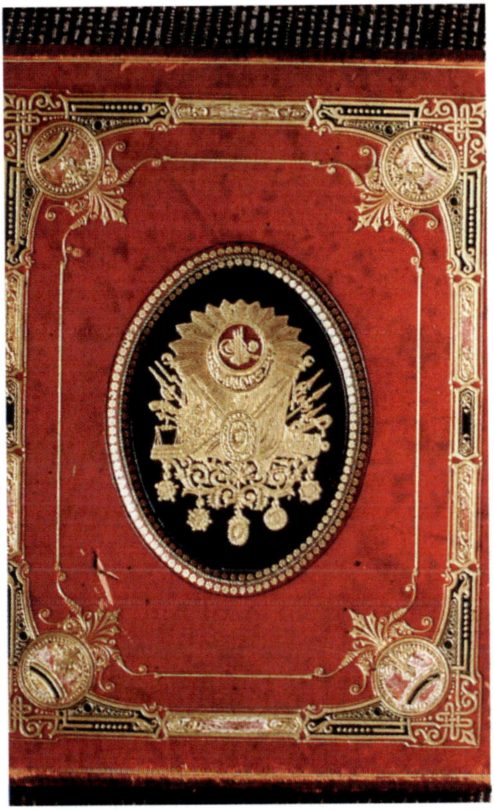

Fig. 5. Gold-ornamented cover of Journal of Hamidiye-i Etfal Hospital (Library of Istanbul University).

facilities of the time. The hospital library had 260 different textbooks on paediatric diseases and surgical disorders. For the case reports, medical statistics and new discoveries a special journal called "*Journal of Hamidiye Children's Hospital*" was published and first issue was printed in August 1900 (Fig. 5).[6,12]

From 1906 to 1907, 87 paediatric surgical procedures had been performed in this surgical unit including urinary stones and tumors (Table 1). Mortality and mortality rates were not higher than the major European Children's Hospitals. Prof Cemil Topuzlu Pasha was the head of this unit and he initiated new

Table 1. List of pediatric surgical procedures in Hamidiye-i Etfal Hospital (1906–1907). (*From Journal of Hamidiye Etfal Children's Hospital, translated from the original manuscript, Library of Istanbul University, Beyazit, with special permmission-*)

Inguinal hernia	24
Urolithiasis	10
Tbc peritonitis	11
Tbc arthritis	9
Hydrocele	8
Osteomyelitis	7
Anal atresia	1
Various	17
TOTAL	87 operations

surgical techniques, instruments and performed successful sophisticated operations.

Children of the visitors and tourists from all over the world and from all religions were treated as free of charge and whole medication and drugs were supported by the hospital; they were accepted as guests of Ottoman Emperor.

In conclusion, Sultan Abdulhamid II (1842–1918) was the founder of first modern children's hospital in the Ottoman Empire. The first modern paediatric surgical unit founded in this hospital.

The Ottoman Empire Circumcision of boys was an important issue. This procedure was maybe the most important event in a man's life. For that reason, the circumcision procedure and the circumcision ceremony of Ottoman princes were celebrated as a festival. Sometimes these festivals lasted more than ten days. The circumcision ceremony of four princes of Sultan Ahmet the third (Ahmet-III) in 1720 was the best known "circumcision ceremony" in Ottoman history. These ceremonies have been illustrated as miniatures in a book called Surname-i Vehbi[12] (Figs. 6a–f).

Modern Times. In 1930's, Prof Akif Şakir Şakar founded a modern clinic in Istanbul Medical Faculty called Department of Paediatric Surgery and Orthopaedics. In 1936 he published first modern

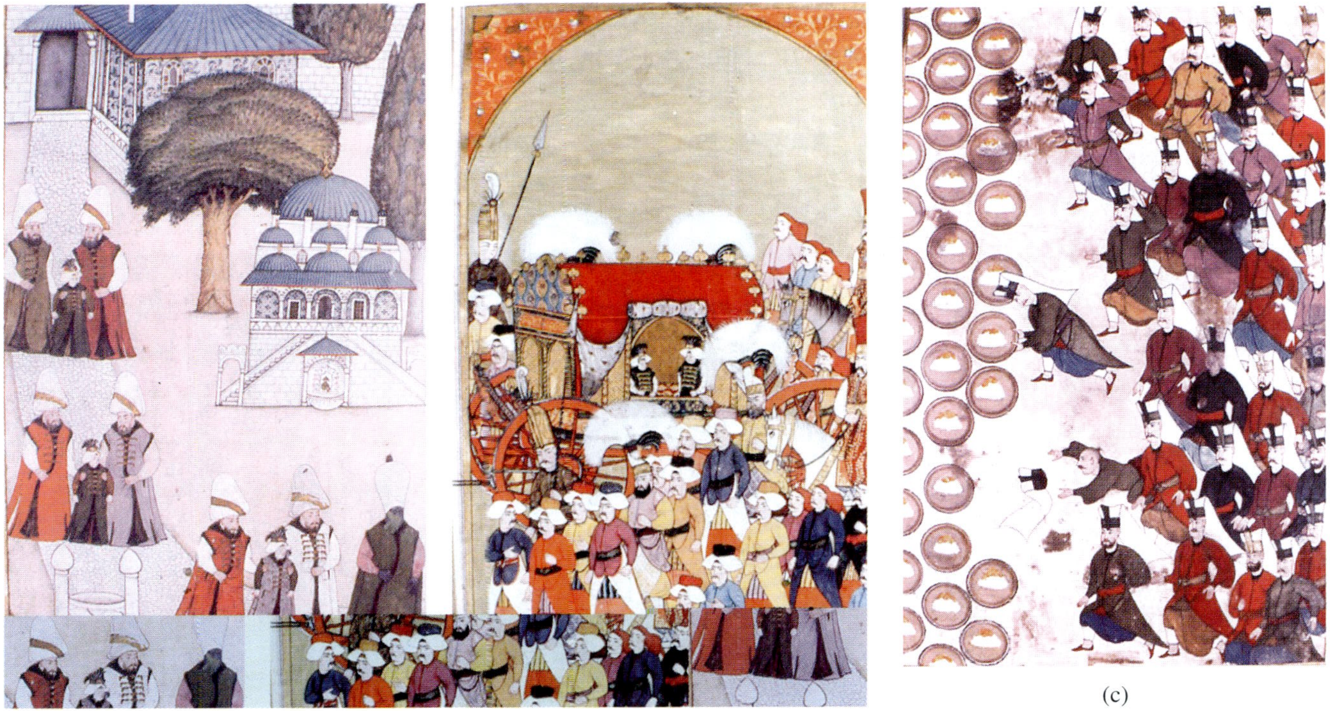

(c)

Fig. 6. Circumcision Festival in Ottoman Palace (Surname-i Vehbi from Topkapi Palace Library). (a) Four princes were on the way to Topkapı Palace for the circumcision procedure. (b) Surgeons and their assistants are on their way to Palace. (c) Lunch for the guests (in the Honor of Princes).

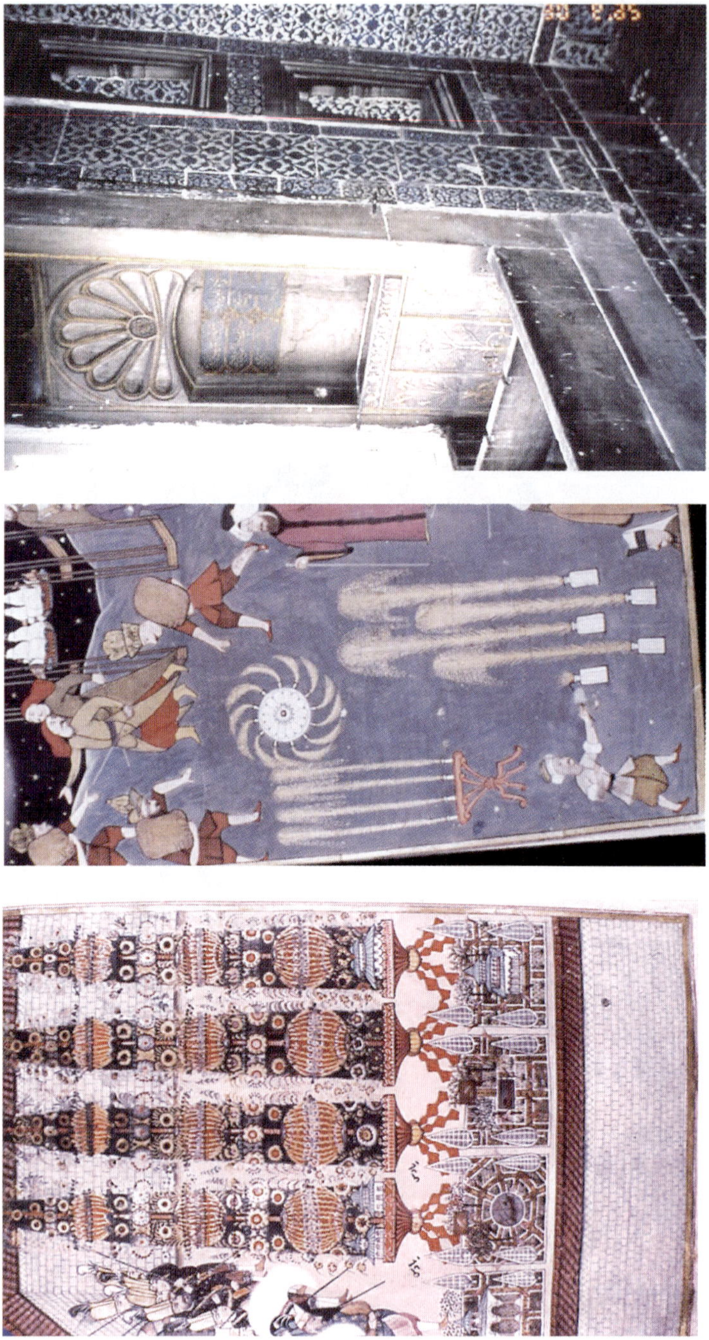

(d) (e) (f)

Fig. 6. (*Continued*) (d) Special colorful huge ornaments called "nahil". These were one of the leading symbols of circumcision festival. (e) Fireworks in the evening of circumcision. (f) Inner view of circumcision room. Notice the special tiles and ornaments and small fountains inside the windows. *The fountains were used to hide the crying voice of circumcised prince.*

paediatric surgical textbook called "*Paediatric Surgery and Orthopaedics, Clinical Lessons for Students and Residents* (in Turkish).[13] Pyloric stenosis, problems related with meningocele and myelomeningocele, orthopedic malformations etc. were the most striking chapters in this book.

In 1934, Munir Ahmet Sarpyener began his work as an Associate Professor in Orthopedics and Pediatric Surgery Department (2nd Clinic) of Hamidiye-i Etfal Children's Hospital. He was one of the initiators of modern pediatric surgery like his colleague Akif Şakir Şakar. He was probably the first one who mentioned "narrow spinal canal" in pediatric age group. In addition, he presented a new surgical technique for the treatment of narrow spinal canal in paediatric cases.[12]

During 1958–1960 period a world famous pediatric surgeon Mr Herbert Eckstein worked in Anakara Medical Faculty and Hacettepe Hospital as well. He was the first modern consultant paediatric surgeon in Turkey and was an expert in pediatric urological operations. He especially worked on stone disease of Turkish children. He was a creative surgeon and especially a nice teacher for Turkish residents.[14–16]

In 1961 a modern pediatric surgery department was founded by Prof İhsan Numanoğlu in İzmir, Aegean region (Fig. 7).[6] Besides, the first modern pediatric surgical training programme was initiated in this unit. In addition to these enormous efforts, he was the first person who succeeded to legalize pediatric surgery as a separate specialization in nationwide basis. In his department he created the first specialized subdivisions such as pediatric urology (Fig. 8), thorax surgery, burn unit, and pediatric intensive care unit. He also wrote a two-volume text book called "*Paediatric Surgery*" (in Turkish), covering whole aspects of pediatric surgery.

On the other hand, in 1963 Prof Akgün Hiçsönmez (Fig. 9) founded a modern pediatric surgery unit in Hacettepe Children's Hospital in Ankara and initiated a training programme.[6,15,16] This unit was very famous with world-known oncology experience, endocrine surgery and pediatric surgical research.

The Turkish Association of Pediatric Surgeons(TAPS) was fonded June 16, 1977, in Ankara by Akgün Hiçsönmez, Münci

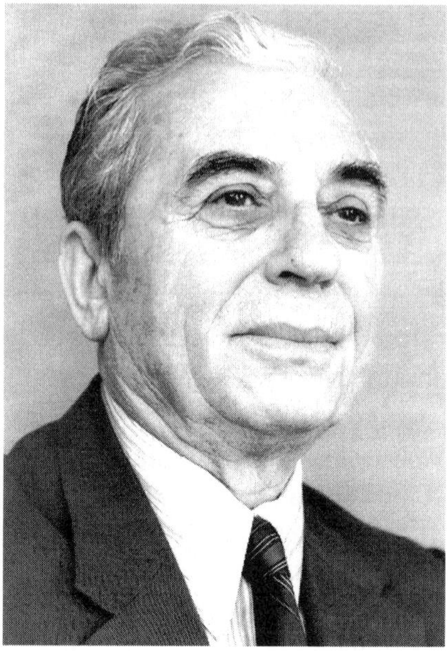

Fig. 7. Prof İhsan Numanoğlu was one of the 2 founders of modern Turkish Pediatric Surgery.

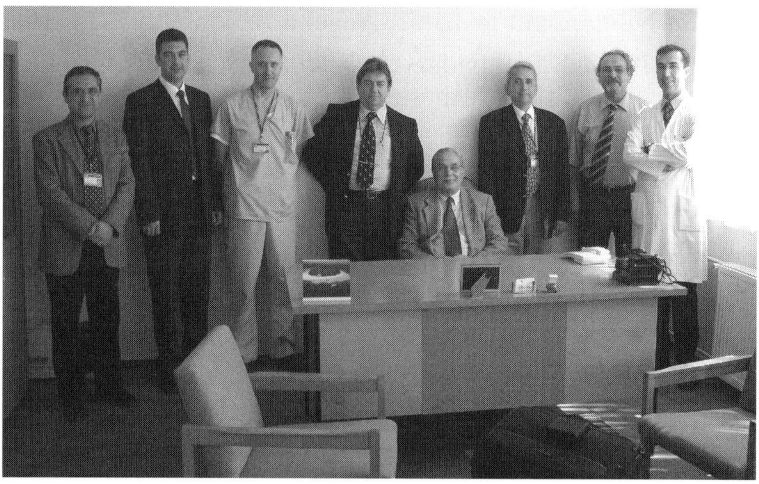

Fig. 8. Prof Acun Gökdemir was the first Turkish Pediatric Surgeon dealing with pure pediatric urology. Gökdemir with his team (April, 2006, İzmir, Aegean Medical Faculty, Department of Pediatric Surgery).

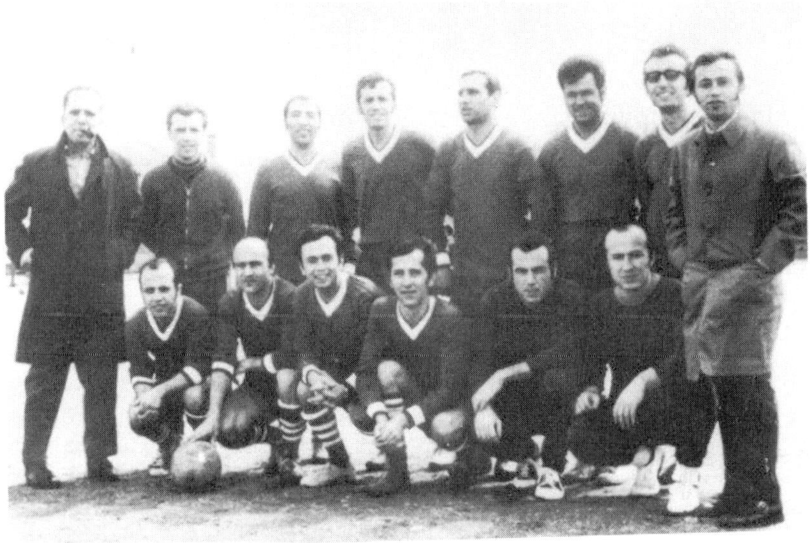

Fig. 9. Prof Akgün Hiçsönmez one of the two founders of modern Turkish Pediatric Surgery. He was also the trainer of unbeaten football team of Hacettepe Pediatric Surgery (Prof Nebil Büyükpamukçu, Prof Işık Olcay, Prof Selçuk Yücesan, Prof Nuri Kale were the stars of this team.

Kalayoglu, Nebil Büyükpamukçu, Naci Gürses, Nuri Kale, M. Ali Altın, Nevzat Uçaner and Halil Atayurt. Prof Akgün Hiçsönmez was elected as the first president of TAPS. In year 2008 T.A.P.S has more than 400 delegates. Since year 1981 T.A.P.S has been organizing National Meetings with International Participations on annual basis. Every year the best research and clinical papers are awarded by İhsan Numanoğlu and Akgün Hiçsönmez prizes. Turkish Association of Paediatric Surgeons (TAPS) hosted 7 world famos Meetings including WOFAPS (1989), BAPS (1997), ESPU (1998), SIOP-IPSO (1998), MAPS, BAPES (2007), and EUPSA (2008). They also hosted 18 international workshops such as: anorectal malformations by Alberto Peña (1990); gastroesophageal reflux by K. W. Ashcraft (1991); hypospadias by J. W. Duckett, H. Snyder and C. Woodhouse (1992); undescended testis and pediatric laparoscopy by J. Hutson and H. L. Tan (1993); bladder exstrophy-epispadias complex; by P. Ransley (1994); J. Gearhardt (1998); intersex, G. Passerini (1995); hypospadias-II; H. Snyder, W. Snodgrass, L. Baskin (2002); undescended testis and related pathologies by F. Hadziselimovich. J. Hutson, D. Cortez, C. Tanyel, A. Hamza, A. Bianchi (2003); pediatric colorectal surgery by K. Georgesson and R. Rintala (2004); paediatric laparoscopy by U. Mustak (2004), A. Najmaldin and B. Ure (2005), BAPES workshop in 2007, etc. In year 2000, 86 pediatric surgeons from Turkey had the opportunity to receive the diploma of European Board of Paediatric Surgery. In 2005 two institutions from Istanbul (Cerrahpaşa Paediatric Surgery) and Ankara (Hacettepe Paediatic Surgery) received a Site Visit Certificate in EUPSA Gdansk Meeting (Fig. 10a,b). In 2006 Part-I

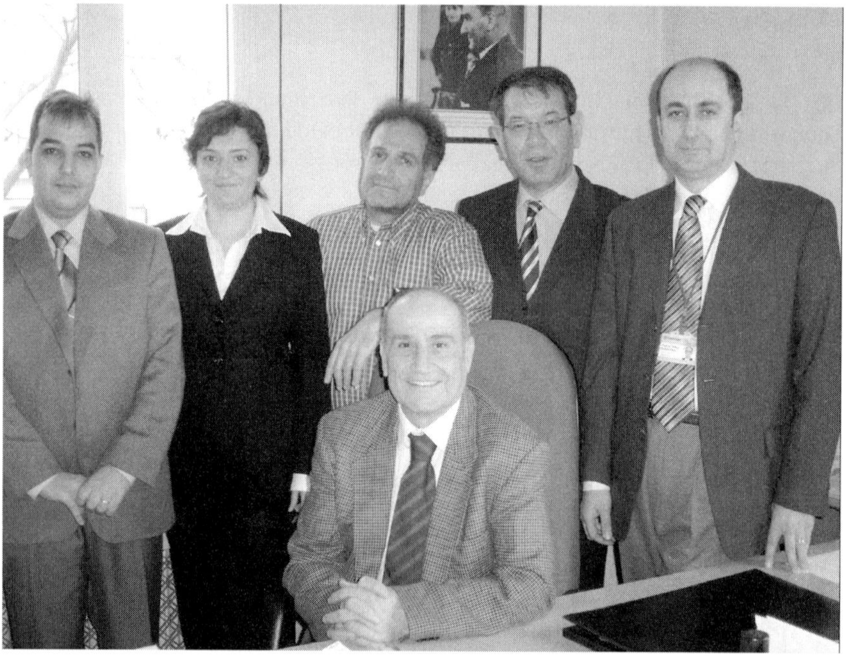

Fig. 10. (a) Prof Nebil Büyükpamukçu was the head of Hacettepe Department of Pediatric Surgery when Hacettepe was certified by UEMS Site Visit. His team in Hacettepe (left to right: İbrahim Karnak, Saniye Ekinci, M Emin Şenocak, Nebil Büyükpamukçu, F. Cahit Tanyel, Arbay Çiftçi). (b) Istanbul-Cerrahpaşa team with observers Yves Aigrain, Gian Battista Parigi, Tolga Dağlı. After a successful site visit.

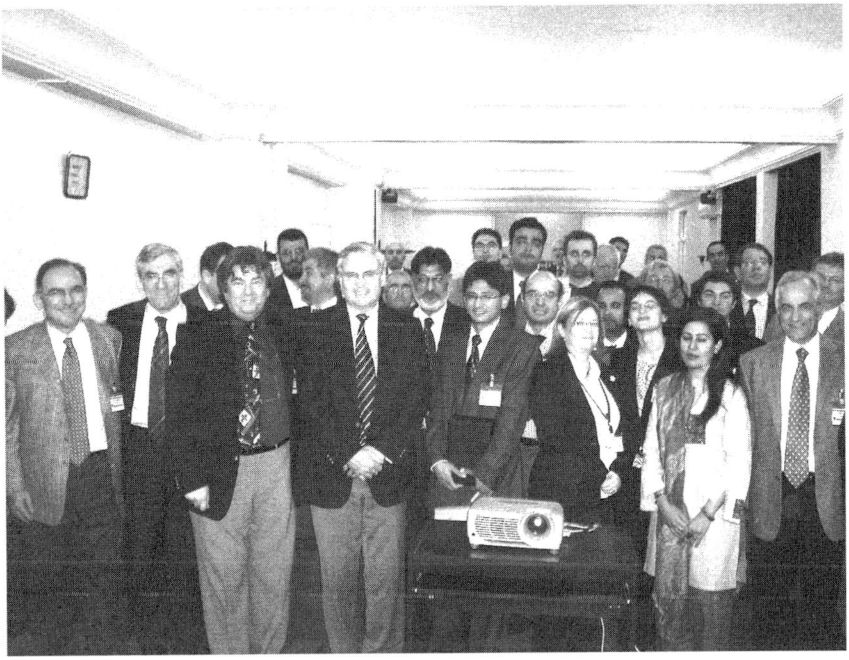

Fig. 11. November 2006, UEMS Board of P Surgery Part-II Exam in Cerrahpaşa-Istanbul. Examiners and candidates together.

and Part-II of European Board Examinations of UEMS has been organized in Cerrahpaşa, Istanbul [Figs. 11].

Turkish paediatric surgeons won eight international prizes in various international meetings (including BAPS, ESPU, AAP). According to the number of publications in three important journals, they were usually in the first 3–5 rows. TAPS has representatives as editorial consultants in "*Journal of Pediatric Surgery*", "*Pediatric Surgery International*", "*European Journal of Paediatric Surgery*" and "*Journal of Paediatric Urology*".

The Turkish Board of Paediatric Surgery (TBPS) has been an active group since October 4, 2000. The constitution of the Board has been prepared by S. N. Cenk Buyukunal, Tolga Dagli, Nebil Büyükpamukcu and Mustafa Melikoglu. Tolga Dagli was the first chairman of TBPS. Today, TBPS has its own log book system, and

Turkish Syllabus Paediatric Surgery. In addition, the Turkish Board of Paediatric Surgery is organizing Board Exams annually (Part-I: Written exam, Part-II: Clinical Exam). The exam has almost the same standards of European Board Exam. The basic standards of Training Paediatric Surgery Centers has already been decided by the council members of TAPS and announced in TAPS website. The website of TAPS **www.tccd.org.tr** is one of the first and most active, functioning pediatric surgical websites in European continent; the first webmaster and the father was Prof Tanju Aktug from Ankara.

For 21 years (1987), TAPS has its own journal called "*Turkish Journal of Pediatric Surgery* (*Pediatrik Cerrahi Dergisi*)". This journal founded by D. Yeker, N. Danismend, O. F. Senyuz and S. N. C Büyükunal, and is already included in E. Medica. During the last ten-year period, S. N. C. Buyukunal and the Presidents of TAPS (biannually) have been the editors of the journal. TAPS has two guide books (published by Cukurova Pediatric Surgery Group) containing the list of publications of Turkish Pediatric Surgeons. TAPS has also published a special Pediatric Surgery Dictionary for the international and Turkish terms of pediatric surgical literature (Güngör Karagüzel is the leading editor).

TAPS has been organizing Annual National Meetings with International Participation for 26 years. E. A. MacKinnon, L. Spitz, A. M. Holschneider, D. Ellis, E.W. Fonkalsrud, J. Waldshmidt, T. Miyano, M. Rowe, O. H. Nielsen, J. Grosfeld, A. Coran, A. Bianchi, P. Ransley, H. Hendren, P. Duffy, R. Carachi, G. B. Parigi, J. Tovar, E. Jaureguilzhiar, M. Hoellwarth, V. Boston, R. Azizkhan, P. Malone, S. Potts, S. Makino, J. Cohen, R. Ohi, K. Georgesson, C. K. Yeung, D. C. Keramidas, D. Lloyd, P. Tam, H. R. Ford, U. Sillen, J. Boix–Ochoa, C. Cywes, A. Hamza, A. Hadidi, E. Elhalabi, P. Puri, J. M. Guys were some of the invited speakers in those 26 National Meetings with international participation.

TAPS members try to attend most of the international meetings with paper presentations. They always try to be the host of international pediatric surgical meetings. We are sure that they will always remain as the active members of pediatric surgical societies such as EUPSA, BAPS, WOFAPS, MAPS, BAPES, ESPU and IPSO.

References

1. Galen (c.130–201 AD). In: *Opera omni*, vol. 10. Kühn, Leipzig, Cnobloch, pp. 1001.
2. Smith ED: The history of hypospadias. *Pediatr Surg Int* 1997;12:81–85.
3. Lascaratos J, Kostakopoulos A, Louras G. Penile surgical techniques described by Oribasius. *Brit J Urol Int* 1999;84:16–19.
4. Büyükünal SNC, Sari N. Şerafeddin Subuncuoğlu,the author of the earliest pediatric surgical atlas: Cerrahiye-i Ilhaniye. *J Pediatr Surg* 1991; 26:1148–1151.
5. Numanoğlu I. Cerrahiye-i Ilhaniye. The earliest known book, containing pediatric surgical procedures. *J Pediatr Surg* 1973;8:547–548.
6. Buyukunal SNC. The past and present of Turkish History of Pediatric Surgery (A project supported by Turkish Association of Paediatric Surgeons, Istanbul-İzmir, 2007. XXVth National Meeting of TAPS, November, 2007, Cesme, İzmir (Invited Lecture).
7. Sabuncuoğlu S. Cerrahiye-i Ilhaniye (3 volume manuscript), Fatih Millet Library, 1460.
8. Topaloğlu B. Islamda Kadın (Woman in Islam). (6th ed.), Yagmur Yayinlari 24, 1975, p. 21.
9. Guzelbey CC, Yetkin H. Gaziantep Şer'i Mahkeme Cilleri'nden Ornekler (Examples from old case reports from Gaziantep Courts) Vol: 81–141, 1729–1825. Gaziantep Kultur Dernegi Yayinlari, Yeni Matbua, Gaziantep, 1970;56:80–105.
10. Akgunduz A. Islam hukukunda sahsi haklarin korunmasi (Personal rights in Islamic Law). In: Akgunduz A. (ed.) *Belgeler Gercekleeri Konusuyor-I-*, Nil Yayinlari, Izmir, 1989, p. 1–13.
11. Baki EA. *Mechul Halk Tarihi, Afyonkarahisar 'da ve XVII-XVIII. Asirlarda (Secret Public History of Afyonkarahisar Region in XVII–XVIII Centuries.* Yeni Matbaa, Afyon, 1951, p. 43–55.
12. Sari N, Büyükünal SNC, Aydın BZ. Developments in child health care during Sultan Abdulhamid-II's reign: Hamidiye-i Etfal Children's Hospital in Istanbul and first modern pediatric surgical department in Turkey. In: *XXXVIII International Congress on the History of Medicine* (Abstract Book, A: 215), 1–6 September, 2002, Istanbul, Turkey, p. 174.

13. *Surname-i Vehbi(XXVIIIth Century Manuscript)*, Library of Topkapi Palace, Istanbul, Turkey (miniatures by Levni).
14. Şakar AŞ. *Çocuk Cerrahisi ve Ortopedi Kliniği Dersleri, Istanbul Tğp Fakültesi Yayınları*, vol. 1, 1936, Istanbul.
15. Say B. Herbert Eckstein. A modest man, a guest surgeon. [Contemprorary issues in pediatric urology, in memoriam H. B. Eckstein]. *Pediatric Cerrahi Dergisi*, 1995;9:3–4.
16. Hiçsönmez A. Pediatric Surgery in Ankara. (Contemprorary issues in pediatric urology, in memoriam H. B. Eckstein). *Pediatrik Cerrahi Dergisi* 1995;9:10.
17. Doğramacı İ. Tribute to Herbert Eckstein. (Contemprorary issues in pediatric urology, in memoriam H. B. Eckstein). *Pediatrik Cerrahi Dergisi* 1995;9:5.

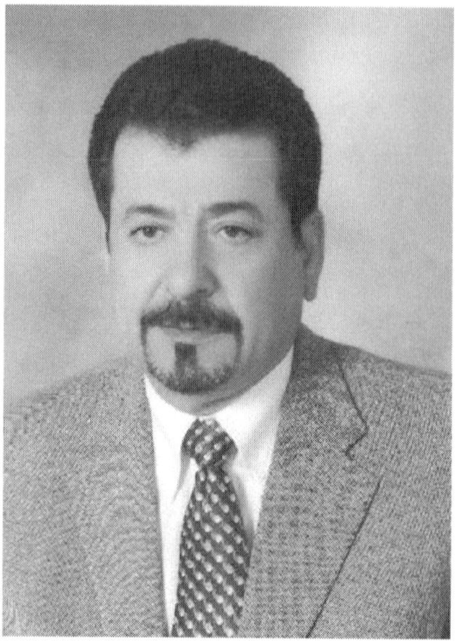

Abdul R. Mustafawi

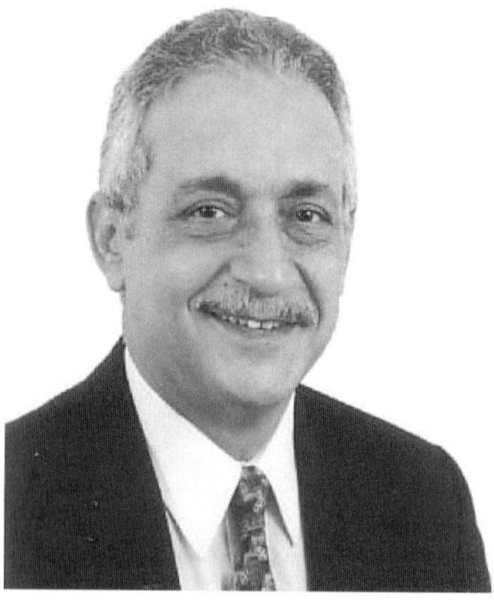

Wasfi K. Jaouni

UNITED ARAB EMIRATES

Abdul R. Mustafawi
Wasfi K. Jaouni

The U.A.E. has a comprehensive, government-funded health service and a developing private health sector. Substantial government investment has enabled the U.A.E. to make major progress in health care, and the country is now ranked 43rd out of 174 industrial and developing countries in the latest UN Human Development Report. Child mortality rates are nine per 1000, comparable to most developing countries, while preventive medicine campaigns have had a major impact on life expectancy, now 76 years for women and 74 years for men. Endemic diseases have been eradicated.

The focus of a network of Government primary health care centres is maternal and child welfare, school health and health education. The public hospitals offer specialised services, including telemedicine links with major hospitals abroad and state-of-the art surgery. The health care infrastructure is upgraded regularly, with a central data base project being prepared. There are plans to double bed capacity in public hospitals over the next ten years.

The Government finances 81% of the cost of health care, but several initiatives towards privatisation have been launched recently.

U.A.E's great strides of development in business have been the envy of many countries. Similarly U.A.E has made great progress in the establishment of the discipline of paediatric surgery with particular progress in the neonatal surgery n the last 15 years. This is a brief glance at paediatric surgery as it is evolving in the States in the U.A.E.

Dubai

In Dubai in 1975 the first paediatric surgical unit was started in Rashid Hospital General Hospital. There were five beds and two places in the SCBU for surgical patients. By 1982–1987 the bed numbers had been increased to 14 and with 4 places in the SCBU. The staff was one Consultant, two Registrars and Senior House Officers.

By 1987 a new hospital was designed and built for Maternity and Pediatric services which was called Al Wasl Hospital (395 beds). Since then the Paediatric Surgery Department has functioned as an independent department. There was a capacity for 35 general surgical paediatric beds along with SCBU which is considered as one of the modern and biggest unit (three ICU beds).

The deliveries in this hospital are around 7500/year and the hospital now serves a population over 3.5 million.

Each year there are from 140 to 150 neonatal operations performed.

The total number of operations annually is 3000 (250 major, 800 intermediate and 2000 minor). The three theatres allocated for paediatric surgery are well equipped and run six operating lists and two minor operating lists per week.

Al Ain

Both Al Ain and Tawam Hospitals are considered to be the major hospitals in the Al Ain Medical District, covering an area of 11,750 Km^2 with a population of more than 325,000 people. Both are considered to be the major hospitals in the Al Ain Medical District, covering an area of 11,750 Km^2 with a population of more than 325,000 people. Taiwan commenced services in 1980 and the Al Ain Hospital was formerly known as Al Jimi Hospital.

Abu Dhabi

The Mafraq Hospital was opened in 1983 and had ten beds allocated to paediatric surgery which also had two beds in the SCBU.

The service has developed and is run by two consultants and supported by three specialist registrars.

The **Shaikh Khalifa Medical Center in *Abu Dhabi*** is another service functioning under the direction of the Health Authority in Abu Dhabi and there is also the **Zayed Military Hospital.**

Total Registered Live Births in UAE is currently around 67, 500. The break down of the births is shown in the table.

Shaikh Khalifa & Mafraq	Abu Dhabi	16331
Tawam Hospital & Al Jimi	Alain & W. Region	10614
Al Wasl	Dubai & N. Emirates	40603

Reorganisation and redirection of the paediatric and other medical services continues as they develop and the capabilities of the medical profession continue to expand.

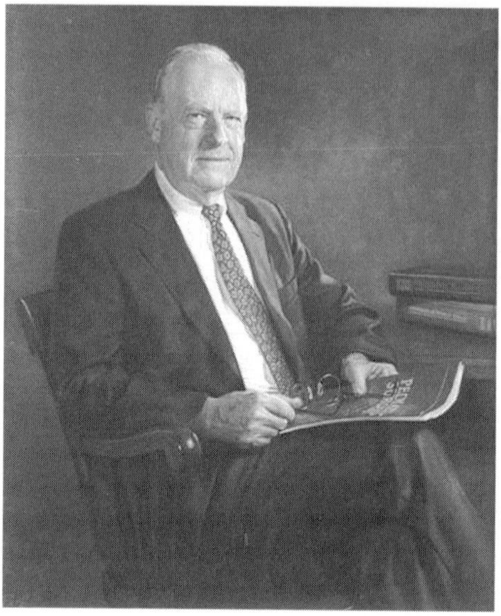

James A. O'Neill Jr.

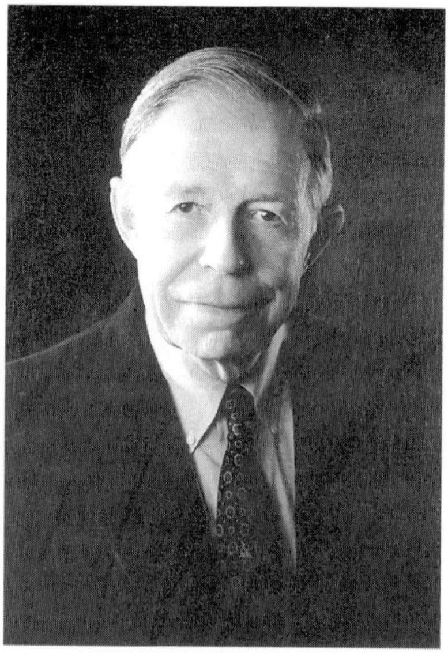

Eric W. Fonkalsrud

UNITED STATES OF AMERICA

James A. O'Neill Jr.
Eric W. Fonkalsrud

Pediatric medicine started prior to the organization of surgical pediatrics in a small way in the 1890's, concomitant with the child advocacy movement and new scientific information related to the specific disorders of childhood. The first children's hospital in the United States was established in Philadelphia in 1855, and more were established in the ensuing years in Boston, New York, Chicago, Seattle, Columbus, Cincinnati and others. The organization of medical pediatrics into a specialty centered around the major children's hospitals, but small children's wards were also developed in general hospitals. The American Academy of Pediatrics (AAP) was established in 1931.[1]

Technology and new instruments stimulated the development of the surgical specialties in the late 1800's, but no surgical specialist concentrated on pediatrics. Additionally, it was not until the late 19th century that surgeons began to limit their practice to surgery. The surgical care of children in children's and general hospitals was provided by adult general surgeons with few exceptions until after World War II. Pediatric general surgery evolved because there was a need. Adult general surgeons doing this work were unable to fulfill the need, and since their work was only ten percent pediatrics, little attention was paid to this aspect of their practice.

Three individuals pioneered pediatric surgery in the United States. Herbert Coe was a general and plastic surgeon at the Children's Orthopedic Hospital in Seattle beginning in 1908, and he limited his practice to pediatric surgery in 1919. Oswald Wyatt established a general surgical practice in Minneapolis after World War I, but in 1927 he became so disgusted with the quality of care provided to infants and children that he obtained additional training in Chicago, subsequently returning to Minneapolis to establish a full-time pediatric surgical practice. Perhaps the most influential of the three pioneer surgeons was William E. Ladd, a well-trained general surgeon in Boston (Fig. 1).[2] He established his general surgical practice including adults and children in 1909 but gradually limited his practice to sick children at the Boston Children's Hospital, where he was made Surgeon-in-Chief in 1927. He had an influence on Dr Coe, who traveled to Boston to observe Dr Ladd in 1920. It was Ladd who had the greatest initial influence on the development of the field. He was the first scientific pediatric surgeon, basing his descriptions of correctable lesions in the newborn on detailed postmortem studies. He stimulated the development of educational programs in pediatric surgery since he felt it was the best way to influence surgical care of the child; he established the first training program in 1937 at Boston Children's Hospital. In 1941, Dr Ladd and his young assistant, Robert E. Gross, published the landmark textbook, "*Abdominal*

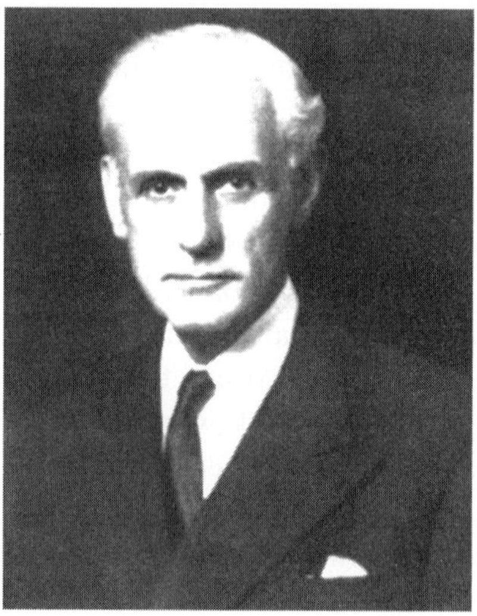

Fig. 1. William E. Ladd, M.D.

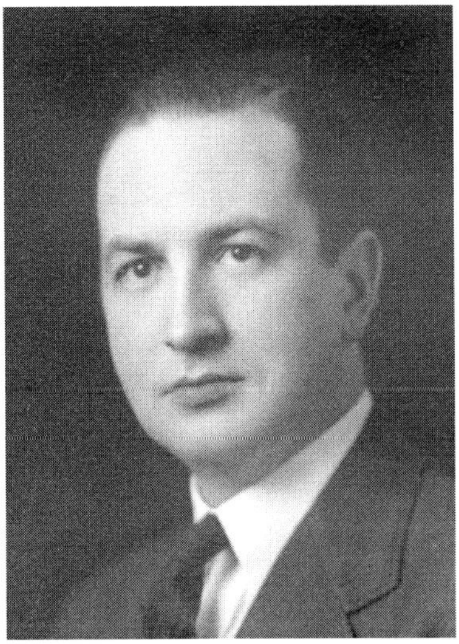

Fig. 2. Robert E. Gross, M.D.

Surgery of Infants and Children", which codified the specialty, and this was updated and expanded to include the chest and urology by Gross in 1953 in "*The Surgery of Infancy and Childhood*" (Fig. 2).[3,4] The first endowed chair in children's surgery, the William E. Ladd Professorship, was established at Harvard in 1941.[5]

Pediatric Surgery Education

The early training for children's surgery in the United States consisted of several months of observation or residency in Boston beginning in 1937. World War II delayed further development, but the war experience defined training needs. In 1945, Gross took over in Boston following Ladd's retirement. The second training program was established in 1945 in Chicago and was followed immediately by new programs in Philadelphia, Boston Floating Hospital, Columbus and Montreal. These educational programs were initiated without any pre-existing guidelines other than the experience and intuition of a small group of surgeons who dedicated their careers to teaching Pediatric Surgery. The latter programs were endorsed without specific guidelines in 1952 by the Surgical Section of the AAP which had only been established in 1948. By 1963 there were eleven approved training programs in the United States whose directors had spent one or more years in pediatric surgery training in Boston.[6]

The most pre-eminent of the new training directors were Robert Gross in Boston, Willis Potts and then Orvar Swenson in Chicago, C. Everett Koop in Philadelphia, and H. William Clatworthy in Columbus (Fig. 3). A few program directors, such as Clifford Benson in Detroit and William Snyder in Los Angeles, were general surgeons who were self-trained but who limited their practice to pediatric surgery. By the early 1960's there were only ten to 12 new pediatric surgeons trained in North America yearly, and there were fewer than 100 pediatric surgeons practicing in the United States and Canada. Pediatric surgical training finally became standardized through the efforts of Clatworthy within the Surgical Section of the AAP beginning in 1965, with formal site visits beginning in 1970. In 1975 the approval function was taken over by the Accreditation Council for Graduate Medical Education, but the Standards for Training in Pediatric Surgery are virtually identical to the ones

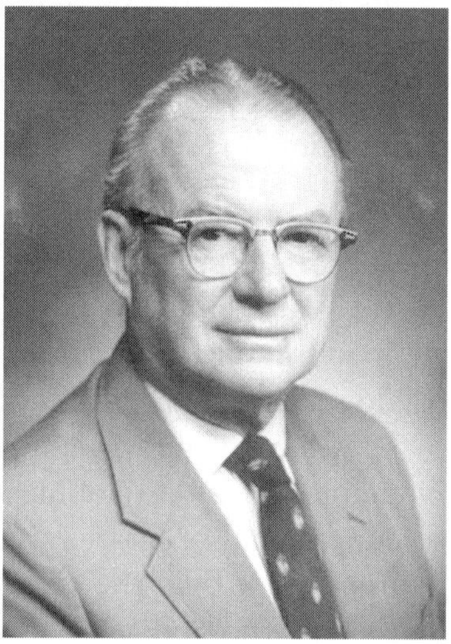

Fig. 3. H. William Clatworthy, M.D.

originally developed by Clatworthy. However, despite these efforts, recognition of the specialty of Pediatric Surgery was slow in coming.

Most general hospitals had one or more adult surgeons who had an interest in operating on children with little or no special training, and their outcomes were often poor. Many influential surgeons held the view that there was little difference in operating on a child compared with an adult, but Hugh Lynn, one of the early Philadelphia-trained pediatric surgeons practicing at the Mayo Clinic, cautioned in 1961, "The adult may be safely treated as a child, but the converse can lead to disaster".[7] By the 1950's, a few untrained general surgeons in university hospitals took a special interest in pediatric surgical care, including Mark Ravitch of Johns Hopkins who went on to make major contributions to the management of chest deformities, intussusception, and other conditions, but his best contribution to the field may be his editorial work and the development of the current leading textbook in the field, "*Pediatric Surgery*".

Pediatric surgery training initially included an extensive experience in all aspects of children's surgery with an emphasis on newborns and neonatal physiology, but also included urology, cardiothoracic, plastic, and head and neck surgery. With the assistance of individuals in the new specialty of neonatology, the survival of premature infants and those with severe malformations increased dramatically over the ensuing years. Parallel developments were key in this process, including the establishment of the first intensive care unit at the Children's Hospital of Philadelphia and the stimulation of the development of pediatric anesthesia. Virtually all of this progress occurred in the major children's hospitals.

By the mid-1960's, only a few beds for children's surgery were available in most university hospitals in contrast to the large number in children's hospitals. The pediatric and neonatal ICU staff were not accustomed to having surgeons participate actively in detailed pre- and post-operative care. It had been the standard practice in university hospitals that general surgeons were not to be trusted to write orders on babies, and this included pediatric surgeons even though pediatric surgical training, beginning with Ladd, included total physiologic care of the surgical child. Pediatric referral patterns were slow to change as well within the community and university hospitals in the United States where most children's surgery was performed. University hospital operating room suites had few rooms modified to limit heat loss by children and few appropriate instruments and supplies for infant surgery. Only a few anesthesiologists in these environments had experience with the special care and equipment necessary for infant surgery. Because recovery rooms were not prepared to take care of post-operative infants, they were usually sent directly to the ward or the pediatric intensive care unit. There was no outpatient or minor surgery for children other than what could be performed in the clinic or treatment room on the ward under local anesthesia. The solution to these problems was the migration of trained pediatric surgeons to university centers.[8]

Eight of the first 24 university pediatric surgeons trained with Clatworthy at Columbus Children's Hospital. Another seven trained in Boston with Gross.[9] By 1969 there were 24 university hospitals with full-time pediatric surgeons as well as some university-affiliated hospitals. The Chiefs of Surgery at many university centers were supportive of pediatric surgical development, but others resisted appointment of pediatric surgeons, because they did not perceive a need. Because these early pediatric surgeons were well-trained in pediatric urology, cardiac, head and neck, and plastic surgery, occasional conflicts arose with these adult surgical specialists. However, following the philosophy of Clatworthy, pediatric surgeons stimulated the establishment of pediatric surgical specialists in these other fields so that the overall quality of care could be ensured, and these conflicts were gradually eliminated. By the 1970's almost all university hospitals had pediatric surgeons who enjoyed the support of pediatric and surgical specialty faculties.

Organizational Changes and Maturation of the Field

Again, it was Dr Ladd who understood that recognition of the field of pediatric surgery would require extensive involvement in national surgical organizations.[2] Through his efforts and those of the individuals mentioned earlier, pediatric surgery slowly gained recognition as a specialty. Clatworthy, in particular, stimulated broad involvement by pediatric surgeons in American Surgery, which included the population of university hospitals by his trainees.

Dr Coe was a capable and effective politician within the AAP. Through his educational and diplomatic efforts, the Surgical Section of the AAP was established in 1948. In 1967, the American College of Surgeons (ACS) recognized pediatric surgery as a sub-specialty, and the following year they established the Advisory Council for Pediatric Surgery. In 1966 the first issue of the "*Journal of Pediatric Surgery*" was published. It was the brainchild of Stephen Gans, and C. Everett Koop was the first Editor-in-Chief. Further maturation occurred with the founding of the American Pediatric Surgical Association (APSA) in 1970, which provided an extensive scientific forum for pediatric surgeons in addition to the Surgical Section of the AAP and the ACS, as well as a route for representation within the ACS and other general surgical organizations.

The last organizational achievement necessary for the validation of pediatric surgery as a specialty was board certification beyond General Surgery. Again, Dr Ladd had the vision to recognize this requirement. He had been a founding member of the American Board of Surgery (ABS) as well as the American Board of Plastic Surgery. It took five attempts between 1955 and 1972 before special certification in Pediatric Surgery was approved by the ABS.[10] There were many individuals involved in the effort including C. Everett Koop, Orvar Swenson, Alexander Bill, Willis Potts, H. William Clatworthy, Lawrence Pickett, Robert Izant, Mark Ravitch and others, but it fell to a Canadian, Harvey Beardmore, to finally accomplish the task. It is likely that the final successful approach to the ABS was helped by the founding of the APSA, spearheaded by Lucian Leape, E. Thomas Boles, Robert Izant, E. Ide Smith, and eighteen other young pediatric surgeons. It is a valid observation that the train of organizational events mentioned above was responsible for the recognition and respectability Pediatric Surgery has in North America today.

Research Contributions Translated to Care

Once established in academic medical centers, including children's hospitals, pediatric surgeons began to expand their interests in research, and broad collaborations were established. Beginning in the 1970's, pediatric surgeons developed extensive research programs in a variety of fields, many supported by the National Institutes of Health (NIH) and other competitive granting agencies. Several pediatric surgeons were pioneers in many areas that were in the forefront of surgical advances during the 20th century, including some of the following. Pediatric surgeons participated in the first organized clinical trial ever performed under the title of Cancer Chemotherapy Group A, which evolved into the National Wilms' Tumor Study, which has served as a model for all subsequent clinical trials. This study was responsible for an unprecedented improvement in the survival of children with Wilms' Tumor. Similar studies with similar results have been accomplished with neuroblastoma, hepatoblastoma, rhabdomyosarcoma, and germ cell tumors.

Pediatric surgeons have been leaders in research in the field of trauma and burns with broad involvement in the study of infection, immunology, nutrition, resuscitation, and wound healing. It is of interest that many of the physiologic observations made by pediatric surgeons studying trauma and burn injury in children have been found to be applicable to the treatment of the newborn and premature infants. The principles of non-operative management of blunt injuries to the abdomen were developed by pediatric surgeons, and this has improved overall survival in both children and adults.

As one might expect, advances in the management of congenital and acquired disorders in infants and children have all been accomplished by pediatric surgeons beginning with Ladd, who has been called "The Father of Newborn Surgery." Pediatric surgeons have also been responsible for advances in what are now associated pediatric surgical specialties, such as H. Hardy Hendren in genitourinary reconstruction, Gross, Potts and many of their early trainees in cardiac surgery, and others. While it is fair to say that a number of advances made in the field of adult general surgery have been tailored for children, such as minimally invasive surgery and transplantation, it is also fair to say that pediatric surgeons have collaborated in producing those technical innovations. Additionally, pediatric surgeons have been responsible for translating established pediatric surgical procedures to adult disorders. One of the best examples of the latter is the modification of endorectal pullthrough for Hirschsprung's disease for the treatment of adults with ulcerative colitis and related disorders.

Pediatric surgeons in the United States and throughout the world have been responsible for basic science advances related to physiology of the newborn, the response to sepsis, enteral and parenteral nutrition, angiogenesis, fetal surgery, transplantation, tissue engineering, and stem cell transplantation. In each instance, these basic science studies have been translated to clinical advances in the surgical care of children. A key factor in the success of pediatric surgeons accomplishing sophisticated basic research has been their access to and collaboration with colleagues with expertise in the basic sciences within university centers.

At this point in time, the specialty of Pediatric Surgery has evolved to a leadership position in American Surgery. Pediatric surgeons are now permanent Directors of the ABS. They hold leadership positions in the ACS, the American Medical Association, the Society of University Surgeons, the Association for Academic Surgery, the American Surgical Association, and many others. Many have served on NIH Study Sections, and C. Everett Koop was the Surgeon General of the United States for eight years. Six have become Chairmen of major Departments of Surgery in university centers. Additionally, pediatric surgery has now become one of the major educational components of general surgical education.

In terms of pediatric surgical practice in the United States today, pediatric surgeons are considered to be the last of the true general surgeons. At the present time, pediatric surgery includes broad aspects of general and thoracic surgery. While pediatric surgeons are no longer routinely involved in urologic, cardiac, and plastic surgery, they have been responsible for training and encouraging specialists in these fields with the satisfaction that the overall surgical care of children has been improved. Over time, pediatric surgery has become more and more attractive to young people as a career despite the long length of training. More than 70 general surgical residents have been competing annually for the approximately 38 residency positions in Pediatric Surgery.

In retrospect, an enormous amount has been accomplished over the last 40 years. There is no doubt that the ensuing years will bring even more advances in the surgical care of children. Most of the organizational aspects of the field have been accomplished. It is likely that future developments will be related to basic science advances in the fields of genetics, proteomics, cellular and molecular biology, oncology, bioinformatics, robotics and advanced imaging, and the evolution of the field of complex systems that will bring about major changes in the way health care is provided. As a balance to these sophisticated technical advances, pediatric surgeons have a tradition of humanistic values and the art of caring, values that will undoubtedly be preserved.

References

1. Pearson HA. The 75th anniversary of the American Academy of Pediatrics. *Pediatrics* 2006;117:1759–1762.
2. Clatworthy HW. Ladd's vision. *J Pediatr Surg* 1999;34(Suppl):32–37.
3. Ladd WE, Gross RE. *Abdominal Surgery of Infancy and Childhood.* WB Saunders, Philadelphia, 1941.
4. Gross RE. *The Surgery of Infancy and Childhood.* WB Saunders, Philadelphia, 1953.
5. Bill AH, William E. Ladd, MD. In Rickham PP (ed.) *Historical Aspects of Pediatric Surgery*. Springer–Verlag, Berlin, 1986, p. 52–59.
6. Randolph JG, Young DG. A brief history of pediatric surgery. In Grosfeld JG, O'Neill JA, Fonkalsrud EW, *et al.* (eds.) *Pediatric Surgery* (6th ed.) Mosby Elsevier, Philadelphia, 2006; p. 3–10.
7. Lynn HB. Details that count in the care of children. *MJ Surg* 1961;101:553–561.

8. Fonkalsrud EW. Pediatric surgery advances into the university hospital. *J Pediatr Surg* 2001;36:409–415.
9. Glick PL, Azizkhan RG. *A Genealogy of North American Pediatric Surgery*. Quality Med, St. Louis, 1997.
10. Johnson DG. Presidential Address: Excellence in search of recognition. *J Pediatr Surg* 1986;21:1019–1031.

Section C

SELECTED BIOGRAPHIES

SELECTED BIOGRAPHIES

Harvey Beardmore (1921–2007)

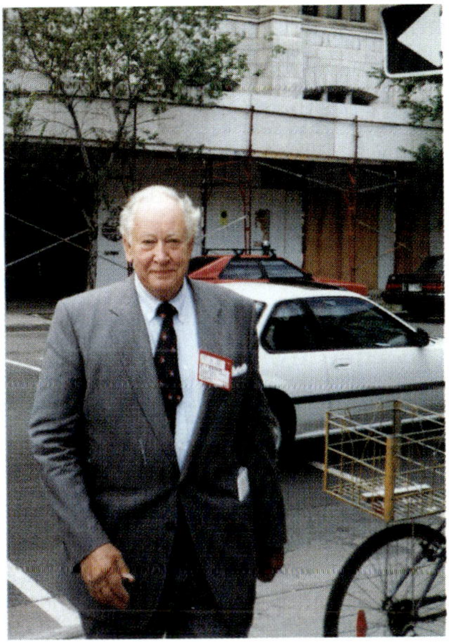

Harvey Beardmore

A McGill graduate in 1946 after having been on military service in World War II, Harvey trained in Montreal and in Boston. He returned to the staff of the Montreal Children's Hospital as a paediatric surgeon in 1953 and had a distinguished though somewhat uneven professional career from then to his retirement in 1995. He made a distinctive and memorable mark on the development of paediatric surgery as has been highlighted by Jud Randolph.[1]

Having been appointed at a time when Montreal had three other recent surgical appointments to the staff, Harvey saw that to make a mark in the speciality it would be important to focus much of his effort outside his own centre and he certainly did become a well-known figure internationally. His pleasant, often amusing interjections at meetings lightened many a rather tedious scientific session and if Mark Ravitch was at the meeting there was sure to be many interchanges between these characters.

The major mark Harvey made was in achieving recognition of the specialty by the American Board of Surgery. The comments expressed when he was being given the Distinguished Service Award by APSA were, "It would be incorrect to imply that this extraordinary event was solely the work of Harvey Beardmore, as clearly many others within the Surgical Section had made similar requests of the American Board of Surgery, but it was Harvey's elegant presentation which finally turned the tide. Dr Harvey Beardmore has been an extraordinary leader in Paediatric Surgery in North America. His name will be invariably linked with our certification of within the American Board of Surgery. I am extremely honoured to present to Dr. Harvey Beardmore on behalf of the APSA's Board of Governors, our Distinguished Service Award."

A founder member of CAPS in 1967 and its first President, Harvey was also elected President of APSA in 1974, the William E Ladd Medal winner in 1986. These are a few of the distinguished Honours which Harvey received and indicated the remarkable esteem he was held in internationally. His eloquent and affable approach and contributions internationally were missed when he retreated from his foremost place in the specialty. Predeceased by his wife Francis his latter years were split between Montreal and his farm with the lake on which he relaxed fishing.

Reference

1. Randolph JG. History of the Section on Surgery. American Academy of Pediatrics. The first 25 years (1948–1973). *J Pedatr Surg* 1999; 34 (5, Suppl 1): 3–18.

DGY

J. J. Mason Brown (1903–1964)

James Johnston Mason Brown was born in St. Andrews on February 20, 1908. He was educated at Edinburgh Academy and the Edinburgh Medical School, graduating MBChB (Hons) in 1931, gaining distinction and the Pattison prize for clinical surgery in his Final Examination. He passed the Fellowship examination of the Royal College of Surgeons of Edinburgh (FRCS Ed) in 1934 and

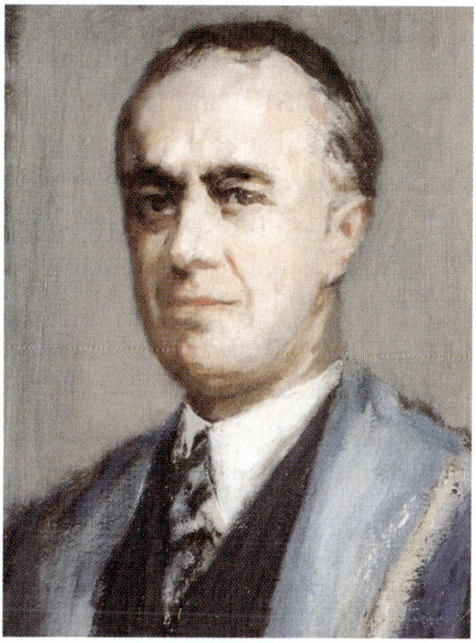

Mason Brown

later held the Syme Surgical Fellowship (1934–1936) and the Crichton Scholarship (1937) in support of research projects into osteochondritis and peripheral vascular disease respectively.

He had been a patient of Prof John (later Sir John) Fraser, in the Royal Infirmary Edinburgh (RIE) as a schoolboy and this experience was a major influence on his career choice. He came under Fraser's influence again, as a medical student and surgical trainee; his early resident posts were with Fraser in RIE and Norman Dott in the Royal Edinburgh Hospital for Sick Children, (REHSC). Fraser, the Regius Professor of Clinical Surgery, is an iconic figure in the development of paediatric surgery in Scotland. He had established his international reputation in the specialty during his period at REHSC (1912–1924) and had published his "*Surgery of Childhood*" in 1926, one of the earliest authoritative texts in the English language. Mason Brown accepted his invitation to become his private assistant and later worked as his clinical tutor and university assistant.

Having displayed a strong interest in the surgical problems of children, Mason Brown was appointed honorary assistant surgeon at REHSC in 1936 to work with Gertrude Herzfeld. Although only a part-time appointment he soon established his reputation as a clinician and teacher of exceptional merit.

Military service (1939–1945), was spent as a surgical specialist, latterly in North Africa and Italy. His unit was selected to provide the field vascular injuries service, Mediterranean area. This service was mentioned in despatches and he was appointed OBE (Military).

On his return to REHSC (1946) he was appointed surgeon-in-charge and Paediatric Surgeon to the Simpson Memorial Maternity Pavilion (SMMP) and to the Western General Hospital (WGH). He was appointed senior lecturer in Paediatric Surgery, later as Reader, and became the first Consultant surgeon in Edinburgh to confine his practice to childhood. Although he was involved in the care of the whole age range, his particular interest was in the newborn child with congenital anomaly and with birth injury. His precise, meticulous, unhurried surgical technique was very appropriate in this group and he was fortunate that, in those days of diagnostic delay, his anaesthetist colleague (Douglas Shannon) regarded anaesthesia as the height of resuscitation.

He had an uncanny knack of getting fractious infants and distressed toddlers to settle (akin to horse-whispering) which made clinical examination and bedside teaching appear so easy and which anxious parents found reassuring. He had the correct words for the occasion whether it was the outpatient clinic, formal lecture or an after dinner speech. His writing had a similar clarity and much of that is included in "*The Surgery of Childhood*" of which he was senior editor, published in 1962.

Jimmie, as he was known by his more intimate colleagues, was a popular and persuasive colleague who although usually mild-mannered and with a well-developed sense of humour, could display great resolve and determination in support of causes he favoured. He was very effective in committee and served the Royal College of Surgeons of Edinburgh over many years as Secretary/Treasurer and then as Treasurer before his election to President in 1962. He was the first paediatric surgeon to be elected to the Presidency of a Royal College.

He had recognised the importance of collegiate activity many years earlier when with his colleagues, Matthew White and Wallace Dennison, in Glasgow he had organised the first meeting of the Scottish Surgical Paediatric Club in Glasgow in 1948. In 1953 he was one of the dozen or so founder members of the British Association of Paediatric Surgeons which has expanded over the years and is now an important international forum. He had been elected to the

Presidency of BAPS from 1964 and was anticipating in particular the Congress in Edinburgh in 1965. Regrettably he died on June 9, 1964 and the anticipated prospect of further significant contributions from him during his dual presidency was lost.

Willie Bisset (1950–2008)

Sir Denis Browne and his Australian Connection (1892–1966)

Denis Browne's Australian origins are of interest in determining the character and personality of this man who had a dominating effect on the development of paediatric surgery in England. To say the least, Browne was a controversial character and a legend in his lifetime. His personality often bristled with venom, especially against orthopaedic surgeons with whom he had disagreements in the management of hip, feet and spinal disease. Yet, in the context of the time he was a giant, in initiating innovative operations and management in a range of paediatric lesions, in establishing an environment which made the specialty possible, against a great deal of opposition in London, and he was a Founder member and a major inspiration for the British Association of Paediatric Surgeons.

His paternal grandfather came from Ireland and was a master mariner, conveying convicts to the early Australian settlement — a large man in every way, over 2 metres tall, masterful and full of strength and energy — and eventually settled in Melbourne in 1838, buying expensive properties in the new colony. He and his wife Eliza (whom he met while she was a passenger on his ship) had nine children. Of relevance were two boys. One, Thomas, wrote a famous bushranging tale "*Robbery under Arms*" under the pen-name of Rolf Boldrewood. He would become an uncle of Denis, but enters the story in another context. His daughter married the first paediatric pathologist at the Royal Children's Hospital in Melbourne, Crawford Morrison, appointed in 1891.

The second son, Sylvester, was Denis' father, also a large and energetic man, and he made a fortune in the mining industry in Western Australia. In 1899 Sylvester married Anne Stawell, whose family played important roles in the history of Victoria, a southern state of Australia. Her father, a barrister, became Chief Justice and Lieutenant Governor as Sir William Stawell, at the time Victoria was becoming independent from New South Wales, 1851. William and his wife produced ten children, all extraordinarily talented variously in medicine, surgery, law, engineering, and one daughter a Lecturer in Classics at Newnham College in Cambridge. So, in his ancestry, from the paternal side Denis Browne inherited strong physical characteristics: his large stature, his courage, his energy, even belligerency, and his capacity for leadership; from his maternal side: the genes of scholarship and high intellect, altogether not a bad start for anyone!

Denis was born in 1892 in Melbourne, where he lived for eight years, before moving with his family to a large sheep "station" (farm) in New South Wales. He was christened Denis John Wolko Browne, the name Wolko being Aboriginal for "big man", an interesting social comment of the times in which the indigenous Aboriginal presence must have been acknowledged and respected in this family, unlike the abuse often directed at these people in other circles. His independence showed itself from birth, temperamental, excitable, his first words said to be a complete sentence hurled with much vigour at his brother! He had private tuition at home until aged 13 years, and on the farm had an idyllic life of riding, shooting, hunting, parties, dancing, swimming and tennis. He was an avid reader, the basis of his intimate knowledge of English literature.

In 1905, aged 13, he was sent to be a boarder at Kings School in Sydney, and from the beginning was a determined individualist. He hated football and cricket, and said so, although he played tennis, and was a brilliant scholar. He actually won a Divinity prize, rather remarkably as he was not known for his piety or saintly behaviour, but he won because of his literary ability that had little to do with theology. He left school a little earlier than planned, after an argument

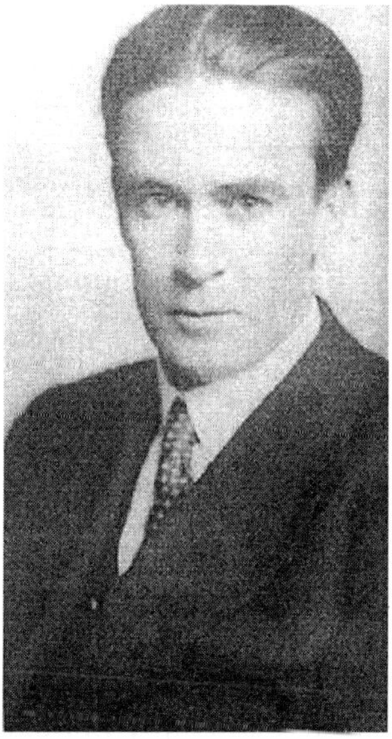

Fig. 1. Denis Browne as a medical student at Sydney University in 1914.

with the headmaster on eschatology! At aged 18, 1910, he began a medical course at Sydney University, a tall, thin, handsome young man (hence the nickname of "Splinter", Fig. 1). He excelled in sport, receiving "Blues" for tennis and shooting, and a team member in athletics, golf, riding and billiards. He was a champion tennis player, representing his State, and later, while living in England, played in the Wimbledon Championship. Because of the War, the course was shortened and the best students were allowed to sit for the final examinations at the end of the 4th year, which he did, and passed.

In 1915, having graduated, he immediately enlisted in the Australian Forces (AIF) and went to the tragic battleground of Gallipoli in Turkey. After some months there he developed typhoid fever and was evacuated home, but after a brief three months he was back in France in 1916 as part of the British Expeditionary Force where he saw out the rest of the war. He was demobilized in December 1919 after serving in an Australian

Auxiliary Hospital in Dartford and Southern General Hospital, Liverpool. In the service hospitals he had met English surgeons, including Thomas Dunhill and Robert Jones, who encouraged him, and so "DB" started surgical training in England, where he stayed. He did not return to Australia until 1965, only 15 months before he died.

A book of Selected Writings of Sir Denis Browne[1] were edited by Harold Nixon, David Waterston and Dr Wink and has interesting observations by ex-colleagues on the man as well as including interesting papers. It is opened by a chapter written by James Crooks — a long term colleague both at Great Ormond Street and at their adjacent private consulting rooms — which starts "Denis Browne was an extraordinary man in whom strength of character and convictions stuck out like rugged and dangerous rocks upon which the unwary might easily founder. Those who understood him — or perhaps it would be better to say partially understood him — admired him almost to the point of idolatry although they must have been aware of the thrust of purpose which would never leave time to admit them to closer friendship. He was an intellectual adventurer, a rebel and a cynic, and he made up his mind from a very early age to take nothing at its face value...."

The Trustees of the Denis Browne Fund established a Medal given annually to an individual to mark an outstanding contribution to Paediatric Surgery. The chosen individuals initially were selected by the Trustees and the Executive Committee of the BAPS but now the responsibility has been passed over to the BAPS although the medal is given to individuals recognised internationally and not only to BAPS members.

E. Durham Smith

Reference

1. Nixon HH, Waterston D, Wink CAS (1983). *Selected Writings of Sir Denise Browne*. Published by the trustees of the Sir Denis Browne Memorial Fund.

Bernard Duhamel (1919–1996)

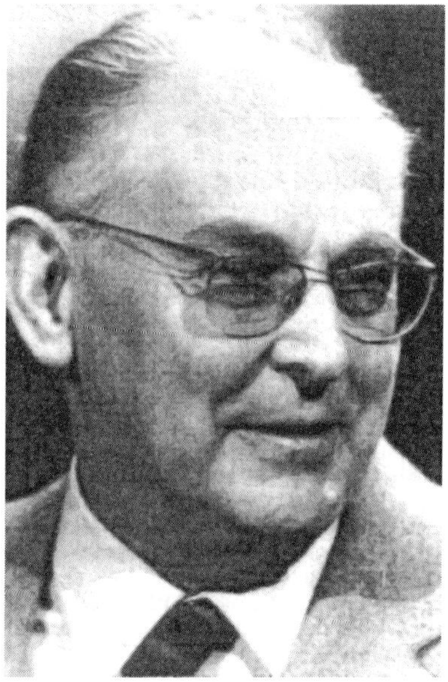

Bernard Duhamel

An interesting tribute to Bernard was written by Robert Pagès in the "*European Journal*" of paediatric surgery more than a decade ago.[1] The first paragraph reads ; "Why" a member of the BAPS once asked me, "Have you French relegated your top pediatric surgeon to a suburb?" "Nobody is a prophet in his own country," I answered, "but you must not forget that the kings who built the kingdom of France over ten centuries were relegated there too!" The city of St Denis, well-known for its basilica and sepulchres of the kings of France, is also a birthplace of modern French pediatric surgery.

An interesting start and clever but evasive answer that has never been analytically answered. Duhamel's name remains very widely known and there remains strong support for his operation which he introduced a short time after Swenson made the initial breakthrough in the surgical management of Hirschsprung is Disease.

Traditional to the time Duhamel initially trained in general surgery before making his move into paediatric surgery after the Second World War. In France as in many other countries the scientific advances had started to raise the opportunity for the emergence of the speciality. Improvements in anaesthesia and the development of non-irritant tubes along with a gradual enlightenment on the fluid balance in surgery of the young patients were two of the factors allowing the further evolution of paediatric surgery. By 1948 Duhamel and Prochiantz achieved success in the correction of oesophageal atresia and his career blossomed in paediatric surgery. He was an outstanding thinker who had a long-term interest in embryology and its relationship to the development of congenital malformations.

By the 1950s he had made many progressive movements forward in the speciality including with Sauvegrain setting up organisational systems for diagnosis and management. By 1953 he had published a book on the subject and made many more contributions to the surgical literature. By 1956 he published his surgical approach to Hirschsprung's disease and from that point on his name has been universally known. He did follow with a modification of his original procedure but the basic approach, for which he was responsible, has remaned through more than five decades. His successor at the *Clinique Chirurgicale Infantile de l'Hôpital des Enfants-Malades* (Denis Pelerin) did present a significant alteration to the Duhamel procedure but this alteration did not stay the course. Pellerin was Duhamel's successor at the above hospital where he became the Chief.

Many other aspects can be cited but only two others will be mentioned in this brief resumé. The introduction of a journal and the formation of a Paediatric Surgical Society are the two aspects I would highlight here. These have had a very significant effect on the development in the specialty in the second half of the 20th century. In each he was a major contributor.

G. Audrey

Reference

1. S R A Tribute to Bernard Duhamel — Fifty Years of Accomplishment in Pediatric Surgery. *Eur J Pediatr Surg* 1997;7:67–69.

Judah Folkman (1933–2008)

Judah Folkman was an outstanding innovative researcher who was enticed into the paediatric field at Boston. Having had a period of training with Chick Koop in Philadelphia he took up his post and was the chief in the renowned Boston Children's Hospital. His earlier research, when working at the National Naval Medical Centre in

Bethesda, continued in the field of angiogenesis. From his work there ensued a series of new drugs in the angiogenesis inhibitors attacking cancer and a number of other less lethal but crippling diseases. He maintained the high standing of the Boston Children's Hospital which had already achieved a high international standing with the clinical work of many of his predecessors including William Ladd and Robert Gross and their trainees and colleagues.

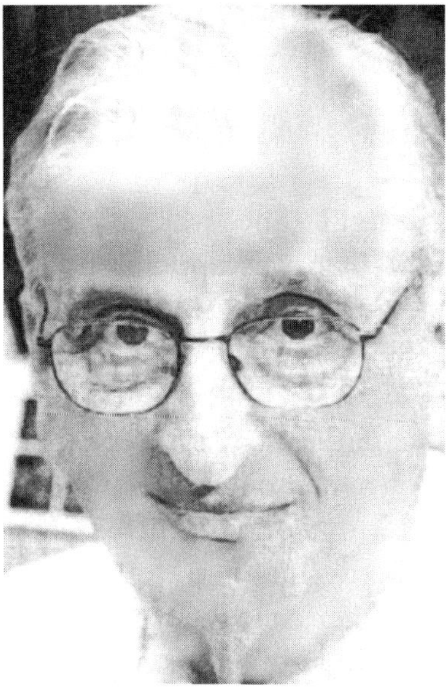

Judah Folkman

An unassuming individual he was noted for the assistance to colleagues in the research field and equally for his patient care and in his attention and consideration for the families to whom he doctored. Having been Chief at Boston for 14 years he then moved to become the Director of the Vascular Biology Program. From student days onwards he received many medals and honours for his distinguished work and held prestigious appointments within the specialty including being president of the American Pediatric Surgical Association.

His reputation out with pediatric surgery is reflected by his election to many societies including National Academy of Sciences, the American Academy of Arts and Sciences, the American Philosophical Society and the Institute of Medicine of the National Academy of Sciences. Moritz Zeigler has written a more detailed obituary[1] which gives greater detail on his outstanding achievements.

Reference

1. Ziegler MM, *J Pediatr Surg* 2008;43:421–422.

DGY

Miss Isabella Forshall (1900–1989)

The backbone of the paediatric surgical service that is widely known at Liverpool was Isabella Forshall. She was a remarkable lady who was appointed as a consultant paediatric surgeon to the Alder Hay Children's hospital in 1947. Her medical training had been at the Royal Free in London. Not a flamboyant character but a determined and efficient character she commanded a high respect from her colleagues because of her diligent care of her patients. A few years later — in 1952 — Peter Rickhan was appointed as her assistant and in time on her retrial he was the "chief" before he became frustrated with the NHS system in UK and the ways of the universities so that he left to head the department in Zurich which he did from 1971 to the time of his retirement in 1983.

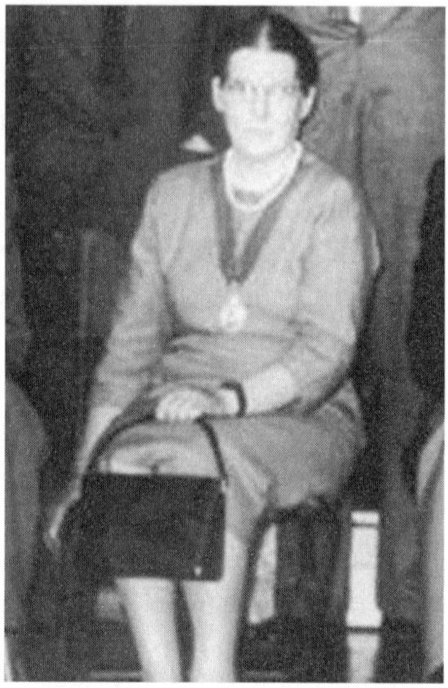

Isabella Forshall

In 1956 Isabella Forshall and Peter Richkam were joined by a third consultant — James Herbert Johnston. Herbie noted that neither Isabella nor Peter had a particular interest in urological problems so he devoted his expertise to this field and was one of the instigators of paediatric urology being considered a speciality. These three surgeons made a very significant impact on the developing specialty of paediatric surgery after World War II. They were responsible for the training of a large number of surgeons from many parts of the world and the Alder Hay became internationally recognised thanks to the solid grounding Isabella had made for the speciality.

As an example of her persistence is that soon after her appointment she insisted on having a set individual as her anaesthetist.

After some discussions Dr Gray who was in charge of the anaesthetic department agreed and designated Gordon Jackson Rees (1918–2001) to take on these duties. The outstanding success of this move had major effects on the delivery of anaesthetics to children and he is listed as the father of paediatric anaesthesia.

The second person elected to be President of the BAPS was Isabella, a unique achievement for a lady at that time. After retiring she moved back south in England and had many years of happy gardening and reading after her strenuous career.

DGY

Steve Gans

See United States of America and Journal of Paediatric Surgery.

Max Grob

See Switzerland.

Jay L. Grosfeld

Born in New York City on May 30, 1935, Dr Jay L. Grosfeld attended undergraduate school at the Washington Square College at New York University where he received a BA in Biology and History. In 1957, he entered medical school at the New York University School of Medicine and graduated in 1961. In 1961, he joined the general surgery resident staff at NYU and Bellevue Hospitals completing his residency training under Dr Frank C. Spencer in 1966.

After serving two years as a Captain in the US Army Medical Corps (1966–1968), he trained in paediatric surgery at the Columbus Children's Hospital, Ohio State University under Dr H. William Clatworthy, Jr. from 1968 to 1970. He returned to NYU as Assistant Professor of Surgery in 1970. In 1972, Dr Grosfeld moved to Indianapolis, Indiana when he was appointed the first Professor and

Director of Pediatric Surgery at Indiana University and the first Surgeon-in-Chief of the Riley Children's Hospital. He pioneered the development of paediatric surgery in the state and set the standard for the surgical care of infants and children.

In 1985 he was appointed Chairman of the Department of Surgery at Indiana University School of Medicine where he served as the Residency Training Program Director in both General Surgery and Paediatric Surgery at Indiana University. He developed excellent training programs and was a role model for his trainees. In 2003, Dr Grosfeld stepped down from the Chair at Indiana University after serving 18 years in that capacity. His tenure was marked by the development of new clinical and research facilities, clinical programs, integration of the Methodist training program with Indiana University and significant growth of the Department of Surgery from 22 to 70 faculty members and a reputation for delivering high quality clinical care.

He is recognized as a superb and sensitive clinician, master surgeon, outstanding teacher, talented administrator, innovative scientific investigator, surgical leader and a staunch advocate for children. Dr Grosfeld has published more than 478 scientific articles in peer-reviewed journals, 118 book chapters and eight textbooks.

Appointments include membership of the American Surgical Association, Society of Surgical Oncology, Society of Surgical Chairmen, Society of University Surgeons and has served as Secretary and Chairman of the Surgical Section of the American Academy of Paediatrics, President of the American Paediatric Surgical Association, President of the Halsted Society, Chairman of the American Board of Surgery (the only pediatric surgeon to serve as chair), Vice-Chairman of the Residency Review Committee for Surgery, Secretary and President of the Central Surgical Association, President of the Western Surgical Association, President of the World Federation of Associations of Pediatric Surgeons, as Governor and a member of the Advisory Councils for both General Surgery and Pediatric Surgery and numerous other Committees, American College of Surgeons and Council Member of the British Association of Pediatric Surgeons.

Awarded the Denis Browne Gold Medal by the British Association of Pediatric Surgeons, named Pediatric Surgeon of the Year at the University of Graz, Austria in 2000, the William E. Ladd Medal by the American Academy of Pediatrics, the Sagamore of the Wabash Award from the late Governor of Indiana, honorary member of 10 overseas surgical societies including Honorary Fellowship in the Royal College of Surgeons of England and the Royal College of Physicians and Surgeons, Glasgow are among his rewards for his outstanding service.

Dr Grosfeld served as Director of Pediatric Surgery and Surgeon-in-Chief of Riley Children's Hospital for 33 years and developed one of the top pediatric surgery training programs in the country. He is Editor-in-Chief of the "*Journal of Pediatric Surgery*", "*Seminars in Pediatric Surgery*", and the renowned two-volume textbook, "*Pediatric Surgery*". He currently is Chairman of the Board of Directors of the APSA Foundation, Secretary-Treasurer of the International Society of Surgery Foundation and is the first pediatric surgeon to be President of the American Surgical Association, the oldest and most prestigious surgical society in the USA.

DGY

Robert E. Gross (1905–1988)

In his early years Gross went to Carleton College in Minnesota as a student who had no clear career direction ahead. While at the college he was given Harvey Cushing's biography of Sir William Osler and that captivated him so that he decided on heading for a medical career. He proceeded to Harvard and from qualifying there MD with Honors there on his progress was impressive and illustrious to become the US doyen of paediatric surgery at the time of its explosion into the surgical scene. Having obtained the George Gorhan Peters Travelling Fellowship he spent some time in Edinburgh before returning to Harvard to be chief resident under Dr Ladd. His career progressed and he became internationally known as one of the most outstanding paediatric surgeons.

What was a high mark in his career was the first and successful ligation of the patent ductus arteriosus in a girl but unfortunately this achievement soured relationships with his chief, Dr Ladd, who was on holiday when this operation was performed. By 1972, Gross had performed this operation on 1610 patients. He was the forerunner for the development of correction of cardiac anomalies by surgery.

The name Gross is quoted many times in this book, indicating the high position he held within the specialty and the major contributions his work and his writings were instrument in the training of paediatric surgeons in so many countries. While Ladd had been responsible for the training of the first generation of paediatric surgeons in the North America Gross, his successor, was responsible for training a large number of the second generation.

Many tributes and awards have been made on his successful career and on the internet accounts such as the one written by Francis Moore and Judah Folkman[1] give some of the details of his achievements. Numerous articles can be referenced from the internet, and give an indication of his standing.

Reference

1. www.nap.edu/html/biomems/rgross.html

DGY

Michael Harrison

See Fetal Surgery

William Hardy Hendren

Qualifying in Boston in 1952 after training at the Massachusetts General Hospital (MGH) from 1950 Hardy completed his surgery training under Edward D. Churchill, MD, former MGH chief of

Surgery. Later Churchill was to be his Chief for a time after further training at the Children's Hospital under Robert Gross. Having trained at the Maas General Hospital and the Children's hospital in Boston he ultimately was appointed as the Robert E. Gross Distinguished Professor of Surgery.

Hardy' base has remained in Boston for his surgical career although his expertise has had him visit and operate extensively throughout the world. It was an interesting climax to his career as he had been Robert Gross's favorite trainee earlier. Hardy did experience the truth in the old statement that seniors who have helped, advised and trained you for your career take a different attitude to you when you become a staff or consultant member and are a risk to them. Hardy who left the Children's for a time made his name establishing the surgical pediatric service in the Mass General Hospital until 1982. He returned in the latter years of his career to be Chief in the Children's hospital and continue his practice there until well into his eight decade.

Genito-urinary surgery was Hardy's special interest and in correcting the anomalies which had affected some children it was not uncommon for him to embark on a major complex operation that would take more than 24 hours to perform — much to the exhaustion of all of his junior staff. He was a surgical enthusiast who was never keen to be separated from his extensive surgical practice. At one point he had to have a colectomy performed and he reluctantly was off his practice for a week before returning to consult and a further week later to operate again. Such was the ability of the man. Could he have survived under European laws of the present century? Fortunately he did not live in modern Europe.

Distinguished and honored in surgical colleges and communities through the world he has had endless Honours. In 2007 — he had the dedication of the W. Hardy Hendren III, MD, Conference Room, located on the eleventh floor of the Warren Building in Boston. To have this Hardy Hendren Conference Room as a memento of him having been the MGH's inaugural chief of Pediatric Surgery in 1960 and forged numerous groundbreaking surgical advances at the MGH until 1982 is a fitting tribute. Today,

Hardy remains on staff at the Mass General Hospital for Children as an honorary surgeon.

DGY

Harald Hirschsprung (1830–1916)

See Denmark.

Dr J. W. Holter (1916–2003)

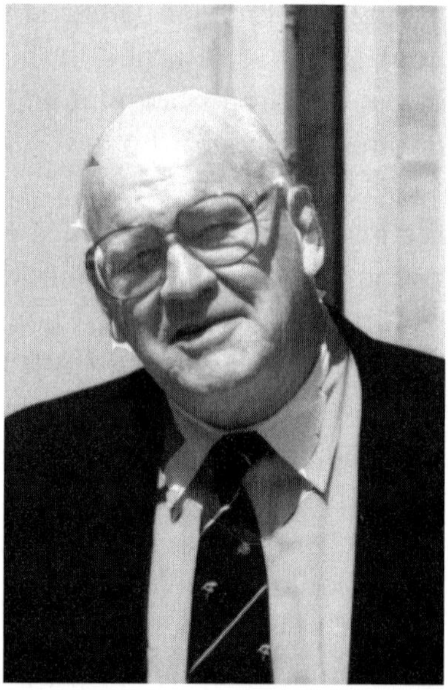

J. W. Holter

Born in 1916 life for John Holter moved along a fairly uneventful path until seven years after his marriage to Mary when they had a son. This highly anticipated happy event was not as had been expected as the couple were faced with the problem of a son with "bad" spina bifida. Their son, Casey, subsequently exhibited the signs of progressive hydrocephalus. As John himself said later in life — "everyone has his or her purpose" and as he indicated Casey's major contribution was to be the stimulus from which his father developed the initial Holter shunt for hydrocephalus. The early work was done in John's garage. Subsequently he expanded into more appropriate premises, soon employing 30 people on various projects as well as the production of shunts.

The problem of progressive hydrocephalus had been an intractable on up to the 1950's despite much effort and energy directed toward developing a successful treatment. One doctor who had been working in that field and under whose care Casey Holter came was a Dr Spitz in Philadelphia. With guidance on the nature of the problem from Dr Spitz, John Holter made the major contribution of developing a valved drainage system using the plastic materials that had become available in the 1950s and which were less irritant to human tissues.

Among his other contributions the Society for Research into Hydrocephalus and Spina Bifida was established by another outstanding character — George Mac Nab — a Scottish surgeon who had practised most of his life in London. He had the support and backing from John who was a regular attendee at the annual meetings of the Society. Even after physical illness made it difficult for him to travel he continued to attend and the Society which remains as a monument to him.

A friendly individual who had time to talk to and listen to the younger generation of doctors and surgeons he was widely respected. His outstanding contribution which transformed the outlook for so many who had hydrocephalus and for the minimising of handicap of these individuals, he will go down in history as the engineer who faced a major challenge, met it head on and succeeded in producing a solution that has been to the benefit of many thousands.

John Holter in his lifetime received recognition in many parts of the world. His death in December 2003 subsequent to a stroke two months earlier leaves the world short of one of the outstanding achievers of the 20th century.

DGY

Morio Kasai (1922–2008)

See Japan.

Charles Everett Koop

Charles Koop was not only renowned in the paediatric surgery field but was also known internationally as the outstanding Surgeon

General of the United States, having been appointed by Ronald Regan to this prodigious post. He was outstanding in his positive contribution to societies when holding the post and used it as well as making it a very active positive drive in the public health field. He was also outstanding in wearing at all his functions in the States the official uniform which the post allows the incumbent to wear.

Having qualified in 1937 BA this was followed by MD in 1941 and his ScD in 1947. Chick, as he was always known (it was supposed to be related to his surname), was appointed in 1948 to be Surgeon-in-Chief at the Children's Hospital in Philadelphia. He has given an interesting account of the early days.[1] His long and distinguished tenure of that office was supported for much of the time by his junior colleague Harry Bishop. Harry, by one means or another, refused any of many possible moves to other centers remaining in this successful partnership in Philadelphia.

Another facet of life in which Chick had was is great support from Elizabeth his wife over so many years. The one major tragedy to strike the family years ago was the loss of a son in an accident — a trial of their faith, which assisted them through that nightmare.

In paediatric surgery there are a small number of names that all paediatric surgeons know and Chick belongs to that small group. Philadelphia became next to Boston in the choice of young trainees wishing to further their career in the specialty and this was only one of the many aspects achieved. Despite the original hospital to which Chick was appointed being old the standard of care and the commitment of the staff was striking to all visitors.

Chick said it was a complete surprise when he received a call from the white House — President Regan inviting him to take over the post of Surgeon General. A medical graduate did not usually occupy this post. It did take a long time before his appointment was confirmed and he was installed but that was accomplished in January 1982. Already he had touched the limelight with appearing in Time as he had strong views on abortion and had written a book on "what ever has happened to the human race" which elicited strong views. Following his appointment it became clear that Chick had a much greater breadth of view than the journalists had been attributing to him and he proved an effective Surgeon General, decreasing the cigarette smoking, alerting the public to the dangers and developing problem of AIDS both nationally and internationally, and to many other public health measures. In consequence of his transfer to public health issues he established the C Everett Koop Institute with the mission "to promote the health and well-being of all people. The Koop Institute works to enhance our understanding of mental and physical health and the prolongation of a high quality of life."

Another nonagenarian who continues to regularly visit his office — it seems that many paediatric surgeons do not understand that three score years and ten are our allotted span. Some of his many achievements are recorded elsewhere in this book.

Reference

1. Koop CE, A perspective of the Early Days of Pediatric Surgery. *J Pediatr Surg* 1998;33:953–960.

DGY

William E. Ladd (1880–1967)

The father of pediatric surgery in North America was born to a wealthy New England family. A keen and effective oarsman, he qualified MD from Harvard in 1906. Despite having had very broad general interests, he focused on children's surgery so that in 1927 he was appointed Chief of Surgery in the Children's Hospital, Boston. In 1936 he became a full-time pediatric surgeon — one of only three in the States at that time. His book on the "*Abdominal Surgery of Infancy and Childhood*" in 1941 was a tremendous stimulus to surgeons interested in the emerging specialty of pediatric surgery. It was the forerunner of the internationally acknowledge "gospel" on the subject subsequently published with the assistance of Robert E. Gross who was to be his successor in Boston.

Ladd was described as a perfect gentleman and left a remarkable group of surgeons who had been trained by him and who proceeded to illuminate the pediatric surgical field in the coming decades. Swenson, Gross, Koop and Hendren are a few of the internationally known names who benefited from training under Ladd. The child was not simply a miniature adult but had their own requirements, physiology and pathology and required special care. His original book on abdominal surgery and his subsequent tome written with his "pupil" Gross are the two most widely read and were major contributions to the international development of paediatric surgery in the twentieth century. Their contribution to the development of the specialty was enormous. William Ladd was a stalwart and his influence, writings and techniques survive these many decades after his retirement and death.

DGY

Jannie Louw (1915–1992)

No mention of South African surgical scene is complete without reference to Jannie Louw. An individual who was in the age when the surgical scene was developing in South Africa despite the subsequent additional problems raised by the political conflicts in the country he maintained his focus on the health of the community and what the surgical sphere could contribute. In the paediatric field — his particular interest — he had an immense effect; the ultimate outcome being the recognition by the Government of the speciality. This was commented on in an editorial for the "*South African Medical Journal*" by Moore, Sidler and Rode.[1] They comment that this "coming of age" was based on the pioneering work of Prof Jannie Louw and others in the 1950's and 1960's.

Head of Surgery in Cape Town, Prof Louw had very wide interests and resposibilities. Not only was he an excellent clinician he was equally successful in training of other inspiring surgeons and in stimulating research. After the Second World War he spent time in London at the Hospital for Sick Children and had close contact with

Denis Browne and the surgical team there. He studied intestinal atresia and recommended what came to be the standard approach with a consequent large drop in the mortality. With Christian Barnard they worked on the aetiology of atresia and showed how intestinal atresia resulted from vascular block.

His early time in London confirmed for him the importance of children's surgery and what could be achieved by meticulous care in the paediatric age group. He did not tolerate individuals who were not willing to put their effort into their profession in the same way in which he drove himself. The result was the emergence of the Red Cross Memorial Hospital in Cape Town and the very high regard there was of the institution that he had been responsible for developing. Trainees from many countries competed for training posts there and this also stimulated the aspiring young surgeons who were able to obtain appointments.

Recognition of his achievements was acknowledged internationally by a large number of surgical colleges and institutions, with his Honorary Fellowship to the Royal College of Physicians and surgeons (Glasgow) in 1970 being stated by him as the start of the flow. After retiring from his clinical work he maintained his teaching commitment for many years and continued to be an excellent teacher. He was a man presented with a small opportunity in difficult circumstances who made light of the problems and worked on to be recognised as a great achiever.

Reference

1. Moore SW, Sidler D, Rode H. Paediatric Surgery: Birth of a new specialty or a coming of age? *S Afr Med J* 2008;98:268.

DGY

Jan Molenaar

See Netherlands and Section A.

James H. Nicoll (1864–1921)

See Day Surgery.

Alberto Peña

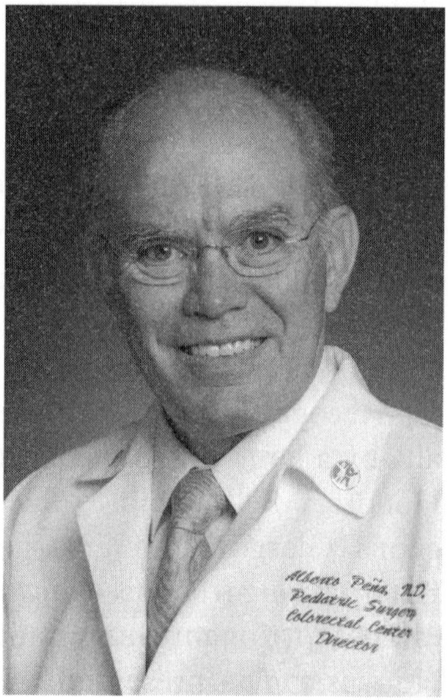

Alberto Peña

Alberto Peña received his medical degree at the Military Medical School in Mexico City, in 1962. Jesus Lozoya–Solis, who trained in Boston with Ladd and Gross, was the dominant figure in pediatric surgery in Mexico City; Alberto Peña was one of his pupils. In discordance with Ladd and Gross, Lozoya believed a pediatric surgeon should be first a pediatrician and secondarily a surgeon and that pattern became prevalent in many Spanish-speaking countries of Central and South America. Alberto Peña was no exception and from 1962 to 1968 he trained first in general surgery and medical pediatrics at the Central Military Hospital, finishing his residency in 1968.

From 1969 until December 1971, he followed his mentor's path at Boston Children's Hospital. Dr Peña moved back to Mexico City as the surgeon-in-chief of the National Institute of Pediatrics from January 1972 until June 1985, when he joined the full-time staff at Schneider Children's Hospital in July 1985. He was the chief of Pediatric Surgery and professor of Surgery at the Albert Einstein College of Surgeons until 2005. He is now director of the Colorectal Center, at Cincinnati Children's Hospital.

Up to the middle of the 20th century, pediatric surgery saw the advent of new surgical techniques designed to treat congenital defects based on detailed descriptions of the basic anatomy of these malformations (esophageal and intestinal atresias, pyloric stenosis, congenital diaphragmatic surgery) allowing the pioneers of our specialty, with relatively small effort, to make remarkable contributions in the field and allowing many previously unfortunate children to integrate into normal life.

One of the few areas of pediatric surgery where detailed knowledge of anatomy was still lacking was anorectal malformations. In 1982, Dr Peña described how the posterior sagittal approach, with the help of an electrical stimulator, can be used for the surgical management of anorectal malformations, named PSARP — posterior sagittal anorectoplasty — an approach and procedure which was to make him well-known internationally. Since 1982 until the present, Prof Peña has been traveling all over the world, lecturing and operating on children affected by this particular malformation.

The recipient of many academic accolades, one is certain none is more important than the gratefulness of all his patients — and their families — who have been the recipients of his gentle hand and expertise, to whom his most meticulously prepared "*Atlas of Surgical Management of Anorectal Malformations*" has been dedicated and the enlightment his many followers have gained by his writings and many demonstrations.

C. A. Hajivassiliou

Conrad Ramstedt (1867–1963)

Conrad Ramstedt, born in 1867, was the third of eight children. There is confusion in the literature, as there was in the family, over the spelling of their name as it seems that by error an additional 'm' was in the name for a time but the position was ultimately resolved and the correct spelling of his name is Ramstedt. He was drawn into pursuing a medical career from his youth, having assisted his father in his practice in his teens. He completed his university studies in 1895. Internationally he is known for his operation on "Pylorospasm"

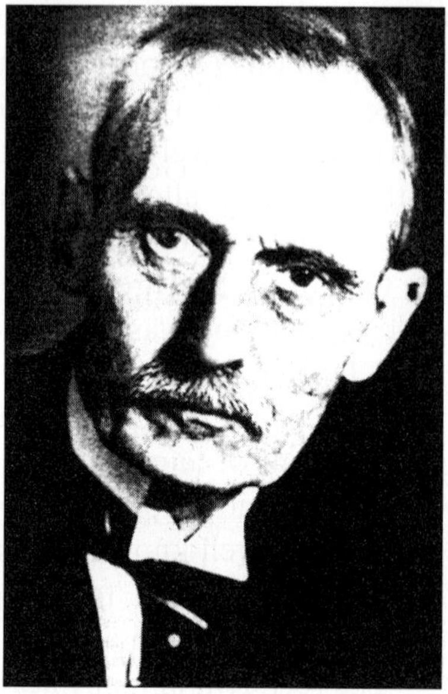

Conrad Ramstedt

now known as hypertrophic pyloric stenosis on which he published six papers between 1912 and 1934.

Although his name is attached firmly to this operation it was not the first successful operation on the condition but his procedure became gradually accepted as the Ramstedt pyloromyotomy throughout the world. Prior to that Styles[1] in Edinburgh had performed the same procedure for the condition but initially without success. Earlier other surgeons had had limited success with other operations, e.g. Nichol who had opened the stomach at laparotomy and dilated the canal using the Loretta forceps. The simpler pyloromyotomy was effective and although numerous approaches have become popular in recent decades the Ramstedt pyloromyotomy has remained the backbone of treatment of hypertrophic pyloric stenosis.

A very active surgeon he retired when he was 80 years old but continued his consultant activities beyond that time. He remained with his vivid strength of mind until his terminal days, dying in 1963 at 96 years of age. An appreciation of Conrad Ramstedt prepared by Götz Borgwardt was published in 1986.[2]

References

1. Mason Brown JJ, Sir Harold Styles and the Surgery of Congenital Pyloric Sterous. *J Roywill Surg Edin* 1955–56;1:316–8
2. Borgwardt G, *Kinderchirurgie* 1986;41:195–200.

DGY

Fritz Rehbein (1911–1991)

Fritz Rehbein was born in Westuffeln in Hessen in 1911. He started his training in surgery, urology, neurosurgery and orthopedics at the University of Goettingen in 1936, which means that his training took place throughout World War II. He delivered his professorial thesis at the same university in 1948 and became Head of the Department of Pediatric Surgery and Pediatric Urology at the Bremen Clinic in 1951. He became professor at the University of Goettingen in 1953.

During his time in Bremen until 1976, he became one of the most prominent pediatric surgeons worldwide, developing numerous surgical techniques, in particular for newborns, which were named after him. During this time, he introduced new techniques for the treatment esophageal atresia, anorectal malformations, Hirschsprung's disease and pectus excavatum. He was one of the excellent clinicians of his time with vast experience, e.g. with more than 500 operations for esophageal atresia, and he influenced not only German pediatric surgery, but the international community considerably.

Many pediatric surgeons from all over the world came to Fritz Rehbein in Bremen to be trained and many of them have become the prominent pediatric surgeons of the following decades in Europe, Japan and other regions.

Prof Rehbein achieved numerous honours, such as the Isabel Forshall Medal of the British Association of Pediatric Surgeons in 1967, the Denis Browne Gold Medal in 1978, the Paracelsus Medal of the German Association of Physicians in 1978, the honorary medal of the German Society of Pediatric Surgery in 1986, he was winner of the Oberniedermayr Memorial Lecture in 1988 and he became *Officier de l'Ordre des Palmes Académiques* in 1970. He was the president of the German Society of Pediatric Surgery from 1964 to 1970, an honorary member of the *Société Francaise de Chirurgie Infantile*, an honorary fellow of the American Academy of Pediatrics and he was a member of the *Akademie der Naturforscher Sektion Chirurgie*, Leopoldina Universität Halle and an honorary member of the Austrian Society of Pediatrics. He, with his secretary

Mrs Arnold, organized and ran a very successful meeting of BAPS in Bremen in 1968. This was the third occasion the BAPS had met in Europe.

The "*Zeitschrift für Kinderchirurgie*", which today is the "*European Journal of Pediatric Surgery*", was founded by Prof Rehbein in 1964 and he was the editor of the journal for many years.

Prof Rehbein was one of Germany's most prominent and innovative pediatric surgeons, who gained international acceptance for his clinical achievements. At his retirement in 1976, a monography "*Pediatric Surgical Operations*" was published and was translated into numerous languages with great success. Prof Fritz Rehbein died in 1991 while taking a walk on the banks of Lake Constance.

B. M. Ure

Peter Paul Rickham (1917–2003)

Born in Berlin in 1917 and educated in Switzerland, Peter had an interesting and varied life as his greatest impact was in the time he spent in Britain. Having moved to England in the 1930s to study medicine at Cambridge and St Bartholomew's Hospital in London he took up his first house post on the surgical side in Chester Royal Infirmary. After active service in the RAMC he trained in paediatric surgery. This included time at the Hospital for Sick Children, London and at the Alder Hey Children's Hospital, Liverpool. Having been appointed in 1953 as a consultant surgeon at Liverpool he was active in the early phase of the development of the British Association of Paediatric Surgeons (BAPS). Peter was the first Treasurer and subsequently he took over the responsibilities of the Secretary from David Waterston to fill the combined post. His strong personality and total commitment to projects in hand were important contributions to the success of that organisation which became an international fatherhood of paediatric surgery.

In Liverpool where Peter had joined Isabella Forshall who had established the Liverpool paediatric school based at the Alder Hay,

Peter's drive assisted in the early development of the neonatal unit in Liverpool, which was one of the first to be established. When the Nuffield Chair of Paediatric Surgery was established in Great Ormond Street Hospital on the retirement of Sir Denis Browne, Peter was a candidate for this appointment. He continued in Liverpool and oversaw the training of many developing paediatric surgeons who came to Britain for training and experience in the emerging specialty.

Contributions to the literature were one of the features by which Peter enhanced and helped in the development of the specialty. Peter was an assistant editor to Steve Gans when he established the "*Journal of Pediatric Surgery*" which was a great contribution to the elevation of paediatric surgery to being a recognised specialty through the world. Peter did find ultimately the structure of the National Health Service limiting and the higher educational system in Britain limiting to his drive. As a result he moved in 1971 back to Switzerland to be the Professor of Paediatric Surgery in the University of Zurich. He retired from this post in 1983 but maintained contact with many of the surgeons he had trained. They with some patients and nurses with whom he had maintained a close relationship met on his celebration of his eightieth birthday.

Recognition for his contribution was international as he received the Denis Browne Gold Medal in the UK, the William E Ladd Medal in the States, Knight Commander of the Grand Cross of the Order of Merit in Germany and *Chevalier of the legion d'Honour* in France.

DGY

F. Soave (1917–1984)

Franco Soave was born on June 14, 1917 in Meta di Sorrento (Naples). He received his medical education at the University of Genoa. After his medical degree in 1943, he moved to Turin where, between 1944 and 1950, he worked as resident in surgery at the

"*Clinica Chirurgica*" of the University of Turin. Between 1951 and 1954 he served as assistant professor of Surgery at the University of Genoa. During this period he was a reserve in the Medical Corps with the ranks of Lieutenant to Major.

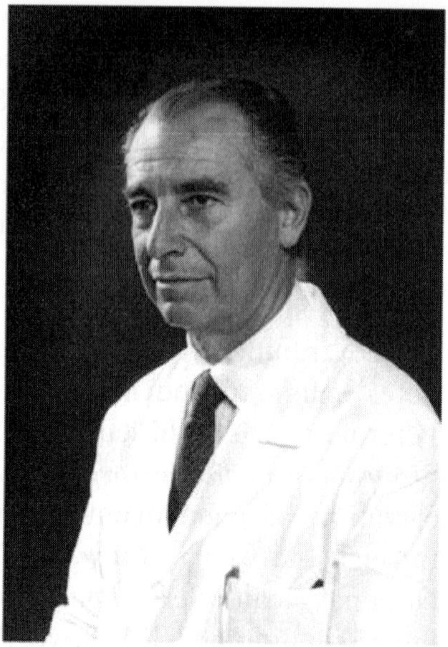

F. Soave

In 1955 he was appointed as Surgeon in Chief at the Gaslini Institute Hospital, and in 1960 as professor of Paediatric Surgery at the University of Genoa, an extraordinary chair. He held both positions until the time of his death (Genoa, September 26, 1984).

As a visiting guest professor in many European countries, Egypt, India, Iran, and Japan, Soave most often lectured and gave surgical demonstrations in the field of colon and anorectal surgery. He was the Windermere Foundation Travelling Professor of Surgery in Australia and he was the overseas guest speaker at the annual meeting of both the Surgical Section of the American Academy of Paediatrics (1971) and the American Paediatric Surgical Association (1984). At the latter, he presented the history of his work in the development of his operation for Hirschprung's disease, as well as his personal method and details of performing the procedure. Among his other international honorary presentations were the Forshall Lecture (1971) and the Oberniedermayr Lecture (1975).

Professor Soave was president of the *Società Italiana di Pediatria* from 1970 to 1972, and was given the Golden Leaves Distinguished Citizenship Award of the City of Genoa and Liguria. He was the Italian representative to the European Union of Paediatric Surgery Associations. Outside of his native land he was awarded honorary membership in the *Società Catalana di Pediatria* (1963), Brazilian Society of Paediatric Surgery (1968), the Surgical Section of the

American Academy of Paediatrics (1971), the Society of Surgeons of India (1974), the American Paediatric Surgical Association (1984); and he was given an honorary degree by the Japanese Society of Paediatric Surgery, a Golden Medal by the University of Wroclaw, as well as being made an Honorary Kentucky Colonel. In recognition of his great contributions the Government of France awarded him its esteemed *Chevalier de la Legion d'Honneur* in 1979.

Soave, an outstanding teacher and a prolific writer, was responsible for more than 160 published papers. They concerned subjects in general surgery up to 1954, and after that date, paediatric medicine and surgery. He had a wide variety of interests and extensive knowledge and experience, but he was best known for his contributions to the management of anorectal and colonic conditions. He served on the Editorial Boards before Progress in "*Paediatric Surgery*", "*Zeitschrift fur Kinderchirurgie*", and the "*Journal of Pediatric Surgery*". The basic principle of Soave's endorectal pull-through for Hirschprung's Disease is bringing proximal normal colon through the aganglionic rectum stripped of its mucosa.

Reference

1. Soave F. Hirschprung's Disease: A new surgical technique. *Arch Dis Child* 1964;39:116.

F. Cozzi

F. Douglas Stephens

Frank Douglas Stephens was born in 1913. He was one of four children of Henry Douglas Stephens and Eileen Cole, daughter of Dr Cole. Douglas's father, Henry Douglas was a paediatric surgeon at the Children's Hospital in Melbourne for 50 years until just after the war. Douglas went to Melbourne Grammar School and then after that went to University in Melbourne and into the Faculty of

Medicine because of the family background in paediatrics and medicine. He attended the University at the age of 17 and spent two years at the Royal Melbourne and one year at the Children's Hospital after completing his undergraduate degree.

When the war broke out in 1939 he joined the medical service in the Australian Army and then for the best part of six years was stationed in the Middle East. He was one of the celebrated Rats of Tobruk during the siege by General Rommel of the Allied Forces in the City of Tobruk in North Africa. He was operating in the hospital in the besieged city when the hospital received a direct hit from an artillery shell, which destroyed most of the hospital.

Douglas was pulled from the rubble by the survivors and as soon as he had recovered he went straight back to operating on all of the other injured soldiers. His commitment to his patients during a time when he himself was a casualty led him to receive the Distinguished Service Order for his efforts.

When the war ended he went back to the Royal Melbourne Hospital for further training and spent half a year at the Children's Hospital before going to England to Great Ormond Street Hospital for Children on a Nuffield Scholarship. While he was at Great Ormond Street he worked with Sir Denis Browne who was at that time one of the senior surgeons in the General Surgery Department. He was inspired not only by Denis Browne but also by Dr Martin Bodian, who was the pathologist at Great Ormond Street at that time. He was able to spend a lot of time helping Dr Bodian in the mortuary doing dissections on post mortems to understand pelvic abnormalities associated with anorectal and urinary tract anomalies. He did not have any formal embryology training beyond that normally provided in medical school, but rapidly became an expert in the field by both reading the books and literature and spending a lot of time looking at children with congenital malformations in the pathology department.

Douglas returned to Melbourne in 1950 and spent a year or two assisting his father who was in private surgical practice and then acquired an appointment at the Children's Hospital where he became the Director of Surgical Research. He had a full-time appointment at the hospital, which was unusual at the time, as most of the other staff members were visiting honorary surgeons. He became head of the urological and pelvic surgery unit in the Department of Surgery and this was staffed by Durham Smith, Robert Fowler, and Justin Kelly. The sub-specialisation which occurred in Melbourne had been fostered by Russell Howard, whose view that the surgeons in the department should all have special sub-speciality interests was a long way ahead of his time. Most other places in the world of paediatric surgeons at that time were full general surgeons.

Douglas had an honorary appointment at The Royal Women's Hospital as well, where he spent time in the pathology department doing mortuary studies of babies that had died with complex pelvic anomalies. Most of his understanding and advances in the understanding of urological and anorectal anomalies came from his dissection of these specimens, which grew into a very large collection.

His first book entitled "*Congenital Malformations of Rectum, Anus and Genitourinary Tracts*" was published in 1963. This was an amalgam of all of the research studies which had been done in the 1950's by his research fellows, mostly based on the collection of specimens which he had built up in the 1950's. He went on to publish a book on anorectal malformations in children jointly with Durham Smith in 1971. This was updated again in 1988. Further, he published a book on congenital anomalies of the kidney, urinary and genital tracts in 1996, jointly with Durham Smith and John Hutson and the 2nd edition of this was produced in 2002.

As he approached retirement in the mid 1970's he was offered a job as a visiting research fellow in the Children's Memorial Hospital in Chicago by Dr Lyle King, and moved to Chicago in 1975. His 12 years in America were marked by a sudden realisation by other surgeons in the world particularly those from the USA that Douglas had made a major contribution into the understanding of the anatomy of urinary tract and anorectal anomalies.

He returned to Melbourne in 1986, to retirement, but then has spent the last 20 years as an Honorary Visiting Surgeon in the Royal Childrens Hospital and has made a significant contribution to the research in the department as well as ongoing teaching of many subsequent fellows with an interest in paediatric urology.

J. Hutson

Keijiro Suruga

See Japan.

Orvar Swenson

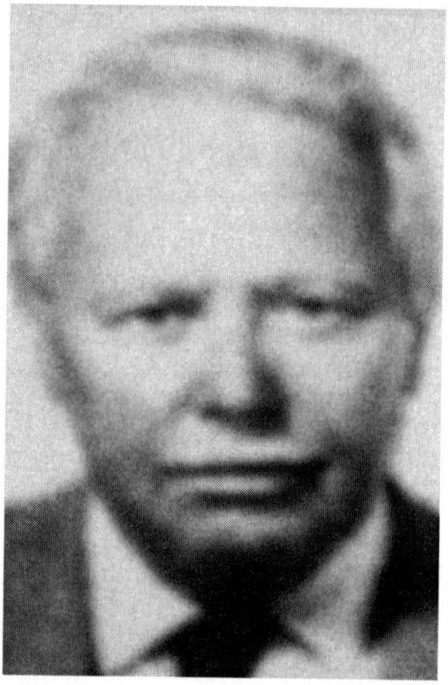

Orvar Swenson

The name Swenson automatically brings to mind the disease identified by Hirschsprung in the nineteenth century. Orvar Swenson was the individual, who along with Alexander (Sandy) Bill focused attention on the correct pathology which was inherent to cause this serious disease in the 1940's. Swenson was the surgeon who initiated the operative technique which changed this disease from carrying about 95% mortality to one which could be "cured". His operation was widely accepted and in many ways the alternatives proposed by Duhamel, Soave, Rehbein and others were modifications of his original approach.

Swenson was another of the generation of surgeons trained by William Ladd in Boston who became highly respected chiefs in the developing centres of pediatric surgery. He moved from the Children's Hospital to the Floating Hospital in Boston where he carried out much of his earlier work. Moving to Chicago he continued to publish valuable papers and books on pediatric surgery. Even in his tenth decade of life he has continued to write and submit papers to the medical journals.

A gentleman who did not have some of the more aggressive instincts of colleagues he continued to train many young surgeons in the specialty. Few if any surgeons have been able to write on their 50 years experience of the management of s single disease as he has done.[1] His contributions to the development of the specialty in Boston Floating Hospital, with help subsequently from John Fisher and his establishment of the Chicago service were major achievements.

Reference

1. Sewnson O. Early History of the Therapy of Hirschsprung's Disease Facts and Personal Observations over 50 years. *J Pediatr Surg* 1996;31: 1003–1008.

DGY

Yoshiaki Tsuchida (1936–2005)

Dr. Tsuchida was born on October 25 1936, in Osaka, Japan. He entered the University of Tokyo, Faculty of Medicine, in 1955. After his graduation in 1961, and a one-year internship, he joined the Second Department of Surgery at the University of Tokyo. There, he met Prof Masanobu Ishida, a founder of the Department of Pediatric Surgery at the University of Tokyo and a Japanese pioneer of Pediatric Surgery. He decided to make Pediatric Surgery his special field of concentration. After receiving his PhD degree, he continued his investigations of alpha-fetoprotein (AFP) assays in pediatric solid tumors, including teratomas, hepatoblastomas and liver diseases. This work resulted in his publication of striking and important quantitative data relevant to the

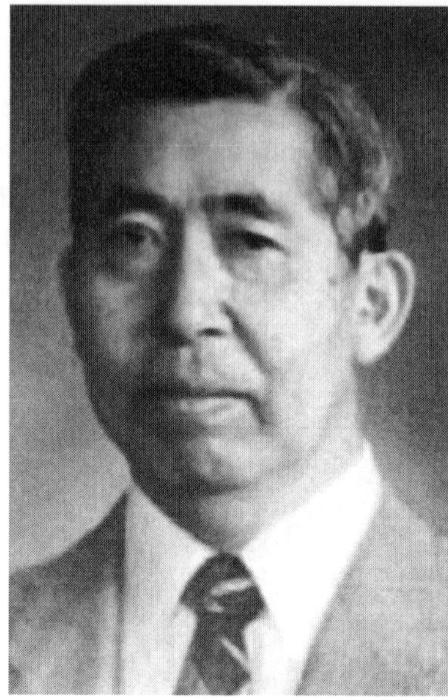

Yoshiaki Tsuchida

normal serum levels of AFP in infants showing the decline until 10 months after birth. This landmark paper has frequently been cited in the literature and has been of great value at the bedside.

Dr Tsuchida was appointed an Assistant in Surgery in 1967, and a Lecturer of Pediatric Surgery in 1975 in the University of Tokyo Hospital. There, his research group established a series of transplantable neuroblastoma xenografts in nude mice, which were used to screen candidate clinical anti-cancer reagents. He then moved to the National Children's Hospital in Tokyo in 1985 as Head of the Department of Surgery. He returned to the University of Tokyo Hospital as Professor and Chairman of the Department of Pediatric Surgery in 1991. For a long time he was the leader of the Japanese Study Group for Advanced Neuroblastoma, and became the President convening the 32nd Annual Meeting of the Japanese Society of Pediatric Surgeons in 1995.

One year before his expected retirement from the University, he was invited to become the Director of Gunma Children's Medical Center, Gunma, Japan. He continued his research at the Gunma University School of Medicine, where his enthusiastic passion to research, his focus to solve clinical problems and to stimulate young pediatric surgeons to undertake clinical research projects was maintained.

Dr Tsuchida published more than 220 papers in English, along with 151 original articles and 16 book chapters. Amazingly, he presented 118 papers at international meetings all over the world. Together with Drs Tadashi Sawada and Minoru Sakurai, he organized the 30th Annual meeting of SIOP in Yokohama as President of the Organizing Committee. Also with Dr Sawada, he established SIOP-Asia, a step forward to internationalism that should never be forgotten.

At his funeral, his wife Mineko said that he was a happy person who devoted himself to his work, regardless of his worsening health condition, despite which he remained actively engaged until his death. Dr Yoshiaki Tsuchida died on June 28, 2005, at the age of 68 after his prolonged illness.

Michio Kaneko
Akira Nakagawara

Max Wilms — A Man and Syndrome (1867–1918)

Dep. Surgical Paediatrics, University of Berne, Inselspital
Freiburgstr. 8, 3010 Berne
Switzerland

Carl Max Wilhelm Wilms was born on November 5th, 1867 in Hünshofen, a small village near Aachen, the second son of the lawyer, Matthew Wilms.

He studied at the universities of Munich, Marburg, Berlin and Bonn, from where he obtained his doctorate degree in 1890 with a study entitled "Resection of the Oesophagus". Wilms' early professional career was as nomadic as his student days, and, as was customary at the time, he embarked on a four-year program as a resident, moving in 1891 to the Department of Anatomy and Pathology at the University of Gießen, where his interest in the manual art of surgery had been aroused.

In 1895 Wilms was appointed pathological anatomist to the Pathological Institute of Cologne under Otto Michael Ludwig Leichtenstern. It was not, however, until 1897 that he began his surgical career under Professor Trendelenburg at the University of

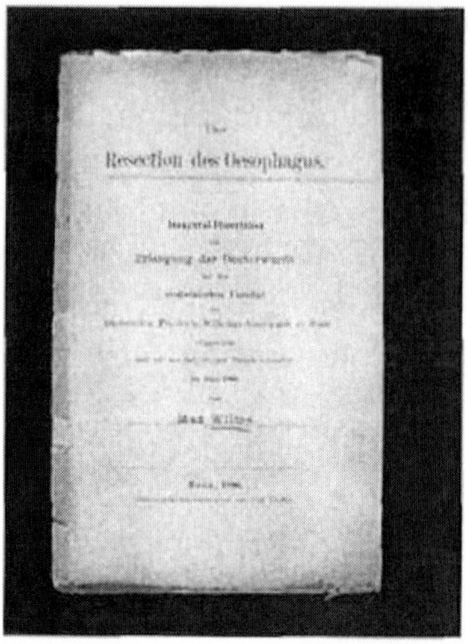

Fig. 1. The original publication of Wilms' thesis 1890.

Leipzig. Trendelenburg was the first physician to have successfully treated an embolus of the pulmonary artery.

In 1899 Wilms became Professor of Surgery in Leipzig where he was described as diligent and highly intelligent, possessing an exceptional working capacity, as well as being a dextrous surgeon. He had a special interest in nephrology and his major contributions were to the fields of the surgical pathology of the kidney, bladder and urogenital tract. Wilms made great efforts to map the pathology and development of tumour cells, and after studying renal tumours comprehensively he proposed the theory that tumour cells are initiated as early as in the embryo. Wilms was only 32 years of age when he published his important monograph on the pathology of mixed tissue tumours "*Die Mischgescwülste*". His book dispelled confusion at the time and his classification provided the foundation for modern concepts concerning this group of disorders.

In 1907, Wilms was appointed Professor of Surgery in Basel and in 1910 he reached the peak of his career when he was called to the Chair at the University of Heidelberg. As a surgeon, Max Wilms established many important developments in the field of paediatric surgery. Regarding his operative techniques, he was far ahead of his time. His name is also eponymously associated with two operations; firstly, perineal prostatectomy through a lateral incision and, secondly, anterior and posterior rib resections used to treat pulmonary tuberculosis.

Soon after his appointment as Chairman of the Department of Surgery at Heidelberg, Wilms published another important paper: "*Ileus; an operative perspective*", a work that was to bring him further international recognition.

In November 1914 in Heidelberg, Wilms married Miss Else Seyferth, who was from Leipzig. She died in her nineties, outliving her husband for a long time. Their home, with great views of the river Neckar and the romantic "Heidelberger Schloss", remains at the foot of the famous Philosopher's Way in Heidelberg.

In May 1918, Wilms was presented with a French prisoner of war who had laryngeal swelling secondary to diphtheria. For Max Wilms, relieving patient suffering was a greater calling than political allegiance, and he saved the French officer by performing a laryngotomy/cricothyroidotomy. Sadly Wilms himself acquired the disease in a severe septic form and died on the 14th May 1918 eight days after contracting the infection.

Wilms was only 51 years old, at the pinnacle of a distinguished career; he died early but his life thus far had been a fulfilling one. He set milestones in the history of German surgery in general and paediatric surgery in particular. He is buried in Cologne but his grave was destroyed during World War II.

What better way to portray this man than to quote from the funeral address of Professor Rost, one of his former students:

> *"There are three qualities that seem to characterise the essence of his nature best. In some respect they are the mainstay of his humanistic and scientific thinking:*
>
> - *First, the love for his work. The hospital, his workplace had become a second home for him. This hard working man was so very much absorbed by his daily work that it proved almost impossible for him to rest or to go on vacation from time to time.*

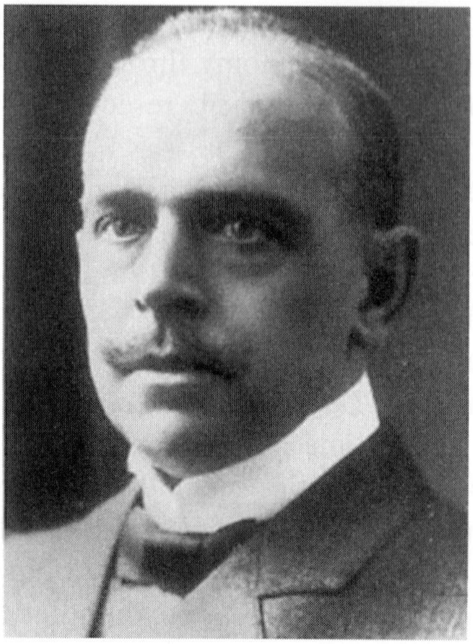

Fig. 2. Max Wilms (1867–1918). Director of the Surgical Clinic of the University of Heidelberg (1910–1918).

- *Second, his exceptional intelligence characterised him as much as his outstanding work. He was a clever man but not in the sense of the ordinary diplomatic shrewdness. In fact, he never was a diplomat and he did not want to be. He was a clever, sensible and intuitive physician.*
- *Third, he possessed an incredible imagination. As a true son of the beautiful Rhine valley, he incorporated intellectual flexibility to an extraordinary extent."*

Z. Zachariou and Roland Daum

Dan G. Young

Dan was born in 1932 and graduated from the University of Glasgow in 1956. In place of National Service Dan served in Ghana on a Special Short Service Commission to the newly formed State before returning to Glasgow via the Liverpool School of Tropical Medicine and then as an Assistant Lecturer in the Physiology Department, Glasgow University. His further surgical training was between Glasgow and the Hospital for Sick Children (HSC), Great Ormond Street, London before being appointed a Senior Lecturer and Honorary Consultant at the HSC and at the Queen Elizabeth Hospital Hackney.

In 1969 he returned to Glasgow as Head of the Department of Surgical Paediatrics, University of Glasgow, based at the Royal Hospital for Sick Children, Yorkhill. The neonatal surgical unit was established in November 1971 on the hospital moving back to new premises on its old site. This was advantageous in concentrating knowledge and experience of the nursing and medical staff. It has been widely recognised. The Unit was refurbished in 1991 and was renamed "The Dan Young Neonatal Surgical Unit" by The Chairman of the Health Board. Over the last 36 years over 14,000 "surgical" neonates have been cared for in the Unit.

He developed a fine Department of Paediatric Surgery, was an excellent educator and role model, and trained many younger surgeons from all continents as well as British graduates. He was appointed Professor of Surgical Paediatrics in the University of Glasgow in 1992. Dan stepped down from his academic leadership role in 1998 but continued to be exceptionally productive as an adviser to many young surgeons in his role as a valued leader in the field. He retired from clinical practice in 1998 but is still active and currently the President of the British Society for the History of Paediatrics and Child Health.

During his professional career, Prof Young has received numerous other accolades. He has served on most local, Scottish and British committees in both the surgical and many on the medical paediatric fields, and was Honorary Secretary of the Society for Research into Hydrocephalus and Spina Bifida and President of the British Association of Paediatric Surgeons (BAPS). Like others selected in this Section he received the Denis Browne Gold medal (1999). In the 1980's he chaired the committee that oversaw the establishment of the Intercollegiate FRCS in Paediatric Surgery in Britain. He has maintained good contact and relationships with surgeons in other specialties through his career and has been an examiner for over 30 years in all in the FRCS and MRCS examinations of the British Royal Colleges as well as being an examiner in the Diploma of Child Health of the Royal College of Physicians and Surgeons.

Internationally he has been of assistance in many countries in establishing the specialty and in consequence has been made an honorary member of many national paediatric associations. With his considerable bibliography of published papers, chapters and textbooks he has also contributed to the literature very actively by being the Editor for the British Isles for the "*Journal of Pediatric Surgery*" for 17 years. The University of Wroclaw, in recognition of his contributions to Polish paediatric surgery development and his international contribution, honoured him with a Doctorate.

Away from his direct clinical and teaching work Dan has been very supportive of handicapped children and their families. He was asked to become the Honorary President of the Scottish Spina Bifida Association (SSBA) 30 years ago and has continued working with them for over three decades. In 2007 the SSBA were able to build a new centre in the middle of Scotland, replacing their three previous offices, and in recognition by the Board of the Association the new more spacious building was named "The Dan Young Building". The staff at this centre is there to give support to the affected individuals and to their families throughout Scotland. With the new technology it is easier to have multidisciplinary clinics using the unit's telemedicine facilities, but the support staff do still have to travel considerable distances from the centre to see families in or near their homes when necessary. This is a charity organisation, now over 40 years old, and is funded by voluntary contributions which have to be raised in support for the affected individuals.

In his "spare" time he will be found either with his family — now married over 50 years to Nan — gardening or curling — a strange sport to which some natives in the cooler countries are addicted.

RC

Jin-Zhe Zhang

In presenting the DB Gold Medal to the President of the Royal College of Surgeons of England Miss Leela Kapila OBE gave the following citation, which is a brief summary of this distinguished and outstanding surgeon's career.

Prof Zhang was born in Ninghe County of Hebei province, recently called Tainjin, on September 25, 1920. He graduated from Yenching University, Peking and then gained an MD from Shanghia Medical College in 1945. He started his surgical training at the Peking Central Hospital and became the Chief Resident at the Medical College Hospital of the Peking University from 1948 to 1950. For the next five years he was Attending Surgeon in Paediatric Surgery at the same hospital. In 1955 Prof Zhang was appointed Chief Paediatric Surgeon and Vice-Director of Beijing Children's Hospital a post he held until 1984 with a gap of four years.

In 1968, during the Cultural Revolution, Prof Zhang was assigned to work as a janitor and had to clean the toilets of his hospital. His wife, a pharmacist at the Hospital of Peking University was sent off to a mountainous village north of the Great Wall to work as a bare-foot doctor and their daughter had to be cared for by the grandparents. The other members of the senior staff were also removed and some disappeared, never to return.

In 1970 Prof Zhang suffered from melaena and was diagnosed to have gastric cancer and a gastrectomy was recommended. There were no fully trained surgeons around so the operation was done under acupuncture with the patient following the procedure in the mirror. When the surgeon said that he could not find the cancer, and asked what he should do as there was no facility for frozen section, Prof Zhang decided to risk losing half his stomach rather than the risk of missing a malignancy. The patient then continued to direct the surgeon in the operative procedure. Clearly the operation was a success and today Prof Zhang feels he is very lucky to have had major surgery under acupuncture.

In 1972 Prof Zhang was liberated and reinstated to his job. The challenge now was to restart the training programme almost single-handedly as there was no tier of middle grade staff.

In 1974, his colleague at the Tainjin Children's Hospital sadly drowned and the bereft junior surgeons, trainees of Prof Zhang sought his help. Hence he visited the hospital one day a month until 2006 when in his own words he felt old and became practically deaf!

During his career Prof Zhang has achieved national and international recognition for his contribution to paediatric surgery. He has published widely, 18 books and chapters, over 200 scientific papers and many presentation to learned societies. His special interests are in Emergency and Ambulatory surgery of children. Regrettably because the pubications were written in Chinese the surgeons abroad were slow to benefit from his wisdom and experiences. The Beijing Children's Hospital with 742 beds has statistics which are astounding. Nearly 2 million children attend the outpatient department per year: 308 cases of intussusceptions seen last year of which 226 were treated as day cases, in comparison to 20 cases seen in Nottingham, all as inpatients. During my last visit to Beijing I was fortunate to have been shown around the hospital by Prof Zhang and learnt a lot about ambulatory care.

Prof Zhang's many outstanding achievements have been rewarded by several awards over the years. In 1989 he received the Model Worker Medal from the Beijing Municipality and a similar honour in 1991 from the Minister of Health. In 2000 he attended the meeting of the British Association of Paediatric Surgeons in Sorrento to receive the Denis Browne Gold Medal, the society's highest honour.

Prof Zhang in addition to his surgical and teaching skills is an accomplished artist in Chinese painting and calligraphy. He enjoys Chinese traditional opera and took part in performances in his youth.

Prof Zhang and his wife Elizabeth Shen En-Lian have four children and their younger son is a paediatric orthopaedic surgeon.

Prof Zhang is now officially a "National Treasure" and a highly respected member of the community. The downside is that even at the young age of 87 years he is not allowed to retire!

Mr. President for all these and many mother contributions to the welfare of children in China and all over the world Prof Zhang Jin-Zhe is more than worthy of the Honorary Fellowship of our College and I have the greatest pleasure in presenting him to you.*

Leela Kapila, OBE

---

* The above oration was given when he was presented for Honorary Fellowship of the Royal College of Surgeons of England.

Section D

ASSOCIATIONS AND JOURNALS

AMERICAN PEDIATRIC SURGICAL ASSOCIATION (APSA)

Dan G. Young

Dr C. E. Koop, one of the surviving initiators of the Surgical Section of the AAP, wrote the following editorial in the *JPS* (*Journal of Pediatric Surgery*) in an editorial in 1971. Since the relatively early establishment of the Section events had moved on substantially and Steve Gans in 1965 had persuaded both the Surgical Section and the BAPS to support the new journal which he was organizing with Dr Koop, the editor-in-chief.

"During the past 20 years regional pediatric surgical associations have sprung up in sections of the continent and in one instance among pediatric surgeons from several countries bordering on the Pacific ocean. However, there never was an American society of those interested in the problems of children standing on its own two surgical feet.

Perhaps had it not been for the excellence of the British Association of Paediatric Surgeons which provided a platform for an international congress in some part of continental Europe each year, the impetus for an American society might have come sooner.

Again it was in Atlantic City, this time in an Italian restaurant, when Jack Campbell, Dale Johnson and Lucian Leape asked this Editor for an historical overview of the development of pediatric surgery in North America and specifically inquired as to the absence of an American Pediatric Surgical Association.

From this inauspicious beginning, and with much work from a number of dedicated, enthusiastic young men in pediatric surgery, there came into being in April 1970 the American Pediatric Surgical Association. In April 1971 it held its first scientific congress in Bermuda under the Presidency of Robert E. Gross. The APSA, as it is now called, was a long awaited arrival, had a very slow delivery, but appears now to be a viable baby. We look forward to a period of rapid growth and development leading to a precocious adolescence and maturity. The Editorial Board and the publishers of the "*Journal of Pediatric Surgery*" look forward to years of happy association with the APSA.

From what may have been a delayed delivery the APSA organisation has steadily grown and has added a progressive international flavour to the annual meetings. It is now a major part of the surgical medico-political scene and individuals who have held the office of President have also had a significant part in the national scene. Examples are the positions held by the first lady president of the APSA — Dr Kathryn Anderson — who has been President of the American College of Surgeons.

With the major changes, partly politically stimulated but also due to the increasing specializing within the practice of medicine major changes such as the accreditation scheme have necessitated the rapid development of medicine in the second half of the 20th century. APSA structure has had a rapid rise to accommodate the evolution.

ARAB ASSOCIATION OF PEDIATRIC SURGEONS

Hayel J. Al-Ejeilat

In 1985, during the BAPS conference in Vienna, a big group of Arab delegates (22 delegates) were attending the conference, representing most of the Arab countries. A meeting was concluded that gathered them all, and a decision was made to create an Arab Association of Pediatric Surgeons. I was given the task of putting the by-laws of the association and preparing for a conference in Amman, Jordan to discuss them. Upon my return to Amman, I started working on the by-laws and had those of the BAPS, the Asian, as well as the APSA associations as a guide. I sent a copy of the provisional by-laws to each of the delegates and got their remarks included. In October 1986, the first Arab Congress of Pediatric Surgery was held in Amman, during which the Arab Association of Pediatric Surgeons was born, and **Prof Sirry Roustom** of Syria was elected as the first president; **Dr Hayel J. Al-Ejeilat** was elected as the first general secretary. The association is still active and is running its activities every two years in each of the Arab countries in turn.

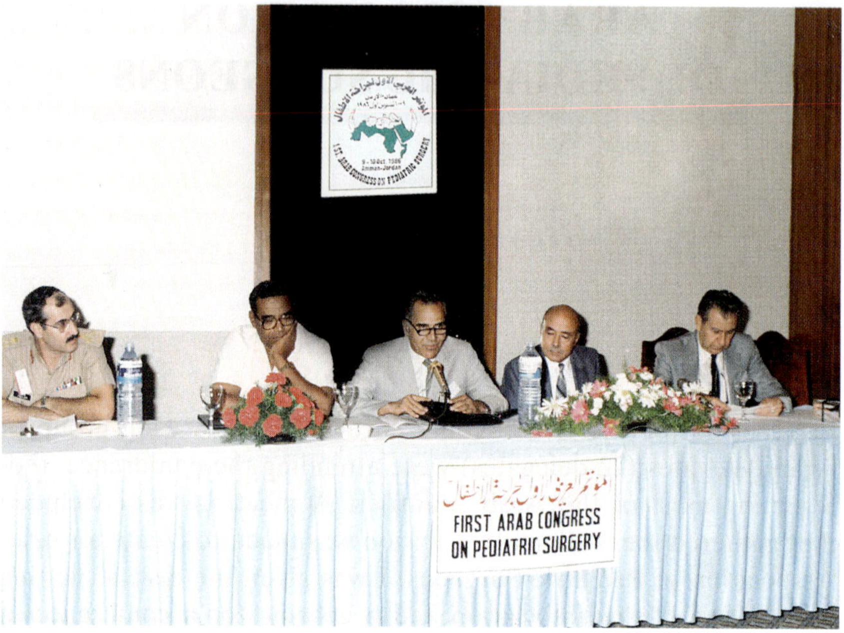

Sitting **left to right**: 1) Dr Hayel Al-Ejeilat (Jordan), 2) Dr Ali Abd Alkarim (Sudan), 3) Dr Aziz Abdelalim (Egypt), 4) Dr Adel Lutfi (Egypt), and 5) Dr Sirry Roustoom (Syria).

AUSTRALASIAN ASSOCIATION OF PAEDIATRIC SURGEONS

E. Durham Smith

The Australasian Association of Paediatric Surgeons, so-named in 1990 after incorporating New Zealand (previously it was the Australian Association of Paediatric Surgeons), the specialist society to which all paediatric surgeons belong, nominates its own members to the Board of Paediatric Surgery of the College. The Board of Paediatric Surgery selects and mentors the trainees and determines the structure of the curriculum. The Association has the autonomy to have its own scientific meetings, but every second year it runs its annual conference within the Annual Scientific Congress of the College, so that inter-disciplinary sessions can be held. Edward Bate, a paediatric orthopaedic surgeon, and Peter Jones became elected Councilors of the College until illness forced the latter's resignation and Edward Bate becoming the Chairman of the Court of Examiners. Patricia Davidson became Censor-in-Chief on Council, one of the toughest jobs in surgery, being the final arbiter in all training matters in all disciplines. Patrick Dewan became a Councillor, and finally, Anne Kolbe became the second paediatric surgical President of the College (2003–2005), and the first woman in any surgical college in the world to be President. This brief analysis should also include the number of senior paediatric colleagues who have played a part on the College State Committees, as Examiners for Fellowship, and as representatives on Council for Paediatric Surgery.

BRITISH ASSOCIATION OF PAEDIATRIC SURGEONS (BAPS)

Dan G. Young

The half century anniversary celebration of the BAPS was recorded in a supplement of the "*Journal of Paediatric Surgery*" in 2003 which was released at the BAPS Annual Congress in Estoril that summer. The early days of the BAPS were recorded by **Sir David Innes Williams** who was recently appointed a consultant in London at the time of formation of the Association.[1] In that initial caucus of 14 surgeons there were six from Scotland as there was much clearer acceptance of paediatric surgery and of paediatric surgeons in Scotland than there was in England where the remaining eight surgeons were in practice. Another interesting fact is that of the 14 surgeons two were female (Isabella Forshall, Liverpool and Rosie Mackay, Edinburgh).

An invitation was sent out to a group of surgeons in Britain who were involved in paediatric surgery. At that time there was a limited number of full-time paediatric surgeons. Erhenpreis recorded that there were only around 60 to 70 paediatric surgeons in the entire world at that time.[2] A significant number of these surgeons — mostly men at the early fifties — and from the formation of the Association it had an international flavour. The first President was Denis Browne who with true Australian drive has often been referred to as the first surgeon in England to devote himself entirely to paediatric surgery. The first Secretary was David Waterston, described by **Denis Browne** as a very good surgeon but a poor secretary, but was very involved in the discussions and agreement to establish an Association.

His personality was such that he was able to allay concern and achieve agreement rather than to create schisms. The third official was Peter Rickham who had been appointed to the staff at Liverpool where Isabella Forshall had established the paediatric surgical service. Peter had significant organising abilities and in 1957 he took over the combined post of Honorary Secretary and Treasurer — a combination of offices which is retained by BAPS members until the present.

In each Annual Congress there has always been held a dinner for those attending and their spouses. Speeches at the end of each of these varied between the serious, the entertaining and the prolonged, but at the second meeting the "speech" by **T. Twistington Higgins** (retired in 1952 from the Hospital for Sick Children in Great Ormond Street) given in Glasgow at the BAPS second Congress in 1955 was:

That sober minded body called the British APS
Concerned to further knowledge for all children in distress
Very wisely came to Scotland where such knowledge has its hame
And to Glasgow where our Matthew is the Pundit of the same

Three days they sat at Glasgow's feet and basked in Glasgow's sun
Three days the laboured woefully to learn the Scottish tongue.
Three days they scoured the Yorkhill braes and gathered
pearls for by
Whiles they toured the Trossachs and drank the College dry.

Three days they lapped up wisdom, inspired by Scottish skill.
From the brain-box to the bladder, Lord God they had their fill!
But let's hear no more of water, whether flowing free or no.
Till ye've dined wi' Scots in Glasgow — the Truth you'll
never know

In all the ends of all the Earth Whaur's Toast that rings sae true?
As "Tae us and ithers like us — and Friends that goes for you"!
So from Greece to Copenhagen, from London to Brisbane
The call runs — "Thank you Glasgow — we'll sure be back again".

The reply given by **Wallace Dennison** as Matthew White was unwell during the meeting:

From the northern wastes of Britain; from provincial Glasgow town
We send our thanks to you, Sir, and salute your great renown
You're an honorary Scotsman and a member of our Club
We like you as a Surgeon and we like you in the pub.

Your presence lent distinction to the British APS
At the recent Glasgow meeting and thus humbly I express
Our deep appreciation of your courtesy and skill
As a firm and tactful Chairman, you nobly filled the bill.

In the absence of our Matthew we accept you without fear
As an honoured Elder Statesman and your presence brings
us cheer.
For the future of our Specialty and for children in distress
We'll rally round your Banner and even back the APS

We tried to do you honour in the lecture named "Yorkhill"
And you gave the cultured lecture with your customary skill
We not only learned of tumours but we heard some common sense,
The plaudits of the audience were, I hope, your recompense.

In the name of Matthew White, Sir, I thank you for your praise
Of Glasgow's hospitality and your liking of our ways.
When next you come to Glasgow what we really hope to see
Presiding jointly over us — M. W. and you T. T.

Many of the international group of paediatric surgeons attended the BAPS and became members of the Association — initial joining fee was one pound sterling. **Ehrenpreis**[2] in his "*100 Years of Pediatric Surgery in Stockholm, with Personal Memories from the last 50 Years*" recording his view on the value of the BAPS which "had grown into a large international body consisting of some 650 members, a hundred of whom worked in the United Kingdom, the rest being overseas members from about 60 different countries". This has resulted in wide expansion of contacts and exchange of methods and ideas as well as giving a family type of atmosphere. This started with Diana Lister — the first employee of the BAPS as a part-time secretary and was enhanced by Dorothy Grant who made a particular point of getting to know new numbers (home or overseas) and making them feel a part of the group.

The officers and executive are all honorary appointments and individuals serve for varying periods. Denis Browne was the first President and was succeeded by Isabella Forshall — probably the first lady President of any of the surgical associations in the UK. The term of President is for two years and has remained at that despite some effort to change it to a one or a three year appointment. The individual elected is involved for four years, being on the executive for one year before and one year after the term of President.

Table 1. Venues of annual meetings.

BAPS Previous Annual Meetings					
1954	London	1955	Glasgow	1956	London
1957	Edinburgh	1958	London	1959	Liverpool
1960	London	1961	Stockholm	1962	London
1963	Sheffield	1964	Rotterdam	1965	Edinburgh
1966	London	1967	Bremen	1968	Liverpool
1969	Dublin	1970	Manchester	1971	Genoa
1972	Glasgow	1973	London	1974	Berne
1975	Newcastle	1976	Sheffield/Warsaw	1977	Oslo
1978	Edinburgh	1979	Marseilles	1980	Oxford
1981	Southampton	1982	Madrid	1983	London
1984	Liverpool	1985	Vienna	1986	Birmingham
1987	Dublin	1988	Athens	1989	Nottingham
1990	Glasgow	1991	Budapest	1992	Leeds
1993	Manchester	1994	Rotterdam	1995	Sheffield
1996	Jersey	1997	Istanbul	1998	Bristol
1999	Liverpool	2000	Sorrento	2001	London
2002	Cambridge	2003	Estoril	2004	Oxford
2005	Dublin	2006	Stockholm	2007	Edinburgh

The initial plan when the Association was being formed was that alternate annual congresses should be in London with the intervening one in the "provinces". The second meeting was held in Glasgow. The rapid involvement of so many surgeons from overseas resulted in an early change to one meeting in three to be held out with the UK while the other two would be in the British Isles. This pattern has been followed broadly since the first meeting was held in Sweden in 1961 (Table 1). The social aspects of the congresses, especially the international contacts, were very beneficial in many ways including the ability to make contacts and arrange training of junior staff in a different environment from their native one.

The Association has continued despite the large increase in the number of paediatric surgeons internationally although it does not have the same degree of international participation compared to the 1960's to 1980's period. Many other Associations have been established around the world and also the political scene in Europe has

Table 2. Denis Browne gold medallists.

1968	R. E. Gross	1969	M. Grab
1970	D. J. Waterston	1971	C. E. Koop
1972	P. P. Rickham	1973	M. Sulamaa
1974	Th. Ehrenpreis	1975	D. Innes Williams
1976	F. D. Stephens	1977	R. B. Zachary
1978	F. Rehbein	1979	O. Swenson
1980	J. H. Louw	1981	A. W. Wilkinson
1982	H. H. Nixon	1983	S. L. Gans
1984	H. W. Clatworthy	1985	R. N. Howard
1986	M. Kasai	1987	0. Knutrud
1988	M. M. Ravitch	1989	B. O'Donnell
1990	J. E. S. Scott	1991	W. H. Hendren
1992	J. Lister	1993	R. K. Gandhi
1994	J. C. Molenaar	1995	J. A. Haller Jr.
1996	E. Durham Smith	1997	J. D. Atwell
1998	J. L. Grosfeld	1999	D. G. Young
2000	J. -Z. Zhang	2001	E. Howard
2002	J. J. Corkery	2003	L. Kapila
2004	L. Spitz	2005	D. Lloyd
2006	P. Puri	2007	A. Coran

changed dramatically since BAPS was born. Planned for 2009 is a combined meeting of EUPSA (European Union of Pediatric Surgical Associations) and BAPS to be held in Graz. The EUPSA is a large organisation since it has metamorphosed into its present form and holds annual meetings now. In the UK during recent years there has been dramatic intervention by the politicians in the training, running and control of the medical profession. A central determination to abide by European laws has had an interesting impact on the services which paediatric surgeons provide, as with others in the medical profession. Training and working patterns has had to undergo major change. Problems like these present major challenges to the BAPS as well as to other Societies and so the problems of today differ substantially from those of the 1950's.

After Sir Denis Browne's death Lady Moira Browne and the Trustees established a Denis Browne Gold Medal to be awarded each year to an individual who had made a significant contribution to the development of the speciality. This award was initially made by the Trustees after consultation with the BAPS Executive Committee but responsibility has now been transferred to the latter body (Table 2).

References

1. *J Pediatr Surg* 2003;38 (Suppl 7). A Historical Review: 1953–2003.
2. Ehrenpreis T. 100 years of pediatric surgery in Stockholm, with personal memories from the last 50 years. *Prog Pediatr Surg* 1986;20:17–23.

CANADIAN ASSOCIATION OF PAEDIATRIC SURGEONS (CAPS): THE FIRST 40 YEARS

Sigmund H. Ein
Arlene Ein

The year 1967 was the 100th anniversary of the founding of Canada and each Canadian was encouraged to develop a centennial project. To that extent, Dr Barry Shandling must be considered both the Godfather and Grandfather of The Canadian Association of Paediatric Surgery (CAPS). On May 8, 1967, he sent a letter to "all surgeons in Canada who spend a relatively large proportion of their time engaged in General Paediatric surgery". The apparent reason for this was because: "Most of us meet annually at the Surgical Section of The American Academy of Pediatrics. There is at present no Canadian Association of Paediatric Surgeons of any kind". He then continued: "During the first week of September of this year, the Canadian Paediatric Society is holding an augmented meeting in the nature of a Centennial celebration, here in Toronto. The annual Alumni Association meeting of The Hospital for Sick Children will take place at the same time. It is hoped that Paediatric Surgeons, whether alumni or not, from across Canada, will attend this meeting".[1]

With his next two sentences, the CAPS seed was planted: "If a Canadian Paediatric Surgical Association is ever to be created, this would probably be a favorable time and place for its inauguration". Dr Shandling then went on to set out, (unbeknownst to him), a charter and raison d'être for CAPS, as we now know it! "Such an

Association could either be quite independent, or conceivably be a Surgical Section of the Canadian Paediatric Society. Annual meetings would be held in different Canadian cities and would foster both professional and social intercourse on an inter-provincial basis. At present, The Royal College of Surgeons annual meeting does not have a program of sustained paediatric surgical interest. Such an organisation would also enable us to speak with more authority on behalf of our specialty where our interests are or might be involved. It is estimated that there were then approximately 30 surgeons throughout Canada "who spend a relatively large proportion of their time engaged in General Paediatric Surgery".[1]

Dr Shandling also suggested that an academic environment should pervade the annual meeting: "If you would like to present a paper at the surgical meeting on Friday, September, the 8th (1967), I would be grateful if you would let me have the title thereof before the end of May (1967)".[1]

The response to his letter was, not surprisingly, uniformly enthusiastic and the attendance at the inaugural gathering on September 7, 1967 was similarly encouraging. The following 28 Canadian Pioneers in the small but growing speciality of paediatric surgery attended this meeting and henceforth were considered The Founding Members of the Canadian Association of Paediatric Surgeons (CAPS): Michael Allen, Toronto; Phil Ashmore, Vancouver; Harvey Beardmore, Montreal; Gordon Cameron, Hamilton; Pierre-Paul Collin, Montreal; Jean Desjardins, Montreal; Jacques Ducharme, Montreal; Fred Duval, Winnipeg; James Fallis, Toronto; Colin Ferguson, Winnipeg; Alex Gillis, Halifax; Frank Guttman, Montreal; Angus Juckes, Regina; Gordon Karn, Montreal; Richard Kennedy, St John's; Murray Kliman, Vancouver; Sam Kling, Edmonton; Russelly Marshall, Vancouver; Stanley Mercer, Ottawa; David Murphy, Sr., Montreal; Herbert Owen, Montreal; Barry Shandling, Toronto; Israel Shragovitch, Montreal; James Simpson, Toronto; Clinton Stephens, Toronto; Stuart Thomson; Toronto, Jacques Turcot, Quebec City and President of the Royal College of Physicians and Surgeons (RCPS) of Canada. An ad hoc Executive Committee under Dr Harvey Beardmore was elected to develop a constitution and by-laws, English and French names of the group, a federal charter, banking arrangements, and aims and objectives for the new organisation.[1]

On January 18, 1968, the first organisational (business) meeting was held at The Royal York Hotel in Toronto. A constitution was discussed and the first President (Dr Harvey Beardmore) and Secretary (Dr Barry Shandling) were elected (Fig. 1). It was decided that the English name would be "The Canadian Association of Paediatric Surgeons"; after extensive correspondence with The Quebec Ministry of Cultural Affaires, the French name chosen was "*L'Association Canadienne de Chirurgie Infantile*". This was subsequently changed to "*L'Association Canadienne de Chirurgie Pédiatrique*". That evening, the first banquet of the Founding Members was held (Fig. 2).[1]

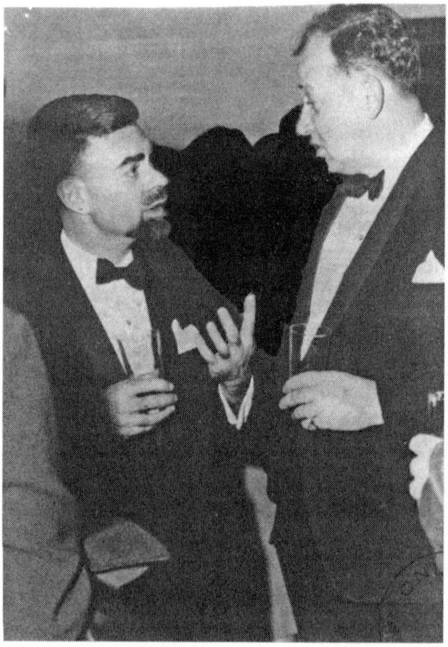

Fig. 1. First Secretary-Treasurer, Dr Barry Shandling and the first President, Dr Harvey Beardmore.

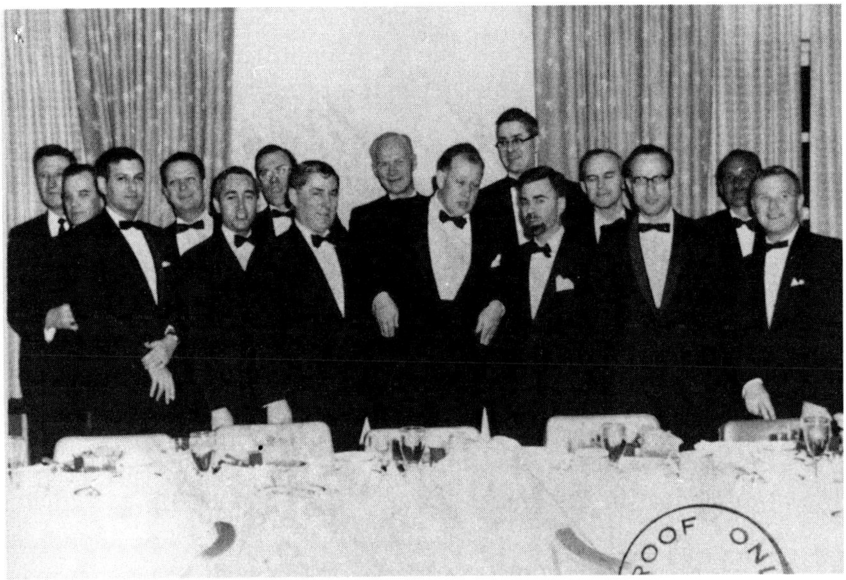

Fig. 2. First Banquet of Founding Members, in Toronto, January 18, 1968. Left to right: Herb Owen, Montreal; Fred DuVal, Winnipeg; Frank Guttman, Montreal; Sam Kling, Edmonton; Jean Desjardins, Montreal; John Burrington, Toronto; Pierre-Paul Collin, Montreal; Clint Stephens, Toronto; Harvey Beardmore (President), Montreal; Jim Fallis, Toronto; Barry Shandling (Secretary-Treasurer), Toronto; Gordon Cameron, Hamilton; Alex Gillis, Halifax; Dick Kennedy, St John's; Stan Mercer, Ottawa.

The objective of CAPS "was to improve the surgical care of infants and children in Canada".[1] "Its areas of interest include all aspects of general and thoracic paediatric surgery with recognition of its unique responsibility to infants born with congenital anomalies and children with malignancies. While its responsibility to paediatric trauma is not unique, it assumes a pivotal role in issues related to paediatric trauma".[2]

On April 3, 1968, the charter was obtained from The Federal (Canadian) Government and the Charter Members received their CAPS Membership.[1] There are five categories of members:

1. **Active** (General, Regular) **Member**: He/she must hold a Certificate of Special Competence in Paediatric General Surgery of

The Royal College of Physicians and Surgeons (RCPS) of Canada, or hold an acceptable equivalent from another country; demonstrate a continuing special interest and competence in the surgical care of infants and children, and must continue to maintain a practice of Paediatric Surgery in Canada. Presently (December 2008) there are 51 Active Members.

2. **Associate Member**: He/she must be non-resident in Canada and have received a substantial portion of their Paediatric Surgical training in Canada; Canadian citizens trained in Paediatric Surgery outside of Canada and the United States; spent at least one year in a Canadian Paediatric Surgical Centre without a Paediatric Surgery Training Program, and Paediatric Surgeons who trained outside of Canada but hold a Certificate of Special Competence in Paediatric Surgery from the RCPS of Canada and are in active Paediatric Surgical practice. These members are ineligible to hold office or serve on Council. This guarantees that CAPS will always be in the hands of Canadians, a topic that was hotly debated during the early years of The Association. There are now 80 Associate Members.
3. **Life Member**: A member who has reached 65 years or has retired from active practice. Such members must apply for Life Membership. Presently there are 38 Life Members.
4. **Honorary Member**: This is granted to those people who have given distinguished service to CAPS, such as visiting lecturers, outstanding guests, visitors and dignitaries to the annual CAPS meeting.[4] By far, the largest number of Honorary Memberships belong to the "*Journal of Pediatric Surgery*" (JPS)/Fred MacLeod Lecturers. On January 23, 1974, at the 6th Annual Business Meeting, it was announced by Dr Colin Ferguson (President of CAPS) that major donors to the Education Fund would be also given Honorary Membership in CAPS. There are presently 45 Honorary Members.
5. **Candidate Member**: These are trainees in Canadian Pediatric Surgical Training Programs or Canadian citizens training in approved Pediatric Surgical Training Programs outside Canada.

On August 20, 1968, Dr Harvey Beardmore received the following letter of incorporation from the law firm Zimmerman and Winters, Toronto: "We submit the following report with respect to the incorporation and organisation of The Canadian Association of Paediatric Surgeons — *L'Association Canadienne de Chirurgie Infantile*. The Association was incorporated ... by letters patent dated the 3rd day of April, 1968. ... In our opinion The Association was duly organised on May 28, 1968. The Board of Directors of The Association consists of six directors of whom three form a quorum for the transaction of business ... The directors and officers of The Association are as follows: Directors: Drs Phillip G. Ashmore, Harvery E. Beardmore, Gordon S. Cameron, Pierre-Paul Collin, Daniel Alexander Gillis, Barry Shandling; Officers: President — Dr Harvey E. Beardmore, Secretary — Dr Barry Shandling ... The Board of Directors may by resolution from time to time admit to membership in The Association persons, societies or companies interested in furthering the objects of The Association. Such a person, society or company may be admitted to membership as a sustaining member or as a general member ... Each sustaining member is required to pay to The Association an annual fee of $25 ... Each general member is required to pay to The Association an annual fee of $10 ... At all meetings of The Association, each member is entitled to one vote ... A seal was obtained for The Association on its incorporation". At the 2007 spring teleconference, CAPS Council ratified the annual fees to be $300, when paid up to January 31 of the meeting year.

Dr Gordon Karn (who had an interest in heraldry) designed the CAPS coat-of-arms (Fig. 3), which was approved by the Royal College of Heraldry in Great Britain: the red and purple colours are also the same colours of the RCPS of Canada and represent the arterial and venous blood met in surgery. The scalpel with the healing serpent of Aesculapius and the figure of a well child combine to symbolise the practice of paediatric surgery. The crest on top is the Canadian Maple Leaf and the founding date (1967) of CAPS. The motto is a quotation in French from Ambroise Paré, a father of modern surgery: "*Je Le Pensay; Dieu Le Guarit*" "I treat him;

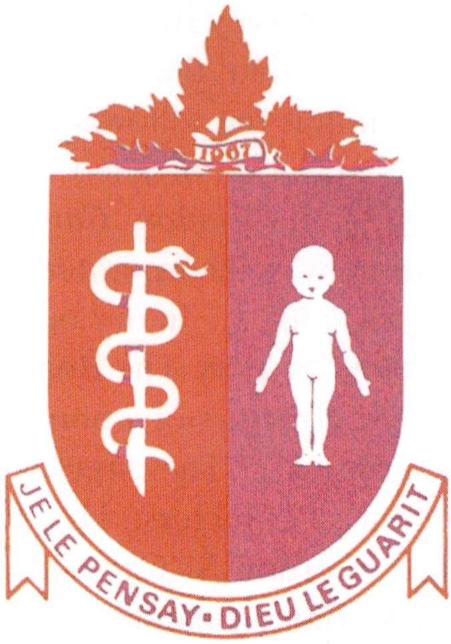

Fig. 3. Canadian Association of Paediatric Surgeons: Coat of Arms designed by Dr Gordon Karn.

God heals him".[1] At the First Annual Meeting on January 22, 1969: "Dr Beardmore then accepted a copy of the proposed crest of The Canadian Association of Paediatric Surgeons together with the motto. Dr Russell Marshall moved that this be adopted as the official crest of The Association. This motion was seconded by Dr Samuel Kling and carried unanimously".

This new coat-of-arms (insignia, logo, crest) held by a wide red ribbon, (to which was added a handsome gold chain, a gift from the British Association of Paediatric Surgeons in 1992) also became the Presidential badge worn proudly throughout each meeting and at other formal Pediatric Surgical functions. Upon handing the Presidential badge over to the new CAPS President every two years at the Annual CAPS Meeting, the new President hands a similar but smaller Past-President's badge on a smaller red ribbon to the outgoing President (who becomes the Immediate Past-President).

At the first Annual CAPS Meeting on January 22, 1969, Dr Colin Ferguson "then took the floor and spoke about the advisability of instituting a paediatric surgical fellowship of The Royal College of

Surgeons. He suggested that a brief be presented to the RCPS of Canada by spring in preparation for the council meeting in June". In 1971, the entire membership resolved that CAPS approve the establishment of a Specialty Certification in Canadian Paediatric Surgery. In February 1973, CAPS finally submitted a second draft: "A Proposal for the Establishment of Paediatric Surgery in Canada as a Specialty within the Specialty of General Surgery" to the RCPS of Canada, from The CAPS Liasion Committee chaired by Dr Ferguson and signed by Drs Beardmore and Mercer.[3]

Concern about the growing number of specialities in the 1970s was first expressed at the RCPS of Canada Council Meeting of January 1974. Moreover, the RCPS of Canada also was concerned that additional specialties would bring about further fragmentation, administrative strangulation and so weakening the College and impending the preservation of unity.[4] This was probably the major concern! Therefore, a committee was formed "to develop a policy for the recognition of new specialties". The committee's suggested guidelines for the recognition of a new specialty was approved by the RCSP of Canada Council in June 1975. Fortunately for CAPS, their application included virtually everyone of the committee's 12 suggested guidelines, so their application was easily approved. The first exam for paediatric surgery was held on November 22, 1976 in Ottawa and the senior author's certificate on that date was number 11, signed by: Dr Robert B. Salter, President; Dr James H. Graham, Secretary; Dr Neil Watters, Chairman, Committee in General Surgery; and Dr Clinton A. Stephens, Chairman, Committee in Paediatric General Surgery; all of the RCSP of Canada. With this Speciality Certification in Canadian Paediatric Surgery, it is impossible to become a member of CAPS and practice pediatric surgery in Canada, without first demonstrating special competence in paediatric surgery by passing this examination.

On June 18, 1969, Dr Harvey Beardmore sent a letter to the CAPS Membership: "Your secretary and I met with The Royal College and we were very enthusiastically received by them as representatives of our new association. We were offered two half days of Paediatric Surgery at the next College meeting in January, 1970, to be held in Montreal and plans are underway to make our "formal" debut as successful as humanly possible. You will be hearing from the Programme Chairman and his committee in the near future, inviting papers".

Also on June 18, 1969, Dr Beardmore sent another letter to the CAPS Membership: "Our relations with the Canadian Paediatric Society are very satisfactory. The President of the CAPS has been invited to present a paper on Paediatric Surgery to a plenary session at their forthcoming meeting in Montreal in July, 1969, and the Canadian Paediatric Society has offered a main speaker to our annual meetings with transportation and accommodation paid by themselves".

It is interesting to note that in spite of the above two good intentions and suggestions of Dr Beardmore, both academic relationships have dissolved.

The Nominating Committee is composed of: The Immediate Past-President as Chair, three Active Members elected from the Membership and one chosen by the Chair. Sixty days before the Annual Meeting, they submit a slate of President, President-Elect, Secretary — Treasurer, 3 Directors, and three members of the Nominating Committee. At the Annual Meeting, the Secretary — Treasurer presents this slate of nominees together with any further nominations received from the membership.

The President holds office for two years, preceded by one year on the CAPS Council as President-Elect and followed by two years as the Immediate Past-President. There have been 20 Presidents of CAPS up to December 2008.

The Secretary-Treasurer is really both the central nervous and musculo-skeletal systems and life blood of CAPS. He/she usually holds office for five years, and is really responsible for running the entire organisation year-round, including the finances, (now also managed by an outside accounting firm). Upon completion of the office, the Secretary-Treasurer is the recipient of a gold lapel pin, the size of which is recognition of inverse proportion to the 24–7 effort. There have been eight CAPS Secretary-Treasurers up to December, 2008.

The Executive consists of the President, Immediate Past-President, Secretary-Treasurer, Director 3rd Year, Director 2nd Year, Director 1st Year, (each appointed in a staggered fashion). The Council consists of the Executive and the President-Elect (chosen during the President's second year in office), Chairs of all Committees (Archives, Bilingual, Constitution and Bylaws, Education and Research, Ethics and Legal, Membership and Credentials, Nominating, Program, Publication, and Trauma, as well as Chairs of the following Specialty Committees: Specialty Committee in Paediatric Surgery of the RCPS of Canada; (which includes the Program Director of each of the 7 (as of December 2008) Canadian Training Programs in Paediatric Surgery and liaison with the American College of Surgeons Pediatric Surgery Committee). The Program and Publication Committees are probably the most important since they decide upon the Scientific Program (and its subsequent publication) of each Annual CAPS Meeting. The Chairs and members of each committee are chosen by the President and Secretary-Treasurer for a three to five year term.

From its inception, CAPS has recognized the importance of education. Therefore, it was decided early to establish an Education Fund, to better achieve its responsibility to education for issues related to paediatric surgery, and in so doing, realise the goals of CAPS. The Fund was established (and continues to exist) through the generosity of donations from medical and non-medical individuals and groups interested in the surgical care of children. It was largely due to the efforts of Drs Colin Ferguson and Jim Simpson that this became a valuable resource. The initial purpose of the Fund was to bring to Canada distinguished paediatric surgeons to participate in the Annual CAPS Meeting, and, if possible, to also travel to some Canadian centres for lectures and teaching the latest concepts and techniques in the art and science of paediatric surgery. To achieve this goal, an annual lectureship was established through the efforts of Dr Jim Simpson. On January 23, 1974, at the 6th Annual CAPS Business Meeting in Montreal, the President Dr Colin Ferguson announced "a very generous donation in the amount of $7500 given by Mr Fred G. MacLeod in the hope to set up an annual lectureship ... known as The MacLeod lecture or The Fred G. MacLeod lecture". Mr Fred MacLeod was a close friend of Dr Jim Simpson and was a Northern Ontario gold miner and prospector who "struck it rich".[5]

Dr Ferguson had also been instrumental in obtaining a donation of $6000 from the Paterson Foundation in Winnipeg, also for educational purposes, in support of CAPS. The list of Visiting Professors from 1969 until the present, sponsored by the Education Fund, reads like a "Who's Who" in paediatric surgery (and other equally famous doctors) locally, nationally and internationally. When the MacLeod Lectureship funds became depleted in 2002, negotiations between the Meeting Coordinator (Arlene Ein) and Dr Jay Grosfeld, Editor of the "*Journal of Pediatric Surgery*" (JPS) enabled JPS to help sponsor this Lectureship, which became known thereafter as the JPS/Fred MacLeod Lecture. Some other endeavors of the Education Fund (which is now called the Education and Research Committee) include: visits of CAPS Members to various centres; sending Chief Residents in paediatric surgery to work in other countries for a few weeks/months, as part of their training in paediatric surgery; supporting the making of instructional media; CAPSNET (a national cooperative effort to generate the best data upon which Canadian paediatric surgeons can make decisions which will affect treatment of all paediatric surgical patients), to name a few.

When CAPS was established in 1967, there were only three Canadian Paediatric Surgery Training Programs: Montreal Children's Hospital (MCH) (established in 1953), St Justine Hospital for Children (Montreal, 1964), and the Hospital for Sick Children (HSC) (Toronto, 1967). As of December 2008, there are five more Training Programs fully accredited by the RCPS of Canada and the Association of Pediatric Surgery Training Program Directors (APSTPD): British Columbia (BC) Children's Hospital (Vancouver, 1986), Children's Hospital of Eastern Ontario (CHEO) (Ottawa, 1987), Issak Walton Killam Hospital for Children (IWK) (Halifax, 1988), Alberta Children's Hospital (Calgary, 2004) and M'Master Children's Hospital (Hamilton, 2008). These eight Programs train from two paediatric surgery residents (Fellows) every year, to one every other year. Since the 1990's, there have been about 50 paediatric surgeons practicing annually across Canada, with an annual requirement for about 2–3 new Pediatric Surgeons. The above eight Canadian Pediatric Surgery Training Programs graduate about five fully trained paediatric surgeons annually, but only two to three are Canadian, and not all of these graduates stay in Canada. This certainly is not "flooding" either the Canadian and/or American paediatric surgery markets, as has been suggested at times by the APSTPD. The support of CAPS continues to be an important ingredient in this ongoing North American debate over the last several decades, since it first raised its ugly head in the late 1980's when Dr Alex Gillis was Chair of the above Speciality Committee in Paediatric Surgery of the RCPS of Canada.

It is generally agreed that the "*Journal of Pediatric Surgery*" (JPS) is the premier journal of paediatric surgery in the English-speaking world. In 1979, Dr Stephen Gans, the founder and 2nd Editor, (after Dr C. Everett Koop), agreed that JPS would be the official journal of CAPS, as it was (at that time) for the other North American and British Paediatric Surgical Associations. Dr Gans wrote in his editorial: "The fact that it (CAPS) is now a viable, healthy, and mature organisation with much to add to the international literature led to the formation of this new partnership. We look forward to a long period of mutual contribution to development, research, education, and practice in the field of pediatric surgery".[6] According to the arrangements made with JPS, the papers presented at the Annual CAPS Meeting are reviewed by the CAPS Publication Committee before being submitted for publication in JPS.

To say that the Annual Meeting is the highlight of CAPS is really an understatement; it is really the heart-beat that has kept CAPS alive. The first Annual Clinical Meeting was held on January 22, 1969 in Vancouver (Fig. 4). Since CAPS initially was more closely aligned with the Royal College of Physicians and Surgeons (RCPS) of Canada than the Canadian Paediatric Society (CPS), the Annual Meeting was originally held in January coinciding with the RCPS Meeting, which was almost exclusively held in the larger Canadian cities like: Vancouver, Montreal, Ottawa, Toronto, Edmonton, Winnipeg, Quebec City and

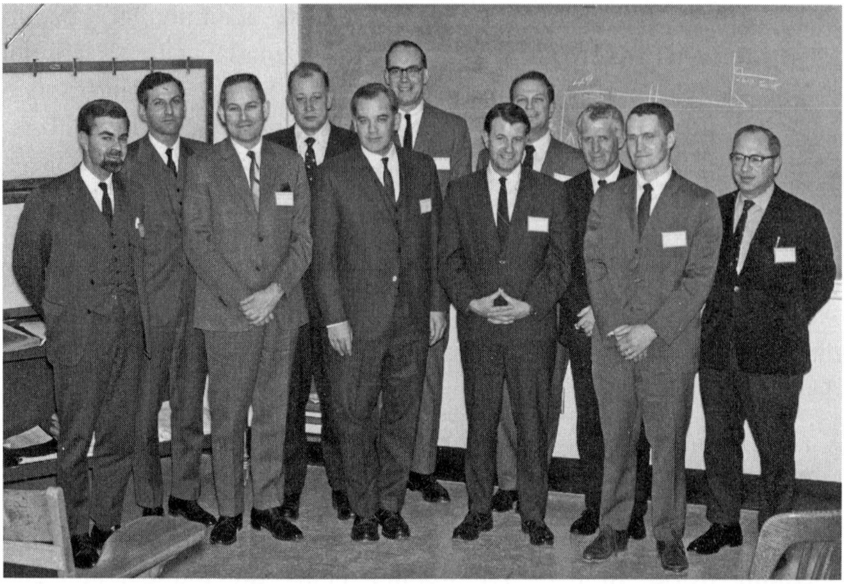

Fig. 4. The first Annual Clinical Meeting, in Vancouver, January 22, 1969. Left to right: Barry Shandling, Toronto; Frank Guttman, Montreal; Don Marshall, London; Harvey Beardmore, Montreal; Fred DuVal, Winnipeg; Phil Ashmore, Vancouver; Graham Fraser, Vancouver; Sam Kling, Edmonton; Russ Marshall, Vancouver; Angus Juckes, Regina; Murray Kliman, Vancouver.

Calgary. In 1986, the 18th CAPS Meeting was held in Halifax and four years later, the 22nd meeting was held in St John's, not in association with either the RCPS or CPS. The CAPS Membership had grown tired of being an appendage of the RCPS Meeting, (which required a second registration fee from CAPS Members, as well as a fee to submit an academic paper) and it was quite apparent that bilateral interest between CAPS and the other specialties (that made up the very large RCPS meeting) was at a low level of mutual disinterest. Moreover, there was an intense desire by CAPS Members to visit smaller, but beautiful areas throughout Canada where paediatric surgery was also being practiced. Finally, it was easy to decide that the Annual Meeting would be even better attended by CAPS Members, their families and our national and international guests and visitors, if it were held between the late Summer (August) and early Fall (September, October).

With this decision, CAPS was on its way to becoming its own boss and directing its own future and style of meeting. Since our 22nd Meeting in St John's, the following locations have provided memorable settings for the subsequent Annual CAPS Meetings: Québec City, Ottawa, Victoria, Toronto, Cheribourg (Québec), Halifax, Banff, Montreal, Montebello (Québec), Vancouver, Niagara-on-the-lake, Winnipeg, and Saskatoon (scheduled for 2010).

The Annual Meeting schedule includes a Council Meeting on Thursday, a Welcome Reception Thursday evening, Scientific Sessions (including a Poster Session) Friday and Saturday, the Annual Business Meeting Saturday afternoon, the Presidential Dinner on Saturday evening, and a third and final Scientific Session Sunday. The 2007 meeting at St John's, was the 39th Annual CAPS Meeting and the 40th Anniversary; there was an excellent clinical program with 39 papers and 15 posters. There were 164 registrants: 34% from out of Canada (35 United States, and 16 outside North America), and the attendance consisted of 50 Regular Members, 21 Associate Members, 82 Resident/Fellow/Nurses, two Life Members and nine Founding Members. During the Scientific Sessions of the CAPS Meeting, there has always been (and indeed continues to be) a major attempt to encourage a free and honest interchange of ideas, no matter how controversial. The CAPS Meeting has always prided itself on being a mostly clinical meeting for both practicing academic and non-academic paediatric surgeons (the so-called silent majority). For that reason, there have always been a minimal number of research papers. It is thus no real surprise that the Annual CAPS Meeting has been described as possibly the best Clinical Paediatric Surgical meeting in North America. This is also in part due to the small attendance and large clinical discussion. As a matter of fact, one of the outstanding benefits of the Annual CAPS Meeting is that the lively and at times outspoken discussion is not published by JPS. A prime example of the latter was the discussion after Dr Donny Marshall presented (informally) his first three cases of peritoneal drainage for preemies with perforated necrotising enterocolitis, on a cold 1975 January day in Winnipeg at the 7th Annual CAPS Meeting. Moreover, what other major international paediatric surgery meeting would dare to have a one hour panel discussion between four senior paediatric surgeons (the President and 3 Life Members), four paediatric surgery residents and the audience? Not only was this very popular, but the CAPS 39th Annual Meeting (40th Anniversary Meeting) ended on a high note with a paper entitled: "Ten Things We Knew 'For Sure' 50 Years Ago," which was an historical discussion between a father and son: Dr Gordon Cameron (a CAPS Founding member) and Dr Brian Cameron (a next generation paediatric surgeon).

The new fledgling Canadian Association of Paediatric Surgery Nurses has also been meeting in association with CAPS for the last few years since its recent inception. This, as well as all of the CAPS meeting activities have been increasingly better organised and coordinated ever since Arlene Ein initially became involved with the Annual CAPS Meeting and soon thereafter became the first Meeting Coordinator in 1990. As with the job of the Secretary-Treasurer, the Meeting Coordinator's task is virtually year-round, not only helping to plan the upcoming meeting, but also planning for the next two or three Annual Meetings that many years in advance. Her experience as a former operating room nurse, being married to a paediatric surgeon, and her involvement with Variety, the Children's Charity, have made her a most valuable and experienced resource for the CAPS Meeting, as well as allowing the local host to actually attend the Meeting. She has instituted many changes in and around the Meeting, including obtaining financial support from 5 to 15 sponsors annually, which has also contributed to the awards for the Resident Best Clinical Research Paper, Resident Best Basic Science Research Paper (Dr Maria DiLorenzo Award) and Resident Best Poster (1st and 2nd Prize for each category).

As of the writing of this chapter (December 2008), CAPS is a strong viable, and thriving organisation. There are now more Canadian paediatric surgeons in training than at any time in the past; they are better trained than ever before, and, like their teachers, skilled and dedicated to the ideals of CAPS — to improve the surgical care of infants and children in Canada.[1]

References

1. Shandling B. The Canadian Association of Paediatric Surgeons. In Morley TP (ed.) Medical Specialty Societies of Canada (ed. 1) Associated Medical Services, Toronto 1991, p. 127–36.
2. Annual Meeting Program. The Canadian Association of Paediatric Surgeons. St John's, NFLD, 2007.
3. Ferguson CC, Beardmore HE, Mercer S. A proposal for the establishment of paediatric surgery in Canada as a specialty within the specialty of general surgery from CAPS to RCPS of Canada, 1973.
4. Shephard DAE. The Royal College of Physicians and Surgeons of Canada 1960–1980: The Pursuit of Unity. RCPS of Canada, Ottawa, 1985.
5. Mrs Jo Simpson. Personal Communication, Aug 17, 1992.
6. Gans SL. Editorial, The Canadian Association of Paediatric Surgeons, *J Pediatr Surg* 1979;14:509–10.

EUROPEAN PAEDIATRIC SURGEONS' ASSOCIATION (EUPSA)

Robert Carachi

The EUPSA was a voluntary body which encompassed 28 countries. Its main concern was for the education and development of paediatric surgeons and to exchange views and ideas on paediatric surgical problems. It had no official standing within the Parliament in Brussels. More recently, it has been involved in the organisation of Scientific Programmes. In the past this union has worked in association with UEMS, since many of the Members belong to both groups. It has allowed countries outside the framework of the UEMS to benefit from the discussions on the scope of paediatric surgery and the training programmes as well as certification programmes. It has evolved from its relatively informal status to being a significant organisation of paediatric surgeons with its own mission statement and complex structure. This initiative was introduced by Professor Michael E. Höellwarth.

Mission statement. The European Paediatric Surgeons' Association (EUPSA's) mission statement is to maintain and promote high clinical standards of surgical care for the paediatric and adolescent patients in European countries, to enhance the capacity of its members to discover, disseminate and apply new knowledge to the benefit of their patients, and to follow the highest ethical standards within the field of paediatric surgery.

Goals. The EUPSA aims to achieve its mission through:

1) The promotion of high clinical standards in all fields of paediatric surgery and in all paediatric surgical centres by:

   a) developing outcome measures, which can be used to assess quality standards;
   b) stimulating the exchange of experience and knowledge between National Associations and between paediatric surgical centers;
   c) promoting and supporting individual scholarships and exchange of specialists between hospitals;
   e) organising workshops and operating teaching sessions; and
   e) establishing high quality training standards in European paediatric surgery in close collaboration with the section of the UEMS and related boards.

2) Supporting the discovery of new clinical and research insights which may lead to prevention, treatment and cure of congenital malformations, trauma, and all paediatric surgical diseases:

   a) committees for special fields in paediatric surgery (e.g. trauma, endoscopy, tumour, intensive care);
   b) organisation of the European Congress of Paediatric Surgery;
   c) sponsoring of awards (best paper, best poster, young investigator award, Journal subscription award, etc.);
   d) sponsoring of invited lectures, and lifetime achievement awards; and
   e) sponsoring of international European collaborative research projects.

3) Friendship and fraternity between all members of the Association:

   a) developing feed-back mechanisms to assess members' wishes and satisfaction in regard to the organisation of the congresses as well as to the administration of the Association;

b) regular communication with and between members by a Newsletter;
c) ensuring that the administration of the Association rotates regularly and includes many members of different countries; and
d) enhancing the active participation of young members representing the future generation of leaders within the administration of the Association.

4) The development of an advocacy role for all fields of paediatric surgery in Europe:

a) supporting all activities to educate the public about the role of paediatric surgeons, paediatric surgical diseases and related achievements;
b) mutual exchange with other professionals and Associations, which have an interest in the field of paediatric surgery;
c) promoting European paediatric surgical achievements worldwide; and
d) enhancing liaison with the National Medical Association, government, members of the parliament, and other opinion formers about the role and importance of paediatric surgery in practice and research.

Having started as an informal meeting it has now progressed over the four decades to hold a large annual scientific meeting and the complexity of the organisation has grown in the structure so that now it has developed to a very large complex organisation.

GERMAN ASSOCIATION OF PAEDIATRIC SURGERY (BRD, WEST-GERMANY)

Alexander Holschneider
Kurt Gdanietz

In 1822, the first Session of the "*Gesellschaft Deutscher Naturforscher und Ärzte*" took place in Leipzig. It was founded by Prof Lorenz Oken, Jena. In 1828 in Berlin, the following sections were part of this association: "*Geognosie, Mineralogie, Astronomie, Geophysik, Chemie, Physik, Botanik, Zoologie, Anatomie, Physiologie*, and *General Medicine*". In the 1850's and 60's surgery was separated from internal medicine, but only in 1875 did paediatrics became an independent speciality. For paediatric surgery in Germany this period took much longer until 1984.

For the *Bundesrepublik* (West-Germany) Prof Dr Anton Oberniedermayr founded 1957 together with Fritz Rehbein (Bremen), Priv Doz Werner von Ekesparre (Hamburg-Duvenstedt), Prof Dr Waldemar Hecker (Munich-Haunersches), Prof Heinz Singer (Munich-Schwabing), Prof Andreas Flach (Tübingen) and Prof Wolfgang Maier (Karlsruhe) and others the "*Arbeitsgemeinschaft Deutscher Kinderchirurgen*" inside the German Association of Surgeons which became in 1963 "*Die Deutsche Gesellschaft für Kinderchirurgie*". In 1972 a professional organisation "*Berufsverband der Kinderchirurgen Deutschlands*" was founded too. In 1977 this professional organisation became a section "*Teilgebiet*" of the professional organisation of the general surgeons. Only in 1967 did paediatric surgery became a clinical section of adult surgery as well and in 1984 finally, an independent speciality. In 1990 the members of the Association of Paediatric Surgeons of the DDR became members of the German Association of Paediatric Surgery.[1–4]

Today (2006) there are 83 departments of paediatric surgery in the BRD (having 81 Mill inhabitants) with 5–83 beds, and 23 Units have 40 or more surgical beds for children. Of these 83 departments, 29 are situated at universities, and 54 at communal or charity hospitals. In January 2001[5] there were 338 paediatric surgeons registered, about 58 settled down as paediatric surgical practitioners, seven were practitioners with cottage-hospital affiliation, 41 did not work as medical doctors, and 239 worked in paediatric surgical units. For further details see website of the German Association of Paediatric Surgery: www.dgkic.de.

The training in paediatric surgery lasts today six years: two years of common trunk training, one year of paediatrics and three years of paediatric surgery. It is finished by an oral exit examination.

Honours of the German Association of Paediatric Surgery

In 1962, the German Association of Paediatric Surgery introduced a lecture to honour Prof Anton Oberniedermayr (1899–1986) which was held every other year. In 1962 a scientific award was founded, the Richard Drachter (1883–1936) award, and a medal to honour Prof Fritz Rehbein (1911–1991). In addition, a special award for Paediatric Urology was introduced, the John–Herbie–Johnston prize. Finally, the Academie for Paediatric Surgery of the German Association for Paediatric Surgery introduced a special award to encourage the rising generation of paediatric surgical scientists, the Ilse Krause (1917–1984) award.

References

1. Windorfer A. 100 Jahre Deutsche Gesellschaft für Kinderheilkunde. *Der Kinderarzt* 1983;14:888–892.

2. Hecker WCh, Witt D. Die Entwicklung der Kinderheilkunde zum selbständigen Fachgebiet. *Der Kinderarzt* 1977;8:1414–1631.
3. Hecker WCh. Die historische Entwicklung der Kinderchirurgie in Deutschland. *Der Kinderarzt* 1979;10:91–94.
4. Hecker WCh. Kinderchirurgie an der Universität. *Der Kinderarzt* 1981;12:1345–1350.
5. Holschneider AM. Pediatric Surgical Reality in Germany and Visions for the Future. *Eur J Pediatr Surg* 2001;11:75–81.

MEDITERRANEAN ASSOCIATION OF PEDIATRIC SURGEONS (MAPS)

Ahmed Hadidi

The Mediterranean Association was established in 1997 by a group of eminent Pediatric Surgeons from the Mediterranean countries who regularly met each other every year in the British and American Annual congresses. It was felt that there is a lot in common among the Mediterranean countries. The Mediterranean people share the same race, social habits and climate. There are many pediatric conditions that are rather endemic in the Mediterranean area.

The first International congress was held in Cairo, Egypt in 1997 where the association is registered as a charity non-profitable organisation. The President was the late **Prof Nabhan Kaddah**, Head of Pediatric Surgery, Cairo University and the secretary General is **Prof Ahmed Hadidi**.

The MAPS executive board committee was established with the following members: **Prof Dr J.-M. Guys** (France), **Prof Dr A. Hadidi** (Egypt), **Prof Dr V. Jassoni** (Italy), **Prof Dr N. Kaddah** (Egypt), **Prof Dr D. Keramidas** (Greece), **Prof Dr L. Siplovich** (Israel), **Prof Dr J. Tovar** (Spain) and **Prof Dr D. Yeker** (Turkey).

Several new members joined the MAPS since its establishment to accommodate almost all the Mediterranean countries including Croatia, Romania, Lebanon, Syria, Libya, Tunisia, Algeria and Morocco.

The current Executive board members include: **Prof Dr J.-M. Guys** (France), **Prof Dr A. Hadidi** (Egypt), Prof **Dr V. Jassoni** (Italy), **Prof Dr A. Nouri** (Tunisia), **Prof Dr L. Siplovich** (Israel),

Prof Dr Vicenç Martinez Ibanez (Spain), **Prof Dr C. Büyükünal** (Turkey) and **Prof Dr D. Zavitzanakis** (Greece).

The Mediterranean Association has already held six successful international meetings:

1) Cairo, Egypt, in October 1997;
2) Genoa, Italy, in October 1998;
3) Corfu, Greece, in October 2000;
4) Izmir, Turkey, in June 2002;
5) Marseille, France, in October, 2004; and
6) Barcelona, Spain, in October, 2006.

The next international meeting of MAPS is due to be held in Tunisia in October 2008.

All these meetings had a large international participation with contribution from all the five continents. World wide experts in pediatric surgery have actively contributed to the success of these meetings and the participation from the Mediterranean countries has been gradually increasing over the years.

Objectives

The objectives of the Association are to serve the children of the Mediterranean Area:

1) to act as an international forum of the Mediterranean pediatric surgeons;
2) to promote the practice, research and the advancement of study in pediatric surgery;
3) to promote and maintain the highest clinical and ethical standards;
4) to encourage and arrange regular meetings for the interchange of ideas and sharing of knowledge and experts; and
5) to foster professional relations with pediatric surgeons throughout the world.

Membership

Mediterranean members. Any fully trained pediatric surgeon who is registered as a medical practitioner with the registering body of their country of practice is eligible for memberschip, provided that:

1) their professional practice is confined to the practice of pediatric surgery or largely engaged in pediatric surgical practice or made a special contribution to pediatric surgery; and
2) the nature of their practice is such as to give them special interest in the subject of pediatric surgery.

Non-mediterranean members. Fully qualified surgeons engaged in pediatric surgery outside the mediterranean area.

Honorary members. Surgeons or others who have made outstanding contributions to pediatric surgery.

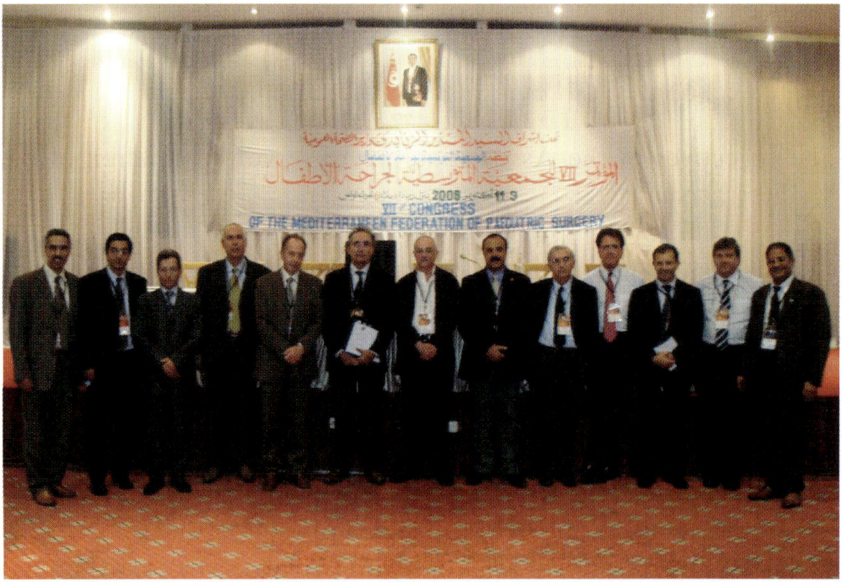

Fig. 1. MAPS meeting in Tripoli 2008.

Senior members. Former ordinary or non-mediterranean members elected on their retirement from active practice.

Associate members.

1) consultants in related specialties other than surgery; and
2) registrars or equivalent trainees in pediatric surgery, general surgery or other surgical specialties.

Candidates for membership are elected by majority vote of the Executive Committee of the Association.

The Mediterranean Association has an active website which contains all relevant information about the association (www.MAPS97.com) (Fig. 1).

PACIFIC ASSOCIATION OF PEDIATRIC SURGEONS (PAPS)

Takeshi Miyano
John R. Campbell

PAPS was bom in I968 with Stephen L. Gans. M.D. (Figure 1) as the attending midwife, drawing its members from those pediatric surgeons living and practicing Pediatric Surgery within the Pacific Rim. The Pacific rim covers a very large area, including the western parts of North and South America, the many Southeast Asian countries and also Australia and New Zealand. Consequently, its membership come from a variety of diverse cultures and background. In the United States candidates for membership must reside west of the continental divide, i.e. those areas that drain into the Pacific Ocean. John R. Campbell (Figure 2) re-told its embryonic period at the 2007 meeting in Queenstown, N, Z. on the occasion of the 40th Anniversary of the founding of this association as follows.[1] Stephen Gans recorded the original thinking and motivation to form this association which now reside in the archives of PAPS.[2]

To Whom it May Concern:

This letter is to explain the background and development for the incorporation of the Journal of Pediatric Surgery as a non-profit Corporation under the laws of the State of California.

In 1966. I initiated steps in organization of the "Western Association of Pediatric Surgery," which was originally intended to be a regional society composed of members in the western states of the United States. In order to save time, complications,

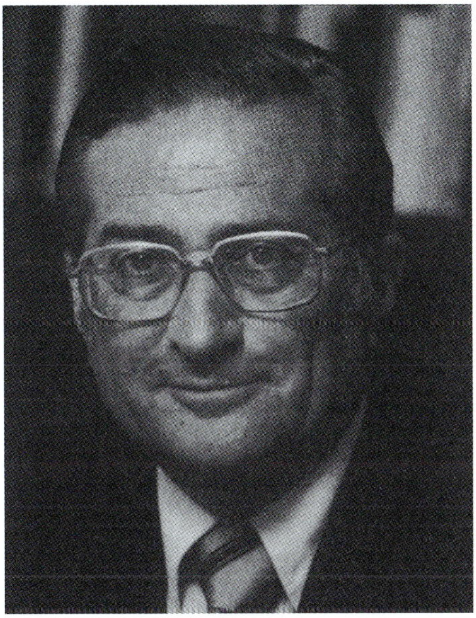

Fig. 1. Stephen L. Gans

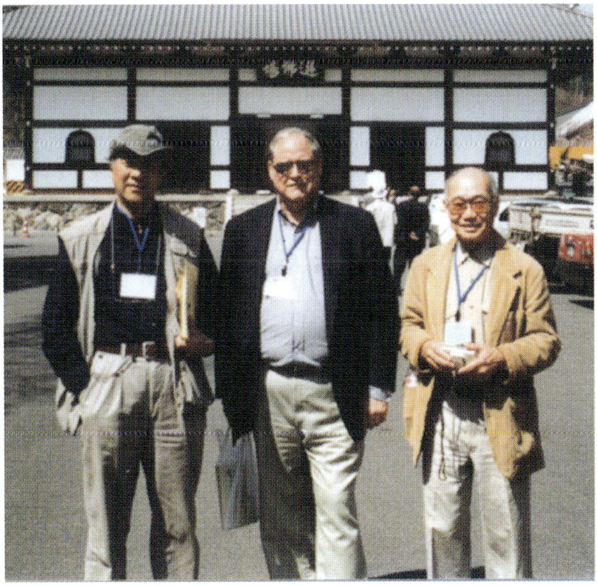

Fig. 2. (L-R.) Takeshi Miyano, John R. Campbell, Walton K.T Shim at PAPS 2001 Meeting in Kyoto, Japan

> and money, I asked the attorneys to change the name of the original corporation to the "Western Association of Pediatric Surgeons," Instead of starting all over again with a new corporation, which they did.
>
> In 1967, an organizational meeting was held in San Francisco, and there it was decided that the name of the organization should he the "Pacific Association of Pediatric Surgeons." Again, 1 asked the attorneys to change the name and this was done with an amendment to the Articles of Incorporation which is also hereby enclosed. Now, the corporation became active and the attorneys prepared the new constitution and by-laws according to the outline and ideas submitted to him by the original organizing committee. He obtained exemption from the Internal Revenue Service for the corporation and also obtained exemption from the Franchise Tax Board in California. He registered the Pacific Association of Pediatric Surgeons with the California Department of Charitable Trust in 1968. All of these activities have been duly kept in a Pacific Associations of Pediatric Surgeons file in the office of the attorneys. Smith und Wilson In Los Angels, California."

After a period of fermentation in the mind of Steve Gans, initial discussion started in 1967 When Sieve Gans recruited Irving "Bud" Meeker to fly with him from Los Angels to San Francisco, California, to meet with Pieter deVries. According to Pieter deVries (Figure 3), Steve. Gans' proposal was to form an association not only only of Pediatric Surgeons who resided within the Pacific Rim, but prominent Pediatric Surgeons from outside of that area, such as his friend, C. Everett Koop. Steve Gans initially wanted to call it the Western Association of Pediatric Surgeons (WAPS). Pieter deVries wanted the association to be smaller, more informal, and to be more specific, a forum where complicated clinical problems could be discussed in detail and guidance offered by west coast colleagues. Pieter deVries summarized this meeting by sayings "Steve was an organizational person, and I was more interested in the daily practice of Pediatric Surgery."[3] Bud Meeker sided wish Pieter deVries

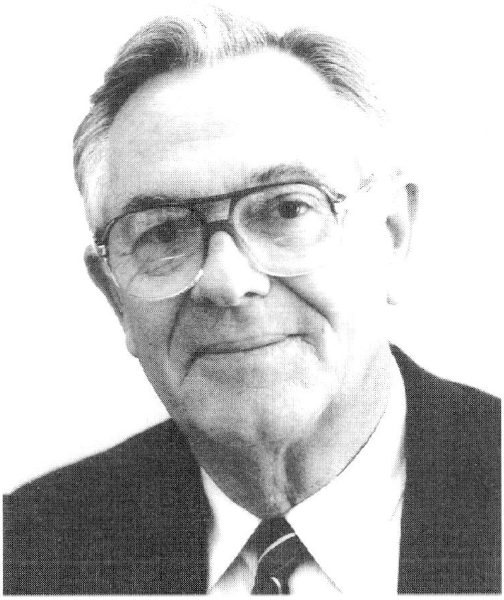

Fig. 3. Pieter A. deVries

and the decision was made to call the association PAPS, rather than WAPS, and to restrict membership to Pediatric Surgeons who lived within the Pacific Rim,

At the same time, there was a growing interest in an international Asian society among Japancsc Pediatric Surgeons, especially by Dr Keijira Suruga (Figure 4). He is undoubtedly considered the prime Asian Contributing to the organization of, and the driving force behind, PAPS in Asia. During the 1960's, he frequently attended the British Association of Pediatric Surgeons (BAPS) meetings, which at that time had the largest number of international participants at any pediatric surgical meeting. It was during a BAPS meetings that Dr Suruga realized that there ware very few, if any Pediatric Surgeons who resided within the Pacific rim attending BAPS meetings. Because of this lack of geographical representation. Dr Suruga flew to Los Angeles to visit with Stephen Gans to discuss the possibility of forming, a new international organization of Pediatric Surgeons primary made up from countries bordering the

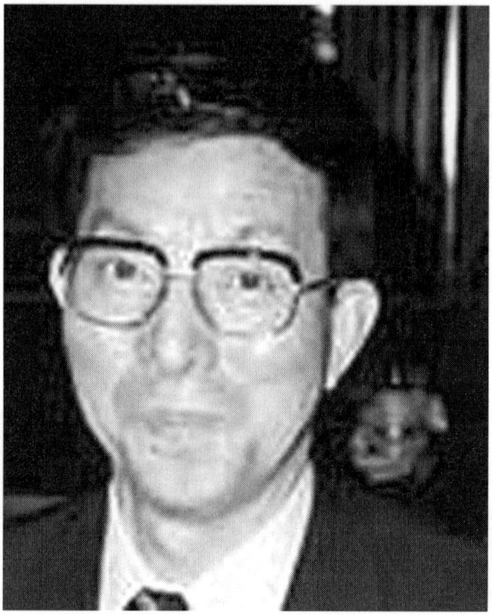

Fig. 4. Keijiro Suruga

Pacific coast. Stephen Gans whole-heartedly agreed and he called Nate Myers (Figure 5), who was the head of division of Pediatric Surgery at the Royal Children's Hospital in Melbourne, to ask for his help and support in garnering interest from Pediatric Surgeons in Australia and New Zealand, and to ask if he would be willing to act as the Australasian organizer, Nate agreed and the three of them proceeded to work on setting up the first inaugural meeting.

Alexander H. "Sandy" Bill (Figure 6) hosted the founding organizing meeting which occurred in 1968 in Seattle, Washington, and then adjourned to Rosario Resort in the San Juan Islands on Orcas Island, Washington, Those attending are shown in Table 1. There, the details of organization were worked out. The original concepts regarding membership in the Pacific Association of Pediatric Surgeons limited membership to those Pediatric Surgeons who lived within the Pacific Rim. For the U.S. that meant those who lived west of the Rocky Mountains — the area that drains into the Pacific Ocean. When members moved east of the Rocky Mountains,

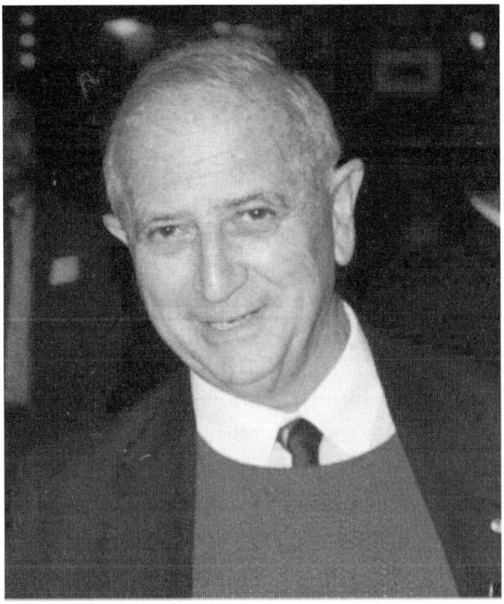

Fig. 5. Nate A. Myers

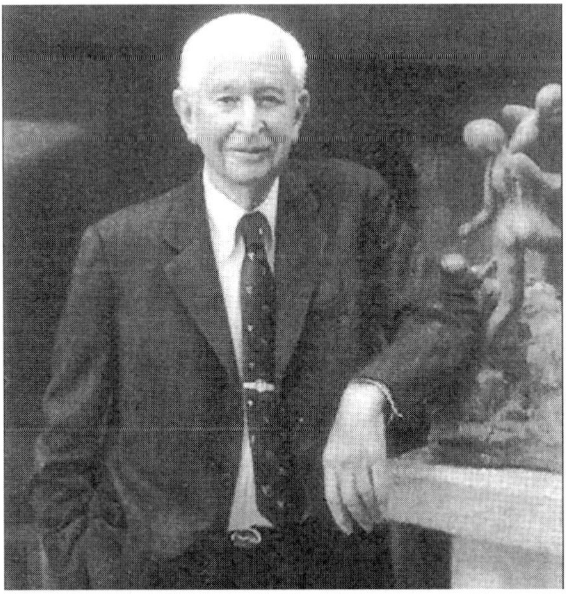

Fig. 6. Alexander H. Bill, Jr.

Table 1. Pediatric Surgeons Attending the Organizing Meeting in 1968 Seattle, Washington, and Orcas Island, Washington, USA.

Stephan L. Gans, Los Angeles, California — Instigator and Organizing Chair
Alexander H. Bill, Jr., Seattle, Washington — Organizing Chair
Phillip G. Ashmore, Vancouver, British Columbia
Chadwick F. Baxter, Spokane, Washington
Jack L. Cahill, Seattle, Washington
Jack R. Campbell, Portland, Oregon
Eric W. Fonkalsrud, Los Angeles, California
Graham C. Fraser, Vancouver, British Columbia
Edward A. Free, Oakland, California
Murray A. Kliman, Vancouver, British Columbia
Jens G. Rosenkrantz, Denver, Colorado
Walton K. T. Shim, Hawaii
John K. Stevenson, Seattle Washington

they maintained their membership, however. These rules were embodied in the concept of keeping the meeting informal so as to encourage frank discussion and to promote social intercourse. Members were free to invite guests. Since venues in the Westerns States were, and still are often limited, guests were invited by a letter to the Organizing Chair requesting the privilege of inviting a guest. An accommodation to this rule was made for meetings in Asia, where large international meetings and invited speakers were what local chairs needed to obtain financial support from their institutions, medical societies, governments and airlines.

The first official meeting of PAPS was held in 1969 at Ojai, California. The founding members are show in Table 2. A complete list of venues and local organizers is shown in Table 3. Presidents, Secretaries and Treasurers are listed in Tables 4–6, Meetings have been held annually without exception. Venues rotated between the west coast of Norih America, Southeast Asian countries, Australia and New Zealand. During the first 20 years, two out of every three meetings were held in North America and Hawaii, the remaining one third taking place in Southeast Asian countries, Australia or

Table 2. Founding Member of the Pacific Association of Pediatric Surgeons.

Stephen Gans — Los Angeles, CA — Instigator	George A. Hyde — San Francisco, CA
Phillip G. Ashmore — Vancouver, BC	Peter Jones — Melbourne, Australia
Chadwick F. Baxter — Spokane, WA	Morio Kasai — Sendai, Japan
Alexander H. Bill Jr. — Seattle, WA	Murray R. Kliman — Vancouver, BC
Patrick L. Brennan — Los Angeles, CA	Lawrence M. Linkner — Phoenix, AZ
John L. Cahill — Seattle, WA	Russell Marshall — Vancouver, BC
John R. Campbell — Portland, OR	Irving A. Meeker, Jr. — Los Angeles, CA
Daniel L. Cloud — Phoenix, AZ	Nate A. Myers — Melbourne, Australia
Douglas Cohen — Sydney, Australia	Jens G. Rosenkrantz — Denver, CO
David L. Collins — San Diego, CA	Lester R. Sauvage — Seattle, WA
Joseph S. David — Orange, CA	Walton K. T. Shim — Honolulu, HI
Alfred A. de Lormier — San Francisco, CA	Durham E. Smith — Australia
Pieter A. De Vries — San Francisco, CA	William H. Snyder, Jr. — Los Angeles, CA
Harry Ditmore — Portland, OR	Jesus Lozoya-Solis — Mexico
Graham C. Frazer — Vancouver, BC	Douglas Stephens — Australia
Edward A. Free — Oakland, CA	John Stevenson — Seattle, WA
Eric W. Fonkalsrud — Los Angeles, CA	Keijiro Suruga — Tokyo, Japan
Lorye Hackworth — Los Angeles, CA	Takashi Ueda — Osaka, Japan
Daniel M. Hays — Los Angeles, CA	Jordan J. Weitzman — Los Angeles, CA
	Mort M. Woolley — Los Angeles, CA

New Zealand. In the last 20 years, they have been held more frequently in Asia than North America, because the proportion of members and participants has increased in Asia, particularly in Japan. A South American venue first occurred in 1979. At the time of this writing PAPS has 411 members representing 22 countries. Japan has the largest number of members with 137 and the United States has the second largest with 126.

The three grandfathers of Pediatric Surgery in North America were William E. Ladd of Boston, Oswald Wyatt of Minneapolis and Herbert E. Coe (Figure 7) of Seattle Washington. PAPS choose to name their honor of Distinction Award, the Coe Medal, after Herbert E. Coe who was the pioneer of Pediatric Surgery in the Western part of United States where PAPS was formed. The Coe Medal Recipients are listed in Table 7.

Table 3. Venues and Organizers.

1968	Founders Organizing Meeting Seattle and Orcas Island, WA, USA	Alexander H. Bill
1969	Ojai CA, USA	Stephen L. Gans Eric W. Fonkalsrud Daniel M. Hayes
1970	Melbourne, VIC, Australia	Nate A. Myers
1971	Hamsun Hot Springs, BC, Canada	Phillip G. Ashmore
1972	Tokyo, Japan	Keijiro Suruga
1973	San Diego, CA, USA	David L. Collins
1974	Salishan OR, USA	Julin R. Campbell
1975	Honolulu, HI, USA	Walton K. T. Shim
1976	Stin Francisco, CA, USA	Alfred A. dc Lorimer
1977	Sydney, NSW, Australia	Douglas Cohen
1978	Osaka. Japan	Takashi Ueda
1979	Mazatlan, Mexico	Rodolfo Franco Vazquez
1980	Colorado Springs, CO, USA	William C. Bailey
1981	Maui, HI, USA	Walton K. T. Shim
1982	Vancouver, BC, Canada	Graham C. Fraser
1983	Fukuoka, Japan	Keiichi Ikeda
1984	San Diego, CA, USA	Timothy G. Canty
1985	Rotorua, New Zealand	R. Stuart Ferguson
1986	Puerto Vallarta, Mexico	Joaquin C. Aspiroz
1987	Rosario-Orcas Island, WA, USA	John L. Cahill
1988	Taipei, Taiwan	Wen-Tsung Hung
1989	Portland, Oregon	Marvin W. Harrison
1990	Kona, HI, USA	Walton K. T. Shim
1991	Hong Kong, China	Htut Saing
1992	Abuquerque, NM, USA	Patrick K. Jewell
1993	Cairns, QLD, Australia	Mervyn M, Lander
1994	Kagoshima, Japan	Hiroshi Akiyama
1995	Hualtuco, Mexico	Giovanni Porras-Ramirez
1996	Singapore	V. T. Joseph
1997	Phoenix, AZ, USA	Joseph T. Zerella
1998	Maui, HI, USA	Walton K. T. Shim
1999	Beijing, China	Jin-Zhe Zhang
2000	Las Vegas, NV, USA	Stephen G. Jolley
2001	Kyoto, Japan	Takeshi Miyano
2002	La Jolla, CA, USA	Harry Applebaum
2003	Sydney, NSW, Australia	Ralph Cohen

(*Continued*)

Table 3. (*Continued*)

2004	Seoul, Korea	Eui Ho Hwang
2005	Vancouver, BC, Canada	Eric M. Webber
2006	Taipei, Taiwan	Jer-Nan Lin
2007	Queenstown, New Zealand	Kevin C. Pringle
2008	Jackson Hole, Wyoming	Rebecka Meyers

Table 4. Presidents Pacific Association of Pediatric Surgeons.

Stephen L. Gans	1969–1970	John R. Campbell	1988–1989
John K. Stevenson	1970–1971	R. Stuart Ferguson	1989–1990
Alexander H. Bill, Jr.	1971–1972	Dale G. Johnston	1990–1991
Keijiro Suruga	1972–1973	Morton M. Woolley	1991–1992
Nate A. Myers	1973–1974	Martin J. Glasson	1992–1993
Jens G. Rosenkrantz	1974–1975	Hiroshi Akiyama	1993–1994
Murray R. Kliman	1975–1976	Giovanni Porras–Ramirez	1994–1995
Daniel M. Hays	1976–1977	Takahiro Ito	1995–1996
Takashi Ueda	1977–1978	Marshall Z. Schwartz	1996–1997
Joaquin C. Azpiroz	1978–1979	Htut Saing	1997–1998
Douglas Cohen	1979–1980	Philip A. King	1998–1999
Walton K. T. Shim	1980–1981	Marvin W. Harrison	1999–2000
Graham C. Fraser	1981 1982	Takeshi Miyano	2000 2001
Keiichi Ikeda	1982–1983	James B. Atkinson	2001–2002
Eric W. Fonkalsrud	1983–1984	Rosslyn Walker	2002–2003
E. Durham Smith	1984–1985	Eui-Ho Hwang	2003–2004
Rodolfo Franco-Vasquez	1985–1986	Stephen G. Jolley	2004–2005
		Jer-Nan Lin	2005–2006
Chadwick F. Baxter	1986–1987	Kevin C. Pringle	2006–2007
Wen-Tsung Hung	1987–1988	Richard Black	2007–2008

Table 5. Secretaries

Jens G. Rosenkrantz	1969–1971	Dale G. Johnson	1985–1988
John R. Campbell	1971–1973	John C. German	1988–1991
Edward A. Free	1973–1975	Marshall Z. Schwartz	1991–1995
George A. Hyde	1975–1977	Marvin W. Harrison	1995–1999
Walton K. T. Shim	1977–1979	Stephen G. Jolley	1999–2001
Pieter A. De Vries	1979–1982	Robert S. Sawin	2001–2004
Wiliam C. Bailey	1982–1985	Harry Applebaum	2004–

Table 6. Treasurers

Eric W. Fonkalsrud	1969–1970	Ann M. Kosloske	1985–1990
Alfred A. de Lorimer	1970–1972	Marvin W. Harrison	1990–1995
Daniel M. Hays	1972–1974	Dale G. Hall	1995–1999
David L. Collins	1974–1977	James B. Atkinson	1999–2001
Ernest B. Haws	1977–1984	Richard E. Black	2001–2007
David Hodge	1984–1985	Kevin P. Lally	2007–

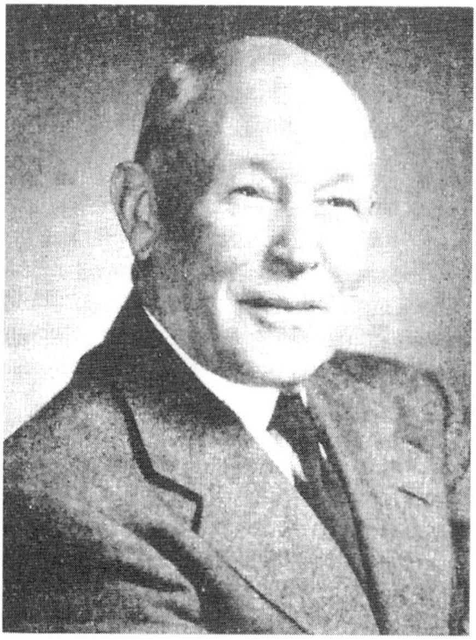

Fig. 7. Herbert E. Coe

Table 7. Coe Medal Recipients.

Mrs Herbert E. Coe	1985	Takashi Ueda	1994
Alexander H. Bill, Jr.	1987	Daniel M. Hays	1995
Morio Kasai	1987	Eric W. Fonkalsrud	1998
Keijiro Suruga	1988	Justin H. Kelly	2001
Nate Myers	1989	Alberto Pena	2002
Stephen L. Gans	1990	Ken Kimura	2003
Morton M. Woolley	1992	Keiichi Ikeda	2008
Durham Smith	1993		

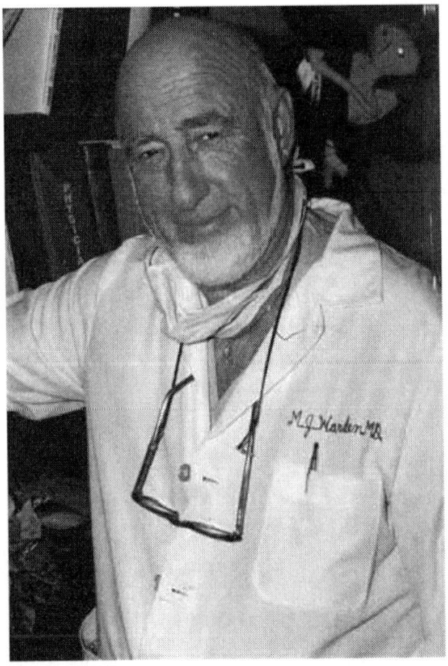

Fig. 8. James M. Warden.

James M. Warden (Figure 8) was the first to suggest that guests from third-world countries be invited and sponsored to attend PAPS meeting. At first he paid these expenses himself, except for the registration fee which was included in the local organizer's budget. The first guest was invited in 1969. With the success of this guest assistance program, it became an integral part of annual meetings, the expenses being born only by voluntary contributions.

Papers presented at PAPS meetings and submitted to the Journal of Pediatric Surgery (JPS) were first published together in 1988, 20 years after it's founding and 23 years after the founding of (JPS). This is especially fitting as Stephen Gans was the founding father of JPS. as well. Since then, JPS has become the official journal of PAPS.

Since PAPS inception one of its highly unique characteristics and special appeal, separating it from other international Pediatric Surgical congresses, is a very informal and friendly atmosphere and familiar attitude during scientific sessions athletic events and formal

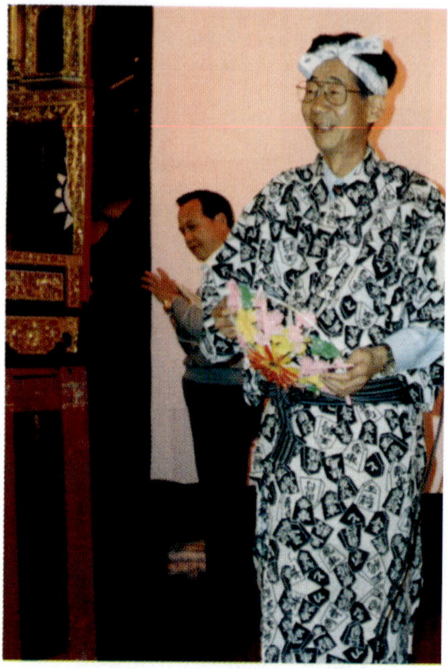

Fig. 9. (L-R) Ezio Okamoto.

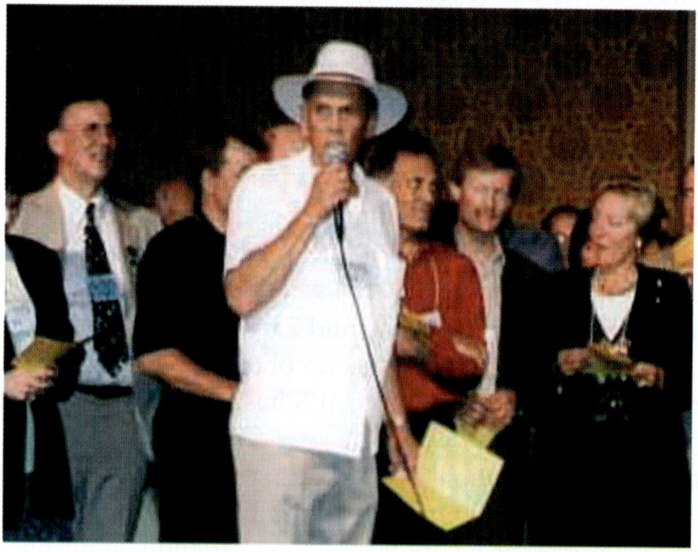

Fig. 10. Chad Baxter Leading a Songfest.

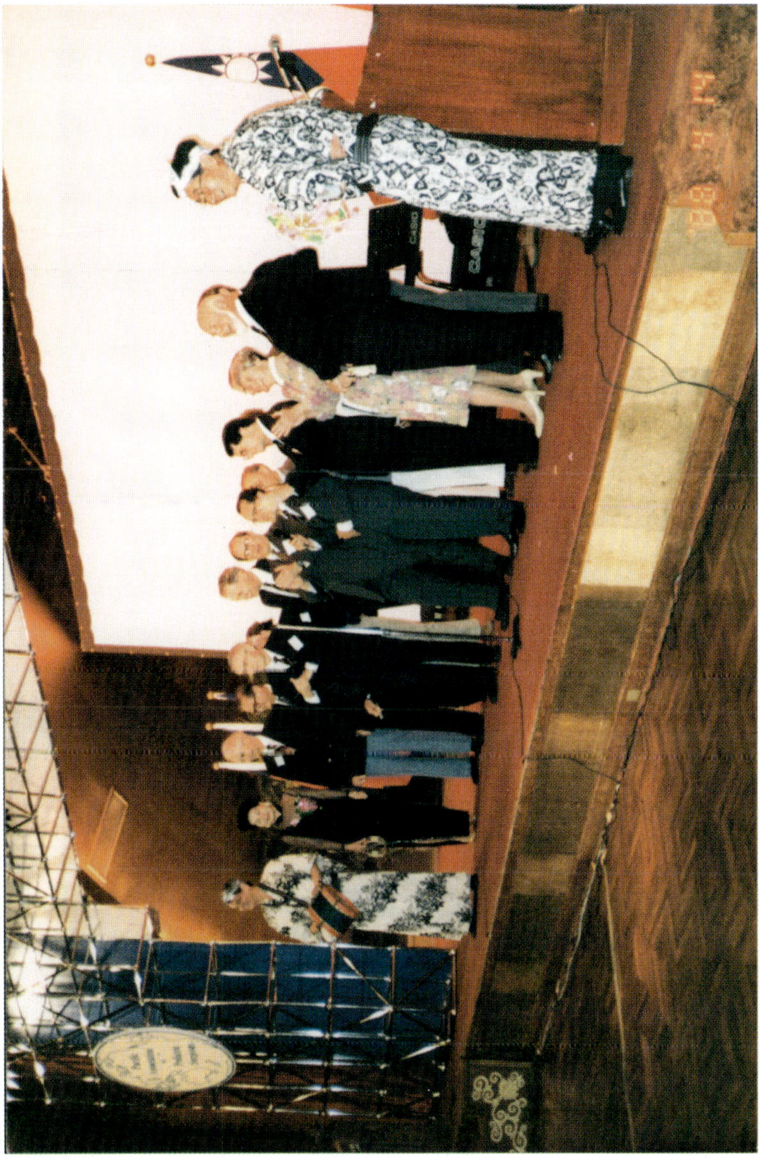

Fig. 11. Traditional Songfest by the American Delegation.

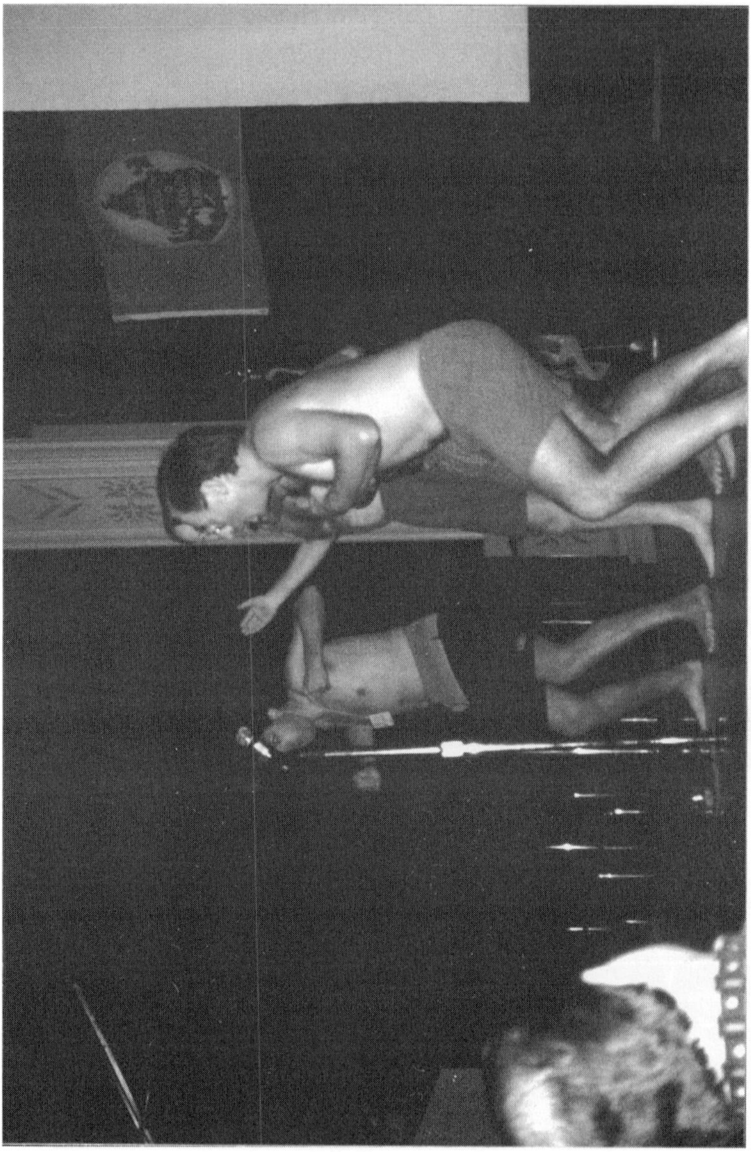

Fig. 12. New Zealand members perform a Mãori Haka or war dance.

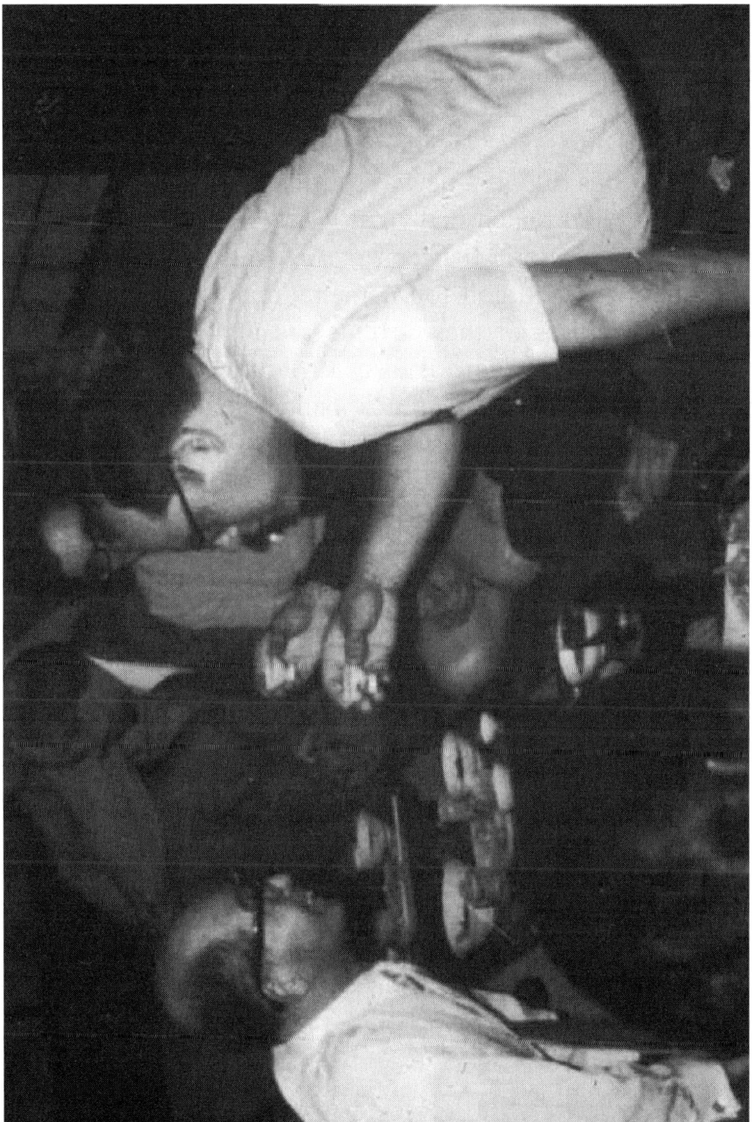

Fig. 13. (L-R) Morio Kasai & John R. Campbell toast Kompai.

and informal social events. Lack of formality between professors and trainees is demonstrated in Figure 9, One way of keeping this light informal mood is through the unwritten rules and customs of PAPS; everyone speaks in colleagues on a first name basis, even during scientific sessions. The infamous "no neck tie rule," is strictly enforced, i.e., neckties arc definitely not be worn at any time during the congress. Chad Baxter (Figure 10) was the first to strictly and playfully police this rule. If a tie was spotted during the congress, he would promptly and unabashedly cut it off, with a pair of scissors, Bonding and camaraderie between participants is fostered though tennis competitions and golf tournaments that are held during the congress. The winners of these events are announced during the annual banquet, where there is also a traditional songfest, where members from each country give a cappella performances unique to their country (Figure 11), and sometime dance (Figure 12).

The result of this informality has been the facilitation of information transfer between both shores of the Pacific. For a long time

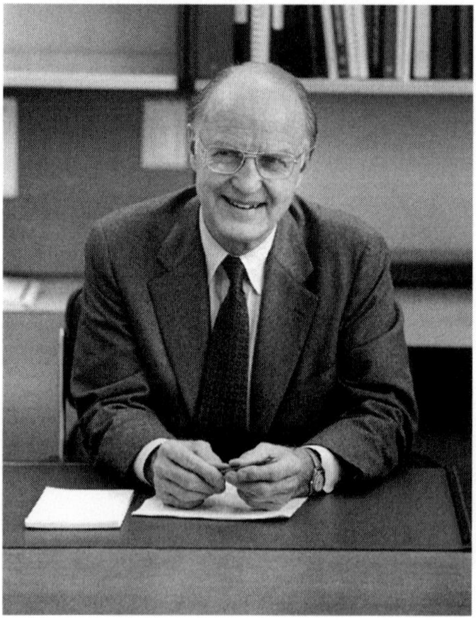

Fig. 14. Daniel M. Hays.

there was disbelief among American Pediatric Surgeons as to the therapeutic value of the Kasai procedure. After the meeting in Tokyo in 1972, several American members traveled to Sendai and met with Dr Kasai and learned from him first hand the principals and techniques of the procedure. We went home with a new understanding and with some success with the procedure (Figure 13). While attending the 1978 meeting in Osaka, we watched Ezio Okomoto perform the procedure and returned home with an even greater understanding and increased success. Dan Hays (Figure 14). after spending a year in Japan wrote a book with Ken Kimura on the Japanese experience with biliary atrcsia.[4]

References

1. Campbell J, History of the Pacific Association of Pediatrlc Surgeons: the First 15 Years (1968–1983). *J Pediatr Surg* 2007;42:1977–1981.
2. Pacific Association of Pediatric Surgeons Archives, Royal Children's Hospital, Melbourne, Australia.
3. Personal comnmnication between Pieter deVries and John Campbell.
4. Hays DM, Kimura K. Biliary atresia — the Japanese experience. Cambridge (MA): Harvard University Press; 1980.

PAN AFRICAN PAEDIATRIC SURGICAL ASSOCIATION (PAPSA)

Heinz Rode

Africa's paediatric surgeons have a wealth of experience and special knowledge of the diseases of Africa, which can differ substantially from those encountered in other regions of the world. These differences include incidents, manner of presentation, patient related factors and predicted outcome. In an attempt to resolve many of these demanding health issues, a group of interested paediatric surgeons from the continent met at the 24th BAPS Meeting in Budapest in 1991 and again in November 1992 in Nairobi, Kenya.

The International Association was formally established in 1992 with specific objectives: to promote the practice, research and advance the study of paediatric surgery specifically in Africa; to promote and maintain the highest clinical and ethical standards; to encourage and arrange regular meetings for the interchange of ideas and sharing of knowledge and experience and to foster professional relations with paediatric surgeons throughout the world.

PAPSA was inaugurated on the March 9, 1994 in Nairobi with 64 members. The World Federation of Associations of Paediatric Surgeons encouraged and supported this new initiative from 1991 and made a major contribution towards the association in 1994. The presidents of PAPSA were J. M. Kyambi (Kenya), N. Kaddah (Egypt) and M. R. Q. Davies (South Africa) and A. Hesse (Ghana). The driving force behind this association and it's development has centred on the secretariat. Single individuals have filled this position with great distinction and service; H. Rode (1994–2002), A. Hadidi (2002–2006), D. Poenaru (2006–present as Secretary-Educator) and E. Elhalaby (2006–present as Secretary-Treasurer). Prof Rode's work in establishing and developing the Association has been exceptional and without his persistence and efforts, what has been achieved may never have occurred. Ahmed Hadidi stabilised and grew the association, and through his input, a strong link with the Egyptian paediatric surgeons was established which significantly helped to steady the tenuous hold the Association had on it's existence at that time. Because of the vastness of the continent and for practical regions, nine regional/country representation has been established to serve on the executive.

Regular biennual meetings were held across the African continent with between 60 and 120 delegates attending. PAPSA Meetings were held in association with WOFAPS in Nairobi 1994, the Egyptian Paediatric Surgical Association in Cairo 1996, the South African Association of Paediatric Surgeons Cape Town 1998, the European African Paediatric Surgical Conference in Cairo 2002 SIOPS in Blantyre 2004, the Egyptian Paediatric Surgical Association Alexandria 2005 and the Kenya Association for Paediatric Surgeon Mombassa 2006. The scheduled 4th Meeting in Abidjan was cancelled due to unforeseen circumstances. These meetings were practical and goal-directed towards the diverse spectrum of surgical pathologies. A more recent addition has been pre-congress workshops. Although in the infancy stage, PAPSA has established a strong African network and is instrumental in disseminating information and setting standards for surgical care.

SCANDINAVIAN ASSOCIATION OF PAEDIATRIC SURGEONS

Ole H. Nielsen

The paediatric surgeons in Scandinavia became aware of each other in the 1950's. They met when visiting at the Great Ormond Street Hospital of Sick Children (the Mecca of European Paediatric Surgery) and at the BAPS meetings, and they began to feel the need for a Scandinavian Association, where the established paediatric surgeons as well as the young trainees could meet and exchange experience and views. In connection with the Rotterdam BAPS meeting in 1964 there was an outing by train to the Philips factories in Eindhoven. Sitting together on the train Gunnar Ekström, Theodor Ehrenpreis, Gunnar Pettersson, Matti Sulamaa and Georg Rabbe Wallgren agreed to found a Scandinavian Association. "Everybody can not travel every year to England or somewhere else in Europe, but to one of the Nordic countries the majority of younger and older paediatric surgeons might go every year." The formal founding meeting was at the Crown Princess Lovisa's Hospital in the autumn 1964 with Matti Sulamaa and G. R. Wallgren from Finland and Ola Knutrud from Norway participating, together with the senior Swedish paediatric surgeons.

It was decided that the first meeting should be arranged in Helsinki in 1965. The founding members concluded the business with a dinner at the famous Opera Cellar, where Theodor Ehrenpreis impressed the party by opening the door with his private key.

The first executive council was:
President: **Gunnar Pettersson**, Gothenburg,
General secretary: Georg Rabbe Wallgren, Helsinki,
Members: **N. O. Ericsson**, Stockholm, **Ola Knutrud**, Oslo, **Tyge Gertz**, Copenhagen.

The association had annual meetings, the venue going on turn between the four countries, with a meeting in Iceland put in at intervals. There was often overseas participation. In later years the increasing amount of international meetings and of sub-speciality societies has forced a decision of going down to biennial meetings, and at present the fate of the association is doubtful.

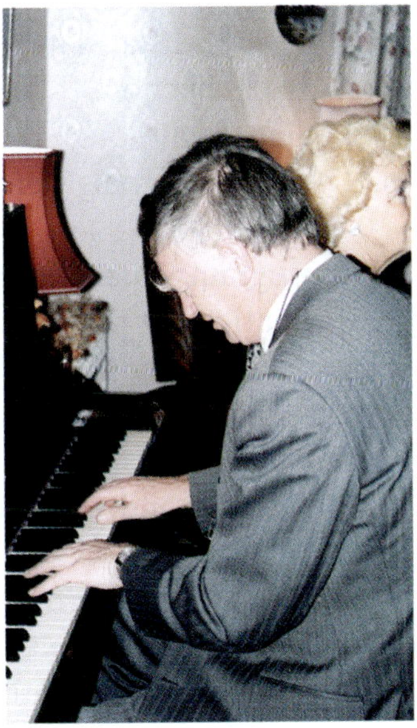

SURGICAL SECTION OF THE AMERICAN ACADEMY OF PEDIATRICS

Dan G. Young

At the same time as the Scottish Surgeons formed their Scottish Surgical Paediatric Club in 1948 (subsequently the name was changed to Society), surgeons in the States moved in the same direction and established the Surgical Section. It continues as part of the American Academy of Pediatrics although it has grown considerably since its inception. The primary goals were:

1) to present a scientific program which will provide state-of-the-art techniques and information for pediatric surgeons; and
2) serve in a consulting capacity to the AAP Board of Directors to make recommendations for educational programs, policy statements and other actions on matters relating to the surgical care of infants, children, adolescents and young adults.

Subsequently the surgeons sought more independence and the American Association of Pediatric Surgeons (APSA) was established as an independent body. Both organisations continue to function and have complimentary roles.

The history of the Section has been recorded in considerable detail by Jud Randolf and John Campbell at the time of the half centenary of its birth. These references are given below and make very interesting reading as does the foreword by Moritz Ziegler. Their papers are followed in the special Supplement to the "*Journal of Pediatric Surgery*" in 1999 by contributions from three individuals mentioned extensively in this book — Bill Clatworthy, Chick Koop and Hardy Hendren.

References

1. Randolf JG. History of the section of surgery, the American Academy of Pediatrics: The first 25 years (1948–1973). *J Pediatr Surg* 1999;34(Suppl)1:3–18.
2. Campbell JR. History of the section of surgery, the American Academy of Pediatrics: The second 25 years (1973–1998). *J Pediatr Surg* 1999;34(Suppl)1:19–37.

UNION OF EUROPEAN MEDICAL SPECIALISTS (UEMS)

Robert Carachi

The History of the UEMS (1958–2008)

On the July 20, 1958, one year after the Treaty of Rome was signed, the representatives delegated by the professional organisations of medical specialists of the six member countries of the European Community (EEC) — created the previous year — met in Brussels and founded the European Union of Medical Specialists (UEMS). The main issue tackled by the UEMS was that of quality, trying to obtain from the European Commission and the Member States, a high level of training for the future Medical Specialists of the six Common Market Countries. By 1962 the UEMS created Specialist Sections for each of the main disciplines practised in the Member Countries. These groups of experts composed of representatives of the National Associations of each specialty carried out a considerable amount of work with the idea of harmonising the Specialist Training, and the criteria for the recognition of Medical Specialists. The first European directives concerning doctors only appeared in 1975 and these were largely inspired by proposals and surveys presented by the UEMS and the Specialist Sections.

Meanwhile, the European Community was enlarging to include the United Kingdom, Denmark, Ireland, as well as Norway and Switzerland. These successive enlargements led to important changes in the UEMS, its statues, and the composition of its various Specialist Sections of which the number gradually increased to 35.

The next important move was the creation by the European Commission of an Advisory Committee on Medical Training (ACMT), a community institution ensuring the link between the European Professional Medical Organisations, the Universities and the National Governments on the one hand, and the Commission on the other. Following this, the Specialist Sections of the UEMS during the years 1980 and 1981, submitted a report explaining the evolution of their specialties. This resulted in the publication of the second and third reports concerning the training of Medical Specialists.

Finally in the 1990s, the UEMS gained a new lease of life by creating European Boards, Working Groups of the Specialist Sections, in order to guarantee optimal care in the field of the specialty concerned by bringing the training of Medical Specialists to the highest possible level. It published the European Charters on the training of Medical Specialists and on the assurance of quality in Specialist Medicine, a key document on the autonomy of practice of Medical Specialists. This highlighted the role and the action needed by the Specialist Sections of the UEMS and progressively opened the UEMS to the countries of central and eastern Europe. At present UEMS has 30 full Members (the 27 EU countries plus the three EFTA countries, Iceland, Switzerland and Norway), plus five Associate Members (Azerbaijan, Croatia, Georgia, Israel and Turkey).

Specialist Sections of the UEMS

These were founded in 1962 and number 39 at present plus seven multidisciplinary joint committees. They are the UEMS commonwealth force and as such, speak with one voice. Their main task is the professional defence of their speciality and harmonisation of the profession at European level. The objectives of the UEMS are laid down in Article 2 of the Statutes which include:

1) to defend at International level the title of the Specialist and his professional status in society;
2) to study, promote, and defend the quality of the comparatively high level of specialist care given to patients;

3) to establish tighter bonds between the national professional organisation grouping together specialists in all fields, to support and coordinate their actions;
4) to contribute to the creation and maintenance of solidarity between European Specialists, particularly between Specialists in the same field; and
5) to study, promote and defend before the international authorities the free movement and the moral and material interests of European Specialists.

Within the UEMS structure there have been developed Boards in each specialty. The European Board of Pediatric Surgery (EBPS) being responsible for recognising training and achievement standards within the specialty in the EC.

European Board of Pediatric Surgery (EBPS)

Aims

- The EBPS shall recommend the standards required for the training of specialists in paediatric surgery and supervise the maintenance of these standards;
- The EBPS shall make proposals for the quality of training and for the syllabus for paediatric surgery;
- The EBPS shall recommend criteria to which training centres in paediatric surgery should conform to be registered as EBPS-approved training centres for trainees tin the specialty;
- The EBPS shall recommend the requirements for quality control or certification as trained in paediatric surgery "European Board Qualification";
- The EBPS shall recommend procedures to facilitate free movement of specialists in paediatric surgery in EEC;
- Within the EEC the free movement of paediatric surgeons or trainees shall be encouraged between member countries; and
- The EBPS may conduct site visits of institutions that have formally agreed to live up to EBPS standards. Site visits will be

carried out only with an agreement of the principle of the visited institutions. Site visits may result in certification as EBPS-recognised training institution. In countries where such sites have already been reviewed, the EBPS will cooperate with such activities.

The Certification Process (Article 3 — Recognition of Qualification (European Board Qualification.) The EBPS shall issue a certificate of recognition of qualification in paediatric surgery to individuals who have attained the requisite training and successfully completed the education requirements specified by the Board.

Only fully trained specialists having undertaken recognised training in a Member State of the EEC, an EFTA country or in another country at a comparable level may apply for this quality control to the EBPS.

European Board Examination in Paediatric Surgery

Many of the other European Boards have introduced the European Postgraduate Examination in their speciality. These include anaesthesiology, intensive care medicine, ophthalmology, plastic surgery and urology; and have been followed by others including paediatric surgery. The EBPS has the authority to organise an examination to certify candidates who have completed their training in paediatric surgery in Centres recognised by the European Board. It is the responsibility of the Examination Board of the EBPS to:

- vet the candidates submitted for registration;
- organise the examination; and
- adjudicate on the results and recommend successful candidates to the EBPS for certification.

Conclusion

The UEMS provides a political structure for medical specialists in Europe to have a common European identity. The mandate from the European Parliament is for the Specialist Groups to set a high standard of professionalism which is ultimately reflected in the best care for the patient. This high standard can only be achieved by good clinical governance, fully accredited training programmes, and trainer, and fully accredited Training Centres, leading to the certification of individuals who have passed through this process. It is anticipated that the search for excellence in paediatric surgery will continue through harmony in the setting of standards fully realising the range of political and geographical needs that exist within each country.

WORLD FEDERATION OF ASSOCIATIONS OF PEDIATRIC SURGEONS (1974–2007)

Jay L. Grosfeld
Jose Boix-Ochoa

The development of pediatric surgery as a distinct specialty was slow in its acceptance. Following World War II, it became apparent that techniques of care and procedures that were used in adults did not always apply to children, particularly the newly born. The advent of antibiotics, vaccines, and newborn intensive care facilities allowed survival of pediatric patients that previously perished many of whom that would subsequently require the expertise of surgeons experienced in the care of infants and children. Progress in the field was influenced by the availability of new technologies including ventilators for babies and that permitted survival of premature infants that prior to that time would ultimately die prenatal ultrasound that improved the early recognition of abnormalities. Organisations representing children's surgeons arose in a few developed countries with advanced medical care including UK, US, Canada, France and Germany. However, there was no specific international organisation that could provide leadership and a voice of support for children's surgeons and develop educational and scientific guidelines for children's care throughout the world. The British Association of Paediatric Surgeons (BAPS) had been in place in the UK since 1953 and included overseas members. The Canadians developed their own organisation (CAPS) in 1967. Although the Surgery Section of the American Academy of Pediatrics had been established in 1948, it was controlled by the pediatricians and was not a separate surgical organisation. The American Pediatric Surgical Association (APSA) was finally established in 1971 to fill this void in the US. Interest in children's surgery expanded many places in the world and it became apparent that an international group representing the various fledgling pediatric surgical associations and societies would be of great value. In 1970, Jesus Lozoya of Mexico and Virgilio Carvalho–Pinto of Brazil raised the interest of a few of the pediatric surgical groups in both developed and developing countries to establish an international organisation for pediatric surgeons. James Lister of Liverpool, UK joined the discussion and served as an organizing catalyst. Others including Harvey Beardmore, Montreal, Canada, Julio Monereo, Madrid, Spain, Keijiro Suruga, Tokyo, Japan, Durham Smith, Melbourne, Australia, Jose Pinus, Sao Paulo, Brazil, Jose Santiago Piñeiro, Buenos Aires, Argentina, and Andrew Wilkinson, London UK also became involved. Discussions were held at the BAPS meetings in Glasgow in 1972 and London in 1973. Andrew Wilkinson of London, UK was the President of the BAPS from 1971 to 1972. In early discussions, it was suggested that Professor Wilkinson might serve as the first President of this potentially new international group to assure that the BAPS would choose to become a member organisation. Drs Lozoya and Carvahlo–Pinto were responsible for putting together a preliminary constitution and the World Federation of Associations of Pediatric Surgeons (WOFAPS) became a reality.

The Constitution specified that membership to WOFAPS involved national associations and societies and not individual members. WOFAPS was established as an international body representing its various constituent associations and societies "organized exclusively for charitable, religious, educational and scientific purposes to improve the care of children throughout the world." The first meeting was held October 15, 1974 in Sao Paulo, Brazil. Dr Carvahlo–Pinto was the host. After a spirited and heated debate surrounded by considerable political intrigue, Dr Harvey Beardmore (Fig. 1) was elected the first President and Mr James Lister was elected Secretary-General (Fig. 2). It was determined that the Presidential term would be three years. Andrew Wilkinson who had

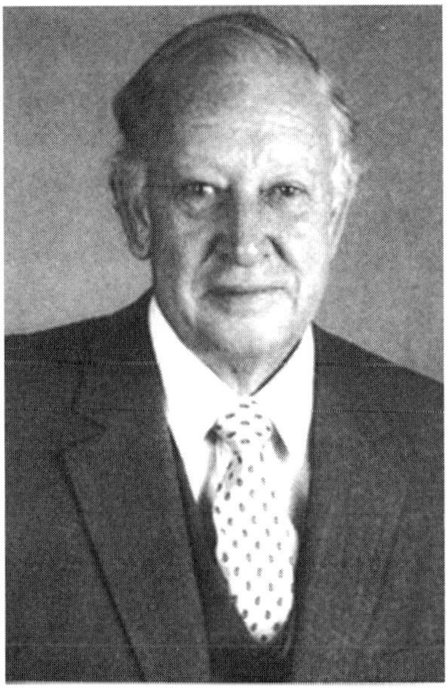

Fig. 1. Photograph of the late Dr Harvey Beardmore, Montreal — the first President of the WOFAPS (1974–1977).

flown to Sao Paulo expecting to be the first President was incensed by the outcome of the election and left the meeting abruptly to return to London. The initial Executive Committee included those members previously noted that were involved in the organisational process (Fig. 3). Initially, only 14 national organisations joined the new group. Mr Lister remained as Secretary-General for nine years (1974–1983).

The next meeting was held three years later (1977) in Barcelona, Spain. Professor Denis Pellerin of Paris, France was elected President (Fig. 4). Prof R. K. Gandhi, New Delhi, India was elected President at the 1980 meeting held in New Delhi. In 1983, Prof Marcel Bettex, Berne, Switzerland became the fourth President of WOFAPS at a meeting in Belgrade, Yugoslavia (Fig. 5). During Bettex's tenure the constitution was amended, Mr Lister resigned as Secretary-General, and Prof Jose Boix–Ochoa of Barcelona was elected to replace him. Boix–Ochoa has served continuously in that

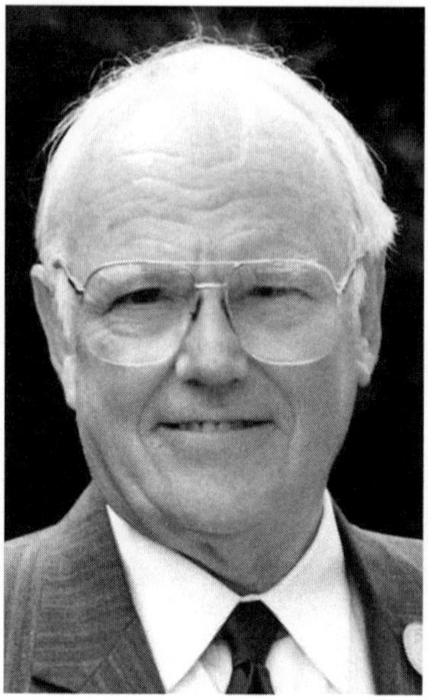

Fig. 2. James Lister, Liverpool, UK — Mr Lister served as the first Secretary-General of the WOFAPS from 1974–1983.

(a)

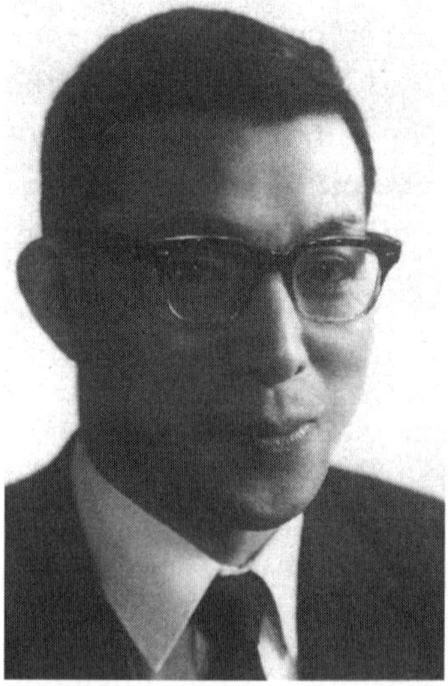

Fig. 3. Some members of the first Executive Council (left to right): (a) Keijero Suruga, Japan, (b) Julio Monereo, Spain, and (c) Durham Smith, Australia.

(b)

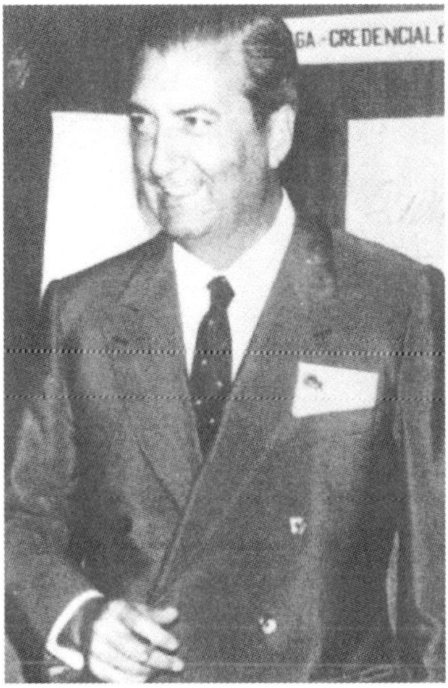

(c)

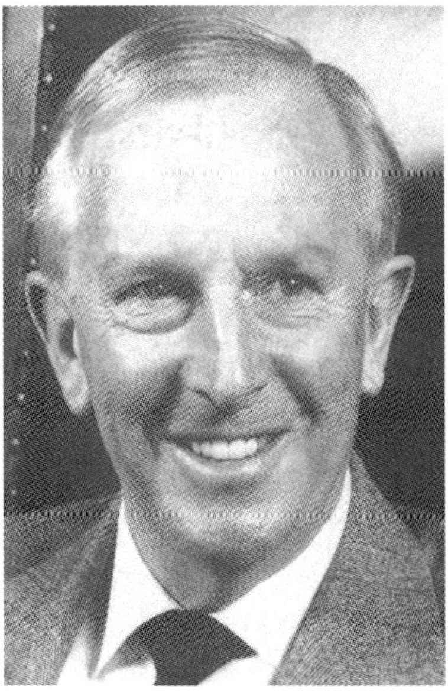

Fig. 3. (*Continued*)

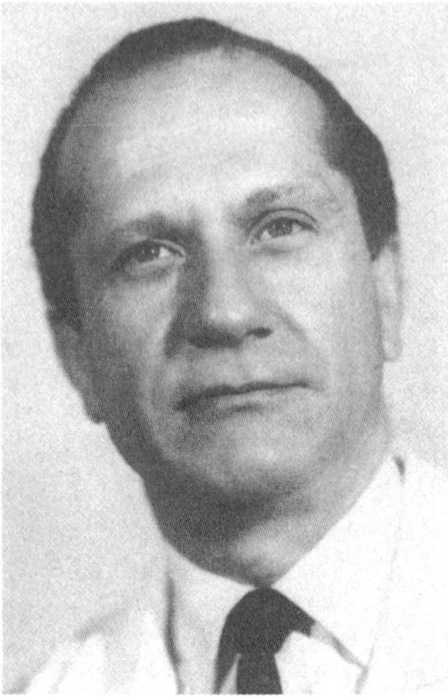

Fig. 4. Prof Denis Pellerin, Paris — the 2nd President of the WOFAPS.

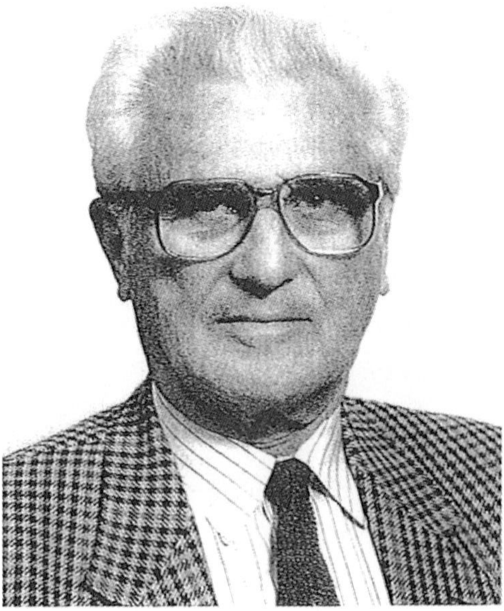

Fig. 5. Marcel Bettex–Berne, Switzerland — the 3rd President of WOFAPS.

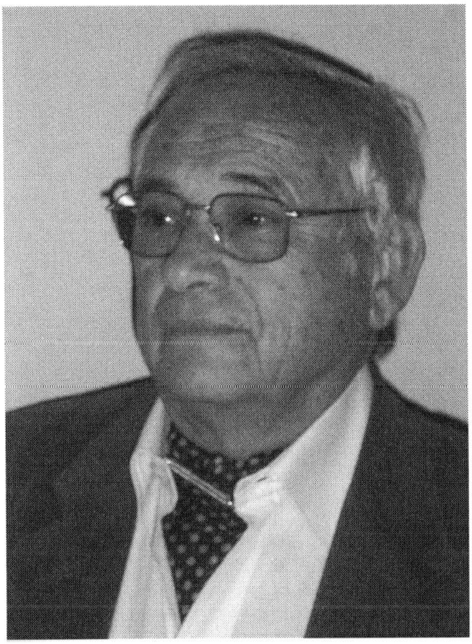

Fig. 6. Jose (Pepe) Boix–Ochoa, Barcelona, Spain. Pepe has been the inspirational leader of WOFAPS and has served continuously as Secretary-General from 1983 until the present time.

position from 1983 until the current time. Influenced by Boix–Ochoa's forward thinking, personal energy and continuity in office the WOFAPS began to establish some credibility (Fig. 6).

As new pediatric surgical organisations began to emerge in nations around the world, they sought entry as a member of WOFAPS. The WOFAPS was invited to hold their Executive Council meetings every three years by a member country's pediatric surgical association. Subsequent meetings were held in Santiago, Chile (1986), Istanbul, Turkey (1989), Hamburg, Germany (1992) and Melbourne, Australia (1995). Jose Ricardo Piñeiro of Buenos Aires, Argentina, Keith W. Ashcraft, Kansas City, MO (USA) (Fig. 7), Wolfgang Meier of Karlsruhe, Germany and Sid Cywes of Cape Town, South Africa (Fig. 8) were the elected Presidents for these respective sites. (Table 1). During these years, the activities of the

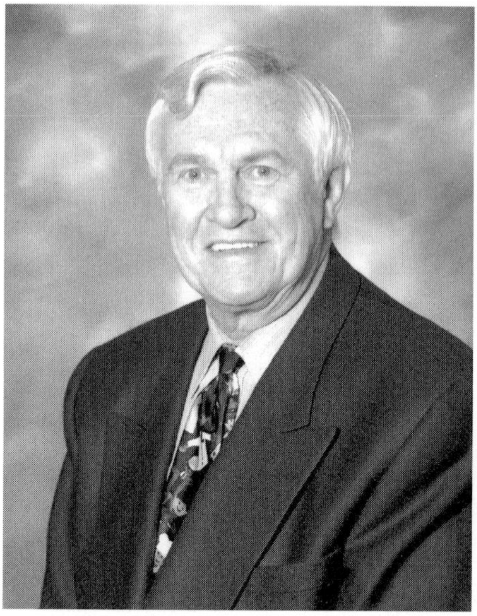

Fig. 7. Prof Keith Ashcraft, Kansas City, MO.

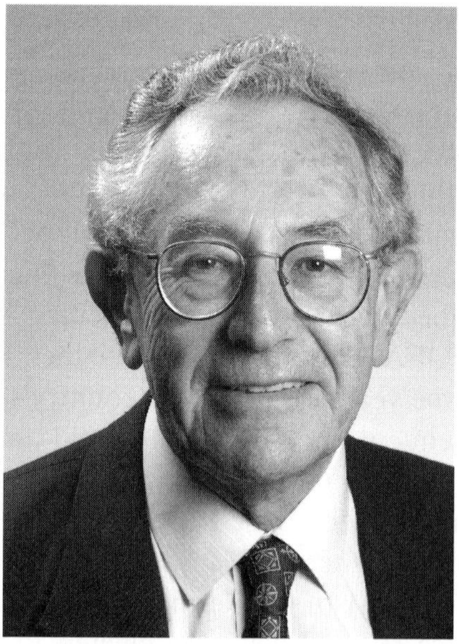

Fig. 8. Prof Sid Cywes, Cape Town, South Africa.

Table 1. The Presidents of WOFAPS and the meeting sites where they were elected.

Meeting site	Years	President
Sao Paulo, Brazil	1974–1977	Prof H. Beardmore (Canada)
Barcelona, Spain	1977–1980	Prof D. Pellerin (France)
New Delhi, India	1980–1983	Prof R. K. Gandhi (India)
Belgrade, Yugoslavia	1983–1986	Prof M. Bettex (Switzerland)
Santiago, Chile	1986–1989	Prof J.R. Piñeiro (Argentina)
Istanbul, Turkey	1989–1992	Prof K. Ashcraft (USA)
Hamburg, Germany	1995–1995	Prof W. A. Meier (Germany)
Melbourne, Australia	1995–1998	Prof S. Cywes (South Africa)
Cape Town, So. Africa	1998–2001	Prof J. Grosfeld (USA)
Kyoto, Japan	2001–2004	Prof T. Miyano (Japan)
Zagreb, Croatia	2004–2007	Prof A. Coran (USA)
Buenos Aires, Argentina	2007–2010	Prof P. Puri (Ireland)

WOFAPS centered on aiding the establishment of the African Association of Pediatric Surgery; and identifying the right representative Pediatric Surgical Association in some countries, especially in India and Portugal where there were two rival groups claiming a leadership role and their intent to join WOFAPS. Diplomacy was the order of the day and subsequently a satisfactory arrangement for each of these countries occurred resulting in membership in the WOFAPS. Through a relationship with WOPSEC, an Italian based group led by Dr Ghinelli and later Dr Georgocopolous, WOFAPS assisted underdeveloped countries, particularly those in Africa by providing volunteers and advice to improve children's surgical care especially for traumatized patients following catastrophic events.

Dr Ashcraft personally hosted visiting surgeons from various developing countries for brief periods in Kansas City in an attempt to expose them to the contemporary pediatric surgical methods of the day. For the first time, regular and frequent WOFAPS news letters were sent to member societies to keep them informed of developments.

Prof Jay L. Grosfeld, Indianapolis (USA) was elected the 9th President of WOFAPS at the 1998 meeting in Cape Town, South Africa that was hosted by Dr Cywes and the South African

Association of Pediatric Surgeons. During his tenure Dr Grosfeld was instrumental in developing the "Declaration of Pediatric Surgery" outlining guidelines for establishment of educational requirements, and providing recommendations for the level of facilities and staffing required to care for ill and injured child and especially the newborn with congenital anomalies (Fig. 9). By this time, 74 national organisations had joined the ranks of WOFAPS. The Declaration of Pediatric Surgery was voted on and ratified at the 2001 meeting of WOFAPS held in Kyoto, Japan in conjunction with the Pacific Association of Pediatric Surgeons (Table 2). The event was attended by the then Crown Prince of Japan (the current Emperor) and Professor Takeshi Miyano of Tokyo was elected the 10th President of WOFAPS (Fig. 10).

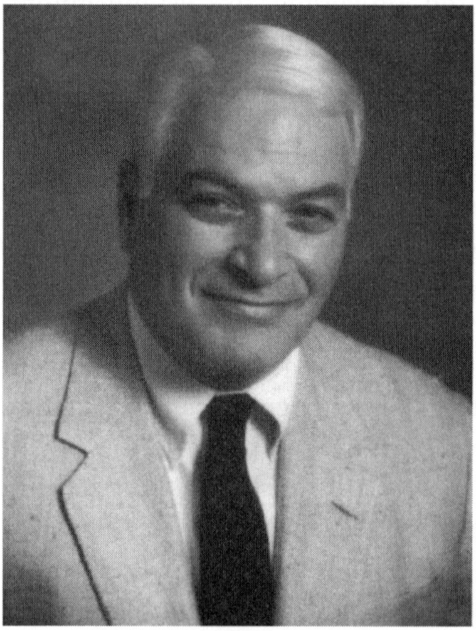

Fig. 9. Jay L. Grosfeld, MD, Indianapolis, IN — the 9th President of WOFAPS (1998–2001) and originator of the Declaration of Pediatric Surgery. Dr Grosfeld was the WOFAPS liaison for the International Surgical Society sponsored International Surgical Week meetings from 1985-to the present day. He is the first President of the recently established WOFAPS Foundation.

Table 2. Declaration of Pediatric Surgery — ratified in Kyoto, Japan in 2001.

- *Children are not just small adults and have medical and surgical problems and needs that are often quite different from those encountered by adult physicians. Infants and children deserve the very best medical care available. Every infant and child who suffers from an illness or disease has the right to be treated in an environment devoted to their care by a pediatric medical or surgical specialist.*
- *Pediatric Surgeons are specially trained physicians with extensive experience and expertise in treating infants and children of all ages (from birth through adolescence) with surgical disorders. Because of their unique training pediatric surgical specialists provide a wide range treatment options and the highest quality care to children.*
- *Pediatric Surgeons diagnose, treat, and manage children's surgical needs including surgical repair of birth defects, serious injuries in children, childhood solid tumors, conditions requiring endoscopy and minimally invasive procedures, and all other surgical procedures in children.*
- *In order to provide the best surgical care for infants and children, complex pediatric surgical procedures should be carried out in specialized pediatric centers with appropriately equipped intensive care facilities staffed 24 hours per day seven days per week. In addition to the trained pediatric surgeons, these facilities should be staffed with other pediatric specialists including radiologists, anesthesiologists and pathotogists. These specialized centers should provide postgraduate education and research.*

In 2004, the first World Congress of Pediatric Surgery was sponsored by WOFAPS and the Croatian Association of Pediatric Surgeons, in Zagreb, Croatia, hosted by Prof Ivan Fattorini. A large attendance guaranteed the success of the meeting. Prof Arnold G. Coran, Ann Arbor, MI (USA) was elected the 11th President of WOFAPS. During the next three years, a number of important changes occurred. The constitution was amended, and WOFAPS was formally incorporated in Philadelphia. as a non-profit, tax exempt 501(c) three organisation by the US Internal Revenue Service approved on January 18, 2007. Dr Coran and his son Michael, a Philadelphia lawyer spearheaded the change (Fig. 11). The WOFAPS Foundation was established under the guidance of Dr Grosfeld as a tax exempt group separate from but embedded within WOFAPS to carry out the charitable, religious, educational,

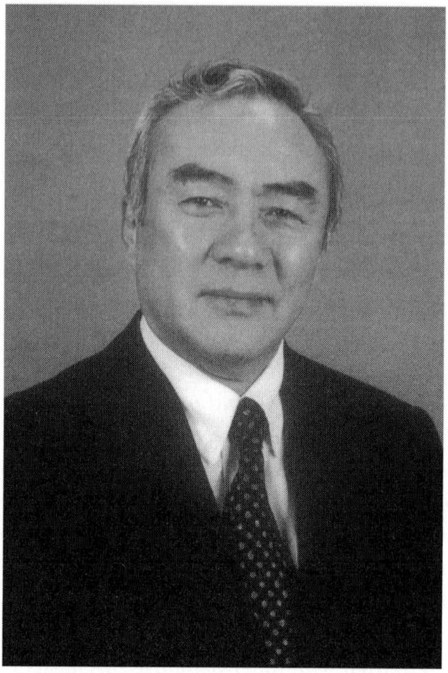

Fig. 10. Prof Takeshi Miyano, Tokyo, Japan. WOFAPS 10th President (2001–2004). Prof. Miyano presided over the 1st World Congress of Pediatric Surgery in Zagreb, Croatia.

and scientific purposes of the Federation. Dr Richard Azizkhan, Cincinnati (USA) was responsible for developing the rules and guidelines for application to and hosting of future Pediatric Surgical World Congresses co-sponsored by WOFAPS.

The 2nd World Congress of Pediatric Surgery and WOFAPS Executive Council was held in Buenos Aires, Argentina, September 9–13, 2007 (Fig. 12). The Pediatric Surgery associations of the Southern Cone Countries of South America (CIPESUR-representing Argentina, Chile, Brazil, Uruguay, Paraguay and Bolivia) were the co-sponsors and Prof Juan Puigdevall was the host (Fig. 13). The IPEG (International Pediatric Endoscopy Group) held their meeting in conjunction with the 2nd World Congress with more than 1500 pediatric surgeons in attendance. The 2007 WOFAPS Executive Council Meeting in Buenos Aires was of note and

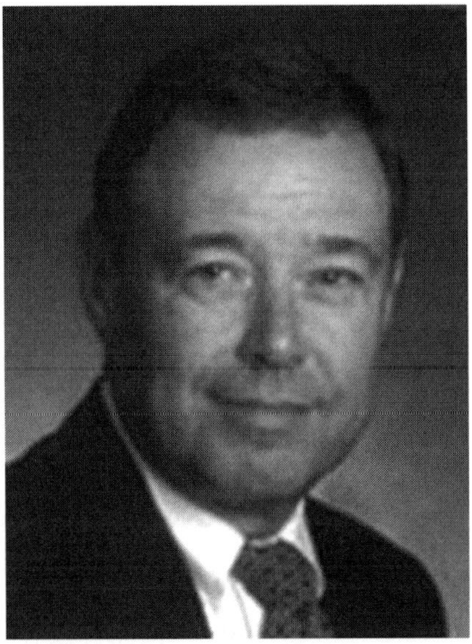

Fig. 11. Prof Arnold Coran, Ann Arbor, MI, (USA) the 11th President of WOFAPS (2004–2011). He was instrumental in changing the by-laws, modifying the Constitution and acquiring corporate status for WOFAPS in 2007 as a legal non-profit, tax exempt entity. He presided over the 2nd World Congress of Pediatric Surgery in Buenos Aires in 2007.

resulted in approval of the new constitution, the rules regarding hosting a World Congress of Pediatric Surgery, and the establishment of the WOFAPS Foundation. The Council approved the addition of representatives of organisations from countries in the Middle East and Africa to the executive council to assure better worldwide-representation. Prof Boix–Ochoa reported that there were now 92 member associations in WOFAPS. This represents 98% of all children's surgical associations worldwide. Prof Grosfeld was elected the first President of the newly formed WOFAPS Foundation with the Board of Directors comprised of Drs A. Coran, T. Miyano, M. Hollwarth, T. Wester, and J. Boix–Ochoa. Prof Prem Puri, Dublin, Ireland was elected the 12th President of WOFAPS and the site of the next world congress and Executive Council meeting in 2010 was awarded to New Delhi, India (Indian Association of Pediatric Surgeons — Prof Devendra Gupta — host).

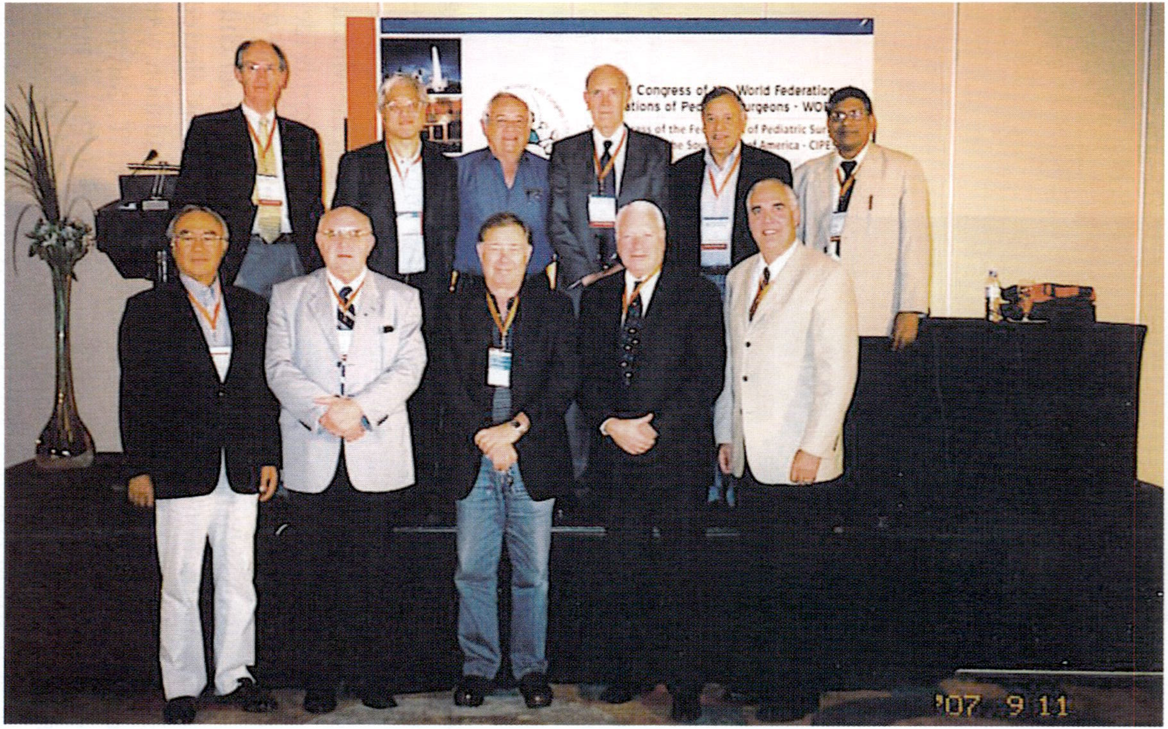

Fig. 12. Photograph of the WOFAPS Executive Council at the 2007 meeting in Buenos Aires, Argentina. Back row, left to right: Alastair Millar, Paul Tam, Pepe Boix–Ochoa, Juan Puigedeval, Prem Puri, Devendra Gupta. Front row, left to right-Takeshi Miyano, Ivan Fattorini, Arnold Coran (President), Jay Grosfeld, and Richard Azizkahn.

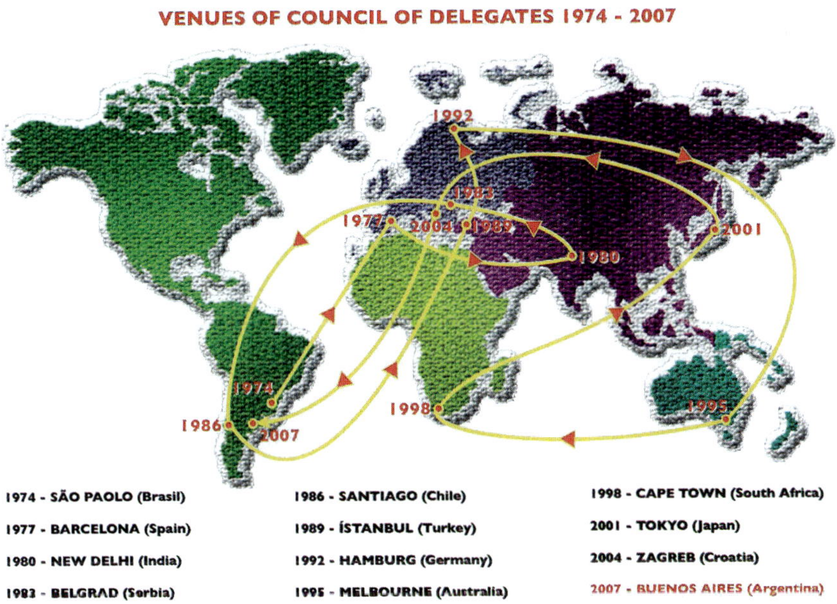

Fig. 13. World map depicting the years and sites of WOFAPS Executive Council meetings. WOFAPS is now comprised of 92 national pediatric surgical societies and associations representing 98% of the children's surgical organisations I the world.

WOFAPS has represented pediatric surgery at-large at the International level. Through the efforts of Prof Boix–Ochoa, WOFAPS has developed a relationship with the World Health Organisation (WHO) in accordance with their goal to improve the care of children and serves in an advisory capacity concerning WHO publications concerning children's surgical care.

WOFAPS has also established itself as the organisation recognized as representing children's surgery in the International Pediatric Association (IPA). Initially, WOFAPS was acknowledged as a nonvoting member of the Executive Council of the IPA in 1983. Through the unrelenting efforts of Dr Boix–Ochoa, in 2001 at the IPA meeting in Beijing, China, constitutional changes were proposed that would assure WOFAPS voting stature on the Standing Committee of the Executive Council of the IPA. This was ratified in 2004 in Cancun, Mexico when WOFAPS was given a permanent seat on the Executive Council of the IPA as a voting member.

Since 1985, WOFAPS has been a participating society in the *Societe de Chirurgie Internationale*-International Surgical Society (ISS-SIC) sponsored International Surgical Week (ISW) Congresses. These meetings occur every other year and are attended by 1500–2000 surgeons representing many different surgical specialties from all over the world. This allows pediatric surgeons to participate in the scientific program and be recognized internationally by their adult surgery colleagues. Dr Grosfeld has served as the WOFAPS liaison and program chairman for these events for the past 22 years. Children's surgeons from various continents join with the local Pediatric Surgical Association in the country hosting ISW to establish the Pediatric Surgical scientific program. These meetings have been held in Paris (1985), Sydney (1987), Toronto (1989), Stockholm (1991), Hong Kong (1993), Lisbon (1995), Acapulco (1997), Vienna (1999), Brussels (2001), Bangkok (2003-cancelled), Durban (2005) and most recently in Montreal (2007). The 2009 meeting is scheduled for September 2009 in Adelaide, Australia. The Australasian Association of Pediatric Surgeons will serve as the host organisation.

The WOFAPS objectives are to improve and maintain the standards of pediatric surgery and promote and integrate these standards throughout the world. The WOFAPS serves as a center for cooperation and interchange of information among pediatric surgical associations, societies and organisations approved by the Federation. The Federation encourages and hopes to maintain high standards of care, ethical practice, education, training, and research in pediatric surgery and its allied sciences worldwide. In the past 33 years, the WOFAPS has matured as an organisation that represents the international body of pediatric surgeons. It is recognized as a formidable group that provides support to the goals and objectives of its member organisations, educational, scientific and clinical recommendations, and an international forum that allows exchange of ideas and exposure to contemporary techniques and methodologies at its world congresses. The newly established WOFAPS Foundation will hopefully provide support in other ways not possible in the past.

JOURNAL OF PEDIATRIC SURGERY

Historical Review of the First 42 Years 1966–2008

Jay L. Grosfeld

During the 1950's and early 1960's, the recognition of pediatric surgery as a specialty was slow in coming. Less than a dozen programs were available at the time to train young physicians interested in children's surgery in the United States (US). There were few organizations that sponsored presentations by children's surgeons at their annual scientific meetings and publication of articles concerning childhood surgery were relatively sparse. In 1962, Dr Lawrence Pickett, the Chairman of the Surgery Section of the American Academy of Pediatrics (AAP) voiced concern that it was difficult to obtain acceptance of papers presented at the annual meeting of the section in adult surgical or pediatric journals (Fig. 1). At the time, Dr Mark M. Ravitch edited a small section in the Journal "*Surgery*" that was devoted to pediatric surgery however, only two or three articles were published each month. Dr Stephen L. Gans was a member of the Publications Committee of the AAP-Surgery Section and was assigned to screen and attempt to expedite publication of manuscripts presented at the meeting (Fig. 2). This was often a thankless job and finding a journal to publish these papers proved a difficult task since there were no journals published in English dedicated to the fledgling field.

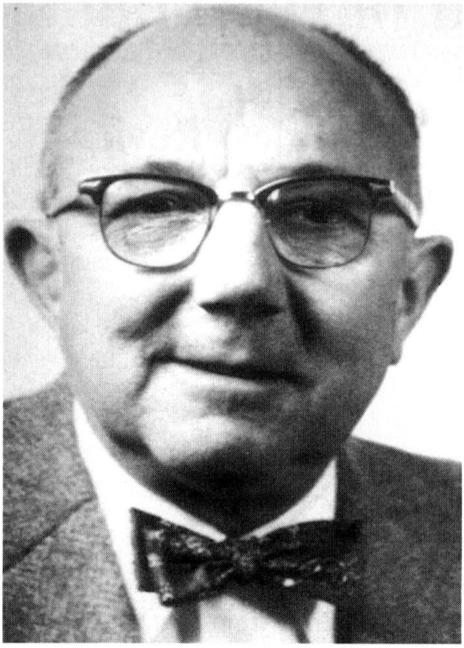

Fig. 1. Dr Lawrence Pickett, Chairman, Surgical Section, AAP 1962.

Dr Gans became convinced that a journal devoted solely to pediatric surgery was needed. He began to canvass children's surgeons about developing a journal and received considerable support to pursue this concept. A number of obstacles were encountered. Numerous efforts to find a publisher interested in a new journal failed because the medical publishers at the time suggested that because pediatric surgery was such a small specialty there was insufficient demand for the journal. In addition, the publishers were hesitant to proceed in developing a journal that had no relationship with a major pediatric surgical organization or society. At the time, the Surgical Section was a component section within the American Academy of Pediatrics and was not an independent surgical society.

Despite the many obstacles encountered, Dr Gans was persistent and began to recruit leaders in the field to serve as prospective members of the editorial board for a journal that did not yet exist. During the July, 1964 meeting of the British Association of Paediatric

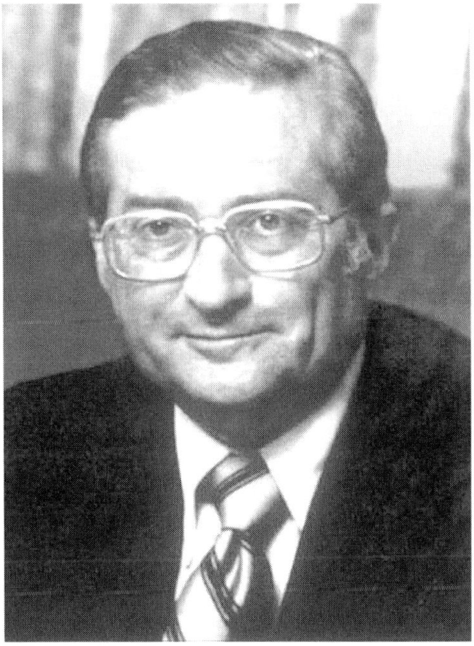

Fig. 2. Dr Stephen L. Gans Publications Committee, Surgical Section, AAP 1962. Dr Gans was the innovator of the "*Journal of Pediatric Surgery*" serving as the 2nd Editor-in-Chief from 1967–1994.

Surgeons (BAPS) in Rotterdam, The Netherlands, Dr Gans continued to pursue the concept of developing a specialty journal and interested children's surgical leaders from abroad to provide additional support (Fig. 3).

On November 15, 1964, Dr Gans met with Mr Henry Stratton of Grune and Stratton Publishers in Seattle, WA and convinced him to publish the "*Journal of Pediatric Surgery*". Dr C. Everett Koop a prominent and well respected leader in the field and Surgeon-in-Chief of the Children's Hospital of Philadelphia at the time, was selected as the first Editor-in-Chief (Fig. 4). Dr Gans was appointed Associate Editor and Prof Peter Paul Rickham of Liverpool, UK, served as Associate Editor for Great Britain (Fig. 5). The rest of the associate editors and editorial consultant Board came from various places in the world (Fig. 6).

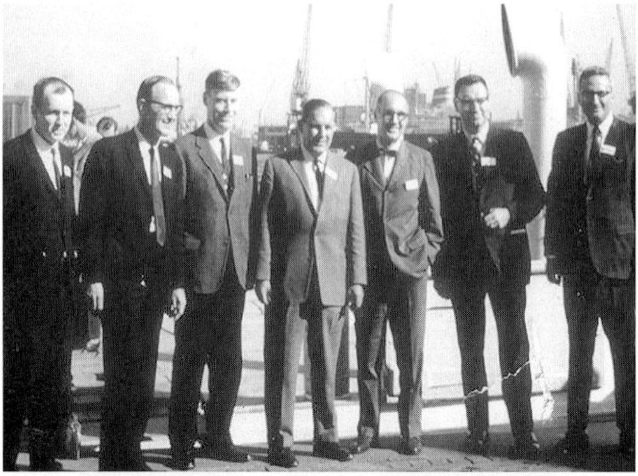

Fig. 3. Photograph of Dr Gans (far right) and a number of pediatric surgeons interested in his concept of developing the "*Journal*". On a pier in Rotterdam, the Netherlands, at the time of the 1964 BAPS meeting, (photograph made available by Mrs Elizabeth Gans).

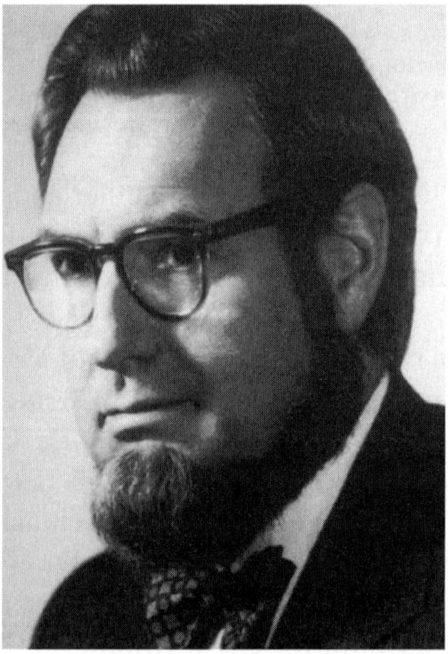

Fig. 4. C. Everett Koop, MD, Philadelphia, PA, the first Editor-in-Chief of the "*Journal of Pediatric Surgery*" (1966–1977).

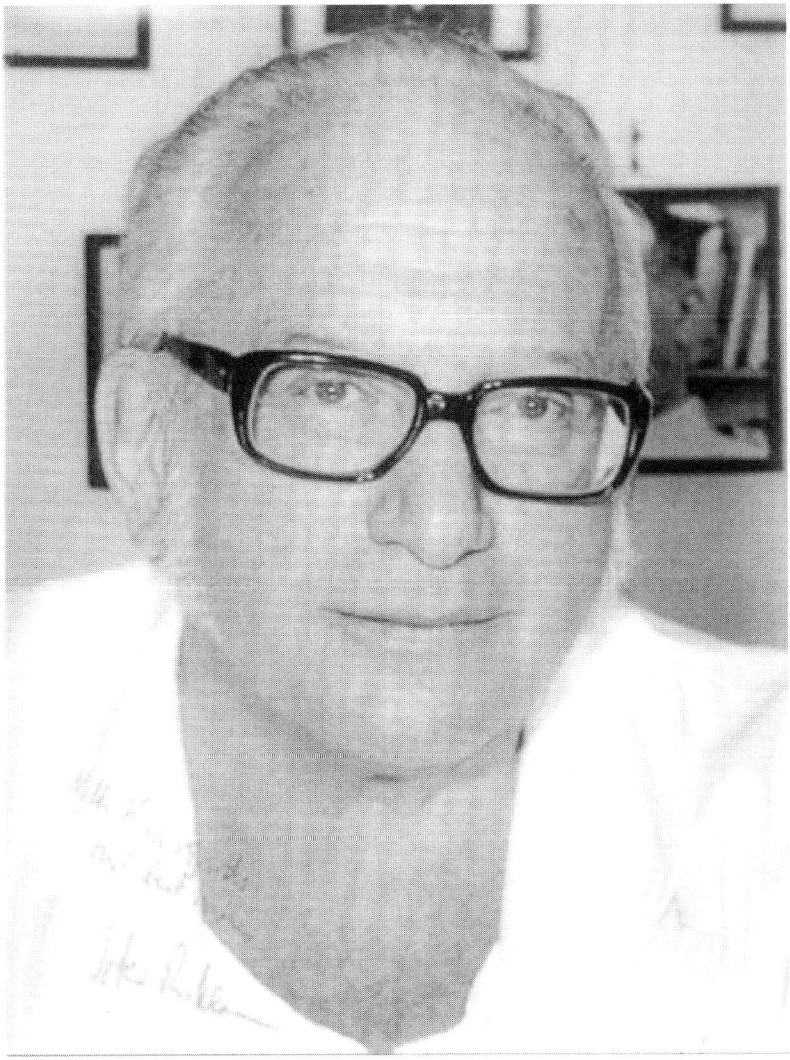

Fig. 5. Prof Peter Paul Rickham. Liverpool, UK, first Associate Editor for Great Britain.

In 1965, Drs Koop and Gans persuaded the BAPS and Surgery Section of the AAP to establish a relationship with the new journal to publish the transactions of their annual meetings. Dr Lester Martin was selected as the Guest editor for the Surgical Section of

Journal of Pediatric Surgery

EDITOR IN CHIEF

C. Everett Koop, M.D., Sc.D. (Med.)
Surgeon-in-Chief, The Children's Hospital of Philadelphia; Professor of Pediatric Surgery, School of Medicine, University of Pennsylvania, Philadelphia, Pa.

ASSOCIATE EDITOR

Stephen L. Gans, M.D.
Chief, Pediatric Surgery Service, Cedars of Lebanon Hospital, Los Angeles; Associate Clinical Professor of Surgery, California College of Medicine; Surgeon-in-Charge of Pediatric Surgery, Los Angeles County General Hospital, Unit II

ASSOCIATE EDITOR FOR GREAT BRITAIN

Peter P. Rickham, M.S., F.R.C.S., D.C.H.
Senior Paediatric Surgeon, Alder Hey Children's Hospital, Liverpool; Lecturer in Paediatric Surgery, University of Liverpool, England

EDITORIAL AND ADVISORY BOARD

Luke W. Able, M.D., *Houston, Tex.*
P. G. Ashmore, M.D., *Vancouver, B. C.*
Clifford D. Benson, M.D., *Detroit, Mich.*
Edward J. Berman, M.D., *Indianapolis, Ind.*
Marcel Bettex, M.D., *Berne, Switzerland*
Tague C. Chisholm, M.D., *Minneapolis, Minn.*
Daniel T. Cloud, M.D., *Phoenix, Ariz.*
George W. Dorman, M.D., *Dallas, Tex.*
Th. Ehrenpreis, M.D., *Stockholm, Sweden*
Colin C. Ferguson, M.D., *Winnipeg, Canada*
Michel Gilbert, M.D., *Miami, Fla.*
W. Hardy Hendren, M.D., *Boston, Mass.*
Robert J. Izant, Jr., M.D., *Cleveland, Ohio*
J. H. Johnston, F.R.C.S., F.R.C.S.(I.), *Liverpool, England*
Vaclav Kafka, Dr.Sc., *Prague, Czechoslovakia*
Benjamin M. Kagan, M.D., *Los Angeles, Calif.*
William B. Kiesewetter, M.D., *Pittsburgh, Pa.*
I. S. Kirkland, F.R.C.S. (Ed.), *Edinburgh, Scotland*
Luther Longino, M.D., *Boston, Mass.*
Jan H. Louw, Ch.M., F.R.C.S. (Eng.), *Capetown, S. A.*
Hugh B. Lynn, M.D., *Rochester, Minn.*
Carlo Montagnani, M.D., *Florence, Italy*
Jorge Roza de Oliveira, M.D., *Lisbon, Portugal*
Denys Pellerin, M.D., *Paris, France*
Lawrence K. Pickett, M.D., *New Haven, Conn.*
Willis J. Potts, M.D., *Sarasota, Fla.*
Fritz Rehbein, M.D., *Bremen, Germany*
William L. Riker, M.D., *Evanston, Ill.*
F. H. Robarts, F.R.C.S. (Ed.), *Edinburgh, Scotland*
Thomas V. Santulli, M.D., *New York, N. Y.*
William K. Sieber, M.D., *Pittsburgh, Pa.*
E. Durham Smith, F.R.A.C.S., *Melbourne, Australia*
Rowena Spencer, M.D., *New Orleans, La.*
Keijiro Suruga, M.D., *Tokyo, Japan*
D. Vervat, M.D., *Rotterdam, Netherlands*
D. J. Waterston, M.B.E., F.R.C.S. (Ed.), *London, England*
Harvey White, M.D., *Chicago, Ill.*
R. B. Zachary, F.R.C.S., *Sheffield, England*

Lester W. Martin, M.D., *Cincinnati, Ohio*
Secretary, Surgical Section, American Academy of Pediatrics

James Lister, F.R.C.S., *Sheffield, England*
Secretary, British Association of Paediatric Surgeons

Fig. 6. Copy of the initial mast head indicating the members of the editorial board of the journal in 1966.

the AAP and Mr James Lister was chosen to serve in that capacity for BAPS (Fig. 6). The *Journal* was to be published 6 times per year. In the first issue published in February 1966, Prof I. S. Ravdin, the Barton Rhea Professor of Surgery at the University of Pennsylvania and a Regent and Past-President of the American College of Surgeons wrote the lead editorial recognizing the progress of the

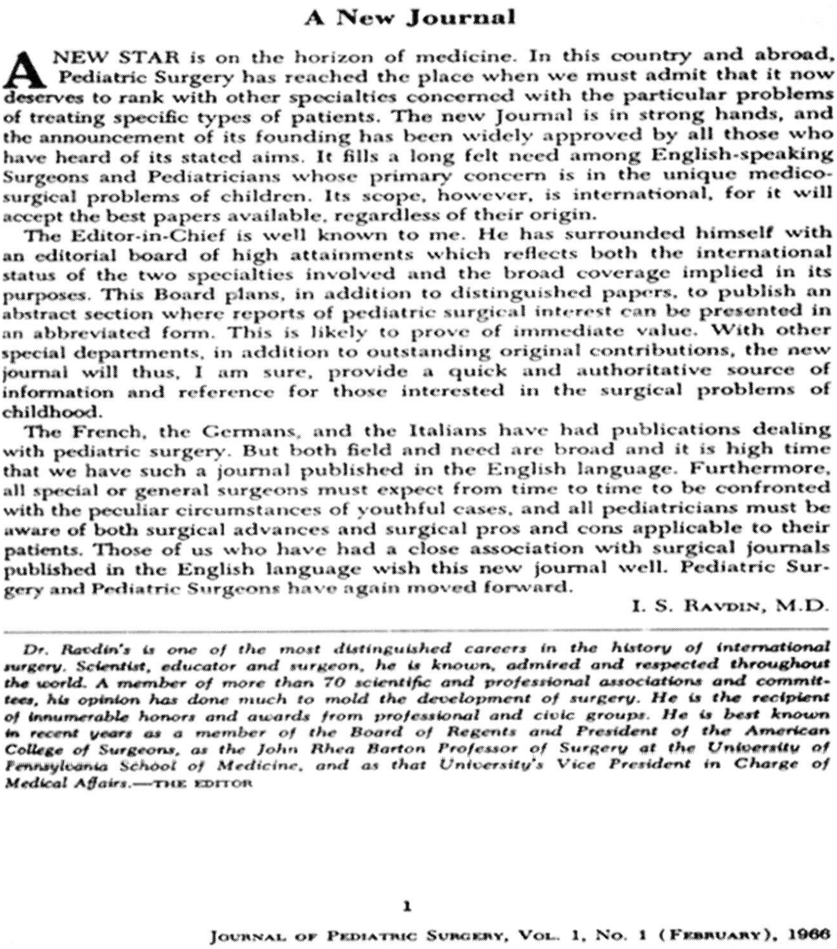

A New Journal

A NEW STAR is on the horizon of medicine. In this country and abroad, Pediatric Surgery has reached the place when we must admit that it now deserves to rank with other specialties concerned with the particular problems of treating specific types of patients. The new Journal is in strong hands, and the announcement of its founding has been widely approved by all those who have heard of its stated aims. It fills a long felt need among English-speaking Surgeons and Pediatricians whose primary concern is in the unique medico-surgical problems of children. Its scope, however, is international, for it will accept the best papers available, regardless of their origin.

The Editor-in-Chief is well known to me. He has surrounded himself with an editorial board of high attainments which reflects both the international status of the two specialties involved and the broad coverage implied in its purposes. This Board plans, in addition to distinguished papers, to publish an abstract section where reports of pediatric surgical interest can be presented in an abbreviated form. This is likely to prove of immediate value. With other special departments, in addition to outstanding original contributions, the new journal will thus, I am sure, provide a quick and authoritative source of information and reference for those interested in the surgical problems of childhood.

The French, the Germans, and the Italians have had publications dealing with pediatric surgery. But both field and need are broad and it is high time that we have such a journal published in the English language. Furthermore, all special or general surgeons must expect from time to time to be confronted with the peculiar circumstances of youthful cases, and all pediatricians must be aware of both surgical advances and surgical pros and cons applicable to their patients. Those of us who have had a close association with surgical journals published in the English language wish this new journal well. Pediatric Surgery and Pediatric Surgeons have again moved forward.

I. S. Ravdin, M.D.

Dr. Ravdin's is one of the most distinguished careers in the history of international surgery. Scientist, educator and surgeon, he is known, admired and respected throughout the world. A member of more than 70 scientific and professional associations and committees, his opinion has done much to mold the development of surgery. He is the recipient of innumerable honors and awards from professional and civic groups. He is best known in recent years as a member of the Board of Regents and President of the American College of Surgeons, as the John Rhea Barton Professor of Surgery at the University of Pennsylvania School of Medicine, and as that University's Vice President in Charge of Medical Affairs.—The Editor

1

Journal of Pediatric Surgery, Vol. 1, No. 1 (February), 1966

Fig. 7. Editorial by Prof I. S. Ravdin published in the first issue of the "*Journal of Pediatric Surgery*", February, 1966.[1]

field and the need for publishing a journal devoted to pediatric surgery in the English language (Fig. 7).[1] The timing of the initiation of the journal was important, as English was commonly accepted as the language of choice for most international scientific symposia and congresses.

The journal was an immediate success. It was quite clear that the time had come for children's surgeons to have their own journal dedicated to the specialty of pediatric surgery. The number of subscribers to the new journal rapidly increased and the volume of manuscripts submitted for publication was far in excess of the designated pages available to publish them. In 1971, the newly formed American Pediatric Surgical Association (APSA) selected the "*journal of Pediatric Surgery*" as its official publication. Robert E. Gross, MD, the first President of the American Pediatric Surgical Association and one of the fathers of Pediatric Surgery in the US, and perhaps the most revered and respected member of the field at the time wrote, "I think the "*journal of Pediatric Surgery*" has done more to advance children's surgery, only here but around the world, above anything else in the last couple of decades" (Fig. 8).

The Journal became recognized as the representative journal of a growing and progressive specialty. The "*Journal of Pediatric Surgery*" promoted recognition of the field throughout the world and gave the specialty additional credibility. It was noted as one of a number of supporting factors in the decision by the American Board of Surgery to issue a Certificate of Special Competence in Pediatric Surgery in 1973. Similarly, at the same time, once Board status was available, the Accreditation Council for Graduate Medical Education (ACGME) Residency Review Committee (RRC) for Surgery became responsible for accrediting pediatric surgery resident

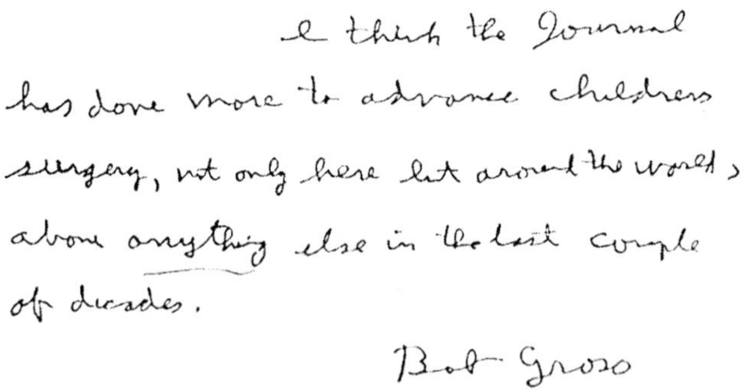
I think the Journal has done more to advance childrens surgery, not only here but around the world, above anything else in the last couple of decades.

Bob Gross

Fig. 8. A hand written note to Dr Gans from Dr Robert E, Gross, the first President of APSA concerning the importance of the "*journal*" to the field of pediatric surgery. (made available from the personal file of Mrs. Elizabeth Gans).

training programs as it had for adult training in general surgery for many years. One of the many criteria used to evaluate accredited training programs was the academic productivity of the faculty and residents and whether their work was published in a peer reviewed journal representing their specialty. The "*journal of Pediatric Surgery*" fulfilled this need.

In 1976, Dr Koop resigned his post as the Editor-in-Chief having served 11 years in that position. He subsequently would go on to serve as the Surgeon-General of the United States from 1981–1989 and continues to participate in health care policy issues today. Dr Koop is currently 92 years old. Dr Gans was appropriately selected as the new Editor-in Chief of the journal. He was an innovative editor and changed the format of reporting publications — strongly emphasizing the peer review process.[2] The journal was one of the first periodicals to employ an abstract and use index words to assist computer information retrieval. An International Abstracts section was added to provide the journal readership with information concerning children's surgical articles published elsewhere. Prof Keijiro Suruga, a longstanding member of the editorial board, was appointed the Editor for Asia (Fig. 9). In 1979, the Canadian Association of Pediatric surgeons (CAPS) agreed to publish the transactions of its annual scientific meeting in the journal. That same year, Prof Michele Carcassone of Marseille was selected the Editor for Europe (Fig. 10).

In June, 1986, Drs. Gans and Jay Grosfeld, then an Associate Editor, met with Mr Thomas Mackey, representing Grime and Stratton Publishers in Orlando, FL to discuss the future of the journal — then it its 20th year of publication. They negotiated an agreement to publish the journal monthly. Finally, the journal had come of age and gained the respect of the publishing world and achieved its place among the other more mature monthly surgical periodicals. In 1988, Prof Daniel G. Young of Glasgow became the Editor for the British Isles and Ireland (Fig. 11). That same year the Pacific Association of Pediatric Surgeons (PAPS) became the fifth surgical society to develop a relationship with the journal serving as the organization's official publication. This expansion into the east

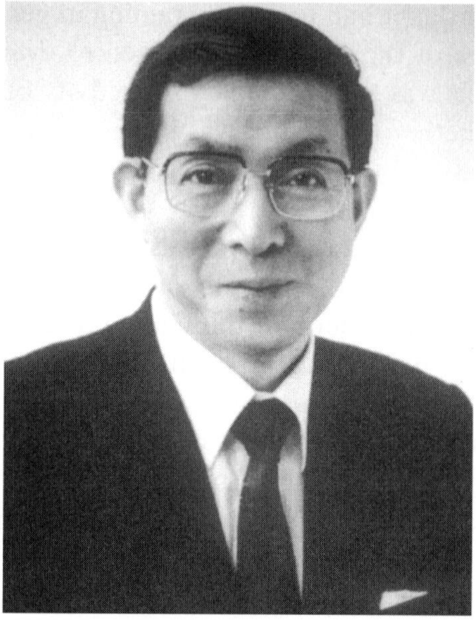

Fig. 9. Prof Kerjiro Suruga, the first appointed Editor for Asia.

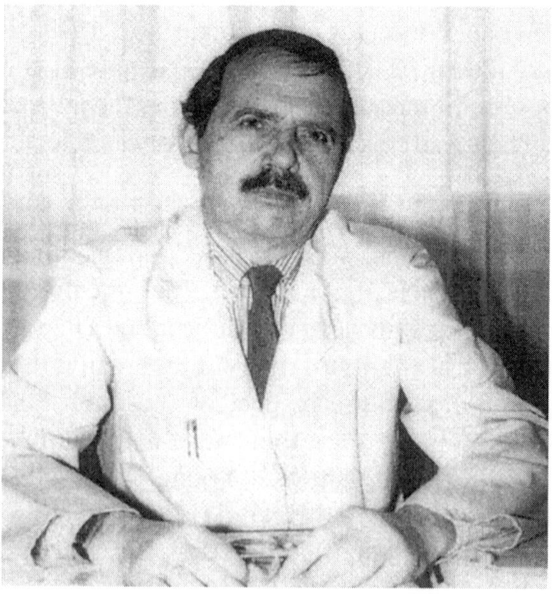

Fig. 10. Prof Michele Carcassone of Marseille, Editor for Europe (1979–1992).

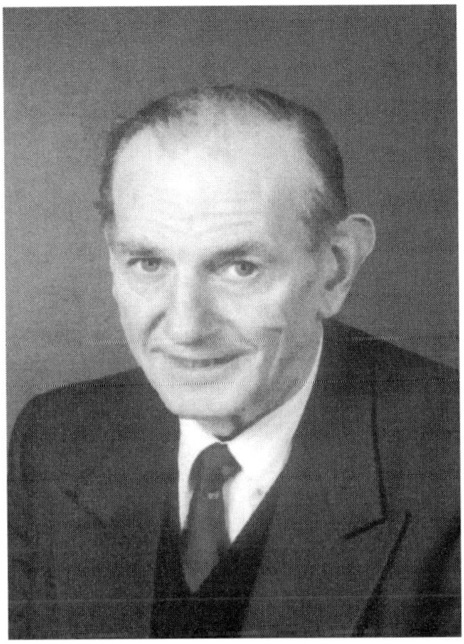

Fig. 11. Prof Daniel G. Young of Glasgow, Editor for the British Isles and Ireland (1988–2005).

further emphasized the international nature of the journal. In 1990 Prof Jan Molenaar of Rotterdam, became the Editor for Europe and in 1992, Prof Takeshi Miyano of Tokyo, replaced Prof Suruga as the Editor for Asia (Figs. 12 and 13).

In 1992, a sister periodical was developed "*Seminars in Pediatric Surgery*" — a quarterly publication that would serve as a valuable bridge between the journal and the various textbooks in the field. Each issue of *Seminars* contained numerous articles concerning a single topic of importance that provided detailed current information in great depth that was usually unavailable in the journals, and was more contemporary than information in textbooks which often had a significant lag period between publication of the new editions. Drs Gans and Grosfeld served as the founding editors of the *Seminars.*

On August 1, 1994, after a valiant battle with bladder cancer, Dr Stephen L. Gans passed away at age 74 years. He had served as

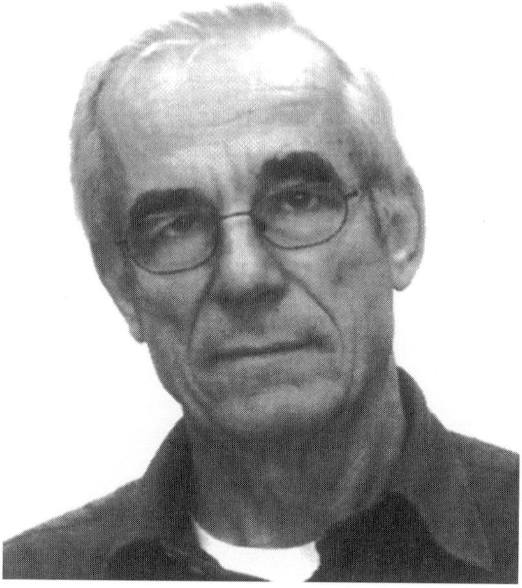

Fig. 12. Prof Jan Molenaar, Rotterdam, Editor for Europe (1992–2002).

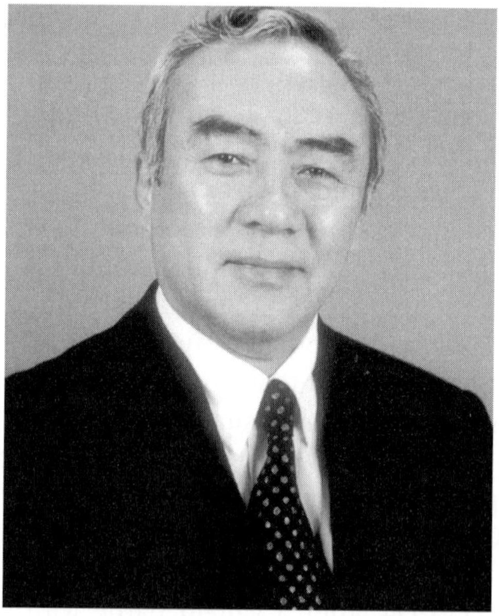

Fig. 13. Prof Takeshi Miyano, Tokyo, Editor for Asia (1992–present).

Editor-in-Chief of the journal for 18 years. He was eulogized for his unrelenting dedication to the specialty and for his efforts to champion, develop and nurture the journal from its inception until the time of his death.[3] He was a visionary in establishing the "*Journal*" and "*Seminars*" — two periodicals that were vital in providing access for publications in the evolving field of pediatric surgery. Dr Gans was also a practicing pediatric surgeon and pioneered minimally invasive "peritoneoscopy" in infants and children in the 1970's as a prelude to the current common use of laparoscopic surgery (Fig. 2).

Dr Jay L. Grosfeld of Indianapolis, a long standing member of the Editorial Board and a recognized and respected leader in the field was selected to succeed Dr Gans as the third Editor-in-Chief of the "*Journal of Pediatric Surgery*" and Editor of the "*Seminars*" (Fig. 14). The "*Journal*" office was moved from Los Angeles to Indianapolis. Over the next few years, the "*Journal*" experienced

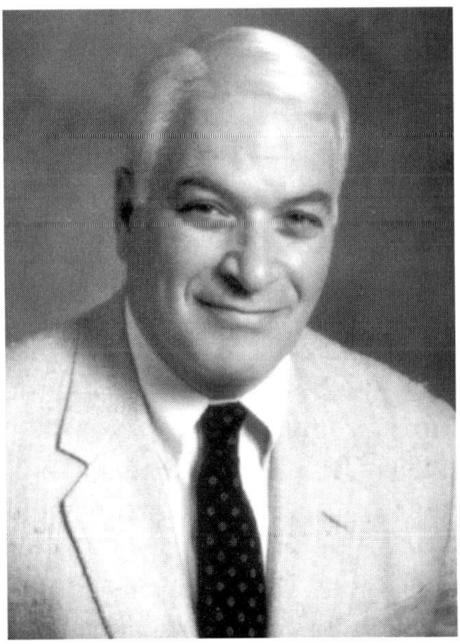

Fig. 14. Prof Jay L. Grosfeld, Indianapolis, the third Editor-in-Chief, Journal of Pediatric Surgery (1994–percent), Founding Editor, "*Seminars of Pediatric Surgery*" (1992–present).

several managerial changes reflective of acquisitions and mergers that affected the publishing world. W.B. Saunders, Columbia Broadcasting System and Brace–Jovanovich Inc, served as publishers. Further mergers with C.V. Mosby and Churchill–Livingston occurred and eventually, Reed–Elsevier became and still is the parent company. These changes were relatively seamless for the "*Journal*", which continued to thrive despite the corporate changes. This was made possible by a group of highly professional and supportive publishers assigned to the "*Journal*" during the past 14 years including Joan Blumberg and Livia Berardi of Philadelphia, and Andrew Berin and Patricia Hogan in New York.

The "*Journal*" transitioned to electronic publishing and developed its own web site (www.jpedsurg.org), with search and linking features to citation resources, a variety of useful databases and access to many other journals produced by the publishers.[4] Subscribers to the journal had online access to full text journal articles and the availability of online only e-publications to facilitate earlier publication of articles.

In 2002, Prof Juan Tovar of Madrid became the Editor for Europe and in 2005 Mr Victoria E. Boston of Belfast was selected as Editor for the British Isles and Ireland (Figs. 15 and 16). Drs John Schullinger (New York) and Steven Stylianos (Miami, FL) serve as Section Editors of the International Abstract section of the journal and Prof Geoff Blair of Vancouver, BC is the editor of the Section on Pediatric Surgical Images.

The Editor-in-Chief (Dr Grosfeld) represents the "*Journal of Pediatric Surgery*" in the Surgical Journal Editors Group (SJEG) whose membership is comprised of editors from all the major surgical journals. The SJEG meets annually and develops important consensus statements regarding common publication problems affecting most surgical journals including for example, duplicate and fraudulent submissions, authorship responsibility, ethical matters, required institutional review for animal and human research, guidelines for prospective randomized studies, and submissions dealing with studies supported by the pharmaceutical industry and technological corporations. Consensus statements concerning these

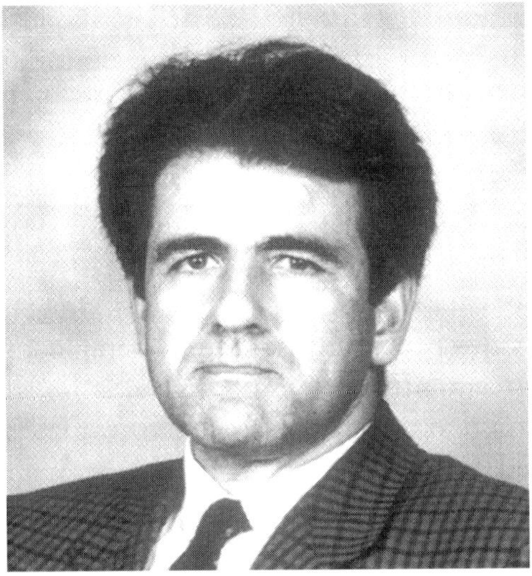

Fig. 15. Prof Juan Tovar, Madrid, Editor for Europe (2002–present).

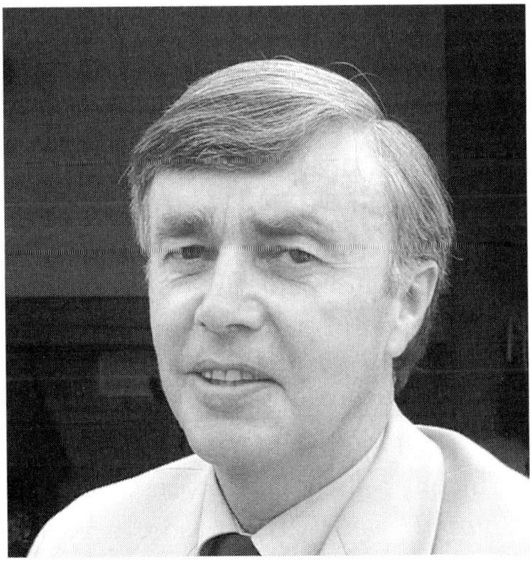

Fig. 16. Mr Victor E. Boston, Editor for the British Isles and Ireland (2005–present).

important issues that are agreed to by the surgical editors are published simultaneously in a specific journal issue by all the participating surgical journals.[5,6]

In 2007, the "*Journal*" initiated electronic submission and review of manuscripts using the Elsevier electronic editorial system (http://ees.elsevier.com/jpedsurg/). This has also provided a significantly enhanced database for the journal editorial board and manuscript reviewers. The electronic system has improved handling of manuscripts, enhanced communications, expedited and improved the efficiency of the review process and obviated most mailing costs for authors, reviewers and editorial management.[7] In general, electronic submission provides prospective authors a simple, efficient and less costly method of submitting their work to the "*Journal*". Of interest is the observation that the change to an electronic system has significantly increased the number of independent manuscript submissions to the "*Journal*" by 30%.

During the past 43 years, the "*journal of Pediatric Surgery*" has matured into the leading periodical in the field of children's surgery. The journal has achieved a balance of high quality clinical and scientific publications that provide contemporary content for the subscribers. The implementation of guidelines for reporting clinical research has aided in the preparation of clinical articles and improved the quality of the content of the journal. This effort was accomplished with the aid of Dr R. Lawrence Moss of New Haven, CT an Editorial Consultant for the "*Journal*".[8,9] The ability to publish new and contemporary information in the field presented at the annual meetings of five major pediatric surgical societies that use the journal as their official site of publication significantly enhances the journal content. The "*Journal*" values its long standing relationship with APSA, BAPS, CAPS, PAPS and the Surgical Section of the AAP and supports and sponsors special Lectures at some of the meetings. The stringent peer review process that has been the hallmark of the I "*Journal*" 's activities, has been kept at an extremely high level thanks to the outstanding group of loyal, knowledgeable and efficient associate editors, editorial consultants and valued external reviewers. The correspondence section of the journal also provides an additional source of peer review in the form of letters to the editor.

In the future, the "*Journal of Pediatric Surgery*" will continue to strive to improve and maintain its position as the major source of new clinical and investigative information in the field and provide its readers with the most contemporary content.

References

1. Ravdin IS. A New Journal. *J Pediatr Surg* 1966;1:1.
2. Gans SL. Recognition in peer review. *J Pediatr Surg* 1993;28:121–122.
3. Grosfeld, JL. 30th Anniversary issue: Journal of Pediatric Surgery 1966–1996. *J Pediatr Surg* 1996;31:1–2.
4. Grosfeld JL. 35th Anniversary of the Journal of Pediatric Surgery (1966–2001): A look into the future. *J Pediatr Surg* 2000;35:1685–1686.
5. Grosfeld, JL. The Journal of Pediatric Surgery enters the age of electronic submission. *J Pediatr Surg* 2007;42:757.
6. Grosfeld JL for the SJEG. Duplicate and fraudulent submission of manuscripts. *J Pediatr Surg* 2001;36:835–836.
7. Surgical Journal Editors Group. Scientific data from clinical trials: Investigator's responsibilities and rights. *J Pediatr Surg* 2002;37:809–810.
8. Moss RL. The Consort Statement: Progress in clinical research in Pediatric Surgery. *J Pediatr Surg* 2001;36:1739–1742.
9. Moss RL, Grosfeld JL. A new standard for reporting clinical research in the journal of pediatric surgery. *J Pediatr Surg* 2006;4–6.

THE EUROPEAN JOURNAL OF PEDIATRIC SURGERY

Alexander Holschneider
Kurt Gdanietz

Forty three years ago, in August 1964, a German journal for pediatric surgery was published for the first time: the "***Zeitschrift für Kinderchirurgie und Grenzgebiete***", edited by **K.-A. Bushe** (Neurosurgical University Clinic Göttingen), **Gerhard Joppich** (Pediatric University Clinic, Göttingen) and **F. Rehbein** (Bremen) (Fig. 1). It appeared quarterly and ran to about 480 pages per year.[1]

This was a time in which demand and interest in pediatric surgery experienced a sharp rise, due to a birth rate of 1.2–1.3 million annually in Germany alone and to the revolutionary successes initially of American and later also of European pediatric surgeons in the treatment of previously incurable, congenital malformations. In 1948 Swenson performed the first successful resection of an aganglionic intestinal segment in Hirschsprung's disease, Denis Browne published his techniques for the treatment of hypospadias (1949) and 1941 Haight carried out the first intrathoracic end-to-end anastomosis for esophageal atresia, Ladd's procedure for malrotation (1933) became known in Europe and the Gross textbook "*The Surgery of Infancy and Childhood*" (1953) became available in Germany. The successful treatments with these techniques had a stimulating effect, so that a forum for the publication of works in Germany was sought for. The pediatric surgeons M. Grob (Zürich), H. Hartl (Linz), F. Meissner (Leipzig), A. Oberniedermayr (Munich), P. P. Rickham (Liverpool), D. Vervat (Rotterdam), the

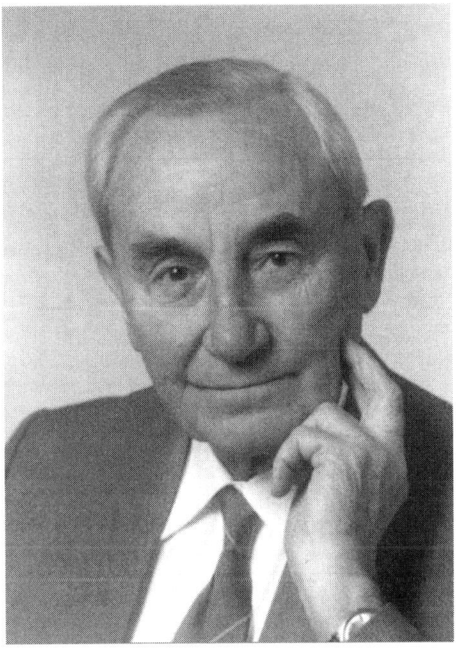

Fig. 1. Fritz Rehbein.

pediatricians E. Rossi (Berne), E. Zweymüller (Vienna), the urologist H. K. Buscher (Hannover), the orthopedist H. Mau (Tübingen), the anesthesiologist J. Van T'Oever (Rotterdam) and the pediatric radiologist E. Willich (Bremen) all contributed to the first edition of the "*Zeitschrift für Kinderchirurgie and Grenzgebiete*" (Fig. 2).

In the foreword the editors emphasized that the one of the aims of the journal was to include papers on pediatric surgery from the Netherlands, Austria, Switzerland, Germany and other countries in a single journal. The scope of the journal was also intended to go beyond the narrow field of pediatric surgery, i.e. the treatment of congenital malformations, and include interdisciplinary fields connected to pediatric surgery such as orthopedics, radiology, anesthesia, urology and neurosurgery. In his introductory foreword Prof Rickham welcomed the appearance of the new journal in the name of the British Association of Pediatric Surgery.

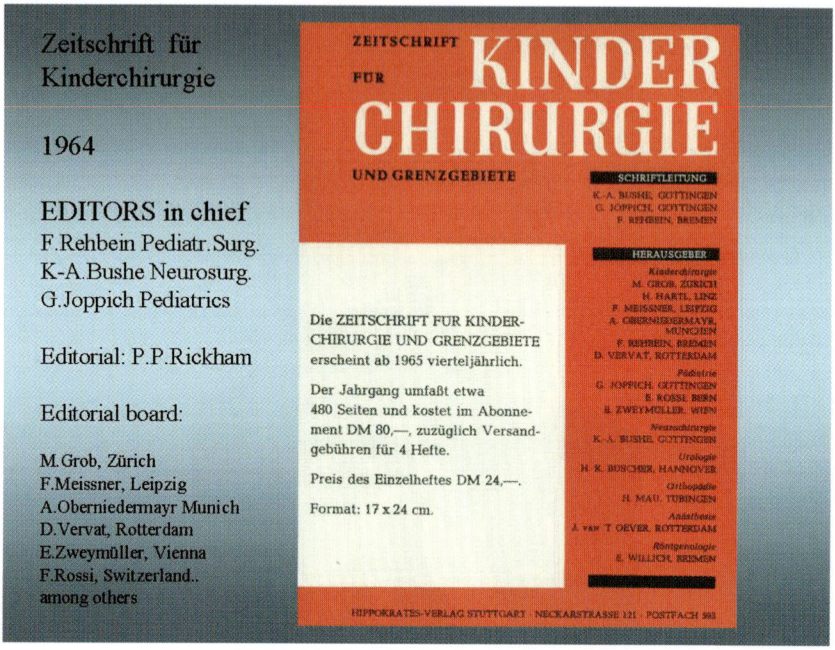
Zeitschrift für
Kinderchirurgie
1964
EDITORS in chief
F.Rehbein Pediatr.Surg.
K-A.Bushe Neurosurg.
G.Joppich Pediatrics
Editorial: P.P.Rickham
Editorial board:
M.Grob, Zürich
F.Meissner, Leipzig
A.Oberniedermayr Munich
D.Vervat, Rotterdam
E.Zweymüller, Vienna
F.Rossi, Switzerland..
among others
ZEITSCHRIFT FÜR
KINDER
CHIRURGIE
UND GRENZGEBIETE
SCHRIFTLEITUNG
K.-A. BUSHE, GÖTTINGEN
G. JOPPICH, GÖTTINGEN
F. REHBEIN, BREMEN
HERAUSGEBER
Kinderchirurgie
M. GROB, ZÜRICH
H. HARTL, LINZ
F. MEISSNER, LEIPZIG
A. OBERNIEDERMAYR, MÜNCHEN
F. REHBEIN, BREMEN
D. VERVAT, ROTTERDAM
Pädiatrie
G. JOPPICH, GÖTTINGEN
E. ROSSI, BERN
E. ZWEYMÜLLER, WIEN
Neurochirurgie
K.-A. BUSHE, GÖTTINGEN
Urologie
H. K. BUSCHER, HANNOVER
Orthopädie
H. MAU, TÜBINGEN
Anästhesie
J. van T OEVER, ROTTERDAM
Röntgenologie
E. WILLICH, BREMEN
Die ZEITSCHRIFT FÜR KINDER-CHIRURGIE UND GRENZGEBIETE erscheint ab 1965 vierteljährlich.
Der Jahrgang umfaßt etwa 480 Seiten und kostet im Abonnement DM 80,—, zuzüglich Versandgebühren für 4 Hefte.
Preis des Einzelheftes DM 24,—.
Format: 17 x 24 cm.
HIPPOKRATES-VERLAG STUTTGART · NECKARSTRASSE 121 · POSTFACH 593

Fig. 2. First issue of the "*Zeitschrift für Kinderchirurgie*", 1964.

More than 40 years with many new developments have passed since then. The number of manuscripts submitted to the "*Zeitschrift für Kinderchirurgie*" steadily increased, so that in the 1970's the Hippokrates publishing company together with the journal's editors decided to turn the quarterly journal into a monthly journal.

By this time the journal had diversified and moved from being a purely German-language based journal to having a European circulation. This was also reflected by the composition of the Editorial Board in 1980. The Board at that time consisted of M. Bettex (Berne), K.-A. Bushe (Würzburg), H. Hartl (Linz), G. Joppich (Göttingen), A. M. Holschneider (Munich). The extended Editorial Board included in addition F. J. Berchi (Madrid), R. Daum (Heidelberg), H. B. Eckstein (London), E. A. Enger (Gothenburg), St. L. Gans (Los Angeles), I. Joppich jun. (Mannheim), V. Kafka (Prague), T. Kitamura (Tokyo), C. E. Koop (Philadelphia), F. Meissner (Leipzig), J. C. Molenaar (Rotterdam), C. A. Montagnani (Rome), R. Morger

(St. Gall), A. Oberniedermayr (Starnberg), J. Prévot (Nancy), H. Sauer (Graz), A. Schärli (Lucerne) and Louise Schnaufer (Philadelphia). The field of embryology was represented by G. Töndury (Zürich), pediatric pathology by D. Harms (Kiel), anesthesia by P. Dangel (Zürich), neurosurgery by W. Th. Koos (Vienna), urology by K. V. Parkkulainen (Stockholm), orthopedics by H. Mau (Tübingen) and gynecology by E. Dreher (Berne). In addition to the journal almost every year a supplement was published dedicated to special important subjects such as traumatology in 1972: "*Der Unfall im Kindesalter — Klinik — Rehabilitation — Prophylaxe*", a complete book with 889 pages.

The broadening of the journal's scope whereby it became an international publication and had an international publisher and Editorial Board must be placed against the fact that the journal was now the official organ of the German, Swiss and Austrian Societies for Pediatric Surgery, and this led to a problem. The number of English language articles increased, the number of manuscripts written in German declined. One important reason for this was that at the beginning of the 1980s, above all in the German-speaking countries, related specialist fields such as urology, neurosurgery, and orthopedics, which at the time of the founding of the journal had felt that the pediatric questions in their field were represented by the journal, had by now founded their own independent pediatric departments and wished to present surgical questions arising with respect to pediatric patients in their particular specialist field in their own journals. (We should not forget that at this point, in Germany for example, pediatric surgery was still classed as a subsidiary branch of general surgery: it only became an independent field in 1994).[2]

In 1980 **Prof A. Holschneider**, Cologne, took over the journal from Rehbein and in 1982 the decision was taken to also publish manuscripts written in English in the "*Zeitschrift für Kinderchirurgie and ihre Grenzgebiete*" and from that point on, the journal's title also included the English subtitle "*Surgery in Infancy and Childhood*". The journal continued to be the official organ of the German, Swiss and Austrian Societies for Pediatric Surgery. In addition, however, the journal also published work from almost all European and many non-European countries. Apart from the well-known Anglo-American periodical "*Journal of Pediatric Surgery*" it was the only international journal in our specialist area. The process of becoming more international, which started in 1982, led to a wish which was increasingly voiced, namely that the journal should be completely transformed and turned into an international journal written in English.[1]

In 1990 Prof Juskiewenski (President of the French Surgical Society) and myself established contact and began talks about a merger of the French journal Zeitschrift "*Chirurgie Pédiatrique*" and the German journal "*Zeitschrift für Kinderchirurgie*". The journal "*Chirurgie Pédiatrique*" had also been founded at the beginning of the 1960s by Bernhard Duhamel and now faced the same sort of problems as the German-language "*Zeitschrift für Kinderchirurgie*" did. With the consent and approval of the French and German Societies for Pediatric Surgery the "***European Journal of Pediatric Surgery***" bearing the subtitles "***Zeitschrift für Kinderchirurgie und Chirurgie Pédiatrique***" was created in 1991. In addition, through discussions and negotiations held with other specialist societies the "*European Journal of Pediatric Surgery*" began to cooperate with other national societies for pediatric surgery (Fig. 3).

When the first issue of the "new" journal, now published bi-monthly, first appeared, it was already the official organ of the Austrian, Belgian, Dutch, French, German, Scandinavian and Swiss Societies for Pediatric Surgery. The former division into the categories anesthesia, embryology, pathology, neurosurgery, oncology, radiology pediatrics, traumatology, orthopedics, urology and pediatric plastic surgery was retained.

The internationalization over the past 22 years continued apace. In 2003 there was a further opening of the journal in the direction of Eastern Europe, when cooperation between the "*European Journal of Pediatric Surgery*" and "*Surgery in Childhood International*" was agreed upon by its former editor (K. Łodziński, Warsaw).

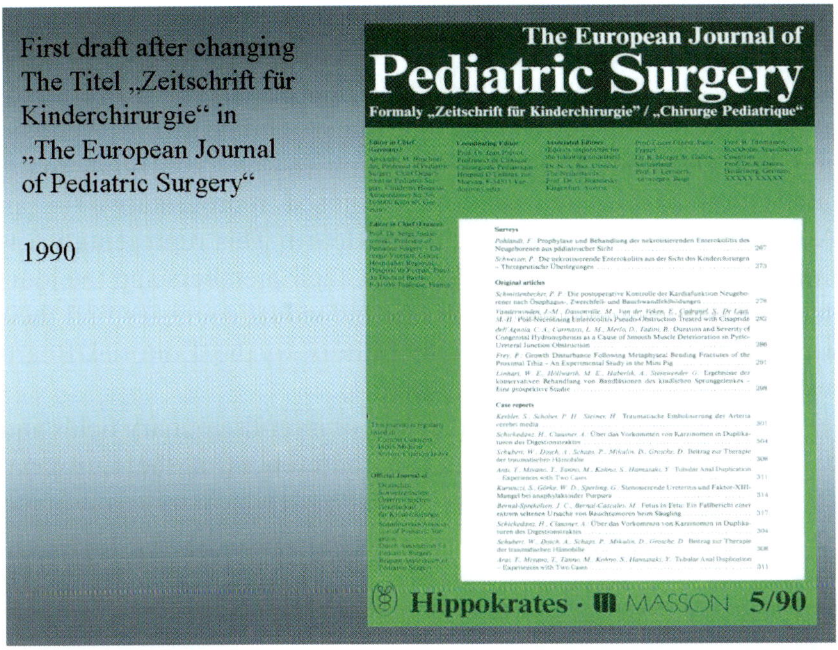

Fig. 3. First issue of the "*European Journal of Pediatric Surgery*" 1990.

At this point "*Surgery in Childhood International*" represented the countries Russia, Hungary, the Ukraine, Lithuania, Slovakia, Poland and the Baltic States. As of 2003 the "*European Journal of Pediatric Surgery*" took over the task of acting as a forum for pediatric surgery for these countries as well. Since then, Prof Kaliciński (Warsaw) has actively reinforced the Editorial Board of the "*European Journal of Pediatric Surgery*", so that from that point on, the journal opened up to the Eastern European countries on a large scale. The journal continued to thrive. Today manuscripts from more than 80 different countries are submitted to the "*European Journal*". The circulation of the journal and its dissemination is also continually increasing. In 2007 the **Prof Benno Ure**, Hannover became editor in chief of the journal and an enlarged editorial board was created with the Editorial Board Members: A. M. Holschneider,

P. Kalicinski (Poland), G. Martuciello (Italy), A. Pierro (UK) and Yann Revillon (Paris).

Today, the "*European Journal of Pediatric Surgery*" still adheres to the concepts laid down at the time of its founding by Prof Rehbein and Prof. Duhamel. The individual countries which contribute to the publication of the journal send a chosen representative — an Associate Editor — to the Editorial Board. This representative is the link between the national societies, their members and the journal. Important manuscripts from the individual countries find their way via the respective Associate Editors to the Editorial Board members and the editor-in-chief (Fig. 4).

The journal continues to take note of interdisciplinary fields and to publish conferences such as the conferences of the European Association of Pediatric Surgeons (EUPSA), which are represented

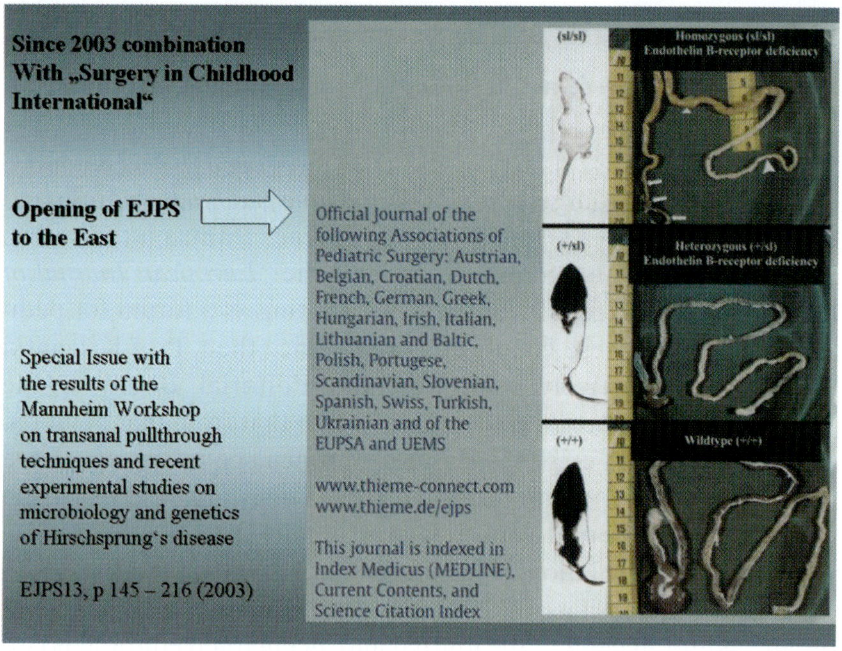

Fig. 4. Recent cover of the "*European Journal of Pediatric Surgery*".

annually in a special issue, but sets up main areas of discussion for others conferences too, such as the publication in May 2003 of the papers of the Mannheim Workshop on the subject "The transanal pull-through technique and recent experimental studies on microbiology and genetics of Hirschsprung's disease". In addition, the journal takes account in its communication of its readers' demand for information while representing the interests of the individual societies. Thus, for example, the members of the French and the German Society's of Pediatric Surgery receive the journal as part of their membership. Since 1999 the "*European Journal of Pediatric Surgery*" is also the official journal of the EUPSA and for the political News of the UEMS (Union of European Medical Specialists — Section Pediatric Surgery) and regularly publishes communications from these bodies. The "*European Journal of Pediatric Surgery*" has thus become a connecting link between the scientific European branch, the EUPSA and the political demands of the UEMS.

The future of the "*European Journal of Pediatric Surgery*" depends — as does the future of every scientific journal — on what sort of active role the members of its Editorial Board and its readers play in the shaping of the journal. What counts is the quality of the contents and the use and recognition of the journal as a scientific forum. As long as the scientific results published in the "*European Journal of Pediatric Surgery*" continue to have a high standard, the use for such a specialist journal will continue to be high. This must be the common goal of all persons involved, i.e. the readers, participants, authors and the different societies.

Besides two other journals have been published in Germany in the past: from 1970–1991 a scientific series entitled "*Progress in Pediatric Surgery*" edited by Peter P. Rickham, Waldemar Ch. Hecker and Jan Prévot. Altogether 27 books appeared first at Urban & Schwarzenberg, later at Springer Publisher, each dedicated to special pediatric surgical topic. After the reunification of both parts of Germany Prof Siegfried Hofmann von Kap-herr/Mainz edited the "*Zentralblatt für Kinderchirurgie*" in German language, which was published from 1990–2002 (Fig. 4).

References

1. Holschneider AM. The European Journal of Paediatric Surgery: 40 years of publication. Editorial, *Eur J Pediatr Surg* 2004;14:145–150.
2. Holschneider AM. Pediatric Surgical Reality in Germany and Visions for the Future. *Eur J Pediatr Surg* 2001;11:75–81.

PEDIATRIC SURGERY INTERNATIONAL

Arnold G. Coran
Prem Puri

The brain child of Pediatric Surgery International was clearly Alois Scharli from Lucerne, Switzerland, who came up with the idea of an international journal of pediatric surgery which would represent the entire world and not have a major focus in any particular continent such as North America. He began to discuss this concept with Springer-Verlag Publishers and with a few pediatric surgeons, namely, Arnold Coran, from the United States, Prem Puri from Ireland, Lewis Spitz from the United Kingdom, Sid Cywes from Africa, Michael Hollwarth from the European continent and Takeshi Miyano from Asia. All these pediatric surgeons agreed that there was a need for this type of pediatric surgery journal, and the publisher agreed to proceed with plans to establish "*Pediatric Surgery International*".

Final arrangements were made for the organization of the journal in 1985. Alois Scharli was appointed Editor-in-Chief, and Arnold Coran was appointed Editor for North America, Lewis Spitz Editor for the United Kingdom, Sid Cywes Editor for Africa, Takeshi Miyano Editor for Asia and Nate Myers Editor for Australia and New Zealand. The first issue, Volume 1, Number 1, was published in March 1986. From March 1986 until May 2003, issues were published every other month. Following the May 2003 issue, Volume 19, Number 3, the Editor-in-Chief and the editors convinced the

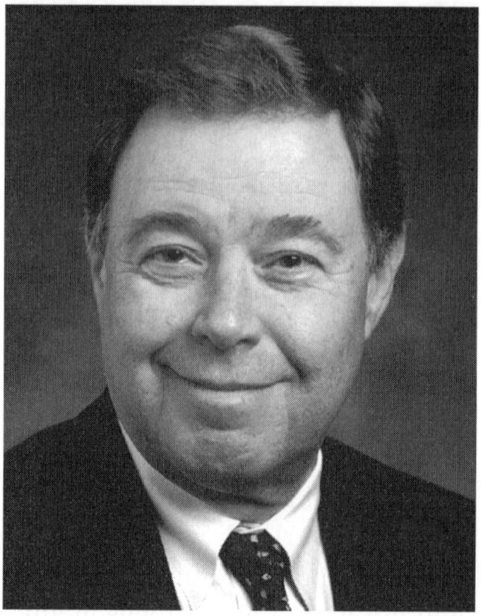

Arnold G. Coran

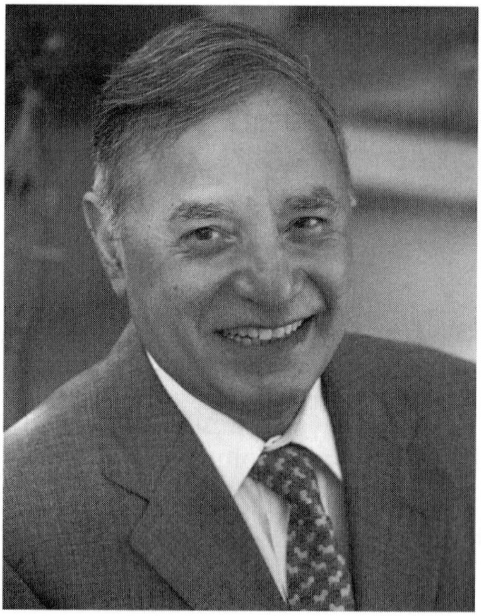

Prem Puri

publisher to move to an issue every month because of the large number of papers being submitted.

Once the Editor-in-Chief and editors were appointed in 1985, an editorial review board was selected from all the continents of the world. Over the years this board has changed as members have retired from practice. In 2003, Alois Scharli stepped down as the Editor-in-Chief, and Prem Puri and Arnold Coran were appointed Co-Editors-in-Chief. The positions of editor for the various continents were eliminated since they were felt to be redundant.

Early issues of the journal contained a large number of case reports with few major original articles and occasional review papers. As the journal matured, the number of case reports published markedly decreased and the number of original articles significantly increased. In addition, relationships between the journal and other societies developed during these past 10 years, such as the Japanese Society of Pediatric Surgeons, the International Society of Pediatric Surgical Research and the Pediatric Colorectal Society. The best papers from the annual meetings of these societies have been published in the journal each year. These various manuscripts have significantly enhanced the scientific quality of the journal.

In summary, "*Pediatric Surgery International*" is a true success story, starting out as a small publication, mainly of case reports, and growing into one of the major international journals of pediatric surgery.

Section E

PAEDIATRIC SURGICAL SERVICES

THE *MARIENTIFT KINDERHOSPITAL*; PEDIATRIC SURGERY IN 19TH CENTURY JERUSALEM

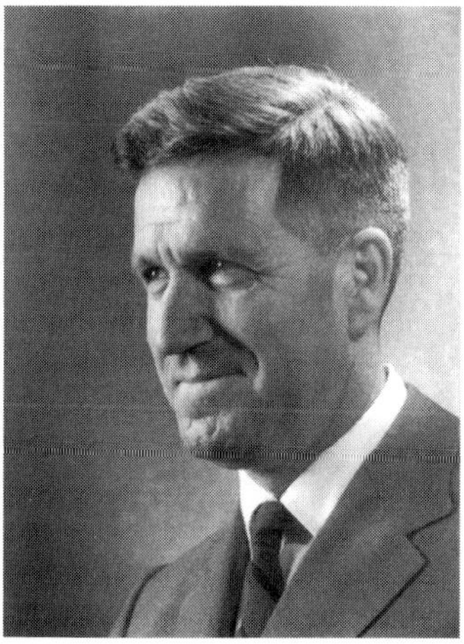

Shemuel Nissan

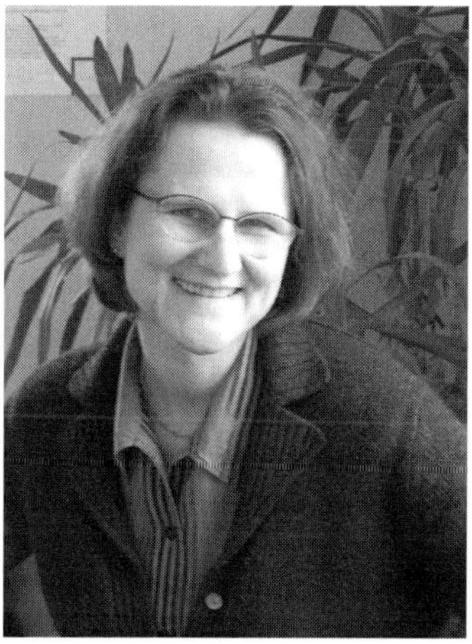

Petra Martin–Fiedler

Shemuel Nissan
Petra Martin–Fiedler

The Deaconess German Hospital

Pediatric surgery in 19th century Jerusalem amounted to one pediatric surgeon and one Children's Hospital. The Jewish and Arab communities in 19th century Jerusalem were medieval societies, which accepted a high mortality rate in children. Into this kind of society a modern, western type children's hospital was implanted. The *Marienstift Kinderhospital* was founded and operated by Dr Max Sandreczky, a

German pediatric surgeon.[1] Until the mid 19th century there had not been any resident physician present in the adjacent countries and the Holy Land.[2] The response of the Jewish and Arab communities to the *Marienstift Kinderhospital* were studied and is recorded.

Dr Max Sandreczky, the son of Karl Sandreczki, was born on the Cycladic island of Syra (today a part of Greece in the Aegean Sea).[3] His father Karl Sandreczki was appointed by Bishop Gobat to the position of secretary of the Church Missionary Society in Jerusalem. Max arrived in Jerusalem when he was 12 years old. After his graduation from the Anglican School in Malta[4] he studied medicine in Munich[5] and Wuerzburg.[6] He joined, as assistant, to Heinrich von Ranke in the newly founded Kinderpoliklinik in Muenchen.

In 1866, when Bismarck declared war against Austria, Max Sandreczky joined the Prussian army and was appointed medical director of the field hospital at Schloss Camenz.[7] There he met his future wife, Johanna Alida Hofs, a lady-in-waiting to Princess Marianna of the Netherlands (Fig. 1).[8]

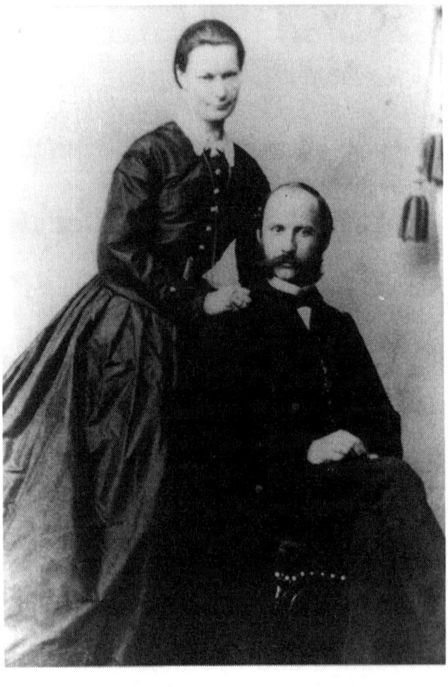

Fig. 1. Johanna and Max Sandreczky, in Nurenberg approx. 1874–1878.

They both arrived at the Holy Land in 1868.[9] He became the first German physician at the Deaconess hospital, Jerusalem. At the Deaconess hospital Max Sandreczky dedicated his time, energy and experience to the care of children. His desire was to establish a children's hospital.

In 1869, in connection with the opening of the Suez canal, the Prussian Crown Prince visited Jerusalem, with his son, the future Kaiser Wilhelm the second. Karl Sandreczki was their guide. Karl, Max and the Prussian consul von Alten, asked the Crown Prince to donate the means to establish a children's hospital in Jerusalem. Promises were made, but nothing came out of it.[10]

The Archduke and Duchess of Mecklenburg–Schwerin

In 1871, the Archduke of Mecklenburg Schwerin and his newly wedded wife, Princess Marie of Schwarzburg and Rudolstadt came as pilgrims to Jerusalem (Fig. 2).[11] The ruling family of

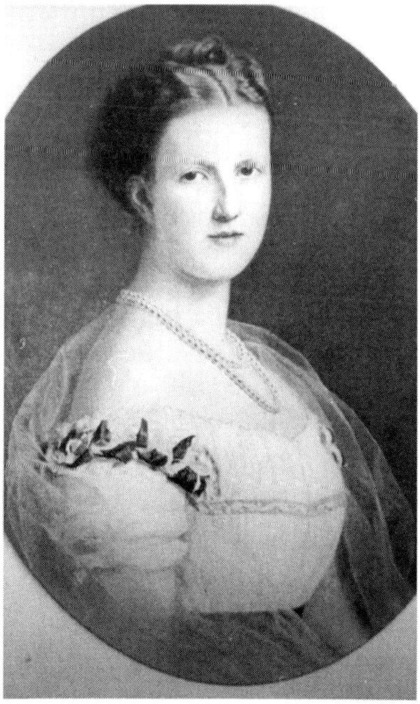

Fig. 2. The Archduchess Maria, from Mecklenburg Schwerin.

Mecklenburg–Schwerin had close relations with the Royal family of Holland. The youngest son of Princess Marie married Wilhelmina the Queen of Holland. When the Archduke and Duchess met Johanna and Max Sandreczky they were very much impressed and agreed to support a children's hospital[12] a year later the hospital was named after the Princess: *Marienstift Kinderhospital.*[13] The agreement was that no proselytism will be attempted on the children and their families. The hospital would serve the children of the Holy Land regardless of religious or ethnic affiliation. Johanna and Max Sandreczky pledged that they would work without a salary.

In a written proposition to the Archduke Sandreczky described the condition of children in the Holy Land: filthy environment, ignorance and apathy of parents and the child mortality reached 50%. The only hospital that took care of children was the German Deaconess, but because shortage of vacant beds,[14] often children were not admitted to the hospital.[15]

Treating children's in a special children's hospital would reduce the high mortality and disabilities attended upon various diseases. In a children's hospital, mothers could be admitted with their children; "rooming in", and the presence of the mother had an important effect on the child. In addition, he felt that children should be kept occupied while at the hospital. For this purpose he brought them all sorts of toys from Schwerin (Fig. 3)[16] while to the mothers he taught them basic ideas of cleanliness and hygiene.[17]

The *Mariestift Kinderhospital* Finances

The hospital was financed by the Archduke and Duchess of Mecklenburg Schwerin.[18] Bismarck allocated some funds to the hospital, remembering the service of Max Sandreczky in Schloss Cmenz, during the war of 1866. They were discontinued because there were only few children of German origin, treated in the hospital.[19] When the hospital ran a deficit, Kaiser Willhelm the second, donated 1500 marks, to cover half the deficit. The remainder was covered by Max Sandeczky.[20] The *Marfienstift* did not have the financial support of an organization, such as the Deaconess movement

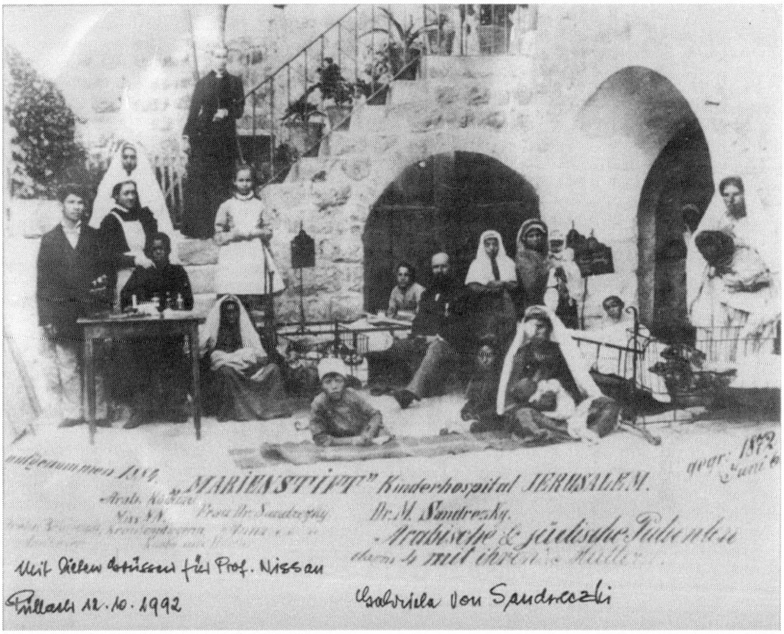

Fig. 3. The *Mariemstift Kinderhospital* court yard. Max and Johanna Sandreczky, and their daughter Anna. Behind a table his Jewish Pharmacist. "Arab and Jewish patients with their mothers". Toys are scattered on the beds.

or the Catholic Church. Max Sandreczky was unable to raise funds for the hospital because he opposed proselytism.[21] However Dr Max Sandreczky managed to gather a fair number of "friends of the hospital" and the budget was balanced.[22]

Max Sandreczky: A Surgeon and Physician

The following is a list of common diseases in the Holy Land during the 19th century: reported in the *Jahresbericht*, Annual report (Fig. 4) for the year 1872–1873: malaria, trachoma, leprosy, rheumatic fever, measles, pertussis, parasitic infestation, smallpox, diphtheria, meningitis, osteomyelitis and gastrointestinal infections. Some of the above he treated surgically; in addition he treated trauma, burns, herniotomies, resections of small bowel, resections of lymph nodes for tuberculosis, tonsillectomy, amputations, repair of cleft lip

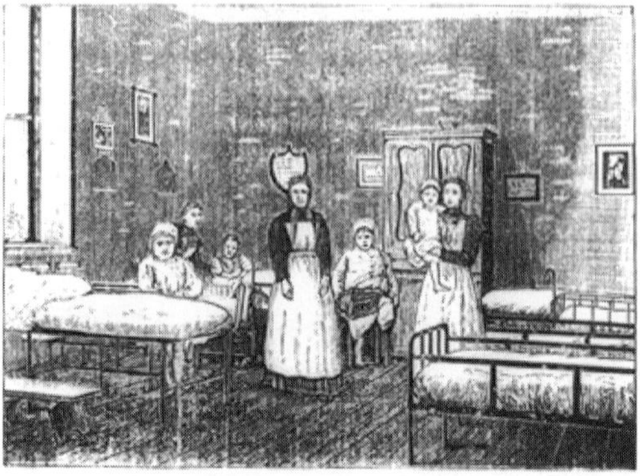

* * * * * *

23. Jahresbericht

des deutschen

Kinderhospitals Marienstift

zu

JERUSALEM.

Für das Jahr 1895.

"Wünschet Jerusalem Glück, Es gehe wohl denen, die dich lieben."

"Die Liebe ist des Gesetzes Erfüllung."

Fig. 4. *Jahresbericht* (annual report). A quatation "Pray for the peace of Jerusalem."

and rectal prolapse.[23] He also treated urinary tract stones, which he removed and tested chemically.[24]

The operations were performed under primitive conditions; inhalation anesthesia was given by his daughters, who were trained for it in Bethel medical center in Bielefeld, Germany. Surprisingly the mortality rate was low. In 1898, nine out of 548 patients admitted died in the hospital. He was highly regarded, as a surgeon and a physician, by his contemporaries, in and outside the country.[25] His concept of leprosy, was very much like ours today.[26] When Rudolf Wirchow sent Paul Langerhans to study leprosy in the Holy Land, Langerhans collaborated with Max Sandrezky and praised him in his publications.[27] In his first annual report, Jahres Bericht in 1872 wrote that the high rate of infection in Arab children was due to the fact that they lived in an unsanitary environment; dirt constituted a good culture media for fungus and bacteria.[28]

Nursing Staff

Sandreczky was unable to recruit nurses from western countries. Organizations such as the Catholic Church, The London Society for Promoting Christianity amongst the Jews, The Deaconess movement, had no difficulty in recruiting nurses from amongst their members. Sandreczky planned to train nursing staff from amongst the graduates of the Lutheran Orphanages. He failed because of the mentality of the local populations.[29] Johanna Sandreczky who was a house keeper of the hospital and three of Max Sandreczky's daughters, who were trained in Bethel in Bielefeld, Germany as nurses, undertook to serve as nurses and anesthetists in the children's hospital.[30]

A Board of Trustees (Kuratorium)

The hospital had a board of trustees that included the German Consul General; the German-Swiss architect Conrad Schick, the Swiss banker Johannes Frutiger, the German Bishop (Probst), and Dr Max Sandreczky.

All of them resided in the street of the Prophets, Jerusalem. When the board of trustees ceased to function, a committee was appointed by the Archduke in Schwerin and directed the activities of the hospital from there.[31]

Patient Population

During the year of 1872, the majority of the patients were Arabs and Ottoman citizens. Some of them came from Gaza, Damascus, Nablus and Jaffa.[32] Soon Sandreczky gained the trust of the Jewish population. No attempt at proselytism was practiced in the hospital. Jewish children were brought to the hospital from as far north as the Caucasus and Safed, from as far south as Alexandria in Egypt, Hebron and Gaza. Naturally they came from neighboring Jerusalem.[33] Max Sandreczky was admired by the Jewish community as a whole, as shown in the bulletin of the General Committee of the Jewish community in the Holy Land ("*Shemesh Tzdaka, The Sun of Charity*"). The only non-Jewish institution or person to whom the committee allocated financial support was Dr Max Sandreczky and the Marienstift Children's Hospital.[34] From the Hebrew press of the 19th century we learn how Max Sandreczky was admired and how the feeling of gratitude of the Jews to him and his institution. This was manifested by a letter to the editor of Hazvi (editor; Eliezer Ben Yehuda), written by a teen-aged boy Yacov Shabtai Sides.[35]

The Building of the *Marienstift Kinderhospital*

The building of the *Marienstift Kinderhospital*, was one of the first buildings built outside the city walls of Jerusalem. It was the property of the Syrian Bishop (Fig. 5). The building appeared on the "Ordnance Survey of Jerusalem", map of Captain Charles Wilson, 1864 (Fig. 6).[36] The building was inadequate for the purposes of the hospital (Fig. 7). Sandreczky made unsuccessful efforts to raise funds for a permanent children's hospital in Jerusalem.[37] His hope was the visit of the KaiserWillhelm II to Jerusalem in 1898. Augusta Victoria, the Kaiser's wife visited the hospital. The Kaiser's camp was located across the road from the hospital (today Prophet's street 29). She was very much impressed.[38,39] The Kaiser gave Dr Max Sandeczky a second decoration, "the red Eagle" but did not contribute to the building of a permanent hospital for children. As soon as the Kaiser left Jerusalem the Pasha, governor of Jerusalem, instructed Sandreczky to close down the Children's hospital. Sandreczky's reply to the Pasha, was that he had served the children of the Holy Land for decades, regardless of religion or ethnic group, with no remuneration. For this he was decorated by Sultan Abdul Hamid the II.[40] No evidence was found that

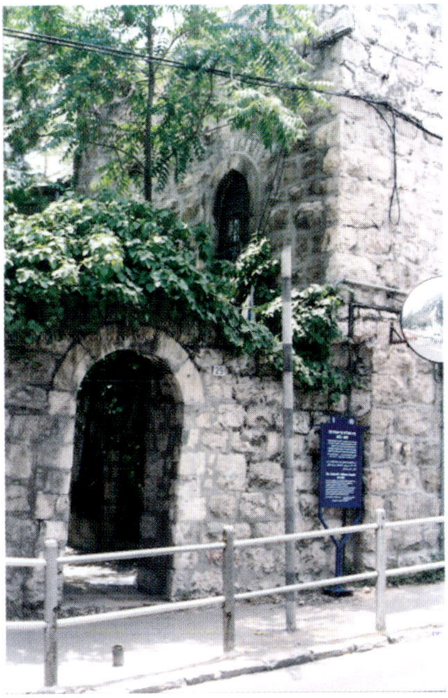

Fig. 5. The entrance to the building of the hospital.

a permit to operate the hospital was given. The hospital continued to function as usual.

The Epilogue

June 22, 1899 — Sandreczky has the belief that life had been given us as a deposit for a certain length of time. At the end of this period one has to return the deposit and stand for judgment. He felt that at the age of sixty he reached the end of the road. He suffered from arthritis, dermatitis and renal colic (according to the family, he also had carcinoma in the stomach). He was unable to care for children the way he had done for thirty two years. At 5 o'clock in the morning he descended to the valley of Jhoshaphat, located between the Mount of Olives and Mount Moria, (Temple Mount) where the last judgment would take place.[41] He entered a burial cave of a priestly family; Bene Hezir, who served in the first and second Temples.

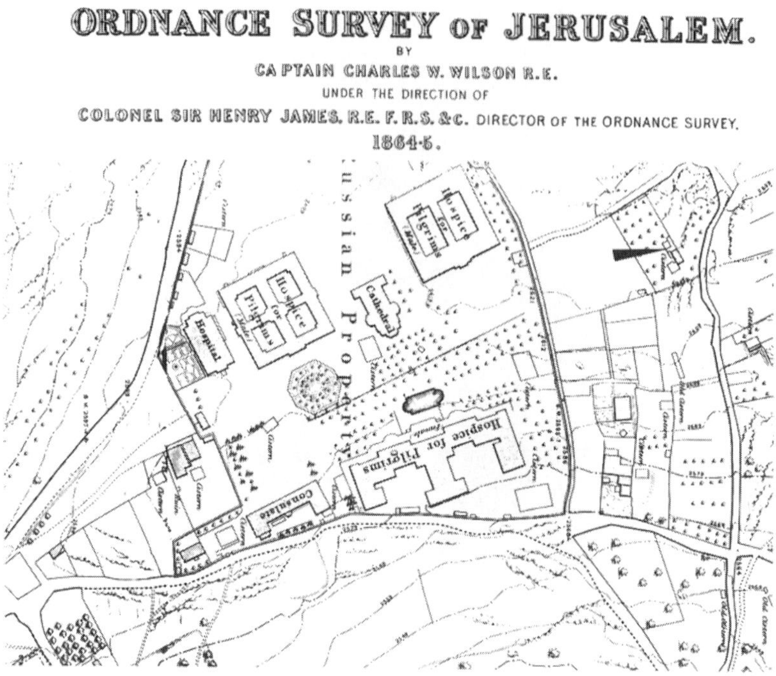

Fig. 6. Wilson's map of Jerusalem, a black pointer on the right directed to the building.

At dawn he "returned the deposit" and took his own life.[42] Sandreczky left a will, asking the German Bishop and his friends in Germany to care for his wife, children and the young pharmacist Wolff Jerusalimsky. He asked that the funeral and the grave stone will be modest: "if you want to place a wealth of flowers on my grave, you can write a servant of the Lord and a lover of mankind."[43]

Neither the Jewish community nor the Christian considered Sandreczky's suicide a mortal sin. They considered it to be part of his illness. Large crowd attended Sandrezky's funeral,[44] services were held at the Redeemer's church in old Jerusalem.[45] He was buried in consecrated ground of the Protestant cemetery on mount Zion.[46] On Sandreczky's tomb stone, inscribed was a quotation from the Sermon on the Mount: "Blessed are the Merciful" (Fig. 8).

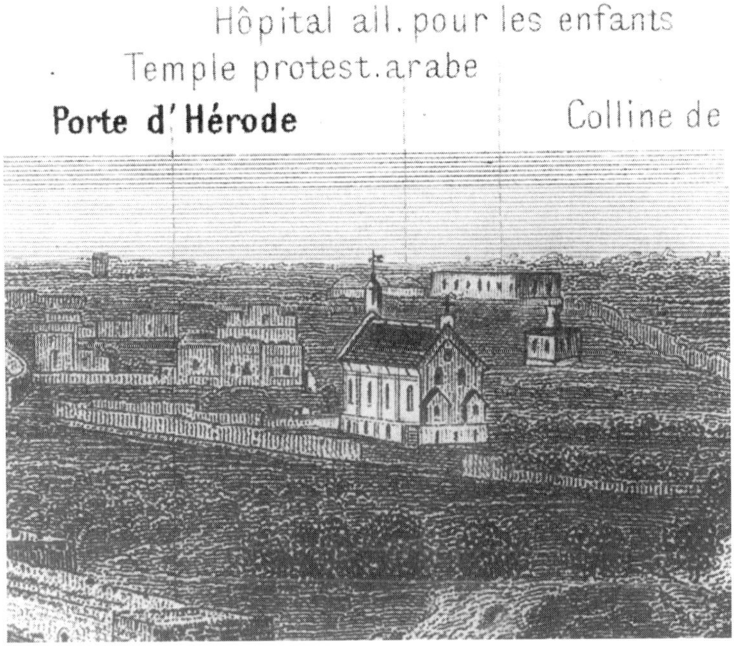

Fig. 7. Panorama of Jerusalem, the Baedeker guide 1875.

The Fate of the *Marienstift Kinderhospital*

Within one year of Sandreczky's death the hospital was closed down.[47] The Archduchess transferred the funds allocated to the *Mariensit Kinderhospital* to the Deaconess Hospital in Jerusalem, for the establishment of "four free beds" for children that were named after her.

In Memoriam of Max Sandreczky and the *Marienstift Kinderhospital*

On June 23, 1996, the Israel society of Pediatric Surgeons and the Israel Council for the Preservation of Historical Monuments, mounted a plaque on the building of the Marienstift Children's Hospital that told the story of Dr Sandreczky and the Children's hospital (Fig. 9). The unveiling of the plaque was in the presence of members of the Israel Society of Pediatric Surgeons, members of the

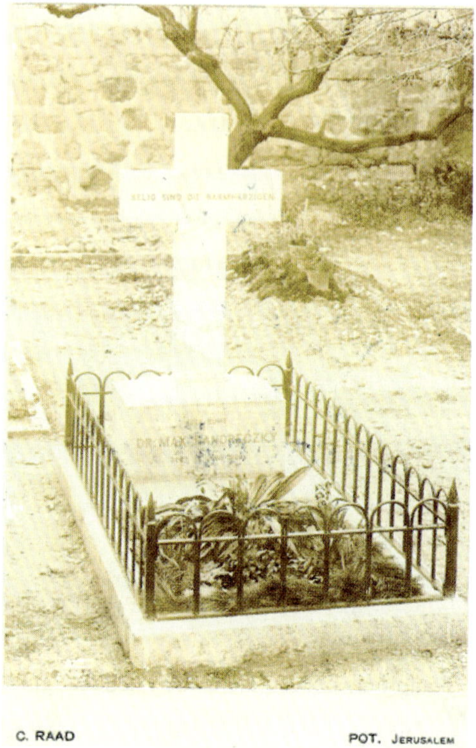

Fig. 8. Sandreczky's grave photographed soon after his death.

diplomatic corps, academic and theological institutions. Mrs Tamar Kolek, the wife of the former mayor of Jerusalem Teddy Kolek, unveiled the plaque (Fig. 10). Ehud Olmert the former mayor of Jerusalem, that followed Mr Teddy Kolek, in response to pleas from Israel, Europe and the United States declared the building of the Marienstift Children's Hospital "an historical monument for preservation".[48]

Discussion

Dr Max Sandusky's specialty was: "Surgeon and Obstetrician". The combination of the two specialties led to Pediatric Surgery. He was motivated to dedicate his life to the care of children by the

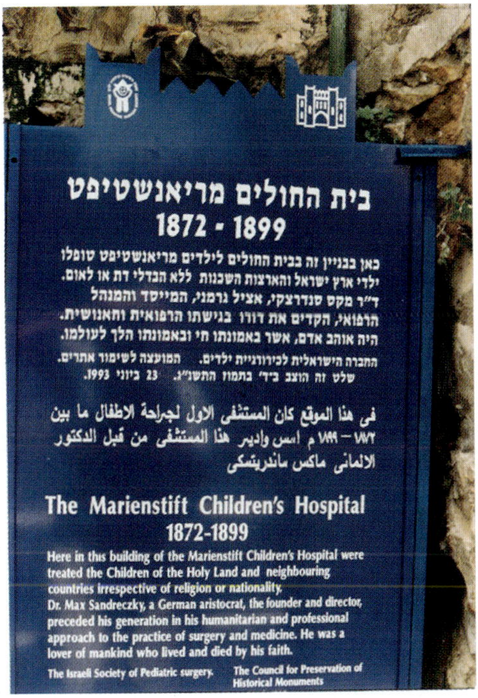
בית החולים מריאנשטיפט
1872 - 1899
כאן בבניין זה בבית החולים לילדים מריאנשטיפט טופלו
ילדי ארץ ישראל והארצות השכנות ללא הבדלי דת או לאום.
ד"ר מקס סנדרצקי, אציל גרמני, המייסד והמנהל
הרפואי, הקדים את דורו בגישתו הרפואית והאנושית.
היה אוהב אדם, אשר באמונתו חי ובאמונתו הלך לעולמו.
החברה הישראלית לכירורגיית ילדים.
המועצה לשימור אתרים.
שלט זה הוצב בד' בתמוז התשנ"ג. 23 ביוני 1993.
فى هذا الموقع كان المستشفى الاول لجراحة الاطفال ما بين
١٨٧٢ — ١٨٩٩ م اسس وادير هذا المستشفى من قبل الدكتور
الالمانى ماكس ساندريتسكى
The Marienstift Children's Hospital
1872-1899
Here in this building of the Marienstift Children's Hospital were treated the Children of the Holy Land and neighbouring countries irrespective of religion or nationality.
Dr. Max Sandreczky, a German aristocrat, the founder and director, preceded his generation in his humanitarian and professional approach to the practice of surgery and medicine. He was a lover of mankind who lived and died by his faith.
The Israeli Society of Pediatric surgery.
The Council for Preservation of Historical Monuments

Fig. 9. The plaque that was placed on the building in Hebrew, Arabic and English.

death of his baby sister and four baby brothers. On a tombstone in the Protestant cemetery on Mount Zion, Jerusalem, the names of these young children, aged two months to two years, are prescribed. Below their names there is a proclamation by the father (Karl Sandreczki): "*Weine Nicht*" (Do not Cry), accepting that five out of 12 of his children died in tender age (Fig. 11).[49] In addition he was influenced by Heinrich von Ranke the director of the *Kinder Poliklinik* in Muenchen, who's assistant Sandreczky became after he completed his medical studies at the University of Wuerzburg.[50] Heinrich von Ranke participated in the Crimean war, taking care of British wounded soldiers. After the war he visited Jerusalem and returned to England, where he was associated with Dr Charles West and Sir William Jenner in building the Hospital for Sick Children at Great Ormond Street.[51]

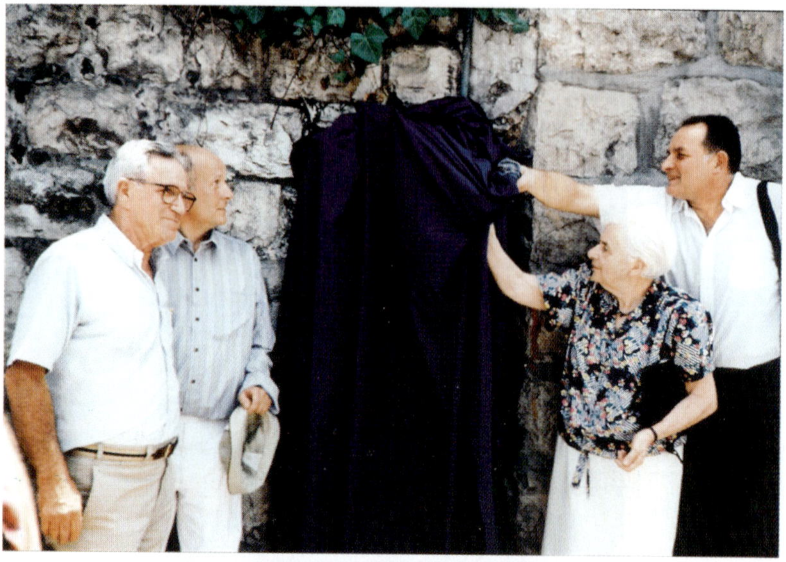

Fig. 10. Mrs Tamar Kolek unveils the plaque. Right to left: the late Shemuel Katz, the president of the Israeli Association of Pediatric Surgeons. Mrs T. Kolk, Mr H. C. Gaitzsch, great-grand son of Max Sandreczky, Shemuel Nissan, Professor of Surgrey (Emeritus) Departments of Surgery and Pediatric Surgery, Hadassah University Hospital Mount Scopus Jerusalem.

William Holt Yates a British physician, from Woburn Place, Russell Square, reported in the Lancet, on March 8, 1843: "and even in modern times, it is a well known fact that until lately, there has not been a single resident practioner to be found, (possessing the slightest claim to respectability), from Gaza to Antioch, from Hebron to Haouran,or from Beyrout to Damascus, Homs and Hamah".

By the first World War in 1914, 19 hospitals were established in Jerusalem alone. Four of them were specializing: the first and foremost *Marienstift Kinderhospital*, where pediatric surgery was widely practiced, the Leprosorium Jesus Hilfe, founded in 1867, the St John Ophthalmic Hospital founded in 1886 and the Psychiatric Hospital Ezrat Nashim, founded in 1896.

Max Sandreczky returned to Jerusalem that he knew from childhood and that he loved. He was fluent in six languages including arabic; this facilitated his work and communication with the citizens

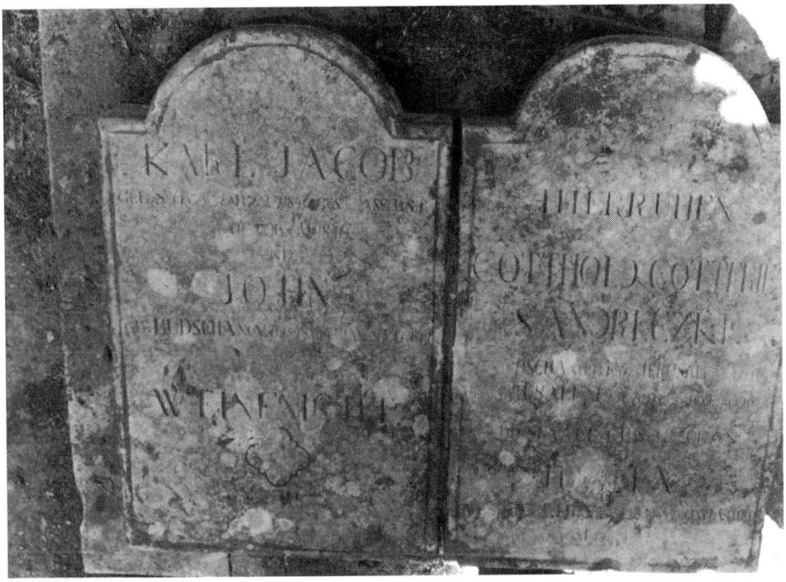

Fig. 11. Inscription on a tombstone under the name of *Sanderczki*, the names of the five Babies that died at a tender age, and the inscription of *Weine Nicht*.

of the land. He and his wife Johanna were motivated by deep religious feelings and compassion expressed by service, sacrifice, and work ethics. In spite of the fact that he was not backed by any organization he managed with his wife and daughters to keep medical and surgical standards that compared favorably with any in the west. He preceded his generation by understanding the nature of leprosy, and infectious diseases caused by bacteria and fungi. He introduced occupational therapy and rooming in for mothers that are greatly appreciated today in the care of hospitalized children. His competence as a pediatric surgeon, and the impressive results in the care of children as well as the lack of ulterior motives such as attempt on proselytism, and financial gain, explain the trust and admiration of both Arabs and Jews. In this sense he was unique in his generation. The demise of the *Marienstift Kinderhospital* following the death of Max Sandreczky was inevitable.[52]

The *Marienstift Kinderhospital* was an advanced western institution that was implanted into a medieval society that was unable to support it. External support was out of the question, because the hospital did not care for patients of any one religion or one ethnic group, nor was there the practice of proselytism. The hospital cared from it's beginning, for the entire children population of the Holy land and beyond. Max Sandreczky was the first and foremost pediatric surgeon in the Holy land. It would take another half a century before a children's hospital would be inaugurated in Israel and pediatric surgeons, who were trained abroad in the USA, the UK and elsewhere will fill the great need for this specialty.

Abbreviations

AOK	Archive of the *Oberkirchenrat*, Schwerin.
BAK	*Bundesarchiv Koblenz*, Department Potsdam, Turkey Abt 09.01 No 39558 (1878–1894). No 39559 (1894–1904);
EZA	*Evangelisches Zentralarchiv*; Berlin Best 56 "*Evangelische Jerusalemsitung*".
FA	Fliedner's *Archiv Diakoniewserk Kaiserwerth Dusseldorf.*
GCA	Israel State Archive; German Consulate Archive, Jerusalem;
MLS	*Mecklenburgisches Landeshauptarchiv Schwerin Grosseherzoglisches Kabinet III* (Signatur 2098 (1872–1896), (Signatur 2100– (1896–1910).
PAAA	*Politisches Archiv des Auswaertigen Amtes*, Bonn.

References

1. Schwake N. *Die Entwicklung des Krankenhauswesen der stadt Jerusalem*, Vol 2 (ed.) Murken, Altrogge Herzogenrath, 1983.
2. Yates WH. Medical News from the East, *Lancet* 1842–1843 1:867–868.
3. Historic Archiv Syra. Birth regisrtration book for the years (1828–1858 No. 214.)
4. Hanauer JE. In *Megron Y Barkai G*. Schiller E (eds.) Ariel Jerusalem (1996), p. 115.
5. Ludwig Maximilians — Universtaets Archiv, Muenchen, Students' register, Winter semester 1864–1865.

6. Koeniglich Bayerische Julius Maximilians Universitet Wuerzburg Students' Register, *Winter semester* (1864–1865).
7. Family Archive, Letter of Hofrat Herrlioch to the director of the Deaconess Institution Berlin, (28.1.1867) "PAAA Spec 154 Abt 22–5 Konst.413" Ausuebung der Artzlichen Praxis.
8. Family Archive, Mastricht Letter of Princess Marianna to Evelyne von der mey (30.10.1867).
9. Wedding certificate of the Protestant Reformed Community Stitswerd "Protocol (1866)" signed Pastor Theodor Uilkens (19.2.1868).
10. Sandrczxki Karl. *Die Anwesenheit des Kronprinzen von Prussen in Palestina von einem Sueddeutschen.* Dundek K (ed.) Berlin, 1870.
11. GCA: file 221 "Reiseangelegenheiten (1842–1872)" Letter of the German Vice Consul E. Ziffos to Consul von Alten Jerusalem. Haifa, (14.3.1872).
12. MLS. Guaranty of the Duke from (29.2.1872).
13. MLS. A letter from the Kuratorium to the Archduke in Schwerin. Jerusalem (8.7.1873).
14. MLS. Max Sandreczky to the Archduke of Mecklenburg Schwerin: "Vorsclag zur gruendung eines Deutschen hospitals fur Kinder in Jerusalem." Jerusalem (26.2.1872).
15. Shemuel Nissan and Petra Martin. A proposal to establish a children's hospital in 19th century Jerusalem. (in Hebrew) *Kathedra* 2003;107: 167–182.
16. MLS. Letters of the Kuratorium to the Archduke. Jerusalem (8.7.1874) and (31.7.1875).
17. MLS: Max Sandeczky to the Archduke of Mecklenbug — Schwerin "Vorsclag zur Gruendung eines Deuschen Hospital fur Kinder in Jerusalem." Jeruslem (26.2.1872).
18. MLS: Jahresbericht (1872–1873) ueber das Kinderhospital Marienstitzu Jeruslem Passau, 1873, p. 8.
19. BAK: letter from the Consul Baron on Muenchhausen "An den Reichkanzler Fuerst von Bismarcck" Jerusalem (15.7.1881).
20. GCA: file 257 "Marienstift (1881–1885)" Letter of the Foreign Office to Consul Dr Reitz Berlin (13.6.1883).
21. BAK: Letter of Sandreczky "Hochvereherter Herr Unter Staatssekretaer" Jerusalem. (12.1884).

22. BAK: 23.Jaheresberichtdes Deutschen Kinderhospitals Marienstiftzu Jerusalem fuer das Jahr (1895). Jerusalem, 1896, p. 3.
23. MLS: Jahrfes-Bericht des Kinderhospitals Marienstift zu Jerusalem fur das jahr (1890) erstattet von Dr Max Sandreczky, p. 4.
24. MLS: Jahresbericht des Deutschen Kindrhospitals zu Jerusalem fuer das jahr (1897). Jerusalem, 1898, p. 21.
25. Hibberd JF: Jerusalem from a doctor's Standpoint American Practioner, 1870, p. 99–100;Karl Baedeker: Palestine and Syria. Leipzig, London, 1876, p. 145.
26. Sandreczky M. A study on Leprosy. *Lancet* 1889;31:423.
27. Paul Langerhans. Lepra und Leproserien in Jerusalem. *Virchow Archiv* 1870;50:453–455.
28. MLS. Jahresbericht (1872–1873) ueber das Kinderhospital Marienstift zu Jerusalem. Passau, 1873, p. 24.
29. MLS. Jahresbericht (1872–1873) ueber das Kinderhospitl Marienstift zu Jerusalem. Passau, 1873, p. 4–5.
30. BAK. 23 Jahrebericht des Deutschen Kinderhospital Marienstit zu Jerusalem fuer das jahr, 1896, p. 5.
31. MLS. Letter of Consul von Alten, Wesser, Schick, Frutiger and Sndreczky to the Archduke. Jerusalem (25.10.1872).
32. MLS. Jahresbericht (1872–1873). ueber das Kinderhospital Marienstift zu Jerusalem Passau, 1873, p. 11.
33. GCA. File 287 Marienstift (1893–1899). Letter from the Kuratorium to the Archduke. Jerusalem (4.9.1882).
34. Shemesh Tzedaka 16, 1895, p. 21. [Hebrew]
35. Hatzvi, 1879, p. 12. [Hebrew]
36. Wilson CW. Ordnance Survey of Jerusalem The Lords Commission of her Majesty's Treasury, London, 1865.
37. BAK. Jaharesbericht des Kinderhospitals Marienstift zu Jerusalem, 1884, p. 4.
38. EZA. 26. Jahresbericht des Deuthschen Kinderhospitals Marienstift zu Jerusalem.edas jhar 1898. Jerusalem, 1899, p. 5.
39. David Yellin. Jerusalem of Yesterday (1896–1904) Rubin Mass Jerusalem, 1972, p. 298. [Hebrew]
40. GCA. 287 "Marienstift (1893–1899) Letter of Sandreczky to the governor of Jerusalem. Jerusalem (12.1.1899, 1895–1899).

41. Joel 3:12
42. GCA. File 823 "Selbsmorde (1895–1901)" A death certificate signed by the German Consul von Tischendorf and the Consulate physician, Dr Einzler. Jerusalem. 22.6.1899.
43. GCA. File 823 "Selbsmorde (1895–1901)" A will no date.
44. Hahvazeleth 37, 1899, p. 291. [Hebrew]
45. EZA. Report of Probst Hoppe in Jerusalem (1899) Aus dem Leben der Gemeinde.
46. GCA. File 258 "Marienstift (1893–1899)" Letter of Consul Rosen Jerusalem, 19/8/1899. Letter of the Kuratorium Jerusalem, 12.8.1899. AOK: Letter of the Kuratorium, Jerusalem 27.8.1901.
47. AOK. Open letter of the Kuratorium in Schwerin, "Giese, Dr Wolff and von Prollius Sachwerin 27.2.1901.
48. Letter from the former mayor of Jerusalem, Ehud Olmert to the authors, 4.6.1996.
49. Das Marientift Kinderhospitalin Jerusalem (1871–1899) Shemuel Nissan and Petra Martin Historia Hospitaliun, Heft 20 (1995–1997).
50. Nissan S, Martin P. Max Sandfeczky: a pediatic surgeon in 19th century Jeusalem, *J Pediatr Surg* 1998;32:1187–1193.
51. Seitz C. Heinrich Ranke zum 70 Geburtztage Muenchener. *Mediziniche Wochenschrift* 1900;47(19):652–653.
52. Kaplan T. Death of an Institution, *Br J Med Psychol* 1991;64:97–102.

JAMES HENDERSON NICOLL — "FATHER OF DAY SURGERY" (1864–1921)

Robert Carachi
Dan G. Young

James Henderson Nicoll was the son of the Reverend James Nicoll, MA, born on September 30, 1863 in Dundee. He was educated at Glasgow Academy and then the University of Glasgow where he graduated MB, CM in 1886 at the age of 23. His first house jobs were under Sir Hector Cameron and Dr McCall Anderson in Glasgow. He decided early he needed to broaden his experience and headed south where for the next four years he undertook his surgical apprenticeship under Sir Frederick Treves in London. He developed a strong interest in urology which was to serve him later in his surgical practice. Sir Frederick Treves was appointed Professor of Anatomy when Nicoll joined him and he became famous because he drained an appendix abscess for King Edward for which he received his knighthood. He is also renowned for being the physician who cared and befriended the much written about elephant man, Joseph Carey Merrick, who had Proteus Syndrome.

Nicoll, as his Houseman, would undoubtedly have cared and been in contact with Merrick and looked after him. It is very likely that the surgical skills were not the only ones that he learned from Sir Frederick Treves but also his humanitarian characteristics. Nicoll (Fig. 1) had an insatiable desire and an innate drive to visit other centres and meet experts in his field of surgery. His knowledge of surgical skills was far advanced for his time because he did not rely

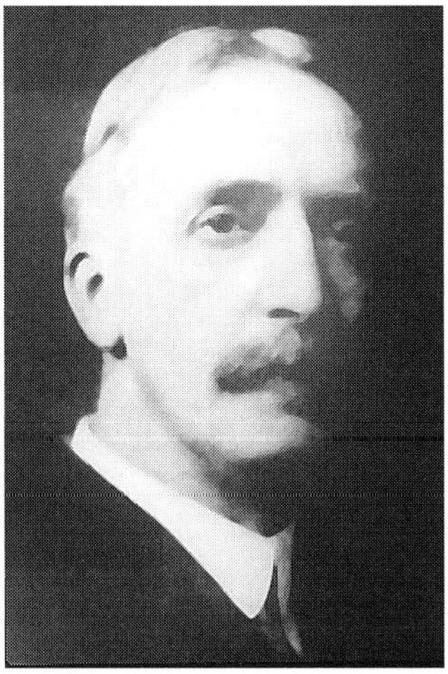

Fig. 1. Prof James H. Nicoll.

solely on his local experience or on book knowledge but sought out well known international figures of those days and visited and worked with them to gain first-hand experience (at his own expense). Following this period in London he toured the continent and visited the surgical centres of excellence. He travelled as far as Moscow before returning to Glasgow.

Nicoll's Appointments

Nicoll returned to Glasgow full of original ideas and was first appointed as a Dispensary Surgeon to the Western Infirmary from 1891 to 1895. He rapidly gained recognition with this appointment both as an excellent surgeon, a teacher, a trainer and a prolific writer. He was renowned for his endoscopic skills in urology and developed an extensive private practice. Although his early interests were in the field of urology he extended this to a more general surgery and in particular to children's surgery.

His surgical skill was matched by his soundness as a diagnostician and his judgement. As an operator he had courage and confidence working quickly and crisply. He developed the concept of

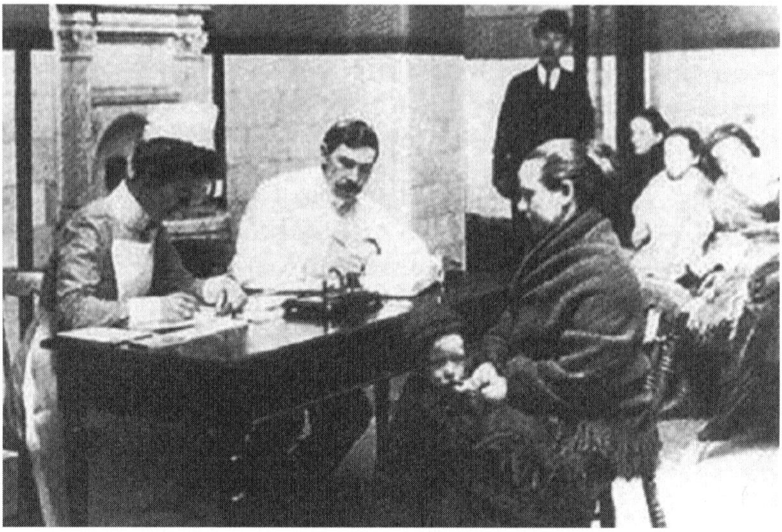

Fig. 2. Dispensary or outpatient department of the Royal Hospital for Sick Children Glasgow.

a team working closely with the bacteriologist and pathologist submitting all specimens for microscopic examination. His skills as a genito-urinary surgeon resulted in 1893 his appointment to the Glasgow Central Dispensary. On his appointment as an extra Honorary Surgeon to the R.H.S.C. Dispensary in 1894 (Fig. 2), a major interest for his life became paediatric surgery. He decided that a great deal of surgery could be done on an out-patient basis rather than requiring admission to a hospital and demonstrated that clearly from his practice.

He was appointed by the Board of the Western Infirmary in 1896 as an Assistant Surgeon, a post he held until 1906 when he was appointed Visiting Surgeon to the Infirmary and retained this post until 1917 when he resigned on being posted to France in August that year.

With the turmoil of the First World War, a large part of the new Sick Children's Hospital was commandeered by the Military Authorities and only a part was allowed to function as a children's hospital. Although Nicoll resigned his post in 1914, he continued to assist and care for the children at Yorkhill during these difficult times until he was dispatched to France in 1917.

Anderson's University

Anderson's University had four Faculties: Arts, Medicine, Law and Theology. It was bequeathed by John Anderson (1726–1796) in his will and the Medical School was founded in 1800. James Nicoll was appointed Professor of Surgery in 1903 until 1908, thereafter taking appointment as a Visiting Surgeon at the Western Infirmary. It is reported that his classes were very popular and attended by a large number of keen medical students who benefited from his precise, lucid, dogmatic lectures.

Besides his clear lectures on surgery and operative surgery he was renowned for new methods to illustrate his lectures. He spent considerable effort and his own money on delivering and using very innovative technology at that time, lantern slides and illustrations to produce brilliant talks. He was a recognised artist and enhanced his lectures with illustrations which gained further respect from all his students.

Nicoll and the "Glasgow Dispensary"

The Glasgow Dispensary opened in October 1888. For over seven decades, the "Dispensary", as it was fondly known, was an outpatients Department of RHSC in West Graham Street (Fig. 2). During that time it treated a total of 750,000 patients who attended a total of 2.7 million attendances.

By the time Nicoll returned to Glasgow the Hospital for Sick Children had been granted its Royal title and the outpatient department at West Graham Street was functioning. It was here that Nicoll made his greatest mark and practised his skills as a surgeon. He adapted this place to his needs. He persuaded the Glasgow Sick Children's Board to extend the premises and operating theatre for him to do his "Day Surgery". On the July 9, 1895 Nicoll donated a sum of money to buy sterilising apparatus for the Dispensary. He never made any fuss about his many donations nor did he seek any publicity.

"The Father of Day Surgery"[1]

His lifetime of work at the Dispensary (Fig. 3) earned him the title of "The Father of Day Surgery". He was appointed as an extra honorary surgeon to the Dispensary in 1894 and remained in post until

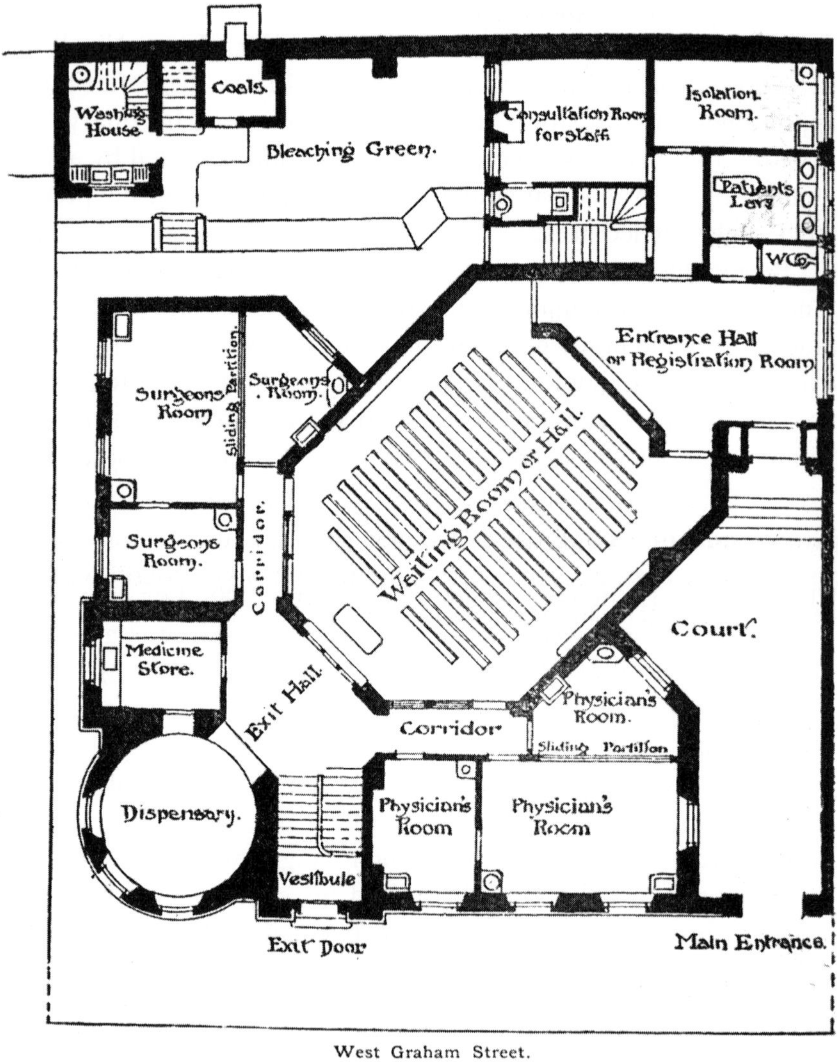

Fig. 3. Plan of the Dispensary.

1914. He refused an offer to become "Visiting Surgeon" to the Royal Hospital for Sick Children in Scott Street and then Yorkhill because of regulations of the Children's Board and because of his dedication to the outpatient care at West Graham Street. (When the new Children's Hospital moved to Yorkhill the clinical staff had to devote their full time to children's work.) He was eventually given the title of Honorary Consultant Surgeon in recognition of his work and elected Director of the "Dispensary" on December 22, 1920. He accepted this office on January 10, 1921 but died seven months later.

Nicoll the Surgeon

From 1894 to 1914 he was surgeon to the Dispensary. The workload at the Dispensary was enormous and Nicoll's report published that between 1899 and 1908, 8988 operations were performed in this "Day Centre" and he personally had done 7392 of them. From Annual Reports of those times 17,833 operations were performed under anaesthesia in the first decade of the twentieth century.

He operated on infants and children with cleft lip and cleft palate and other conditions like mastoid empyema, spina bifida, fractured skull and hypertrophic pyloric stenosis. Nicoll was the forerunner of the paediatric surgeons in the West of Scotland. His paper in the "*British Medical Journal*" in 1900 on the treatment of pyloric stenosis and subsequently his report of a series of patients in the medical journals showed that Nicoll was well ahead of his time in performing successful operations for this condition.[2]

Spina Bifida and Day Surgery

Spina bifida was another area in which Nicoll was active. In 1902 Nicoll wrote, "On reviewing an extensive list of cases with spina bifida, hydrocephalus and hydro-encephocele treated by operation in hospital and private practice I am convinced of a growing belief that infants fare at least as well in the care of their mothers as in the ward of a hospital". In this article he stated very clearly that day case surgery was beneficial.

The resignation of Nicoll in 1914 was because of the First World War. Nicoll volunteered to continue to assist at the Sick Children's Hospital which had been considerably upset as a large part of the hospital was commandeered and used by the military and only a small part allowed to function as a children's hospital. Normality ultimately returned in 1920 when the children's hospital became fully functional as a children's unit. Nicoll continued to work in the Sick Children's Hospital from 1914 to 1917 when he was dispatched to France but returned the following year due to having contracted dysentery. Ill health limited his contribution to medicine in his remaining years.

Nicoll the Academic

He published over 100 papers was a prolific writer and he audited his clinical work. He was an original thinker and published his views on a number of topics. He published in the "*British Medical Journal*" and the "*Glasgow Medical Journal*" as well as contributing many case reports to the Royal Medical Chirurgical Society of Glasgow. In 1900 he published the first successful operation for pyloric stenosis (Fig. 4) a full 12 years before Rammsted reported his operation of pyloromyotomy. In 1906, in the "*Glasgow Medical Journal*", a predecessor of the "*Scottish Medical Journal*", he reported his series of patients treated for this condition.

The Domiciliary Nursing Service

The domiciliary nursing service that had been started in 1888 was supported very vigorously by Nicoll and the system of nurses visiting and checking the patients post-operatively was a vital part to allow him to operate in the Dispensary. He took an active part in teaching the nurses and ensuring that they looked after his patients properly. These sisters and nurses often gave help and support to families as well as caring for the post-operative needs of the patients. It is

A

B

C

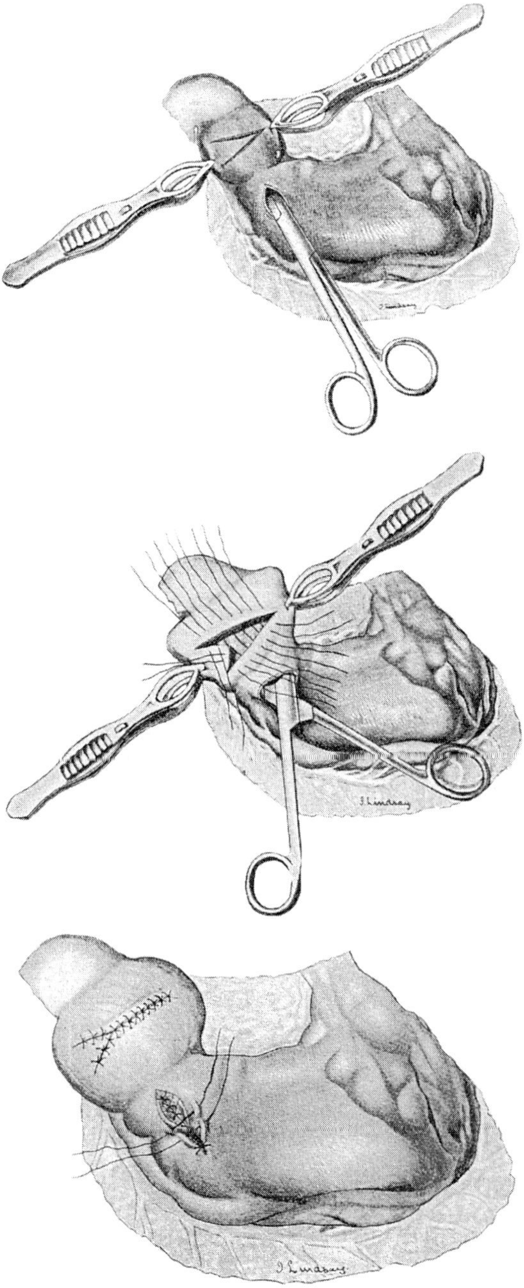

Fig. 4. Pyloric Stenosis: Loretta–Nicoll Operation — Steps A, B and C.

notable that Nicoll supported this service financially. In the Minutes of the Board Meeting a disagreement between Nicoll and the Board was recorded. Nicoll had rented a house close to his work where patients and their families could be kept temporarily post-operatively for nursing staff to care for them before they departed long distances to get to their homes. He had established the "House Hotel" for his patients. He organised a body of outdoor visiting nurses, who were devotedly attached to this work.

As a result of Nicoll's extensive Day Surgery practice (Table 1) he enunciated his conclusions in the "*British Medical Journal*" on September 18, 1909 where he stated:

- Much surgery done in hospital was a waste of resources! The cost of day case surgery was one tenth of in-patients.
- The concept of bed rest was impractical in children. An unnecessary but careful selection was needed for day case surgery.
- Nursing Sisters were employed to visit children at home.
- Separation of the child from the mother was harmful and day case surgery minimised this.
- Turn over of patients in day case surgery was more rapid by reducing the anaesthetic time.

Table 1. Dispensary Operations 1906.

Abscesses	455
Amputations	14
Curetting bones	85
Circumcision	564
Excision of Glands	134
Spina Bifida	5
Tonsils and Adenoids	86
Hernia	25
Cleft Palate	23
Harelip	62
Miscellaneous	542
Total	1,995

Nicoll the Man and the Politician

He was an eager connoisseur in art and was a contemporary of Sir David Young Cameron (1865–1945), the landscape artist and etcher. He was the owner of a large art collection which included many of Cameron's landscapes, and etchings by Whistler as well as a fine collection of paintings by Hornel. He was a man of charm and grace, liked by all his colleagues medical and nursing and "children were devoted to him and he to them". He never married, remaining a bachelor till the end. He was a successful accomplished surgeon, a great teacher innovator but most of all was known in all circles as a "forebearing, tactful and kindly friend", and "a great philanthropist". He never took long holidays but settled for weekends with close friends of his. He enjoyed walking in the countryside and was knowledgeable about nature. Apart from medicine, his other passion was art and he was a member of the Glasgow Art Club.

In 1911 he was appointed a Justice of the Peace for the County and the City of Glasgow.[4] He was also appointed as Secretary of the West of Scotland Board of the BMA and for years was the Vice President of the Section of Surgery at BMA meetings.

The Cross of the Legion of Honour

In 1915 the Minutes of the University Court recorded the intimation from the French Ambassador in London that President Poincaré, Rector of Glasgow University, had nominated James H. Nicoll as his assessor on the University Court. Nicoll served for the next five years. In 1920, the Minutes of the Court recorded a cordial congratulation to Nicoll on hearing that he had been acknowledged by the French President with the Cross of the Legion of Honour.

Formal recognition of his excellence as a teacher and academic was recorded in the Minutes of the University Court. Another vignette in Nicoll's life is connected with the Minutes of the University Court that he had donated £5000 to establish a Lectureship in collaboration with the Western Infirmary. Whether this was a personal gift or one by benefactors no one will know but he often made donations in his life time and made little demonstration about it which reflected some of his reticence and his West of Scotland upbringing.

While he was serving in France during 1918 he contracted dysentery which caused prolonged ill health. He was very popular and his early death made a deep impression on the whole community in Glasgow but most of all on the medical profession. This occurred on 15th August 1921 at his home in 4 Woodside Place. He was only 57 years old.

In 1944 his sister-in-law made a bequest of £1000 to the Royal Hospital for Sick Children to commemorate the name of J. H. Nicoll called the James H. Nicoll Nurses Fund. It was set up to award each nurse who completed her training to get a bronze medal and a gilt and silver medal were awarded to the best two nurses of the year (Fig. 5).

His tombstone in the Necropolis overlooking his beloved City and its people has the following words inscribed "From the grave … He speaketh". Hebrews 11 verse 4 — a fitting epitaph for such a great

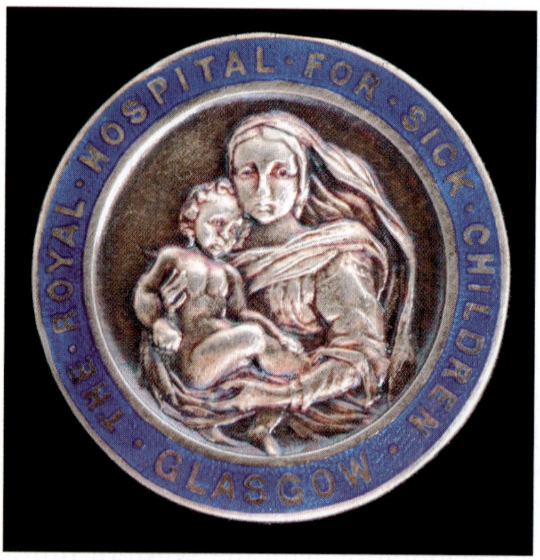

Fig. 5. RHSC badge given by Nicoll's sister-in-law.

man who has to be admired for his work and contribution. In his life he never sought fame.

Conclusion

James Nicoll, a Glasgow surgeon, was making significant contributions over a hundred years ago to the advancement of medicine and surgical knowledge. As a paediatric surgeon he was a forerunner of the West of Scotland tradition of paediatric surgeons. As an educationalist he was ahead of his time in illustrating his lectures which were greatly admired and attended by medical students and nursing students in Glasgow. He spared no expense in using the latest technology of the time to make his talks artistic and interesting. As a pioneer in surgical innovation he acquired skills and ideas from his enthusiastic visits abroad earlier in his career and reported on these widely. He was a medical politician and clashed with authorities on a number of occasions in his zeal to develop and help the nursing profession and develop his ideas of day surgery which were completely contrary to the established practice at the time. As a scientist he was a great observer. He contributed and documented his excellent results — a tribute to his skills, hard work and prolific operations and his ultimate aim to give the best care for his patients.

The main reason why Nicoll should be remembered today is for his advocacy in the practice of **day surgery**.[3]

References

1. Young DG, Carachi R, James H. Nicoll. Father of Day Surgery. *Scot Med J* 2006;50:48–50.
2. Nicoll JH. Congenital hypertrophy stenosis of pylorus with an account of a case successfully treated by operation. *Brit Med J* 1900;2:571–573.
3. Nicoll JH. The surgery of childhood: a plea for the more extensive use of the outpatient department for operation in children. *Brit Med J* 1913;2:792–793.

ENDOSCOPY AND ENDOSCOPIC SURGERY IN CHILDREN

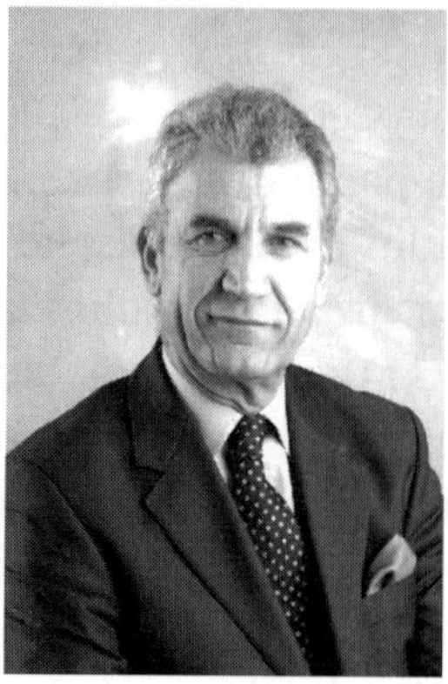

Azad Najmaldin

Introduction

Since its inception, one of the major issues in medicine has been the visualisation of internal anatomy and execution of surgical procedures within tissues plains, body cavities and lumen of hollow organs. The use of the tube and speculum in medicine dates from the earliest days of civilisation in Greece, Egypt, Mesopotamia and China. Techniques were developed in parallel in many countries as time went on, but the pace of changes accelerated during the second half of the nineteenth and throughout the twentieth century. Because of geographic, economic and political constraints, language barriers and difficulties with communication that existed in the past, it is difficult to be certain of the exact sequence of events.

Until the middle of the 20th century, and still is in many parts of the world, paediatric surgery was part of general surgery. It is, therefore, hardly surprising that early history contains very little if any specific references to paediatric endoscopy. This chapter highlights some of the participants in the development of endoscopy and endoscopic surgery as a whole with emphasis on paediatric surgery as deemed appropriate.

Early Days

The earliest description of endoscope and endoscopic examinations came from Greeks — the Kos school led by Hippocrates (460–375 BC). They described a rectal speculum that is remarkably similar to the instrument that is in use to today. Similar items that were used to access the ear, nose and rectum, and a three-bladed vaginal speculum were discovered in the ruins of Pompeii. The Babylonian Talmud written in 500 AD, describes a tube made of lead (siphopherot) that was used as a vaginal speculum.[1,2] Others had used hollow reeds or bamboo shoots to access natural orifices of the human body.

Natural light or its reflection were used to inspect the concealed areas of the body. There is good evidence to suggest that the insides of early pyramids and tombs were decorated not using the light of candles or oil lamps but under the illumination of sunlight directed down tunnels and importantly, bent around corners using mirrors. This clearly was simply the delivery of light and not its collection and re-direction to a viewer. An Arabian physician, Abul Kasim of Cordoba (980–1037 AD), and later Giulio Ceasare Aranzi (1530–1589 AD) were credited to have attempted to use the reflection of natural light to illuminate and examine body cavities and internal organs such as the cervix.[3]

Modern Era

Modern endoscopy started in the early nineteenth century by Phillip Bozzini (1773–1809), a physician born to an aristocratic Italian family but he practiced in Frankfurt. Bozzini introduced an endoscope

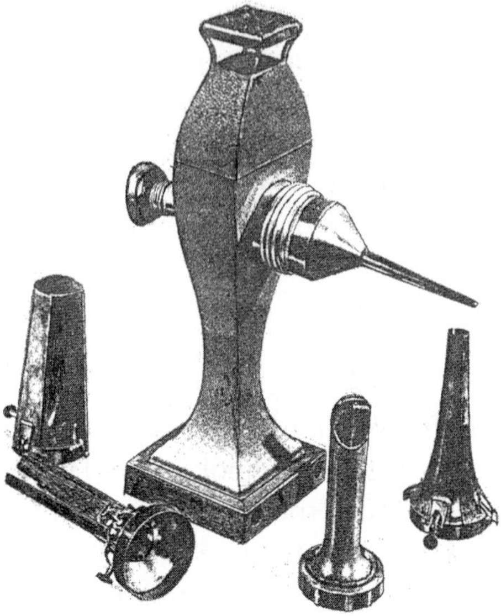

Fig. 1. Bozzini's Light-Conductor 1806 (from History of Endoscopy vol V–VII, by Matthias A Reuter, Hans J Reuter, Rainer M Engel).

named Lichtleiter (light conductor). It consisted of elongated thin funnels of different sizes that could be used for inspecting the bladder, vagina, rectum, nose, throat and ear; a stand carrying a wax candle that was covered in shark skin to prevent burns, and a concave mirror to reflect light and protect the user's eye (Fig. 1). Visualisation would have been very limited and probably rather unpleasant. In 1806, he presented his invention to the Academy of Medicine of Vienna who rejected it as a "magic lantern" and Bozzini was ridiculed for undue curiosity. Although there is no evidence that this instrument was ever used on a patient, it laid the foundations for others to build upon.[4,5] Many simultaneous yet independent attempts at modifying this or developing similar instruments continued by enthusiasts including Pierre Segalas of Paris in 1826, John Fisher of Boston in 1827, and Francis Cruise of Dublin in 1865.

In 1853, Antonin Desormeaux of Paris (1815–1894) described the first serviceable endoscope which consisted of a kerosene lamp burning alcohol and turpentine held in a reservoir, chimney to

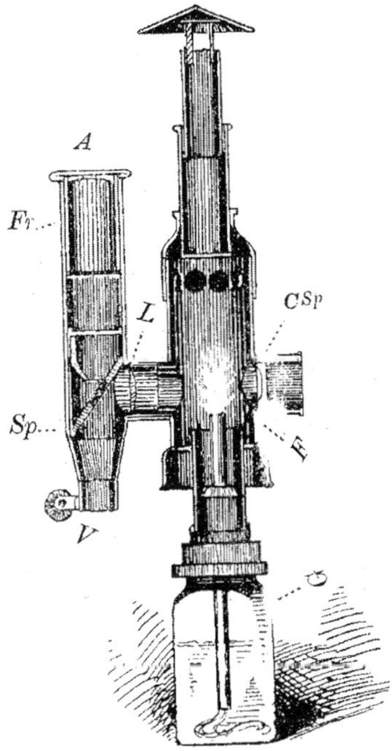

Fig. 2. Desormeaux Endoscope 1853 (from History of Endoscopy vol V–VII, by Matthias A Reuter, Hans J Reuter, Rainer M Engel).

enhance the flame, and a concave mirror and lens to reflect and condense the beam to achieve a clear view.[6] This elaborate instrument was used to view (Fig. 2) and probably for therapeutic measures within the urethra, bladder, cervix, uterus, oesophagus and even stomach, but the major complications were burns.[6,7] Desormeaux presented his instrument to the Academy of Medicine in Paris in 1865 and used the term "endoscopy" in an article published in 1868.

In 1868, Alwin Bevan announced an illustration of an oesophagoscope which was constructed of a straight tube, 4 inches in length and 3/4 of an inch wide with a moveable piece served for easy introduction, mirror attached at its proximal end for observation and a candle light or magnesium lamp served as a light source. He recommended the gadget for the diagnosis of stricture and malignant ulcers and removal of foreign bodies.[7] In the same year Adolf

Kussmaul (1822–1902) from Freiburg, demonstrated the possibility of inspecting the stomach with a rigid tube and kerosene lamp using a professional sword swallower as his subject.[8]

Electric Light Era

The greatest problem with the early endoscopes was illumination. Julius Bruck, a dentist in Breslau, realised that to light up a room one must carry the lamp inside. In 1867, he examined the oral cavity of the patient using a platinum wire heated with an electrical current. Because of the risk of burning, he later developed a water jacket for cooling the heated platinum wire.[9] Interestingly, this device was used inside the rectum to transilluminate the bladder. This idea impressed Max Nitze (1848–1906), a urologist from Berlin. First working with Wilhelm Deicke and Louis Beneche, optical technicians in Berlin, then Joseph Leiter, a well known instrument maker in Vienna, in 1879 Nitze produced the first practical endoscope (Nitze–Leiter cystoscope).[2,10] This instrument consisted of a metal tube with lenses to magnify the field of view and light provided by electrically heated platinum wire loop sheathed in a goose quill and cooled by a separate cold water circulation. Later he added separate channels within the cystoscope which allowed surgical procedures to be performed using purpose-made instruments.

Following Thomas Edison's (1847–1931) discovery of the incandescent light bulb in 1880, in 1883 David Newman from Glasgow was the first to place the light bulb at the distal end of the Nitze. At the time the electrical bulb became the most reliable source of light, and was less likely to damage tissue by heat but too bulky to pass through the male urethra.[9]

By 1889, Boisseau De Rocher of France, separated the optical component (telescope) from the operating and irrigating channel. This principle allowed the use of different telescopes and operating instruments and easy bladder irrigation, thereby the complexity of the diagnostic and therapeutic measures increased.[9]

Stimulated by the famous Viennese surgeon, Theodor Ch. A. Billroth and the instrument maker Joseph Leiter, in 1881 Johann

Von Mikulicz–Radecki, a physician in Vienna (1850–1905) developed a system similar to Nitze cystoscope for examining the oesophagus and stomach. At first he used an overheated platinum wire to create light at the tip and a separate water circulation for cooling. Shortly after he replaced the wire with an electric bulb and made the version of the scope that could be angled by 30° in its distal third which became a clinically usable oesophagoscope and the start of flexible endoscopy (Fig. 3).[11] It took another 55 years (1936) before Wolf, an instrument maker, and Schindler, a physician from Berlin, designed a semi-flexible gastroscope which was 1.2 cm wide, 77 cm long and contained 48 lenses.[4]

In 1854, Manuel Garcia of London, used the laryngeal mirror for laryngoscopy. In 1898, Gustav Killian of Freiburge, developed and

(a)

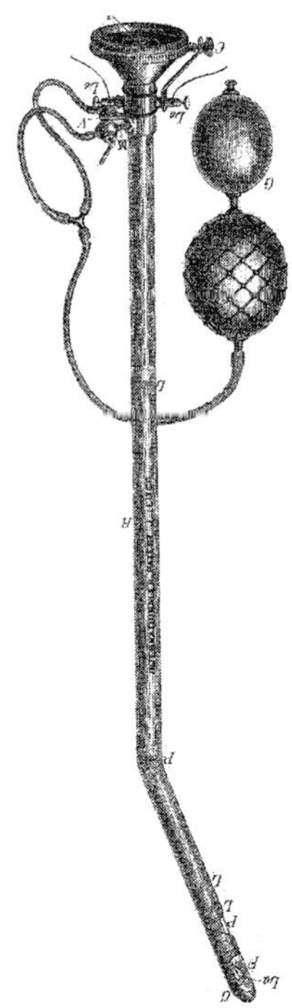

Fig. 3a. Mikulicz-Leiter Gastroscope 1881 (from History of Endoscopy vol V–VII, by Matthias A Reuter, Hans J Reuter, Rainer M Engel).

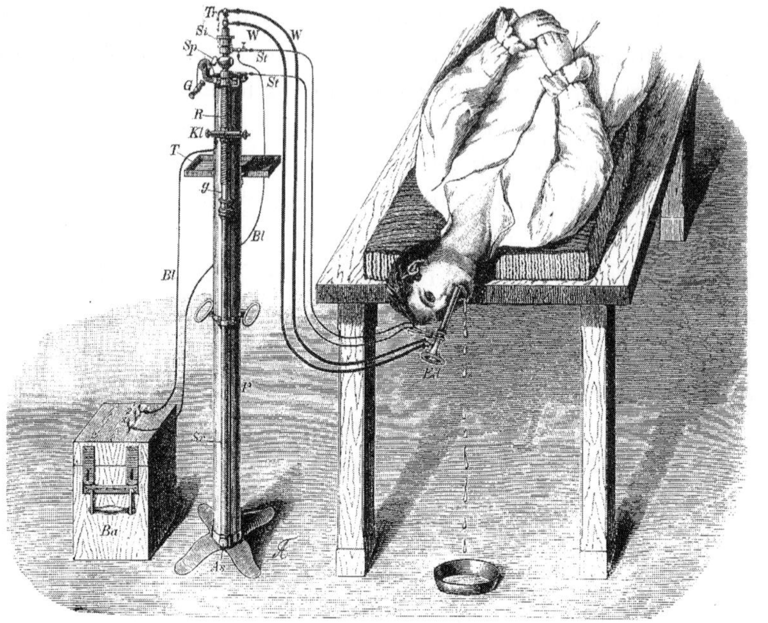

Fig. 3b. Mikulicz Gastroscopy.

successfully used a bronchoscope with the light source being augmented by a head mirror.[12]

The rapid progress and successful use of the endoscopes in general and cystoscope in particular, prompted physicians and surgeons of that time to use the same instruments to view other areas of the body namely: pelvic cavity, abdomen, pleural space and intracranial spaces. In 1901, von Ott, a gynaecologist from St. Petersburg, used a culdotomy, head mirror, speculum and incandescent lamp to view the pelvic cavity of the patient and named the procedure "ventroscopy".[13] In 1902 George Kelling of Dresden examined the abdominal cavity of a living dog using a cystoscope and cotton filtered air and named the procedure 'celioscopy'.[14] In 1910, Christian Jacobaeus, Professor of Medicine in Stockholm, coined the terms laparoscopy and thoracoscopy (*Laparothorakoskopie*) and carried out both diagnostic and therapeutic procedures in humans in large numbers.[15] In the same year, 1910, Victor Darwin Lespinasse

(1878–1946), a urologist from Chicago, performed the first intracranial intraventricular endoscopy and coagulation of the choroid plexus for the treatment of hydrocephalus in two children. One of his patients's died post-operatively, but the other survived for five years.[16]

In 1924, Christoph Zollikoffer of Switzerland, used CO_2 to insufflate the abdominal cavity which made internal electrical coagulation a safe procedure.[17]

The late 19th and early 20th century European and American urologists popularised endoscopy for diagnosis and treatment of genito-urinary diseases. While in the 1930s and 1940s, gynaecologists popularised culdoscopic and laparoscopic procedures. At first, the techniques were executed primarily under opiate sedation and/or local anaesthesia for diagnostic purposes often in small clinics throughout Europe and parts of America. As complications of the procedure mounted and complexity of the procedures increased, the importance of general anaesthesia as well as better instrumentation and refined techniques were strongly emphasised.

Rod-Lens and Flexible Fibreglass

The use of a glass rod to transmit light into the viewing chamber from an external light source was described by D. Smith in 1889.[18] Almost four decades after, in 1926 John Logie Baird, who invented the television, patented the idea of transmitting images through a flexible glass cable. In 1930, Heinrich Lamm demonstrated that bundles of flexible glass fibres can transmit light effectively.[19] These major discoveries were not appreciated until the early 1950s when Harold H. Hopkins (1918–1994), a physicist at the University of Reading, England, who invented the zoom lens in 1948 made, two fundamental breakthroughs. The first was the development of a flexible fibre imaging device which was essentially the first prototype flexible gastroscope in 1954.[20] The other was the invention of a glass rod optical system in 1959.[21] The traditional Nitze endoscope system consisted of a long tube of air with a number of thin glass lenses. The Hopkins' system consisted of a tube of glass with thin lenses of air which provided cleaner and brighter images and more realistic colours.[22] Unfortunately, no one in England showed

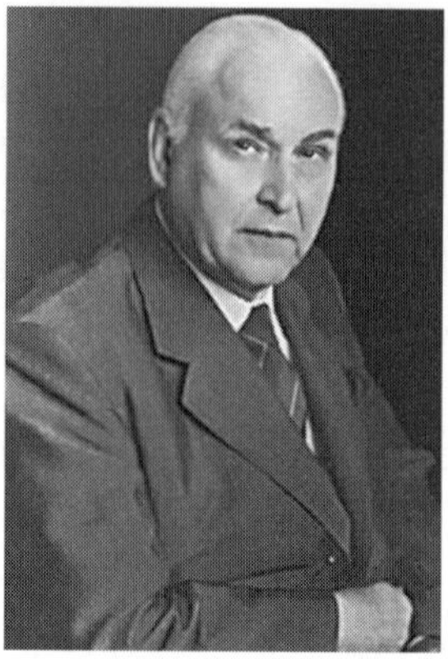

Fig. 4. Karl Storz (courtesy of Mrs S Storz).

an interest in the Hopkins invention and the Americans disapproved it. Six years later, in 1965, Hopkins presented his new optical system at a photographic exhibition in Klon and within days a contract was written between Karl Storz (Fig. 4), then a German instrument maker and Hopkins for the production of the Storz-Hopkins endoscope.[23] This partnership revolutionised the art of endoscopy as a whole.

Six decades after the introduction of the flexible gastro-camera (see Photography and Camera) and a few years after Hopkins flexible fibre imaging device, in 1957 Basil Hirschowitz, a South African who was training as a gastroenterologist in the USA, in collaboration with Wilbur Peters and Larry Curtis, a physicist, and after discussion with Harold Hopkins of England, developed the first clinically usable flexible gatroscope.[24] This home-made instrument which featured a distal light bulb and flexible glass fibres to transfer visual images was used to perform the first successful flexible gastroscopy on a patient who happened to be the wife of a dental student with a duodenal ulcer. The distal light bulb allowed poor illumination and images and colour distortion (Fig. 5).

In 1960, Karl Storz visited a congress in Holland and was impressed by the displayed Hirschowitz's flexible gastroscope which was 4m long and 2cm in diameter. Storz realised that the same system (flexible fibre transmitting image) could also be used for the purpose of light transmission. The following day, he rushed to the

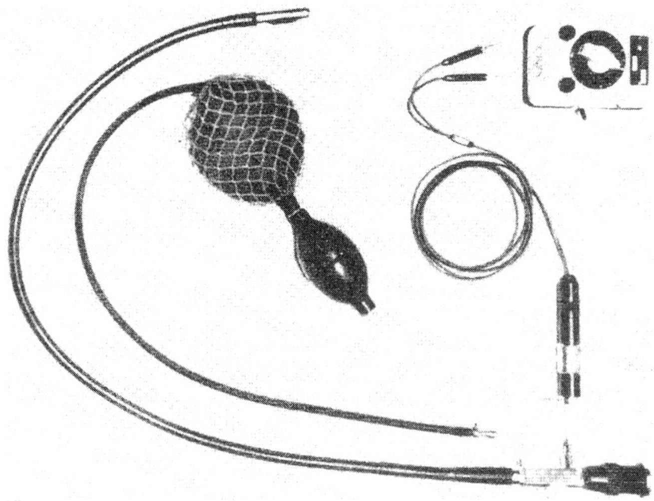

Fig. 5. Hirschowitz Flexible Gastroscope 1958–1962 (from History of Endoscopy vol V–VII, by Matthias A Reuter, Hans J Reuter, Rainer M Engel).

patent office in Stuttgart and licensed the idea of a fibroptic light transmission coupled with Hopkins rod-lens optical system.[23]

In May 1961 Hirschowitz published a paper in "*The Lancet*" and stated that flexible endoscopy is the method of choice for upper gastrointestinal investigations[24] and by 1969, endoscopic examination of the entire colon (colonoscopy) became a reality.[25]

Photography and Camera

The importance of documentation, teaching and training and ergonomics have been acknowledged by surgeons, scientists and instrument makers since the introduction of the endoscope.

In 1874, S. Theodore Stein (1840–1892), a physician and physicist from Frankfurt, modified existing cameras to photograph the inside of the urethra and bladder.[26] In 1893 Max Nitze took photographs through the cystoscope and published the first atlas of pathology a few years later.[27]

By the late 19th century adequate examination of the stomach was still hindered by the problems of image and light transmission as well as the difficulty of negotiating rigid instruments through natural anatomic bends. In an attempt to overcome these problems Lange and Meltzing developed the idea of multiple photographic exposures to visualise the interior of a stomach as an alternative to visual exposure (gastroscopy). In 1898, they introduced flexible "gastro-camera" and published the results of its use in 15 patients.[28] This rather curious instrument which was presented as the first flexible gastroscope, had a rigid head which consisted of a film magazine for a miniature film roll which was pulled after each exposure, mini camera head and an electric bulb. The rest of the gastroscope was made of a rubber tube for electric wires, air insufflation and pulling mechanism for the film transport.[4] The gastro-camera was capable of producing 50 exposures per examination.

In 1938, Henning and Keilhack produced the first colour pictures from the stomach using a semi-rigid gastroscope and an over-heated filament.[29]

The use of a television camera probably originated from France and was introduced by Soulas using a studio camera during a bronchoscopy in 1956.[30] In 1962 George Berci and associates introduced the first black and white miniature TV camera for endoscopy.[27,31] The camera was 350 gm in weight and 4.5 × 12 cm in dimensions, excluding the lens, and had 350 TV lines (3.5 MHz). The next major breakthrough came from Bell Laboratories in the USA who produced lightweight, low-powered, highly sensitive, charge-coupled camera devices in 1969. This meant that incoming optical images can be converted into electronic impulses and projected onto TV screens. Ten years later, this technology was incorporated into endoscopy and the modern era of video endoscopy began.[27,31]

Endoscopic Surgery and Paediatrics

The impetus for the development of endoscopy and endoscopic surgery was firmly in the hands of urologists (endoluminal), gynaecologists (laparoscopy) and gastroenterologists (flexible endoluminal), and the paediatric surgeons seem to have had very little if any involvement until the early 1970's.[32] The reason being: paediatric surgery as an independent speciality hardly existed before then, at the same time, there were no miniaturised endoscopes and instruments to use in infants and children. With the advent of the Hopkins new rod-lens system and flexible glass fibre for transmitting image and light it became possible to miniaturise endoscopic instruments for use in infants and children. No one has contributed more widely to the early development of paediatric endoscopy than Stephen L. Gans and George Berci from Los Angeles, both in the design of instruments and identifying clinical indications for laryngobronchoscopy, oesophagoscopy, cystourethroscopy, sigmoidoscopy and even laparoscopy.[33] Their achievements would not have been possible without the support and contribution from the industry in particular that of Karl Storz.

Paediatric intraluminal endoscopy became a routine practice worldwide in the 1970's (rigid endoscopy) and 1980's (flexible endoscopy). During the same period, however, laparoscopy and thoracoscopy remained, primarily as a diagnostic measure, in the hands of a few dedicated surgeons.[32,34–36]

The advent of laparoscopic cholecystectomy in the late 1980's, was the single most important stimulus to the development of therapeutic laparoscopic surgery. Within a few years, the practice had mushroomed across the various specialities and paediatric surgery was not an exception.[37] The feasibility, safety and benefits of therapeutic laparoscopy and thoracoscopy in children was introduced by Alain, Montupet and Valla from France, Schier from Germany, Tan from Australia, Najmaldin from England, and Lobe, Georgeson, Rothenberg and Holcomb from USA, and Yeung from Hong Kong. The application of fetoscopic surgery was addressed by the Harrisons Group from California in 1992.[38]

Together with these technical developments came the introduction of organisation, teaching and training courses and journals aiming to promote the importance, and high standard and safety of the new technique.[39] In 1990, the first paediatric endoscopic group, *Group d Etude de Coeliochirurgie Infantile* (GECI), was formed in France, and the president was Alain. In 1992, the first paediatric laparoscopic surgery symposium was organised by Shier and Waldeschmidt in Berlin. In 1992, the first teaching and training laparoscopy course was organised by Tan Hudson, Harvey and Najmaldin in Melbourne. In 1993 the Leeds Annual International Paediatric Endoscopic Surgery Workshop started by Najmaldin. In 1994, the international paediatric endosurgery group (IPEG) was formed (President Willital) and its first conference was held in Florida in 1995. In 1996, the British laparoscopy group was convened by Johnson in Leicester and in 1999 the British Association of Paediatric Endoscopic Surgeons was born in Leeds (President Najmaldin). In 1997, a dedicated journal "*Paediatric Endosurgery and Innovative Techniques*" (editor, Lobe), went into production. In 1999, a comprehensive paediatric laparoscopic and thoracoscopic textbook was published (editors Bax, Georgeson, Najmaldin and Valla). In 2005, the first comprehensive operative endoscopy and endoscopic surgery book was published (editors Najmaldin, Rothenberg, Crabbe and Beasley).

Latest Developments

Telerobotic surgery is the latest major advancement set to change the practice of endoscopic surgery both in adult and paediatric surgical practice.[40] The technique has been introduced to extend the capabilities of surgeons and address the difficulties (view, precision, dexterity, ergonomics) encountered with the introduction of endoscopic surgery. In the late 1980's an industrial robot "PUMA" was used to hold instruments for neurosurgical stereotactic biopsies. At the same time, The Imperial College in London developed a robot for prostatic surgery, and in California a machine was developed for orthopaedic surgery. In early 1990's, the NASA Research Centre found interest in the idea, and became of the main driving force behind the development of telerobotic surgery.[41] The early devices, AESOP and ENDOASSIST, were camera manipulators. ARTEMS had two arms and a control station. Subsequently, more comprehensive machines Zeus and da Vinci with multiple arms and a control console were developed.[41,42] The da Vinci is now the only system available in the market for use in laparoscopy and thoracoscopy.

The application of telerobotic surgery in children is documented by Heller from Germany; Olsen from Denmark, Peters, Lobe, Irish and Mehan from USA, Najmaldin from England and Anderberg from Sweden.[41,43]

Conclusions

Endoscopy and endoscopic surgery are the product of a collaborative effort by surgeons and physicians from all disciplines as well as scientists, engineers and industry from many countries over a long period of time. As medicine evolved technical advancements improved the surgical views and surgeons' capabilities. The wide variety of modern rigid and flexible endoscopes and the introduction of the high definition computer chip camera and robotics allow routine diagnostic examination and complex therapeutic procedures with minimal morbidity and have greatly facilitated teaching and training of surgeons. With the recent development in genetic and biomedical engineering and nanotechnology, the only certainty is that endoscopic innovation is no longer assured.

References

1. Rosin D. History. In: Rosin D. (ed.) *Minimal Access Medicine and Surgery*. Radcliffe Medical Press, Oxford, 1993, pp. 1–9.
2. Gordon A. The history and development of endoscopic surgery. In: Sutton C, Diamond MP (eds.) *Endoscopic Surgery for Gynaecologists*. Saunders, London, 1993, pp. 3–7.
3. Gotz F, Pier A, Schippers E, Schumpelick V. The history of laparoscopy. In: Gotz F, *et al.* (eds.) *Colour Atlas of Laparoscopic Surgery*. Thieme, New York, 1993, pp. 3–5.
4. Lau WY, Leow CK, Li AKC. History of endoscopic and laparoscopic surgery. *World J Surg* 1997;21:444–453.
5. Bozzini PH. Lichtleiter eine Erfindung zur Anschauung innerer Teile und Krankheiten. *J Prak Heilk* 1806;24:107.
6. Desormeaux AJ. *Endoscope and its Application to the Diagnosis and Treatment of Affections of the Genitourinary Passages. Chicago, Med J.* 1867.
7. Bevan L. The oesophagoscope. *Lancet* 1968;1:470.

8. Kluge F, Seidler E. Zur Erstanwendung der Osophago-und Gastroskopie: Briefe van Adolf Kussmaul und Seinen Mitarbeitern. *Med Hist J* 1986;21:288–307.
9. Belt AE, Charnock DA. The history of the cystoscope. In: Cabol H. (ed.) *Modern Urology*. Lea & Febiger, Philadelphia, 1936.
10. Nitze M. Beobachtung-und Untersuchungsmethode fur Harnohre. Harnblase und rectum. *Wein med Wochenschr* 1879;29:649.
11. Mikulicz J. Uber Gastroskopie and Oesophagoskopie. *Verth Dtsch Ges Chir* 1882;10:81–85.
12. Margulies DK, Shabot MM. Fiberoptic imaging and measurement. In: JG Hunter, JM Sackier (eds.) *Minimally Invasive Surgery*. McGraw-Hill, New York, 1993, 7–14.
13. von Ott DO. Ventroscopic illumination of the abdominal cavity in pregnancy. *Zhenskikh Boloznei* 1901;15:7–8.
14. Kelling G. Zur Coelioskopie. *Arch Klin Chir* 1923;126:226.
15. Jacobaeus HC. Kurze Ubersicht Uber Meine Erfahrungen mit der Laparothorakoskopie. *Munchen Med. Wochenschr* 1911;58:2017.
16. Grant JA. Victor Darwin Lespinasse: A biographical sketch. *Neurosurgery* 1996;39:1232–1233.
17. Zollikofer R. Zur Laparoskopie. *Schweiz Med Wochenschr* 1924;54:264.
18. Marlow J. History of laparoscopy, optics, fiberoptics and instrumentation. *Clin Obstet Gynaecol* 1976;19:261–275.
19. Fourestier M, Bladu A. Vulmiere J. Perfectionnement de I Endoscopie Medicale. *Presse Med* 1952;60:1292.
20. Hopkins HH, Kapany NS. A flexbile fiberscope using static scanning. *Nature* 1954;76:864–869.
21. Gow JG. Harold Hopkins and optical systems for urology — an appreciation. *Urology* 1998;52:152–157.
22. Berci G, Forde KA. History of endoscopy: What lessons have we learned from the past? *Surge Endosc* 2000;14:5–15.
23. Linder TE, Simmen D, Stool SE. Revolutionary inventions in the 20th century — The history of endoscopy. *Arch Otolaryngol Head Neck Surg* 1997;123:1161–1163.
24. Hirschowitz BI. A personal history of the fibrescope. *Gastroenterology* 1979;76:864–869.
25. Wolff WI. Colonoscopy: History and development. *Am J Gastroenterol.* 1989;84:1017.

26. Stein S. *Das Photo-Endoshop*, Part 3, Berl. Klin. Wochenschr, 1874.
27. Berci G. History of endoscopic surgery. In: Greene FL, Ponsky JL (eds.) *Endoscopic Surgery*. Saunders, Philadelphia, 1994, pp. 1–5.
28. Lange F, Meltzing S. Die Photography des Mageninnern. *Munch Med Wochenschr* 1898;50:1585.
29. Henning N. Keilhack H. Fan Benphotography der Magenhole. *Dtsch Med Wochenschr* 1938;64:1328.
30. Soulas A. Televised bronchoscopy. *Presse Med* 1956;64:97.
31. Berci G. Paz-Partlow M. Electroic imaging in endoscopy. *Surg Endosc* 1998;2:227.
32. Gans SL. *Pediatric Endoscopy*. Grane and Stratton. New York, 1983.
33. Gans SL, Berci G. Advances in endoscopy of infants and children. *J Pediatr Surg* 1971;6:199–223.
34. Kusch NL, Timchen KO. Laparoskopiia u detei. *Vestn Khir* 1969;102: 92–94.
35. Rosenberg D. Gognat M. La Coelioscopie dans L'enfrance et L'adolescence. *Gynaecol Pract* 1971;22:531–539.
36. Rodgers BM, Ryckman FC, Moazam F, Talbert JL. Thoracoscopy for intrathoracic tumours. *Ann Thorac Surg* 1980;31:414–420.
37. Najmaldin A, Rothenberg S, Crabbe, Beasley S (eds.). *Operative Endoscopy and Endoscopic Surgery in Infants and Children*. Hodder Arnold, London, 2005.
38. Estes JM. MacGillivary TE, Hedrick MH, Adzick NS, Harrison MR. Fetoscopic surgery for the treatment of congenital anomalies. *J Pediatr Surg* 1992;27:950–954.
39. Najmaldin A. Skills training in paediatric minimal access surgery. *J Pediatr Surg* 2007;42:284–289.
40. Cadierre GB, Himpens J. Feasibility of robotic laparoscopic surgery: 146 cases. *World J Surg* 2001;25:1467–1477.
41. Najmaldin A. Paediatric telerobotic surgery: Where do we stand? *Int J Med Robot* 2007;3:183–186.
42. Satava RM. Surgical robotics: The early chronicles: A personal historical perspective. *Surg Laparosc Endosc Percutan Tech* 2002;12:6–16.
43. Najmaldin A, Antao B. Early experience of telerobotic surgery in children. *Int J Med Robot* 2007;3:199–202.

A NEW LIGHT — THE DEVELOPMENT OF IMAGING TECHNIQUES

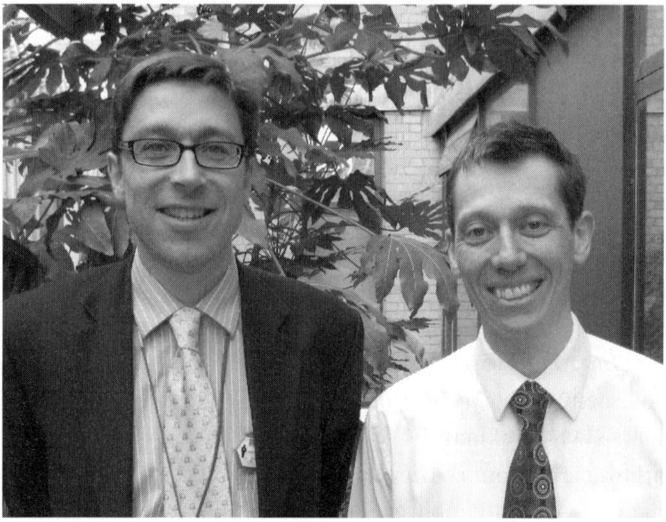

Greg Irwin
Michael S. Bradnam

Introduction

Radiology as a specialty came into being due to a series of significant discoveries, principally in the field of physics. A succession of innovators have taken novel scientific phenomena, and from them developed strategies to image the human body. In the case of X-rays, the discovery of their existence was followed by an evaluation of their potential for imaging within just a few days.

Paediatric radiology as a separate sub-speciality is relatively new, although the first clinical X-ray taken in America, on the February 3, 1896, was of a 14-year-old boy's wrist. The first book specifically concerned with paediatric radiology was published in 1910.

In the 1940's John Caffey described the association of multiple long bone fractures and chronic subdural haematomas, creating the debate which first established the existence of physical child abuse. Radiology continues to have a prominent role in the investigation of this condition. Caffey published his landmark textbook "*Pediatric X-Ray Diagnosis*" in 1945, which now continues in its eleventh edition.

The Society for Pediatric Radiology (SPR) was founded in America in 1958, electing Edward Neuhauser as its President, and was followed by the establishment of the European Society of Paediatric Radiology (ESPR) in 1963. Paediatric neuroradiology emerged as the first formal sub-speciality of paediatric radiology during the late 1960's. A recent initiative by the SPR is to reduce the radiation burden to children undergoing CT scans, as they are inherently more sensitive to the effects of ionizing radiation. This is readily achievable by altering the CT scanner tube current.

The X-Ray

X-rays were discovered on the November 8, 1895 by Wilhelm Conrad Röntgen, working in Wurzburg, Germany. Perhaps appropriately for the father of radiology, the discovery was made in a darkened room. He was performing experiments with cathode ray tubes, where streams of electrons pass across a vacuum, in much the same way as in a conventional television. The electrons in his experiment collided forcefully with the metal of the anode within the vacuum tube. The tubes were entirely covered so that no light could escape, but nonetheless Röntgen observed that a screen several feet from the tube began to fluoresce when the current was applied.

It was apparent that some sort of invisible ray was being emitted by the tube and shining upon the screen. These he termed 'X'-rays, the designation 'X' was intended to be a temporary name, indicating that the nature of the ray was unknown. He immediately began to investigate the properties of this new form of ray. His earliest experiments investigated the ability of the X-rays to cast a shadow from various objects interposed between the tube and the screen, and recorded the results upon a photographic plate. Rather than stopping all of the X-rays, objects were shown to be variably transparent. Paper, wood and cloth were penetrated easily, and also various metals to differing degrees.

One of the first recorded X-rays of a living human was performed on the hand of Röntgen's wife Anna-Bertha. Due to the low output of the unmodified tube, the exposure time was in the region of 30 minutes. By contrast, a modern hand X-ray exposure time is in the region of milliseconds. These early X-rays immediately showed their potential in medical investigation, successfully localising glass and metallic foreign bodies in various patients, facilitating their removal.

Röntgen's paper entitled "On a New Kind of Rays" (*Über eine neue Art von Strahlen*) was immediately published in December 1895. News of his discovery quickly spread, and Röntgen became famous and bestowed with many honours, including the Nobel Prize for Physics in 1901.

What is believed to be the first medical X-ray department in the world was set up in Glasgow Royal Infirmary, Scotland, in March 1896, by Dr John Macintyre (Fig. 1). Röntgen had sent a copy of his paper to Lord Kelvin in Glasgow in early 1896, who passed it on to Dr Macintyre's group, along with necessary apparatus. Some of the examinations attributed to this department include the first X-ray depictions of a bullet, and of a coin in the oesophagus (Fig. 2).

Due to the long exposure times, early radiographs were much more successful in imaging the peripheral skeleton than the chest or abdomen, where movement artefact and the thickness of the tissues spoiled the images. Improvements in X-ray tube design allowed for shorter exposures, as did advances in the construction of the film plates. Fluoroscopy was achieved by the examiner holding a fluorescent screen between his eyes and the patient, all the time directly in the path of the primary x-ray beam (Fig. 3).

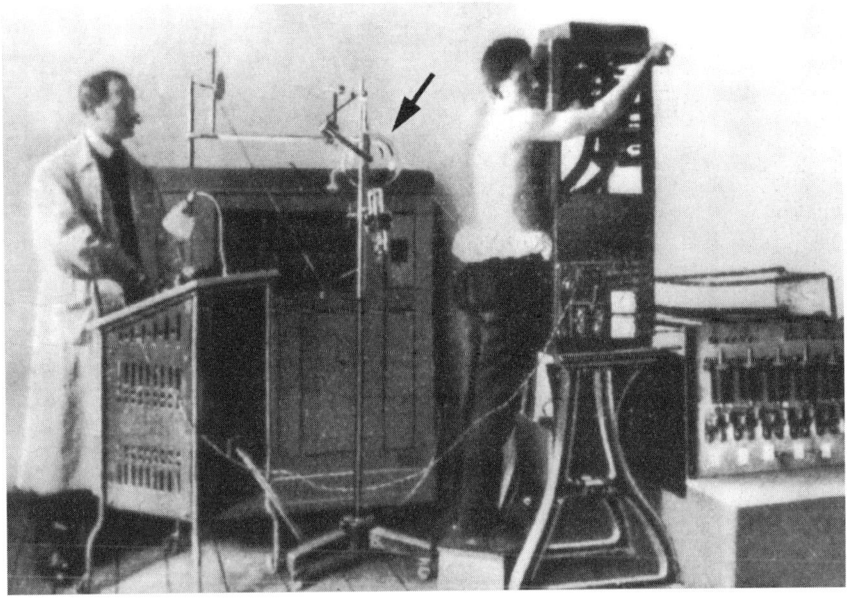

Fig. 1. An early photograph, probably late 1890s, of a chest x-ray being taken in Glasgow Royal Infirmary. Note the x-ray tube (arrowed) is completely unshielded, and is bathing the whole room in x-rays. Image courtesy of NHS Greater Glasgow and Clyde Archives.

Although there were many early reports of skin damage, the harmful effects of radiation were not initially fully appreciated. Many early X-ray workers suffered burns, lost fingers, hands or eyes, or succumbed to radiation induced cancers. The "Martyrs Memorial" to 169 who lost their lives was dedicated in 1936, outside the Röntgen Institute of St. George's Hospital in Hamburg.

Modern X-ray set ups still use X-ray tubes based on the same design. They are however, heavily shielded, and include collimators to enable the area irradiated to be minimized. Films have been replaced with digital sensors, and the processed images are sent electronically to picture archiving and communications systems (PACS). The images are then immediately available for reviewing at multiple geographically separate locations. Currently a National PACS system is being installed across the whole of Scotland, on which all imaging modalities are stored.

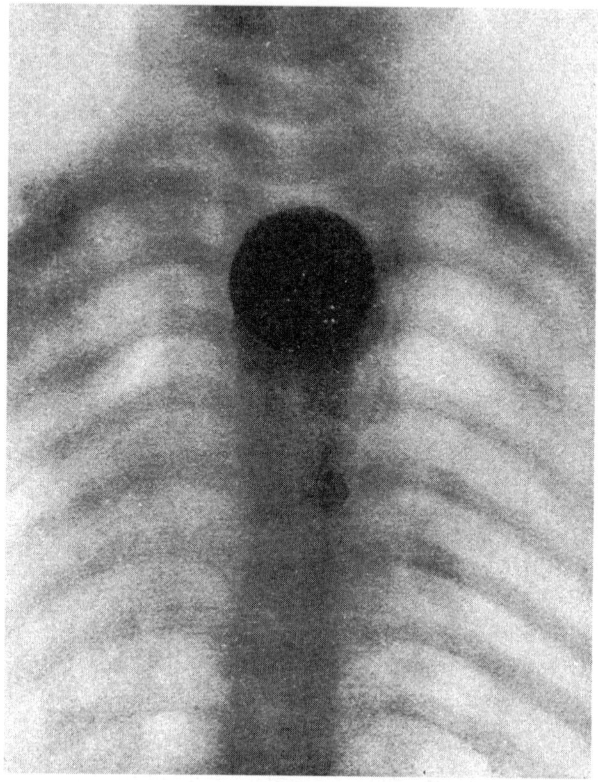

Fig. 2. An X-ray of a half penny impacted in a child's upper oesophagus, taken by Dr John Macintyre. The image was exhibited at the Royal Society in June 1896. Image copyright of Medical Illustration, Glasgow Royal Infirmary, used with permission.

Ultrasound

Medical ultrasound has its roots in the development of SONAR (Sound navigation and ranging). In the First World War, experiments were under way to develop sonar for submarines. It was known that bats could navigate by listening for the echoes of the high frequency sound waves they produced, and it was hoped to replicate this principle under water. The recent sinking of the RMS Titanic by an iceberg in 1912 had added impetus to the project.

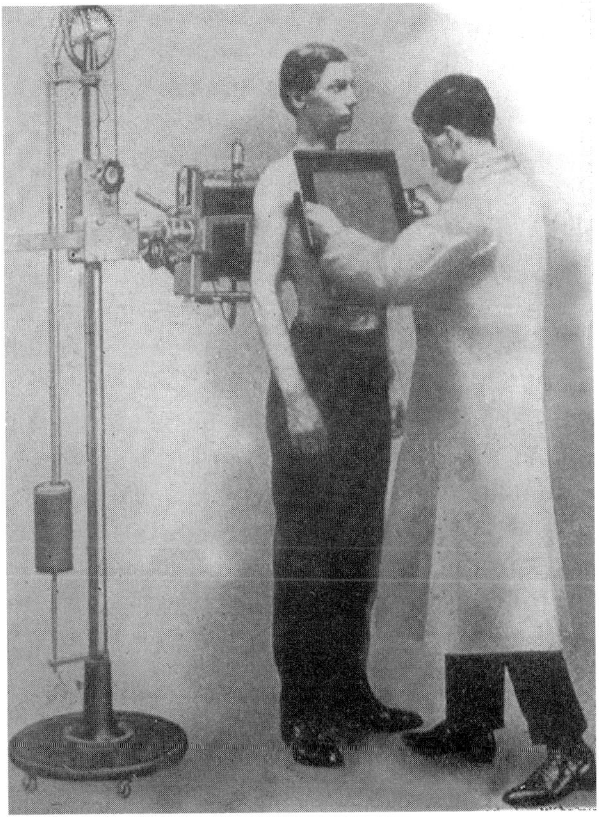

Fig. 3. A 1905 image of fluoroscopy. The X-ray tube is behind the patient. The examiner is standing directly in the primary X-ray beam, observing the movement of the heart and diaphragm on the fluorescent screen he is holding. Image courtesy of NHS Greater Glasgow and Clyde Archives.

An early system developed in 1914 by Fessenden was partially successful, but limited in its direction finding ability due to the low frequency of the sound waves it used. High frequency sound waves (hence ultrasound) were produced with quartz crystals glued between steel plates by the French physicist Paul Langévin, using the piezoelectric effect. This is where crystals are caused to change size and vibrate by passing electrical currents through them and *vice versa*. This produced a short "chirp" of high frequency sound underwater. By timing how long it took the echo to return, and knowing the speed of sound in water, it was possible to determine the distance from the source of the sound to the source of the echo. In practice, this gave the distance from the ship to the submarine/seabed/iceberg. The pulse echo technique was developed using radio waves rather than sound waves in the development of RADAR (radio detection and ranging).

A parallel field of study was in the use of ultrasound to detect otherwise invisible flaws in metal. The Second World War meant that several groups were investigating the technique at the same time in different countries. Wartime also proved the catalyst for further sonar development.

The application of ultrasound to medicine was initially confined to attempts at therapy, rather than diagnosis. High frequency ultrasound generated heat, which was used in many conditions as symptomatic treatment. The destructive force of high energy sound waves were also used as a neurosurgical tool for ablation of parts of the brain.

Working in America in the late 1940's, George Ludwig began animal experiments using metal flaw-detector equipment to identify foreign bodies, such as gallstones surgically implanted into dogs. His work established many fundamental concepts of diagnostic ultrasonography.

Ian Donald (Fig. 4), an obstetrician and gynaecologist working in Glasgow, Scotland, assisted by John MacVicar conducted experiments on the freshly removed tumours from human patients. The ultrasound device was provided by Tom Brown a local boilermaker, where it was used to check the integrity of metal welds. It was immediately apparent that different traces were produced by different masses, and further experiments on *in vivo* tumours were planned. Difficulties were encountered in transferring the industrial equipment to clinical usage. Initially a small bucket of water with a latex bottom was placed on the patient's abdomen, which itself was smeared with lubricating jelly to exclude air. The ultrasound probe was then applied to the surface of the water. Subsequently, direct application of the probe to the skin, with olive oil as a coupling film, proved less hazardous. There was an early clinical success, where a

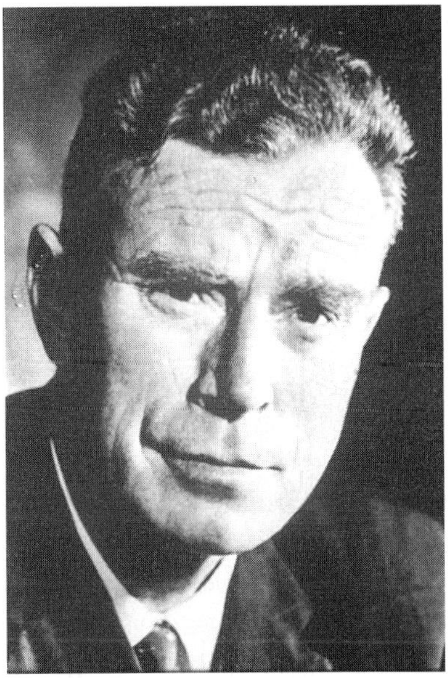

Fig. 4. Ian Donald.

middle-aged women thought to be dying of a gastric carcinoma with ascites, was instead shown to have an enormous ovarian cyst. This was removed, and the patient made a full recovery. It is noted in his memoir however that after this Donald was "inflicted with horrid specimens of her grandchild's attempts at cooking by way of an expression of gratitude".

Donald went on to publish a landmark paper in the "*Lancet*" of June 7, 1958 "Investigation of abdominal masses by pulsed ultrasound (Fig. 5)". His co-worker James Willocks went on to establish the utility of biparietal measurement of the fetal skull to measure growth.

From the mid 1960's there was a rapid increase in the use of diagnostic ultrasound, matched with great enhancements in the scanning machines. Early commercial machines were large and cumbersome, with either large fixed gantries or articulated probe arms. Original (A mode) scan displays were simply blips on an oscilloscope trace, although accurate measurements with these systems were possible. More advanced electronics needed to be developed before

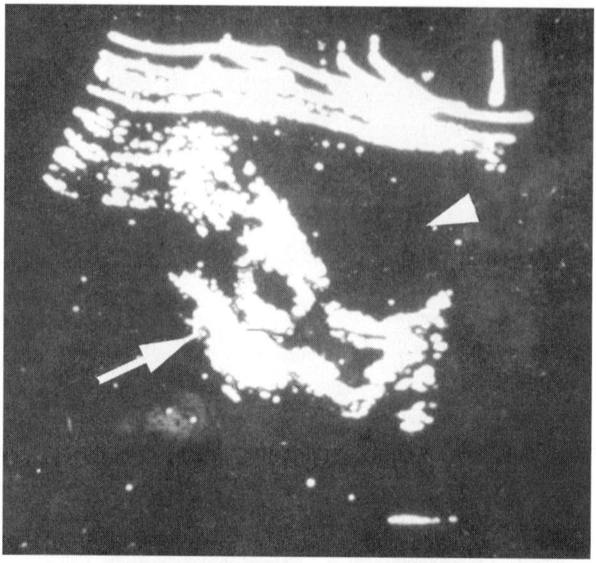

Fig. 5. 1963 ultrasound performed by Prof. Ian Donald, showing a fetus in utero (arrow) using the urinary bladder (arrowhead) as an acoustic window. Image courtesy of NHS Greater Glasgow and Clyde Archives.

cross-sectional (B mode) images with grey scale could be produced. The next major innovation was that of real time scanning, which relied upon mechanical rotating or oscillating transducers to quickly sweep back and forth across the area of interest, building up a moving picture. These in turn have been superseded by electronic phased array transducers. Doppler techniques have developed in parallel to grey scale imaging, and from the outset have allowed investigation of the movement of heart valves, and the flow of blood in peripheral vessels. The power of modern computers has enabled the recent addition of 3D scanning which uses advanced surface shading and volume rendering (Fig. 6).

Computed Tomography (CT)

Sir Godfrey Hounsfield was an English engineer who invented the CT scanner. He grew up on a farm in Nottinghamshire, the youngest

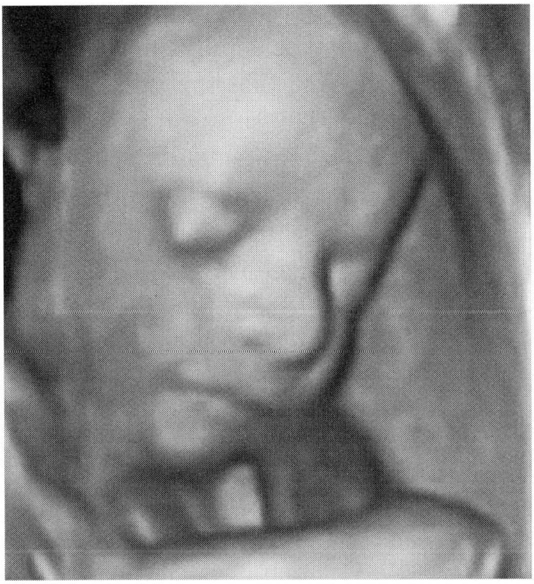

Fig. 6. Modern 3D ultrasound of a fetus of 20 weeks gestation. Image courtesy of Cara Duguid.

of five children. He was free to pursue his interests in electrical and mechanical devices, even constructing a home made glider, in which he launched himself from the top of haystacks. During the Second World War he joined the Royal Air Force, as a radar mechanic instructor. Joining EMI in 1951, he initially continued his work on radar and guided weapons. He subsequently led the design team building the first all transistor computer to be built in Britain.

He had the germ of the idea that was to become computerised tomography in 1967, whilst walking in the countryside. He realized that "you could determine what was in a box simply by taking readings at all angles through it." In practice this required a minicomputer to reconstruct a picture from X-ray measurements taken through the body at a multitude of different angles. The computer was essential as there would be hundreds of thousands of calculations to be made.

Initial tests with gamma rays were too slow, but even switching to X-rays still required a scanning time of nine hours. The first scan of human tissue was performed on a preserved human brain from a local hospital museum, and successfully showed differentiation of grey and white matter. Fearing that the preservation process had enhanced the images, Hounsfield substituted fresh bullocks' brains (Fig. 7). In scanning through the carcasses of pigs, problems were encountered as each picture took a day to acquire, during which gas bubbles formed and expanded within the tissues.

Faster prototypes were produced, and the first patient was scanned on the October 1, 1971 at Atkinson Morley's Hospital in South London. The patient had a suspected brain lesion, and the scan demonstrated a frontal cyst. The next step was a machine capable of scanning the body, and a larger and faster scanner was produced capable of taking a picture in 18 seconds. The first body images produced in the body prototype were of Hounsfield himself.

Hounsfield proposed a scale for measuring the relative absorption values in CT, from 1000 for bone, 20–40 for tissue, 0 for water and –1,000 for air. These Hounsfield units remain the standard unit for CT imaging density. He was awarded the Nobel Prize (in Physiology or Medicine) in 1979 and shared the honour with Allan

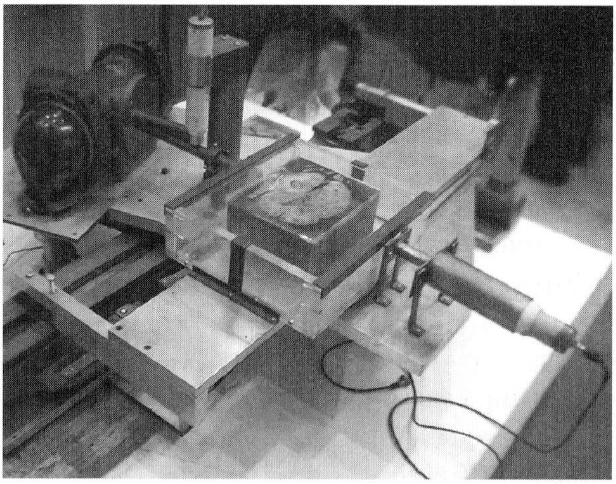

Fig. 7. Hounsfield's prototype for the CT scanner. Note the section of brain in the centre of the image. Image by courtesy of Philip Cosson.

Cormack, a South African physicist of Scottish descent. Hounsfield received a Knighthood in 1981.

Magnetic Resonance Imaging (MRI)

MRI is a complicated imaging technique, and the history of its development is no less complex. In many ways it is well suited to investigate children, giving fantastically detailed images with unparalleled soft tissue contrast. However, the machine is expensive and apt to induce claustrophobia, and the long scan times may require sedation or general anaesthetic for younger patients. The use of strong magnetic fields precludes scanning of patients with certain metallic implants, but the absence of ionising radiation secures it a place in the arsenal of the paediatric radiologist.

Expressed simply, placing the body in a strong magnetic field causes the hydrogen nuclei of the water molecules found throughout the body to line up. A brief radio wave is applied, which pushes these protons out of alignment. When the protons flick back into line, they release energy which is detected and localised by the scanner. Areas with lots of water release relatively more energy, and the scanner is able to build up a cross-sectional picture of the body, depending upon the amount of water, and therefore the amounts of energy released.

MRI was initially termed Nuclear Magnetic Resonance (NMR). Working independently in the 1940s, Felix Bloch at Stanford University, and Edward Purcell at Harvard University, found that some nuclei in a magnetic field absorbed radio frequency range energy, and emitted this energy upon returning to their original state. Their discoveries in nuclear magnetic absorption earned them a joint share in the Nobel Prize in Physics in 1952. NMR spectroscopy was used by physicists to investigate the properties of small samples in high strength magnetic fields, rather than to produce anatomical images.

In the early 1970s, Raymond Damadian found that normal and cancerous tissue could be separated *in vitro* according to different physical parameters using NMR. This raised the possibility of non-invasive tumour characterisation, and in 1974 Damadian constructed a scanner with the intention of analyzing the whole body.

In 1973 Paul Lauterbur, a Professor of Chemistry at the State University of New York published a paper in "*Nature*" describing an imaging technique for the spatial localisation of two capillary tubes of water inside a narrow tube of heavy water. The introduction of gradients allowed two-dimensional images to be produced. Reportedly, he was eating a hamburger at the time when the idea occurred, and he jotted it down on the napkin. The development of this idea resulted in the award of the Nobel Prize in Physiology or Medicine 2003, shared with Sir Peter Mansfield. Mansfield is a British Physicist who further developed the utilisation of gradients, and showed how the signals could be mathematically analysed to develop a useful imaging technique. He discovered how fast imaging could be performed with the echo planar technique, and laid the basis for functional MRI.

By 1980 Edelstein and Hutchison at the University of Aberdeen in Scotland had developed a practical two dimensional imaging technique, dubbed "spin-warp imaging" and the world's first clinical diagnostic MRI service was started at the Aberdeen Royal Infirmary in August of that year.

Nuclear Medicine

Nuclear medicine uses radioactive isotopes to image the body and to treat disease. As the isotopes can be attached to various pharmaceutical compounds, analysis of a wide range of physiological function and anatomy is possible. Two important applications of nuclear medicine in the field of paediatric radiology are imaging of the renal tract and oncology.

The 1903 Nobel prize for physics was shared by Henri Becquerel, Marie and Pierre Curie, for their work in the discovery of radioactivity. Whilst investigating a possible connection between Röntgen's X-rays and natural phosphorescence in 1896, Bequerel discovered by chance that uranium emitted radiation that exposed photographic film. Marie and Pierre Curie continued his work, discovering polonium (named after Marie's native Poland) and radium.

Unfortunately, some early applications of radioactivity included the addition of radioactive compounds to water as a cure-all, and to toothpaste promising "radioactive brilliance."

The use of radioactivity in imaging required the use of tracers with a short half life, to limit the potential for side-effects. In 1937 iodine-131 was created, followed by the production of technetium-99m in 1938, which remains the most commonly used isotope in nuclear medicine. These and many other isotopes were created using a cyclotron, an apparatus which accelerates charged particles to great speed in a vacuum chamber and fires them at a target. The cyclotron was invented and developed by Ernest Lawrence, later to receive the Nobel prize in Physics for his work. It is no coincidence that his younger brother John Lawrence became a pioneer in the field of nuclear medicine. It is notable that all of this work came from one centre, the Berkeley Laboratory in California.

The use of isotopes in imaging was revolutionised in the 1950's by the invention and development of the first clinically successful scintillation camera by Hal Anger, also working at Berkeley. The design principle of his gamma camera was so successful that it is still the basis of most of those used today. The technology has evolved to form the basis of single photon-emission computed tomography (SPECT) and positron emission tomography (PET) which permit cross-sectional imaging, analogous to CT. SPECT uses standard nuclear medicine tracers but PET uses a different class of short-lived tracers which emit positrons, also produced in a cyclotron. It is the need for an accessible cyclotron which has slowed the introduction of PET. In 2008 there are approximately 1500 PET centres in the United States of America, however in the United Kingdom the modality is only emerging as a highly specialized regional service. The most widely used PET tracer is currently fluorine-18 fluoro-deoxy-glucose (FDG), which produce images of tissue metabolism.

The images produced in nuclear medicine are generally of low resolution, and these can now be enhanced by combining the images with high resolution CT techniques, hence SPECT/CT and PET/CT. The fused images produced by these complementary techniques combine functional information with anatomical detail, and these can be used to improve the localization of certain disease processes and enhance diagnostic accuracy. The primary application of PET in children is in oncology, where it particularly useful for the diagnosis and staging of disease, as well as for assessing the response of individual treatments.

Selected References

1. Regarding Röntgen. *Nobel Lectures, Physics 1901–1921*, Elsevier Publishing Company, Amsterdam, 1967.
2. Rotch TM. *Living Anatomy and Pathology: the Diagnosis of Diseases in Early Life by the Roentgen Method.* Lippincott, Philadelphia, USA, 1910.
3. Calder JF. *The History of Radiology in Scotland, 1896–2000.* Dunedin Academic Press, Edinburgh, UK, 2001.
4. Griscom NT. History of pediatric radiology in the United States and Canada: Images and trends. *Radiographics* 1995;15(6):1399–1422.
5. Willocks J, Barr W. *Ian Donald — A Memoir.* RCOG Press, London, UK, 2004.
6. Donald I, MacVicar J, Brown TG. Investigation of abdominal masses by pulsed ultrasound. *Lancet* 1958;7;1(7032):1188–1195.
7. Kirks DR. Eugene W. Caldwell Lecture. Pediatric imaging: the oldest radiological subspecialty comes of age. *Am J Roentgenol* 1999;172(2): 291–299.
8. Odelberg W (ed.) Sir Godfrey Hounsfield. In: *Les Prix Nobel. The Nobel Prizes 1979*, Nobel Foundation, Stockholm, Sweden, 1980.
9. Burrows EH. *Pioneers and Early Years: History of British Radiology.* Colophon, Alderney, Channel Islands, 1986.
10. Rosenbusch G, Oudkerk M, Ammann E (eds.) *Radiology in Medical Diagnostics: Evolution of X-ray Applications 1895–1995 (English language edition).* Blackwell Science, Oxford, UK, 1995.

11. Anger H. A new instrument for mapping gamma-ray emitters. In: *Biology and Medicine Quarterly Report UCRL*, 3653 pp. 38 (University of California Radiation Laboratory, Berkeley), 1957.
12. Slovis I. *Caffey's Pediatric Diagnostic Imaging: 11th ed.* Mosby, Philadelphia, USA, 2007.

FETAL SURGERY

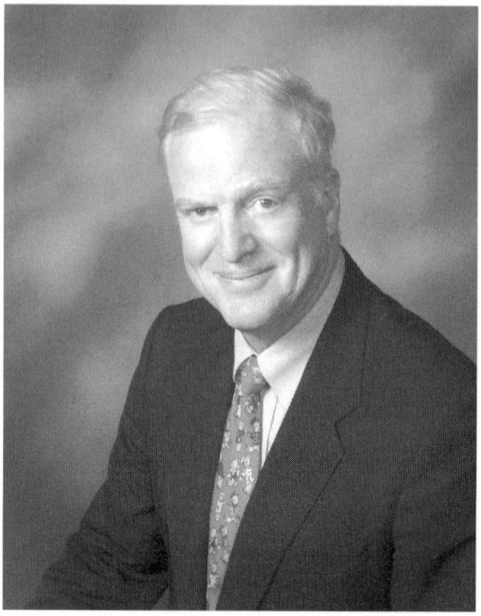

Michael R. Harrison

PART I: History of the Fetus as a Patient

The concept that the fetus is a patient, an individual whose maladies are a proper subject for medical treatment as well as scientific observation, is alarmingly modern. It was not until the last half of the last century that the prying eye of the ultrasonographer rendered the once opaque womb transparent, letting the light of scientific observation fall on the shy and secretive fetus.

Historically, we approached the fetus with a wonder bordering on mysticism. Enid Bagnold's description in "*The Door of Life*" captures the awe engendered by a scene that no one had actually witnessed.

> "Hanging head downwards between cliffs of bone was the baby, its arms all but clasped about its neck, its face aslant upon its arms, hair painted upon its skull, closed, secret eyes, a diver poised in albumen, ancient and epic, shot with delicate spasms, as old as a Pharaoh in its tomb."

Whether this reverence is a reflection of our profound wonder at the "miracle" of differentiation of a fertilized egg into a human infant, or a clandestine Darwinian mechanism to ensure the survival of the species, it has certainly hindered investigation of fetal physiology and precluded any consideration of fetal therapy. Only in the last few decades have techniques for visualizing, monitoring, measuring, and prodding the fetus begun to alter our perceptions of the living human fetus. Only now are we beginning to consider the fetus seriously — medically, legally, and ethically. Now that our perspective is undergoing radical change, it is instructive to trace the medical history of our approach to this, our most reticent patient.[1]

Early attempts to describe the fetus. In attempting to explain how the fetus was related to the child, the Greek and Roman thinkers conceived the idea of the homunculus — a miniature person living and growing within the mother before birth. This concept undoubtedly evolved from practical experience in animal husbandry and from observation of aborted human and animal fetuses. The fetus was seen to grow in resemblance to the child as gestation progressed. In the absence of "modern" biologic information, the homunculus provided a very good explanation for, at least, the older fetus.

The homunculus, a purely descriptive explanation, was sometimes carried to a wonderfully whimsical extreme. Lawrence Sterne, in "*The Life and Opinion of Tristram Shandy, Gentlemen*" (Book 1, Chapter 2), had his hero soliloquize:

> "The homunculus, sir, in however low and ludicrous a light he may appear, in this age of levity, to the eye of folly or prejudice; to the

> eye of reason in scientific research, he stands confessed — a being guarded and circumscribed with rights. The minutest philosophers who, by the by, have the most enlarged understandings their souls being inversely as their inquiries), show us incontestably, that the homunculus is created by the same hand — engendered in the same course of nature — endowed with the same locomotive power and faculties with us; that he consists, as we do, of skin, hair, fat, flesh, veins, arteries, ligaments, nerves, cartilages, bones, marrow, brains, glands, genitals, humors, and articulations; — is a being of as much activity — in all senses of the word, as much and as truly our fellow creature as my Lord Chancellor of England. He may be benefited, he may be injured, he may obtain redress; in a word, he has all the claims and rights of humanity...
>
> The work of Charles Darwin had an indirect but significant impact on our scientific and philosophical attitude toward the fetus. His ideas about the evolution of species provided a macroscopic view of reproduction that posited a progression from seed to infant, as well as from generation to generation. Before his view of procreation and speciation became generally known, the relation between the seed and the infant was a religious matter, a continuum accepted on faith. This may account for the derivation of the current religious doctrine that links copulation directly with procreation and, thus, ascribes the sacredness of life to the conceptus or homunculus from its very beginning. Darwin's ideas demystified the role of reproduction. In "*The Descent of Man*", he wrote, "Man is developed from an ovule, about 125th of an inch in diameter, which differs in no respect from the ovules of any animal."

At the dawn of the 20th century, the fetus was shedding its metaphysical trappings in favor of biologic description. Still, the concepts of inheritance and evolution did little to explain exactly how the seed became an infant, and work on the development of the human fetus remained entirely descriptive during the first part of the 20th century. In the 1920s, Minkowski examined human fetuses obtained at cesarean operations by placing the recently delivered fetus in warm saline solution. Hertig and Rock studied aborted fetuses at various stages of gestation and were able to piece together the morphology of embryonic and fetal development. This descriptive information was supplemented by the study of animal fetuses in various species, an undertaking that also blossomed and bore fruit in this century (Figs. 1 and 2).

Experimental fetal observation. Since early observations of the human fetus were limited to an occasional aborted "homunculus", fetal developmental anatomy and physiology had to be derived almost exclusively from observations made on animals. This is undoubtedly how Hippocrates arrived at the brilliantly intuitive proposal that the fetus urinated in utero and that amniotic fluid consists of fetal urine, an observation confirmed only during the last

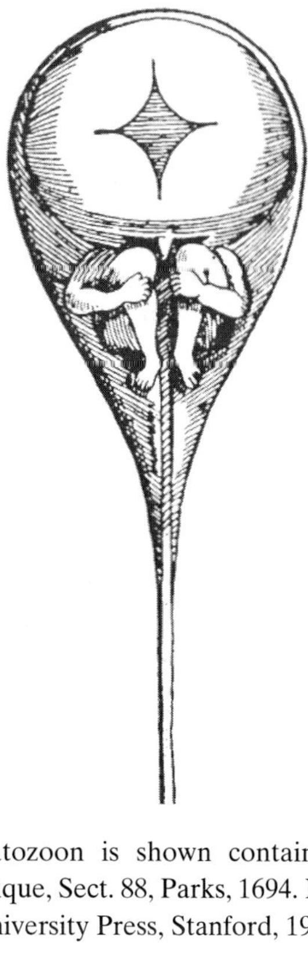

Fig. 1. A human spermatozoon is shown containing a homunculus. (From Hartsoeker. Essai de Dioptrique, Sect. 88, Parks, 1694. In: Meyer AW (ed.) *The Rise of Embryology*. Stanford University Press, Stanford, 1939.)

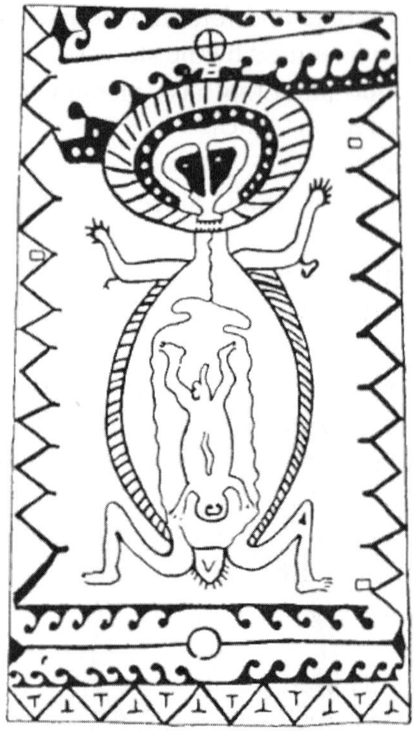

Fig. 2. A fetus is displayed on a painted and carved door from Dutch New Guinea. (From deClercq FSA and Schmelz JDE. Ethographische Beschrijving van de Westen Noordkust van Nederlansch, New Guinea. In: Needham J (ed.) *A History of Embryology*. Abelard–Schuman, New York, 1959, pp. 19).

century. Andreas Vesalius must be credited with the first truly analytic observations on the living mammalian fetus. At the time when Galen's dogmatism reigned and before the circulation of blood was discovered, Vesalius described in "*De Humani Corporis Fabrica*" (1543) the anatomy of the fetoplacental unit and the experimental preparation on which observations were based:

> "Quite pleasing is it, in the management of the fetus, to see how, when the fetus touches the surrounding air, it tries to breathe. And this dissection is performed opportunely in a dog or a pig when the sow will soon be ready to drop her young...the naked

> fetus attempts and struggles for respiration and thereupon, when the coverings are punctured and broken, thou shalt see that when the fetus breathes that pulsations of the arteries of the fetal membranes and the umbilicus stop. Up to this moment, the arteries of the uterus are beating in unison with the rest of the arteries outside of itself".

This remarkable description based on direct observation of a dissected living fetus, marked the beginning of scientific fetal observation.

It was not until the 19th century that experimental animal preparations were used to make physiologic observations on the living mammalian fetus. Bichat in 1803 was the first to study fetal movements. Zuntz (1877) and later Preyer (1885) studied intact fetal guinea pigs suspended in warm saline. They noted that the fetus must be kept in warm physiologic salt solution and that a fetus, once allowed to breathe, could not be returned to its mother and survive.

Experimental fetal observation blossomed in the 20th century, at first reluctantly, and then with a crescendo of enthusiasm. By 1920, the first successful fetal operations had been performed: Mayer removed guinea pig fetuses from the uterus and placed them in the maternal abdominal cavity — a few guinea pigs survived for several days. Graham Brown studied fetal movements in the cat, and Lane in the rat. In the 1920s, Swenson demonstrated the first experimental *in utero* manipulation, and Nicholas established the possibility of normal delivery after *in utero* surgery.

In the 1930's and 1940's, experimental fetal observation gained momentum. Barcroft introduced the most productive fetal experimental model when he described operations on the lamb fetus using spinal anesthesia. Surgery was performed through a small uterine incision, without removing the fetus. Hall's work on development of the nervous system in the fetal rat and Barron's work on neurologic development in the fetal lamb extended the techniques for fetal surgery, including the use of purse string sutures to avoid the loss of amniotic fluid.[2]

Experimental fetal intervention to study fetal malformations. The first major dividend from experimental fetal manipulation came when Jost demonstrated that removal of the fetal rabbit testes had a profound influence on subsequent sexual development.[3] In the 1950's, Louw and Barnard produced intestinal atresia, similar to that seen in human neonates, by interrupting the mesenteric blood supply in fetal puppies.[4] This contribution was important, although it was less glamorous than Barnard's later work with cardiac transplantation, because it not only established the ischemic pathogenesis of neonatal intestinal atresia, but also demonstrated the feasibility of simulating human birth defects by appropriate fetal manipulation.

In the 1960's and 1970's, experimental fetal surgery was used to simulate a variety of human congenital anomalies: coarctation of the aorta in the puppy,[5] intestinal atresia in the rabbit,[6] congenital diaphragmatic hernia in the lamb,[7] congenital hydronephrosis in the rabbit[8] and lamb,[9] and congenital heart disease in the lamb.[10] Perhaps more important, the development of a chronically catheterized fetal lamb preparation led to intensive investigation of fetal cardiovascular, pulmonary, and renal physiology.[10,11] Experimental fetal surgery proved to be more difficult in the primate, where uterine contractility and preterm labor were more difficult to control. However, in the last two decades, advances in surgical and anesthetic techniques and in the pharmacologic control of labor have made experimental manipulation of even the primate fetus feasible (Fig. 3).[12]

By the late 1970's, a variety of experimental fetal models were used widely to study both normal developmental physiology and the pathophysiology of several congenital defects. These models proved to be both descriptive and predictive. For example, removal of a piece of diaphragm not only produced a lesion that mimicked the human analog (congenital diaphragmatic hernia), but also produced the associated developmental consequence (i.e. pulmonary hypoplasia).

Once the pathophysiology of certain congenital anomalies has been clarified, these models may be used to explore treatment.

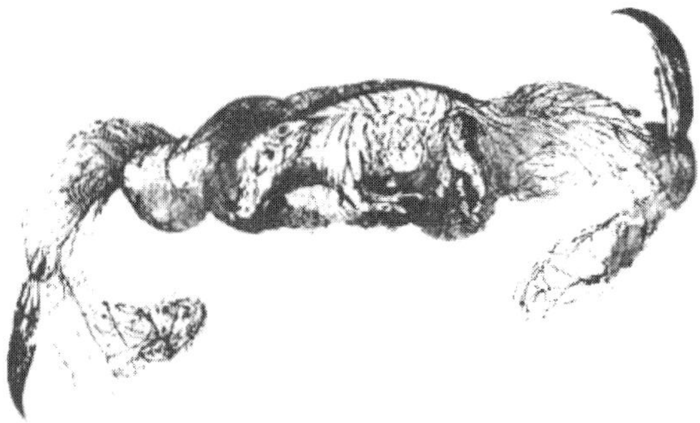

Fig. 3. Dissection of the living mammalian fetus marks the beginning of scientific fetal observation. (From Adelmann HB [trans.]. The Embryological Treatises of Hieronymus Fabricius of Aquapendente. 2; The formed fetus. Copyright 1942 by Cornell University. Used by permission of the publisher, Cornell University Press.)

For instance, the fetal lamb model of congenital diaphragmatic hernia has been used very successfully to explore various types of fetal intervention aimed at reversing pulmonary hypoplasia: total repair *in utero*, maternal steroid treatment, and more recently tracheal occlusion.[13] Now that fetal malformations like diaphragmatic hernia can be detected prenatally, fetal experiments designed to explore the pathophysiology of correctable congenital anomalies assumes some practical clinical significance. Our ability to detect malformations clinically and our ability to study them experimentally raises the questions of what medical treatments can be applied to ameliorate these abnormalities.

The fetus demystified. The fetus could not be considered a patient until it was demystified — until the origin and development of the fetus from embryo to neonate could be explained scientifically. It is only with the development of molecular biology in the last century that we have been able to bridge the conceptual gap between the seed and the full developed and marvelously complex human infant, between subcellular events like DNA-directed enzyme synthesis and subsequent complex biologic functions like the digestion of food.

Modern molecular biology provided the conceptual framework for linking the seed to the infant: the seed contains a microscopic blueprint encoded for DNA for the future individual. We can now be confident that there is an explicable order in the differentiation of the seed into the individual, even if we do not know exactly how the microscopic blueprint is acted out in the orchestrated ballet of fetal development.

Although molecular biology provided a conceptual framework that demystified fetal development, the fetus could not be a patient until his or her ailments could be diagnosed. The ability to diagnose fetal disorders evolved slowly. Fetal activity felt by the mother or palpated by her physician was the first crude measure of fetal well-being. Then the fetal heartbeat, detected at first by auscultation and later by sophisticated electronic monitors, was found to reflect fetal stress and distress. Later, minute amounts of gestational hormones were detected in maternal blood and urine. These levels correlated with the condition of the fetus. Then came amniocentesis: analysis of the constituents of amniotic fluid made possible the prenatal diagnosis of many inherited metabolic and chromosomal disorders and permitted assessment of fetal pulmonary maturity and the severity of fetal hemolytic reactions.

But the development that had the most profound effect on our approach to the fetus was the introduction of a safe, non-invasive imaging technique that permitted direct visualization of the living fetus. X-rays were recognized as being potentially harmful to the developing organism. Plain X-rays yielded little information, and introduction of radiopaque materials into the amniotic fluid (amniogram) increased the risk of premature rupture of the membranes or preterm labor without yielding much more diagnostic information. Sonography was then developed. This technique enabled accurate delineation of normal and abnormal fetal anatomy with considerable detail and later on "live" moving pictures. Unlike previous techniques, ultrasonic imaging appears to have no harmful effect on the mother or on the fetus.

The sonographic voyeur, spying on the unwary fetus, finds that he or she is surprisingly active and does not at all resemble the passive parasite that we had imagined. The sonographer sees the fetus kicking and rolling, breathing in peculiar cyclical bursts, swallowing enormous quantities of amniotic fluid, and emptying its bladder. The sonographer can even see the rhythmic motion of the heart and its valves. Fetal parts can be measured to assess fetal growth, and an increasing number of anatomic malformations can be accurately delineated. Sonography can be used to guide needle punctures of the amniotic cavity for amniocentesis, or needle aspiration of fetal urine, ascites, and cerebrospinal fluid.

Real-time sonography can guide the safe acquisition of fetal blood and other fetal tissues (e.g. skin, liver, muscle). Such samples enable the diagnosis of fetal hematologic disorders and enzymatic defects that cannot be detected by amniocentesis alone. In addition, the newest non-invasive imaging technique, nuclear magnetic resonance, promises not only definition of fetal anatomy but actual chemical definition of fetal tissue without being invasive.

Early attempts to treat fetal disease. Although we are only now beginning to attempt fetal treatment, the idea is not new. Hydrops fetalis, associated with maternal Rh sensitization, was the first fetal disorder to be treated successfully. In the early 1960s, treatment of the neonate with severe hydrops fetalis was so discouraging that Liley attempted to transfuse the fetus *in utero*. He demonstrated that intraabdominal infusion of blood ameliorated severe hydrops, thus inaugurating fetal intervention.[14]

A little-known side to this story marked a rather inauspicious start for more invasive fetal treatment. A logical refinement in the treatment of the erythroblastotic fetus was complete exchange transfusion. This required direct access to the fetal circulation, which prompted the first in utero fetal operations. In the early 1960's, obstetricians in New York and Puerto Rico exposed several fetuses through uterine incisions to cannulate femoral and jugular vessels for exchange transfusion. The overall experience was apparently discouraging. Reports are sketchy and this approach was quickly abandoned and lay dormant for the next decade. Surgical exposure of the living fetus would have to await development of better anesthetic agents and surgical techniques, but this initial experience at least raised the possibility of fetal surgery.[15]

The next fetal disease to be approached therapeutically was the devastating respiratory distress syndrome of prematurity. Through a combination of clinical experience with severely premature infants and laboratory experiments using fetal lamb and rabbit preparations, surfactant deficiency was established as being the physiologic basis for respiratory distress syndrome. Effective treatment could then be devised. Glucocorticoids administered to the fetus via the mother increase fetal surfactant production, hasten fetal lung maturation, and ameliorate the respiratory distress syndrome. Glucocorticoid therapy to induce fetal lung maturation, combined with improved methods of respiratory support for tiny premature infants, has greatly reduced the mortality caused by this condition.

It is now apparent that there are other fetal disorders that not only can be diagnosed *in utero*, but also can be treated by prenatal administration of appropriate medications or hormones. The severe developmental consequences of congenital hypothyroidism, for example, might be prevented by giving thyroid hormone to the fetus. Furthermore, certain other fetal deficiencies can be treated by providing blood cells, hormones, or medications.

By the 1980's, we were ready to take the next step, which is the correction of fetal anatomic defects. Although many fetal anatomic malformations can be detected by sonography, only selected cases warrant consideration for intrauterine therapy because only a few have a compelling physiologic rationale for prenatal correction. Congenital hydronephrosis, diaphragmatic hernia, and obstructive hydrocephalus are examples of malformations in which a simple anatomic lesion interferes with organ development and, if the anatomic defect is corrected, fetal development may proceed normally. The physiologic rationale for in utero correction of these lesions was defined, and the feasibility of *in utero* correction was established.[16,17]

How the fetus became a patient in our lifetime. It is important to recognize that it is only during our professional lifetime, and really only in the last decades of this century, that the fetus has become a patient. We now know that the fetus has disorders that can be diagnosed and treated, and how society can now accept the fetus as an unborn patient. How did such a remarkable shift in attitude toward the fetus occur in such a short time?

The impetus for fetal treatment came from two fields of endeavor that developed rapidly during the last two decades. Neonatologists and surgeons traced the pathogenesis of the problems they treated after birth back to the fetus, and obstetricians, geneticists, and sonologists developed the ability to accurately diagnose human fetal disease.

Clinical frustration provided the impetus for unraveling the pathophysiology on neonatal malformations, such as congenital diaphragmatic hernia, hydronephrosis, and hydrocephalus. Pediatric surgeons and neonatologists were frustrated by caring for newborn babies with problems that were discovered "too late to correct." This is the same frustration that all physicians feel when they discover a disease process that has already gone too far, whether it is a cancer that has already metastasized or the ulcer that has perforated. The same frustration makes all healers say, "If only we had been here a little earlier, we might have changed the course of that disease." When physicians responsible for neonates who died with a diaphragmatic hernia or hydronephrosis realized that the disease process was already at the final stage of birth, they began to ask whether the course of the disease might be changed if something could be done earlier. Both diagnosis and treatment would have to be before birth. The questions then became, "Can the lesion be diagnosed before birth, will intervention have the desired effect, and can it be done?" Thus, clinical frustration in dealing with uncorrectable neonatal diseases led to the experimental studies in which a model of the human disease was created in fetal animals to study the pathophysiology of the process, to test whether the damage seen at birth was irreversible if corrected before birth, and to establish the feasibility and safety of in utero intervention.

While "baby doctors", like pediatric surgeons, were exploring certain life-threatening neonatal problems that might lend themselves to correction before birth, obstetricians, geneticists, and sonographers were developing the techniques of prenatal diagnosis and were finding fetuses with similar defects. Although prenatal diagnosis by amniocentesis was aimed initially at potentially fatal fetal diseases, the development of sophisticated new imaging techniques allowed accurate delineation of other anomalies that were often found serendipitously during ultrasonography performed for obstetrical indications.

Thus, physicians primarily concerned with management of the mother and fetus through pregnancy (e.g., perinatologists, geneticists, obstetrical sonologists) could detect fetal lesions, such as hydronephrosis and hydrocephalus, and they could begin to wonder what they could for the fetus and how they could best manage this pregnancy. Physicians interested in all phases of fetoneonatal development began sharing information and ideas about how the fetal condition might determine the place, timing, and mode of delivery. Detection of fetal defects also led to serial sonographic studies that defined the naturally history and pathophysiology of an increasing number of human fetal diseases, including hydronephrosis, diaphragmatic hernia, hydrocephalus, and non-immune hydrops. Fetal medicine was established.

Thus, the impetus provided by the neonate who had an uncorrectable disorder at birth and the fetus who had a birth defect detected before birth led to the realization that many fetal diseases may require medical management before birth. Although neither impetus was sufficient in itself to justify fetal intervention, together they spurred the necessary clinical and experimental studies that would lead to successful fetal treatment. When the baby's physician and the mother's physician together began to define the naturally history of the disease by serial sonographic examination of untreated human fetuses and to study the pathophysiology and feasibility of fetal intervention in experimental animal models, the stage was set for a full consideration of the fetus as a patient. Fetal treatment is the flowering of more than a decade of clinical and experimental work in prenatal diagnosis and feto-neonatal physiology by physicians of diverse specialties and backgrounds (Fig. 4).

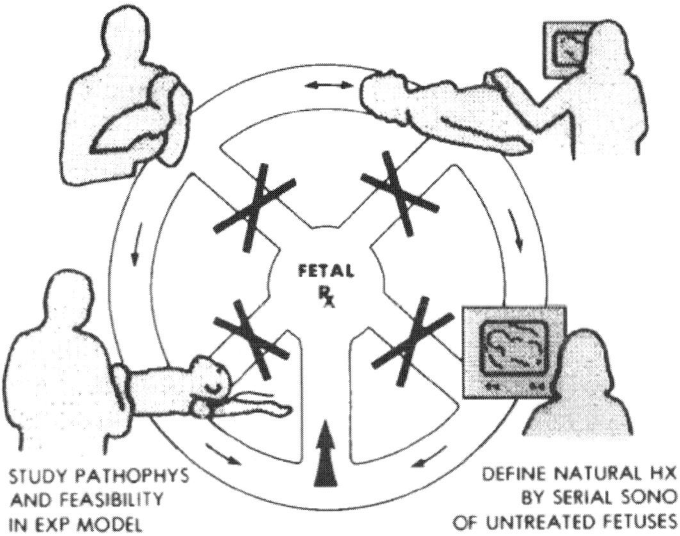

Fig. 4. The impetus of fetal treatment came from pediatricians and surgeons who were frustrated by diseases that were already uncorrectable at birth and from obstetricians and sonographers who were seeing fetuses with potentially correctable defects before birth. However, before fetal treatment could be implemented, the pathophysiology of the disorder and the feasibility of repair had to be established experimentally, and the natural history of the disease in the untreated human fetus had to be defined by serial sonography.

The maturation of fetal therapy. New technologies usually start in a single, highly committed center, and initially remain confined to a relatively small number of centers with the interest, expertise, and resources to achieve reasonable results. This was fetal therapy in the 1980's. In this phase, registries are often useful. Such was the case for the initial registries sponsored by the International Fetal Medicine and Surgery Society (IFMSS) for cases of hydronephrosis and hydrocephalus treated with shunts. But as technologies like fetal treatment diffuse out to less experienced centers, the value of multicenter registries decreases. Such proved to be the case for attempted registries for fetal metabolic diseases and cardiac arrhythmias.

In the 1990's, it became clear that for fetal therapy to progress it would be necessary to determine the efficacy of intervention through properly controlled clinical trials. But they have proven incredibly difficult to execute. Two multicenter trials comparing vaginal to cesarean delivery for gastroschisis have not succeeded despite considerable effort. Single-center trials are much easier logistically. The first successful controlled trial compared open fetal surgical repair of diaphragmatic hernia to optimal post-natal care. It was successfully completed despite incredible logistical and bureaucratic challenges. This trial provided a definitive answer to a difficult question, and prevented further attempts at total repair of diaphragmatic hernias in fetuses without liver herniation. By stopping open fetal surgical repair, it directly spurred development of a new approach to reversing pulmonary hypoplasia by temporary tracheal occlusion. Subsequently, temporary tracheal occlusion was tested in the second successful randomized controlled clinical trial. The results of this trial led to further refinements in the technique and a successful non-randomized trial in Europe by the Eurofetus group. This group also performed a non-randomized but very informative trial comparing laser ablation to amnioreduction for twin-twin transfusion syndrome. The success of the Eurofetus group has inspired formation of the North American Fetal Therapy Network (NAFTNet) to further multi-institutional trials in the U.S. and Canada. The latest and most ambitious trial is the Management of Myelomeningocele Study (MOMS) comparing prenatal to postnatal repair of myelomeningocele. This trial is ongoing at this time.

We can find and define many birth defects *in utero*. As diagnostic abilities improve, so also does our ability to select for treatment only fetuses who will benefit from intervention. We must refine our ability to measure fetal organ function so that we do not have to make important clinical decisions based on morphologic criteria alone. Treatment of several fetal disorders has proved to be feasible, but a great deal of clinical and laboratory expertise will be required to determine which procedures are safe and effective. Treatment of more complicated congenital anomalies will expand as techniques for fetal intervention improve. However, this progress will require a great deal of work, both experimental and clinical.

The short but eventful history of the fetus as a patient reassures us that fetal treatment offers new hope for the fetus with a correctable defect, and reminds us that there is considerable potential for doing harm. We know that innovative fetal treatment must be fully tested in the laboratory, carefully considered in the light of current diagnostic and therapeutic uncertainties, honestly presented to the prospective parents, and finally undertaken only with trepidation. It is now clear that because a procedure can be done does not mean that it should be done and that a fetal abnormality of any type should never be treated simply "because it is there," and never by someone who is unprepared for this fearsome responsibility. In the early harrowing days of fetal treatment, no one could be sure whether the enterprise would succeed or die. We can now be confident that the enterprise itself has succeeded as reflected in the robustness of professional societies like the IFMSS, the Fetus as a Patient Society, the Eurofetus group, and the North American Fetal Therapy Network, and the proliferation of professional journals like "*Fetal Diagnosis and Therapy*" and "*Ultrasound in Obstetrics and Gynecology*", and of textbooks like "*The Unborn Patient: Prenatal Diagnosis and Therapy*" (now in its third edition), "*Ultrasound in Obstetrics and Gynecology*", "*Maternal and Fetal Medicine*", "*Fetal Therapy*", and "*Intensive Care of the Fetus and Newborn*". As the number of professionals devoted to fetal treatment increase, and the number and quality of fetal treatment teams and centers around the world continues to grow, the banner for fetal Surgery in the 21st century should read "Proceed with Caution...and Enthusiasm."

PART II: Personal Perspective: The UCSF Fetal Treatment Center

The field of fetal surgery is too young (<30 years), too varied (open surgery, fetoscopic surgery, image-guided surgery, etc.) and too multicultural (obstetricians, pediatricians, surgeons, etc.) to have a coherent history. That will come with the perspective of time. So rather than try to objectively ascribe credit (and blame) to individuals and institutions around the world, I will instead describe the microcosm of my own institution and its role in the development of fetal surgery.

Making a coherent story out of the long, tortuous, and often tumultuous history of fetal therapy at the University of California, San Francisco (UCSF) has proven a daunting task. For lack of a better organizing principle, I have decided to encapsulate the relevant factual material (dates, names, procedures, etc.) in a few tables that provide a quick overview of the San Francisco experience. I will reserve the running text for my personal, less objective, and perhaps more controversial perspective.

Why San Francisco? A fault zone becomes an epicenter. I came to UCSF straight from pediatric surgery fellowship in January 1978 because I thought it offered at that time the best opportunity of any place in the world to develop fetal surgery. I had been nourishing a crazy idea about fixing surgical defects before birth since the first month of surgical internship at the Massachusetts General Hospital nine years earlier. In July 1969, as a green and naïve surgical intern, I assisted Dr Hardy Hendren repair a newborn baby with congenital diaphragmatic hernia who subsequently died. I was so green and naïve that it seemed obvious to me that the baby died because the lung was too small, and the lung was too small because it was not able to grow adequately before birth, and that the only way to save the baby after birth was to fix the anatomic defect before birth. In that first month of internship, I wrote a short protocol for an animal experiment that would test this hypothesis by creating and repairing diaphragmatic hernias in fetal dogs (most surgical research was done in dogs in those days). I never got to do the experiment, but held on to the idea through seven years of surgical training and two wonderfully productive years of research at the Laboratory of Immunology at NIH, where I became fascinated by fetal immunology and the problem of why the mother doesn't reject the foreign fetus, a problem which remains unsolved to this day. I also had a brief six-month interlude of pediatric surgery training in Oslo, Norway, where my determination to pursue fetal intervention was reinforced by studying the mortality of congenital diaphragmatic hernia in a medical care system that allowed me to document that many babies with diaphragmatic hernia died before they ever reached the tertiary center, a phenomenon I dubbed the "The hidden mortality." This work suggested that the natural history of a disease discovered before birth may not be the same as when the same problem is studied after birth simply because the most severe cases do not survive to be studied. This phenomenon turned out to apply to many fetal diseases (e.g., cystic hygroma).

With these embryonic concepts about fetal treatment bubbling in my head, I was thrilled to learn about the exciting work in fetal physiology going on at UC San Francisco using the fetal lamb model. A trio of brilliant pediatric cardiologists (Drs Abraham Rudolph, Michael Heymann, and Julian Hoffman) and their colleagues at UCSF and the Cardiovascular Research Institute (CVRI) were using the fetal lamb model to unravel developmental cardiovascular physiology. All three were expatriates from tumultuous South Africa. Al deLorimier, the first and, at that time, only UCSF pediatric surgeon, had used their fetal lamb model to study the physiologic consequence of a surgically created diaphragmatic defect. I took the job in San Francisco (my first and only faculty position) specifically because I thought I could tap into this exciting experimental animal research and the techniques and science behind it to see whether fetal intervention made physiologic sense (i.e., would correcting a defect have the desired effect) and to develop the techniques that would make fetal surgery safe and feasible. This proved to be the case.

Experimental models: Physiology in lambs, feasibility in monkeys. Within months of arriving in January 1978, I was able to commandeer an excellent technician, Judith Jester, who had experience in the fetal lamb model in the CVRI. We embarked on a series of experiments creating and correcting diaphragmatic hernia, then urinary tract obstruction, and then hydrocephalus — the first three in a long series of diseases which I thought might be fixable in human fetuses. In each case, we simulated the disease by surgical intervention, studied the consequences of the intervention on development of the target organ system, then corrected the lesion and studied the developmental consequences of correction. This pattern of investigation formed the basis of the fetal intervention enterprise for the next two decades and helped establish the fetal lamb model as the most widely used and widely accepted method of testing the physiologic rationale for fetal intervention in a host of diseases.

But the fetal lamb model had one grave deficiency, it was simply too easy to get away with fetal intervention in the lamb because (as we used to say) the sheep uterus was too dumb to contract in response to an insult like an incision or trocar. This property made it ideal for testing fetal pathophysiology, but completely inadequate for testing the safety of intervention for both mother and fetus and for developing techniques that would allow access to the fetus without precipitating preterm labor. We decided early on that success in the fetal lamb model would not be enough to justify human intervention; instead we would have to prove that a proposed procedure was safe for mother and fetus in the nonhuman primate model before we could offer it clinically. For that reason, we went right on to fetal surgery experiments in rhesus monkeys first at UCSF and then at the Primate Colony at the University of California, Davis, where we could follow the operated mothers for years and study the effect of intervention on fertility and reproductive potential. Availability of the facilities both at UCSF and at Davis for sheep and monkey work played a crucial role in the development of fetal surgery. To get a feel for the magnitude of this enterprise and its role in launching fetal surgery, in the 1980's we operated on more than 2000 fetal lambs and 500 fetal monkeys. A very considerable part of the effort and cost of launching fetal surgery was the many millions of dollars invested in this research, all of which had to be raised through almost continuous (and painful) grant writing.

However, the most important element in launching the enterprise of fetal surgery in the 1980's was the investment of talent and time by a small group of bright, ambitious, and resourceful research fellows. The effort expended was prodigious. For example, every procedure done in Davis required a full day, including several hours to commute back and forth, many hours to arrange the veterinary aspects of the intervention as well as the hours devoted to the surgery itself, and the many, many hours devoted to follow-up of the animals. The bottom line: clinical fetal surgery was made possible by a huge volume of translational research done in our laboratory by the Fetal Treatment Center research fellows. The fellows provided an indispensable pool of talent, enthusiasm, and good humor. Needless to say, they contributed a fabulous amount of hard work in doing the experiments, writing them up, and presenting the results at meetings. They have made immense contributions to the field over many years. Many of them have gone on to successful careers for which I am immensely proud. There is no way to recognize all the talents and personalities in this short piece other than to provide a table of the fellows with a chronological listing of their time in the lab and their projects. On a personal note, I view the people listed in Table 1 as my most important (and certainly most enjoyable) contribution to the enterprise of fetal surgery.

A serendipitous clinical coalition. It was obvious from the beginning that this enterprise could never get off the ground unless a few clinicians from widely disparate backgrounds and specialties learned to work closely together in ways that had really not been achieved previously. The development of fetal surgery at UCSF was largely due to a happy coincidence: a very talented and brilliant obstetrician/geneticist, Dr Mitchell Golbus, an exceedingly skilful, thoughtful, and personable sonographer/radiologist, Dr Roy Filly, and a pediatric surgeon, myself, managed to hit it off. We were all relatively young junior faculty who were still naïve enough to think that we could do something that had not yet been seriously attempted. We played off each other. Mickey was seeing a growing number of fetal anomalies in his prenatal diagnosis clinic and his AFP screening and genetic counselling program. Roy Filly, with his delightful colleagues, Peter Callen and Ruth Goldstein, were establishing the premier fetal ultrasound unit and describing the natural history of a wide variety of fetal malformations. And I was constantly bugging everyone about the possibility of fixing some of these

Table 1. The UCSF fetal treatment center research fellows.

Fellow	Dates	Primary Projects	Where Are They Now?
Donald K Nakayama	1981–82	Correction of congenital hydronephrosis *in utero* Management of the fetus with an abdominal wall defect Correction of congenital hydrocephalus *in utero* Fetal surgery in the primate	Professor and Chief of Pediatric Surgery University of North Carolina Chapel Hill
Philip L Glick	1982–84	Correction of congenital hydronephrosis *in utero* Correction of congenital hydrocephalus *in utero* Fetal cardiac surgery: Surface cooling & rewarming of the fetus Correction of CDH *in utero*	Professor of Surgery Children's Hospital of Buffalo
Thomas M Krummel	1983–84	Correction of congenital hydronephrosis *in utero* Correction of congenital hydrocephalus *in utero* Fetal cardiac surgery: Surface cooling & rewarming of the fetus Correction of CDH *in utero*	Professor and Chair of Surgery Stanford University Medical Center
N Scott Adzick	1983–85	Fetal cardiac surgery: Surface cooling & rewarming of the fetus Use of uterine stapling device for fetal surgery Fetal wound healing Fetal CCAM/*in utero* pneumonectomy Correction of CDH	Professor and Surgeon-in-Chief Children's Hospital of Philadelphia

(*Continued*)

Table 1. *(Continued)*

Fellow	Dates	Primary Projects	Where Are They Now?
		Development of a fetal renal function test Correction of fetal urinary tract obstruction Maternal outcome after fetal surgery	
Alan W Flake	1984–86	*In utero* stem cell transplantation Transamniotic fetal feeding Auxiliary transplantation of the fetal liver Resection of fetal teratomas	Professor of Surgery The Children's Hospital of Philadelphia
Sheldon J Bond	1985–87	Intervention for obstructive uropathy Resection of fetal teratomas Use of absorbable stapling device for hysterotomy & C-section	Associate Professor of Surgery Kosair Children's Hospital, Louisville
Loie Sauer	1986–87	Compensatory renal growth following fetal nephrectomy Neonatal model of heterotopic heart transplantation in swine	Redwood Empire Surgical Group
Asteria Albert	1987	Intervention for obstructive uropathy Use of absorbable stapling device for hysterotomy & C-section	Associate Professor of Pediatric Surgery Hospital Sant Joan de Deu
Timothy M Crombleholme	1987–89	Fetal intervention for obstructive uropathy: Early clinical experience and prognostic indicators *In utero* hematopoietic stem cell transplantation Reduced size lung transplantation in neonatal swine	Professor of Surgery Children's Hospital of Cincinnati

(Continued)

Table 1. (*Continued*)

Fellow	Dates	Primary Projects	Where Are They Now?
Michael T Longaker	1987–91	Fetal wound and fracture healing *In utero* creation and repair of fetal cleft lip and palate Maternal outcome after fetal surgery	Professor of Surgery Director of Children's Surgical Research Stanford University Medical Center
Jacob C Langer	1987–89	Prenatal treatment for gastroschisis & abdominal wall defects Cystic hygroma	Professor and Chief of Surgery Hospital for Sick Children
Russell W Jennings	1989–92	Nitric oxide inhibition of preterm labor Development of fetal radiotelemetry monitoring device Neonatal lung transplantation Fetal wound and fracture healing Fetal intraosseous access for fetal circulation access	Associate Professor of Surgery Children's Hospital
David J Whitby	1990–91	Fetal wound healing *In utero* creation/repair of fetal cleft lip and palate	Consultant in Plastic Surgery Booth Hall Children's Hospital
Colin Ia Bethel	1990–93	*In utero* stem cell transplantation	Chief of Pediatric Surgery New Jersey Medical School Doctor's Office Center
H Peter Lorenz	1990–93	Fetal wound healing *In utero* creation/repair of fetal cleft lip and palate	Associate Professor of Surgery Plastic and Reconstructive Surgery Stanford University Medical Center

(*Continued*)

Table 1. (*Continued*)

Fellow	Dates	Primary Projects	Where Are They Now?
James E Estes	1990–92	Development of endoscopic fetal surgery techniques Chronic fetal vascular access Fetal wound healing Fetal A-V pacing for complete heart block	Assistant Professor of Surgery Division of Vascular surgery Tufts-New England Medical Center
Brian W Duncan	1988–91	*In utero* stem cell transplantation, including collection and banking of human fetal HSC *In utero* creation and repair of craniosynostosis	Assistant Professor of Surgery Division of Pediatric CT Surgery Cleveland Clinic Foundation
Henry E Rice	1991–94	*In utero* stem cell transplantation, including collection and banking of human fetal HSC Chronic fetal vascular access	Assistant Professor of Surgery Division of Pediatric Surgery Duke University Medical Center
Marc H Hedrick	1991–93	Perinatal intervention for congenital high airway obstruction Fetal temporary tracheal occlusion for severe CDH Chronic fetal vascular access	Chief Scientific Officers & Medical Director MicroPore Biosurgery, Inc.
Thomas E Macgillivray	1991–93	Fetoscopic surgical techniques Chronic fetal vascular access Vascular changes with *in utero* correction of CDH Management of fetal lung lesions	Assistant Professor of Surgery Division of Cardiothoracic Surgery Massachusetts General Hospital
Eileen Natuzzi	1991–94	Nitric oxide synthase activity and preterm labor	Vascular Surgery Private Practice
Marcelo Martinez-Ferro	1992–93	Perinatal intervention for congenital high airway obstruction	Pediatric Surgeon Nat'l Pediatric Hospital "JP Garrahan"

(*Continued*)

Table 1. (*Continued*)

Fellow	Dates	Primary Projects	Where Are They Now?
Kerry M Sullivan	1992–94	Fetal wound healing Fetal temporary tracheal occlusion for severe CDH Creation and repair of myelomeningocele in fetal sheep	Pediatric Surgery Attending Kaiser Permanente Medical Center
Andrea P Metkus	1993–94	Treatment of CDH cost analysis Sonographic predictors of survival for CDH	Gen. & Vascular Surgery Private Practice
Erik D Skarsgard	1993–94	Fetal endoscopic surgery Fetoplacental circulation	Assoc Prof and Chief of Pediatric Surgery Children & Women's Hospital of BC
Martin Meuli & Claudia Meuli-Simmen	1993–95	Creation and repair of myelomeningocele in fetal sheep Fetal wound healing	Pediatric Surgeon & Neurosurgeon University Children's Hospital Zurich Switzerland
John F Bealer	1993–95	Fetal endoscopic tracheal occlusion for severe CDH	Pediatric Surgeon Rocky Mountain Associates University of Colorada
Mark A Stringer	1994–95	Correction of CDH *in utero* Prenatal diagnosis of esophageal atresia	Consultant in Pediatrics (Pedi Surgeon) St. James University Hospital Leeds. United Kingdom
Steven W Bruch	1994–95	Treatment of prenatally-diagnosed genetic disease using cationic liposomes Prenatal treatment of pericardial teratomas	Clinical Assistant Professor of Surgery, Division of Pediatric Surgery, University of Michigan, CS Mott Children's Hospital

(*Continued*)

Table 1. *(Continued)*

Fellow	Dates	Primary Projects	Where Are They Now?
David L Gibbs	1994–96	Fetal endoscopic tracheal occlusion for severe CDH Long-term neurodevelopmental outcome after fetal surgery	
Eric J Stelnicki	1994–96	Role of homeobox genes in fetal wound healing *In utero* creation and repair of fetal cleft lip and palate *In utero* creation and repair of craniosynostosis	Plastic and Reconstructive Surgery Joe DiMaggio Children's Hospital Craniofacial Center
Karen J Vanderwall	1993–96	Fetal endoscopic tracheal occlusion for severe CDH	
Kelli M Bullard	1994–97	Fetal wound healing Clinical trial of fetal surgery for severe CDH	Assistant Professor of Surgery, Division of Colorectal Surgery University of Michigan
George B Mychaliska	1994–97	*In utero* hematopoietic stem cell and hepatocyte transplantation Banking of fetal liver hematopoietic stem cells EXIT procedure	Assistant Professor of Surgery, St Louis Children's Hospital
Darrell L Cass	1994–97	Fetal wound healing	Assistant Professor of Surgery Division of Pediatric Surgery Baylor College of Medicine
Joy Graf	1994–97	EXIT procedure Nitroglycerin and necrotizing enterocolitis	Assistant Professor of Surgery Perinatal & Pain Management Div UC Davis Medical Center
Richard Beech	1996–98	Fetal endoscopic tracheal occlusion for severe CDH	

(Continued)

Table 1. (*Continued*)

Fellow	Dates	Primary Projects	Where Are They Now?
Koshi Asabe	1998–99	Fetoscopic tracheal occlusion for severe CDH	Pediatric Surgery Faculty Fukuoka Children's Hospital Fukuoka Japan
Francois Golfier	1996–97	*In utero* hematopoietic stem cell transplantation for treatment of genetic diseases	
H Tamiko Housley	1996–97	Creation and repair of myelomeningocele in fetal sheep & rabbit models Treatment of obstructive uropathy *in utero*	Private Practice — Urology Reno Nevada
Gerald Lipshutz	1996–98	Fetal gene transfer by transuterine injection of cationic liposomes	Transplant Fellow University of California, San Francisco
Corbett Wilkinson	1997–98	Repair of myelomeningocele *in utero*	
John B Lopoo	1997–99	Fetal endoscopic tracheal occlusion for severe CDH *In utero* repair of fetal cleft lip and palate	Pediatric Surgery Fellow Northwestern University Medical Center Children's Memorial Hospital
Tatsuo Ohkubo	1997–00	High-efficiency retroviral transduction of fetal liver CD38-CD++ cells for *in utero* and ex utero gene therapy	Pediatric Surgery Faculty Jikei University School of Medicine Tokyo Japan
Toshio Chiba	1997–00	Fetal endoscopic tracheal occlusion for severe CDH	Pediatric Surgery Faculty Nat'l Children's Medical Research Center Sendai, Japan

(*Continued*)

Table 1. (*Continued*)

Fellow	Dates	Primary Projects	Where Are They Now?
Bettina Westerburg-Paek	1997–00	High frequency ablation of fetal tumors Repair of fetal myelomeningocele *in utero* Chronic fetal vascular access	Resident Department of Obstetrics and Gynecology University of Washington, Seattle
Seok Joo Han	1999–00	*In utero* surgical intervention for fetal anomalies	Pediatric Surgery Faculty Yonsei Univ College of Medicine Seoul Korea
Alfredo Acosta	1999–00	*In utero* surgical intervention for fetal anomalies	Pediatric Surgery Faculty University of Manila, The Philippines
Krishna Granholm	1999–00	*In utero* hematopoietic stem cell transplantation for treatment of genetic diseases Fetal endoscopic tracheal occlusion for severe CDH	Chief of Pediatric Surgery Karolinska Institute Stockholm, Sweden
Crystine Lee	1999–01	*In utero* hepatocyte transplantation	General Surgery Resident University of California, San Francisco
Lourenco Sbragia	2000–01	Fetal lung growth including stimulation of pulmonary cell cycle progression and type I cell differentiation after tracheal occlusion	Pediatric Surgery Faculty Campinas State University Brazil
Jyoji Yoshizawa		Fetal Lung growth including stimulation of pulmonary cell cycle progression and type I cell differentiation after tracheal occlusion	Pediatric Surgery Faculty Jikei University School of Medicine Tokyo Japan
Kuojen Tsao	2000–02	Role of HOX genes in angiogenesis & liver regeneration Selective reduction by radiofrequency ablation in TTTS	General Surgery Resident University of Cincinnati

(*Continued*)

Table 1. (*Continued*)

Fellow	Dates	Primary Projects	Where Are They Now?
Roman Sydorak	2000–02	Chorionic membrane separation after fetal surgery Fetal lung growth including stimulation of pulmonary cell cycle progression and type I cell differentiation after tracheal occlusion	Pediatric Surgery Fellow University of California, Los Angeles
Jeng-Chang Chen	2000–02	*In utero* hematopoietic stem cell transplantation	Pediatric Surgery Faculty Chang Gung Children's Hospital Taiwan
Pierre-Yves Mure	2000–02	*In utero* intervention for fetal obstructive uropathy	Pediatric Surgery Faculty Debrousse University Hospital
Steven Fowler	2001–03	Role of HOX genes in angiogenesis & liver regeneration	General Surgery Resident, Cedars-Sinai Medical Center

problems and telling them about our ongoing experimental work on fetal intervention.

All this information (the clinical problems, the experimental rationale, the natural history of fetal disease) came together every week at the noon OB/Neonatology conference, which was originally set up to coordinate high-risk deliveries, but eventually became the heart and soul of the fetal treatment enterprise. I began to attend this weekly meeting as an outsider (a pediatric surgeon), and then started presenting neonatal surgical cases in order to stimulate discussion about whether a particular defect could be found and perhaps even dealt with before birth. The noon conference proved fertile ground for new ideas posed by Roy Filly's sonographic diagnoses, Mickey Golbus's screening techniques, and my experimental work. Every new clinical problem and every new proposal for management was vetted, argued, and discussed by superb neonatologists like George Gregory, Rod Phibbs, Joe Kitterman, and Sam Hawgood, and savvy perinatologists like Russ Laros and Bill Parer, as well as CVRI scientists and researchers, all of whom regularly attend this weekly noon meeting. I am convinced the fetal treatment enterprise would not have developed at UCSF and cannot develop elsewhere unless surgeons, perinatologists, sonologists, cardiologists, neonatologists, and a whole host of other folks sit down in the same room once a week and wrestle with the ongoing clinical cases. This simple mechanism of a weekly multidisciplinary meeting, like a tumor board, provides excellent clinical care, allows new ideas to be discussed and argued, and, most important, allows professionals from widely different backgrounds and temperament to work together. As the UCSF Fetal Treatment Center evolved, we kept the weekly meeting tied to the noon OB/Neonatology conference so that everyone could attend, and it remains today, 25 years later, the most interesting, informative, and stimulating meeting on everyone's agenda.

The first cases: Clinical necessity meets experimental rationale. While we continued to study a variety of fetal diseases in animal models, including diaphragmatic hernia, urinary tract obstruction, gastroschisis, hydrocephalus, intrauterine growth retardation and the possibility of feeding undernourished fetuses through the amniotic fluid (transamniotic fetal feeding), the first disease to attract serious attention as a possible target for fetal intervention was fetal hydronephrosis, specifically bladder outlet obstruction in a male with posterior urethral valves. It was one of the first and easiest diseases to detect sonographically, and we had a pretty good feel for the course of the disease before and after birth. We could prove in the laboratory and then demonstrate in human fetuses whom we followed without intervention that a severe obstruction would produce oligohydramnios, pulmonary hypoplasia and, of course, renal failure. We thought it would be the easiest disease to treat because all we had to do was decompress the bladder before birth in the same way that it was decompressed after birth, either with a catheter shunt or with a surgical opening. Our bright young surgical research fellows proved that obstruction led to pulmonary hypoplasia and renal dysplasia, which could be ameliorated by decompression before birth. We discussed many clinical cases at our weekly meeting and finally came across one that seemed appropriate for repair. The first successful fetal intervention for urinary tract obstruction was placement of a double pigtail shunt (the Harrison fetal bladder stent developed with Cook Urologic) in a procedure that taught us how to orchestrate and utilize the talents of perinatologist (Mickey Golbus), sonographer (Roy Filly), and surgeon (myself). That boy and his family continue to communicate from their home in Florida 25 years later. Almost simultaneously we did our first open fetal surgery, a desperate case with complete oligohydramnios locking the fetus in a position where the only way to decompress the completely obstructed bladder at 18 weeks' gestation was through a hysterotomy and open vesicostomy. The procedure worked, but the fetus never made urine, undoubtedly because the intervention was too late and the kidneys were already dysplastic. So both the catheter-shunt and the open surgery for urinary tract obstruction were introduced simultaneously. Fortunately, both were technical successes and demonstrated feasibility and initial safety for mothers. Of course, the techniques, the shunts, and most important the selection criteria have greatly improved through a vast amount of work initiated at

UCSF and continued very successfully around the world over the next two decades.

Meanwhile, Bill Clewell in Denver was preparing to do the first shunt for hydrocephalus. We continued studying hydrocephalus in both a sheep and monkey model, but did not pursue clinical application, focusing instead on other defects including diaphragmatic hernia.

A fledgling fetal enterprise and the founding of IFMSS: 1981–1985. With a growing number of catheter-shunts and the first open fetal surgery for obstructive uropathy at UCSF, and with the first news of catheter-shunt interventions for hydrocephalus in Denver and then in several other centers in the United States, it became clear that fetal surgery was not only off to a fast start, but a precarious and vulnerable one. After publication of these first cases attracted considerable media attention, I began to worry that the enterprise of fetal therapy had great potential for disaster, e.g., a media frenzy and meltdown similar to that which accompanied the first heart transplants.

Recognizing that this fragile enterprise could easily be destroyed by too much exposure and that the enterprise would have to be nurtured very carefully in terms of dealing with ethical issues and public perception, we at UCSF and the other early practitioners around the world made a concerted and conscious effort to band together, share information, talk about new techniques, discuss treatment, hammer out ethical guidelines, and agree on some standards for intervention. How was this accomplished?

In early 1981, I went to the Kroc Foundation (McDonald's Corporation) to ask if they would sponsor a symposium at their beautiful ranch in Santa Ynez near Santa Barbara on the California coast. They agreed to sponsor a meeting in which we could invite 24 experts from anywhere in the world (all expenses paid) for a five-day meeting in this beautiful setting. There was a frank, open, and honest discussion of every aspect of this embryonic enterprise from physiology to genetics to techniques of intervention. There was also frank discussion about and acceptance of self-imposed "rules to live by": peer-reviewed publication before media exposure, attempting intervention only for lethal diseases in which the pathophysiology and natural history were understood, and strict adherence to ethical guidelines. It was a fabulous meeting with Sir William Liley as the inspirational keynote participant, and a very multidisciplinary collection of practitioners, which has characterized the IFMSS ever since. This meeting set the style, tone, and character of future meetings of the IFMSS, famous for its open and frank discussions, its informality, its lack of structural organizational rigidity, and its wonderful ambience. It also spawned the tradition of setting up future meetings; Bill Clewell agreed to host the next one in Aspen, Colorado, where the organization was officially named, and the cycle of yearly meetings initiated. Discussion of a journal spearheaded by Maria Michejda and Kevin Pringle led, after several sessions, to the founding of the journal "*Fetal Diagnosis and Therapy*" as the official voice of the IFMSS.

Perhaps the most important precedent set at this first meeting, and reinforced in subsequent meetings of the IFMSS, was that the participants willingly shoulder the heavy responsibility for stewardship of the enterprise. At that first meeting, we created a framework for fetal intervention (e.g., requirements for undertaking fetal intervention and strictures about publishing all cases good or bad before they appear in the media), and published this framework as a consensus in the "*New England Journal of Medicine*", which set a high tone and a high standard for coming years. A registry for fetal interventions was established and later, spearheaded by Frank Manning, the early results with shunts for hydrocephalus and hydronephrosis were published, again in the "*New England Journal of Medicine*". This widely referenced document laid out much of the collective thinking, but most important, led to a voluntary moratorium on shunts for hydrocephalus that held for almost two decades, something for which the international fetal medicine community can be proud.

1985–1990: The best of times, the worst of times. Fetal therapy at UCSF was conceived and developed experimentally beginning in 1978, and came to fruition clinically in 1981. It was initially a thriving, bawling, vibrant, and rapidly growing enterprise with the exploration of many new therapies: decompression for obstructive uropathy and hydrocephalus, surgical treatment of severe sacrococcygeal teratoma and cystic adenomatoid malformation of the lung, pacing for congenital heart block, transamniotic fetal feeding (TAFF) for intrauterine growth retardation, and, perhaps most exciting, hematopoietic stem cell transplantation for a variety of diseases. There was exciting work on the technical aspects of fetal access and control of preterm labor.

In the mid-1980's, we hit some serious snags. Perhaps the most ambitious undertaking was trying to help babies with congenital diaphragmatic hernia. The initial concept was simple: total surgical repair would allow room for the lung to grow. This worked experimentally, but when first attempted in 1984, we encountered the terrible (and ultimately unfixable) anatomic problem of liver herniated into the chest. Attempts to solve this terrible problem proved immensely frustrating and discouraging. For babies without liver herniation, our surgical techniques eventually proved successful (1986), and it looked like the first real breakthrough for fetal surgery. After a few successful cases established proof of concept, we applied to the National Institutes of Health to do a trial comparing open fetal surgery for total repair of diaphragmatic hernia to the standard intensive therapy after birth (including ECMO). I believe the decision to test this novel therapy up front was a pivotal point in the fetal therapy enterprise. NIH funding put the clinical enterprise on the map, and the conduct of the trial was a "coming of age". The trial took the enterprise through an agonizing transition from a promising bouncing baby to a petulant, awkward, controversial, and often ugly adolescent. The first CDH trial illustrates this perfectly. On the surface, the trial appeared to be a straightforward trial with a disappointing but interesting result: open fetal surgical repair worked in those fetuses who did not have the liver herniated, but was no better than postnatal care. But the most important thing was just getting the trial done. Behind the scenes, getting the trial done was a nightmare. I'll illustrate with just one anecdote.

Getting this first fetal surgery trial through the NIH review process and through our own rapidly hardening Committee on Human Research process took two years of immense effort. But the real problem came up after the protocol was finally in place and working. Ongoing experimental work suggested that nitric oxide was important in labor and that the use of nitroglycerin might be the key to controlling preterm labor after hysterotomy for fetal surgery. After pushing this concept extremely hard in the laboratory and getting excellent data in monkeys, we began using nitroglycerin for the mothers during fetal surgery. Although it clearly worked to relax the uterus, in our enthusiasm we overused nitroglycerin drips and, for the first time, had significant (but fortunately transient) sequelae in the mothers, some of whom developed significant pulmonary edema. After a frantic search for the cause, it turned out that the propylene glycol used to solubilize nitroglycerin was responsible and, of course, this approach was abandoned. But in the course of testing and then abandoning nitroglycerin drips, we had a terrible falling out with our Committee on Human Research. The CDH trial became the lightning rod for the anxiety and even hostility of the CHR. The trial was stopped while committees investigated the enterprise. Although eventually re-opened and successfully completed, digging out of this hostile quagmire proved to be a true nightmare and really hurt our team. The worst part was that we had our first very serious falling out among team members. A few obstetricians, who were rightly upset by what they viewed as a real threat to he mothers from these desperate attempts to fix doomed fetuses, lost confidence in the enterprise, became downright hostile, and almost killed the enterprise.

At the time, the UCSF Fetal Treatment Program was an informal working group with no official structure or recognition. While the surgeons, sonographers, anesthesiologists, and some perinatologists remained supportive, several perinatologists led by Mickey Golbus, who was extremely upset with the direction of the diaphragmatic hernia trial, became fervent adversaries. At one point in the darkest days of this period, when the CHR had suspended our protocols and the NIH had launched an investigation, Mickey Golbus and several other obstetricians called a meeting of the Department of Obstetrics and Gynecology and asked me to appear at that meeting to decide the fate of the program and the future of fetal therapy. I asked our then-Chairman of Surgery, Haile Debas, to come as he was well aware of the situation and the hostility, but he forgot and I ended up at that 7am meeting by myself. I felt like Horatio at the bridge, outranked, outgunned, and trying to hold together an enterprise that could have died that day. Fetal therapy at UCSF and arguably the course of fetal therapy in the world was altered that morning by capitulation. I admitted we had very significant problems, apologized, outlined a course of recovery, and then offered to disband the Fetal Treatment Program — end it that very day. This was accomplished. The clamoring rebellion was put down and the dissenters appeased. That same day I changed the lettering on all the stationery from "Fetal Treatment Program" to "Fetal Treatment Center," reorganized the players to include old and new supporters and to exclude adversaries, which unfortunately included the very talented Mickey Golbus. It was a painful transition but necessary, and actually proved to strengthen the enterprise at UCSF going forward.

1990–Present: Fetal therapy comes of age. The three basic trends set in motion in San Francisco in the turbulent times continue to this day:

(1) the move from anatomic repairs to physiologic manipulation, e.g., from complete anatomic repair of diaphragmatic hernia to tracheal occlusion to promote fetal lung growth;
(2) the move from open surgery by hysterotomy to less invasive fetoscopic techniques (Fetendo); and
(3) the move from clinical descriptions and retrospective analysis to proper randomized controlled trials.

Since this most recent history is well documented in the literature, I will not elaborate on UCSF's role, except to point out the increasingly important role of trials in our field. I have already discussed the incredible difficulties we encountered in our first NIH-sponsored trial on open complete repair of CDH. This struggle continued in our second NIH-sponsored controlled randomized trial comparing temporary tracheal occlusion to postnatal repair for diaphragmatic hernia. This trial in turn led to refinements in technique and a successful non-randomized trial in Europe by the Eurofetus group. This same Eurofetus group has also completed a very informative trial on laser ablation for twin-twin transfusion syndrome. But our experience in struggling to do a proper randomized trial paid off when we wanted to submit another NIH grant to test whether fetal surgery for MMC was effective. I believe submission and funding of this trial was pivotal in the development of the field because it spurred the development of a three center trial (UCSF, CHOP, Vanderbilt) that, while agonizing to negotiate and implement, will have a profound effect not only on deciding whether this intervention is the right thing to do, but also (inadvertently) on determining how many fetal surgery centers are needed, how they should be organized and staffed, and who will pay for fetal intervention.

While our work at UCSF continued full-speed ahead in the 1990's, the world-wide fetal treatment enterprise was now in full swing and advances came from many centers. I will condense this brief overview of the field into two tables. Table 2 lists "milestones" in fetal therapy (with an admittedly parochial UCSF slant) just to summarize contributions from our San Francisco team. Table 3 gives my perspective on where we stand in fetal therapy now. I developed this "report card" as a way to grade (subjectively) the two-decade-long efforts of the entire fetal treatment community (not just UCSF) to help fetuses with the few conditions targeted for treatment. I grade our efforts to understand the pathophysiology (often through experimental research), to delineate the natural history of the disease, and select which fetuses will benefit from intervention, and finally our success in treating the condition in human fetuses.

The people who made the UCSF FTC. Whatever the UCSF Fetal Treatment Center has accomplished is directly attributable to the talented, hardworking professionals attracted to this exciting enterprise in this wonderful city over the last three decades. Many of my professional colleagues played prominent roles in the development

Table 2. Milestones in fetal surgery.

Intrauterine transfusion (IUT) for Rh disease	(New Zealand)	1961
Hysterotomy for fetal vascular access – IUT	(Puerto Rico)	1964
Fetoscopy – diagnostic	(Yale)	1974
Experimental pathophysiology (Sheep model)	(UCSF)	1980
Hysterotomy & maternal safety (Monkey model)	(UCSF)	1981
Vesico-Amniotic shunt for uropathy	(UCSF)	1982
Vesico-Amniotic shunt for hydrocephalus	(Denver)	1982
Open fetal surgery for uropathy	(UCSF)	1983
Int'l Fetal Medicine and Surgery Society founded	(Santa Barbara)	1982
CCAM resection	(UCSF)	1984
1st Ed., *Unborn Patient: Prenatal Diagnosis & Treatment*	(UCSF)	1984
Intravascular transfusion	(London)	1985
CDH open repair	(UCSF)	1989
Anomalous twin — cord ligation, RFA, etc.	(London)	1990
NIH Trial: Open repair CDH	(UCSF)	1990
Aortic valvuloplasty	(London)	1991
SCT Resection	(UCSF)	1992
Laser ablation of placental vessels	(Milwaukee, London)	1995
EXIT procedure for airway obstruction	(UCSF)	1995
Fetoscopic surgery (Fetendo)	(UCSF)	1996
CDH — Fetendo clip → balloon	(UCSF)	1997
Myelomeningocele — open repair	(Vanderbilt)	1997
NIH Trial: Fetendo balloon CDH	(UCSF)	1998
Resection of pericardial teratoma	(UCSF)	2000
Resection of Cervical teratoma	(UCSF)	2001
NIH Trial: Open repair myelomeningocele	(UCSF, CHOP, Vanderbilt)	2002
NIH Trial: Twin-Twin Transfusion Syndrome	(CHOP, Perinatal Network)	2002

of the Center: Mickey Golbus, Russ Laros, Bill Parer, Bob Jaffe, Robert Ball, Per Sandberg, and Mary Norton in Perinatology; Roy Filly, Peter Callen, Ruth Goldstein, Vickie Feldstein and Fergus Coakley in Radiology/Sonology; Sam Hawgood, Joe Kitterman,

Table 3. Fetal surgery report card.

Life-Threatening Defects	Effect on Development	Report Card: Patho-physiology	Report Card: Selection	Treatment	Report Card
Urethral	Hydronephrosis → Renal failure	B+	B	Percutaneous cathether	B
Obstruction	Lung hypoplasia → Pulmonary failure			Fetoscopic vesicostomy	B
				Open vesicostomy	C–
CCAM	Lung mass → Fetal hydrops/demise	B	B+	Open pulmonary lobectomy	B
CDH	Lung hypoplasia → Pulmonary failure	B	B–	Complete repair	C
				Temp tracheal occlusion:	D
				Open Balloon	C → A (Trial)
SCT	High output failure → Fetal hydrops/demise	B	B	Resect tumor	B
				Fetoscopic vascular occlusion	C–
				Radiofrequency ablation	C+
TTTS	Vascular steal	C+	C	Open fetectomy	D
	through placenta → Fetal hydrops/demise			Fetoscopic laser ablation of vessels	C → A
				Serial amnioreduction	C →A (Trial)
Anomalous Twin					
Aqueductal	Hydrocephalus → Brain Damage	D	D	Ventriculo-amniotic shunt	F
Stenosis				Open ventriculo-periitoneal shunt	D
Complete Heart	Low output failure → Fetal hydrops/demise	B	C	Open pacemaker	D
Block				Percutaneous pacemaker	D

(*Continued*)

Table 3. (*Continued*)

Life-Threatening Defects	Effect on Development	Report Card: Patho-physiology	Report Card: Selection	Treatment	Report Card
Pulmonary/Aortic stenosis	Outflow obstruction → Ventricular hypo/hyperplasia	C	C+	Valvuloplasty	D → B
Tracheal atresia/stenosis	Overdistension by lung fluid → Hydrops/demise			Tracheostomy	C
				Ex utero intrapartum treatment	B–
Non-Lethal Defects					
Myelomeningocele	Spinal cord damage → Paralysis, neurogenic bladder, bowel	C+	B–	Fetoscopic coverage	D
				Open repair	C→A (Trial)
Cleft/Lip and palate	Facial defect → Persistent deformity	C–	C–	Open repair	F
Metabolic Cellular Defects					
Stem cell/ Enzyme defect	Hemoglobinopathy → Anemia, hydrops	C	B	Stem cell transplant	C+
	Immunodeficiency → Infection			Gene therapy	D
	Storage disease → Retardation				
Predictable organ failure	Hypoplastic heart, kidney, lung → Neonatal organ failure	C	D	Induce tolerance for postnatal organ transplant	?
					?

Rod Phibbs, and Robert Keller in Neonatology; Mark Rosen and Chico Cauldwell in Anesthesiology; Al deLormier, Scott Adzick, Alan Flake, Craig Albanese, Rusty Jennings, Diana Farmer, and Hanmin Lee in Pediatric Surgery; and Michael Heymann, Julian Hoffman, Abe Rudolph in Cardiology.

But a very special and important team member deserves special attention — the incredibly talented and hardworking coordinators who actually run the program day in and day out, help patients, schedule tests, arrange transportation and lodging, coordinate the complex ballet of fetal surgical procedures, struggle with insurance authorizations, etc. We have been blessed with wonderful nurse coordinators: first, Lori Howell (now at CHOP), then Jody Farrell (the bedrock of our program and key player in our complex randomized trials for CDH, MMC, and TTTS), and more recently, Tamara Ryan and Rachel Perry and their assistant Bev Motta. Stephanie Berman has been a stalwart in the psychosocial care of our patients in this most difficult time in their lives.

The fabulous fellows — our most important product. The heart and soul of the UCSF Fetal Treatment enterprise has always been the bright young people from a variety of backgrounds who come to attack clinical problems in the research lab, and thus drive the development of new therapies. It is not an exaggeration to say that all the advances in fetal treatment bear the fingerprints of a research fellow, or often many fellows.

In the interest of space, I have listed all the research fellows in chronological order, the projects they worked on, and where they are now. Obviously, many have made stunning contributions during their time in the lab, and many went on to amazingly productive careers. I will refrain from bragging about their accomplishments. I could go on forever with stories and anecdotes. Suffice it to say that these talented young fellows are the most important "product" of the UCSF Fetal Treatment Center. I believe they are the future of our field, and I am immensely proud of what they have and will contribute to fetal surgery.

References

1. Harrison MR. Unborn: Historical perspective of the fetus as a patient. *The Pharos* 1982;45:19.
2. Rosenkrantz JG, Simon RC, Carlisle JH. Fetal surgery in the pig with a review of other mammalian fetal techniques. *J Pediatr Surg* 1965;3:392.
3. Jost A. Sur la différenciation sexuelle de l'embryon de lapin. I: Remarques au sujet de certaines operations chirurgicales sur l'embryon. II: Experiences de paraboise. *CR Soc Biol* 1946;140:461.
4. Louw JH, Bernard CN. Congenital intestinal atresia: Observations on its origin. *Lancet* 1955;2:1065.
5. Jackson BT, Piasecki GJ, Egdahl RH. Experimental production of coarctation of the aorta in utero with prolonged postnatal survival. *Surgical Forum* 1963;14:290.
6. Blanc WA, Silver LA. Intrauterine abdominal surgery in the rabbit fetus: production of congenital intestinal atresia. *Am J Dis Child* 1962;104:548.
7. deLorimier AA, Tierney DF, Parker HR. Hypoplastic lungs in fetal lambs with surgically produced congenital diaphragmatic hernia. *Surgery* 1967;62:12.
8. Thomasson BM, Easterly JR, Ravitch MM. Morphologic changes in the fetal kidney after intrauterine ureteral ligation. *Invest Urol* 1970;8:261.
9. Beck AD. The effect of intra-uterine urinary obstruction upon the development of the fetal kidney. *J Urol* 1971;105:784–789.
10. Heymann MA, Rudolph AM. Effects of congenital heart disease on fetal and neonatal circulations. *Prog Cardiovasc Dis* 1972;15:115.
11. Assali NS (ed.). *Biology of Gestation.* Academic Press, New York, 1968.
12. Suzuki K, Plentl AA. Chronic implantation of instruments in the neck of the primate fetus for physiologic studies and production of hydramnios. *Am J Obstet Gynecol* 1969;103:272–281.
13. Harrison MR, Bressack MA, Churg AM, deLorimier AA. Correction of congential diaphragmatic hernia. II: Simulated correction permits fetal lung growth with survival at birth. *Surgery* 1980;88:260–268.

14. Liley AW. Intrauterine transfusion of the foetus in haemolytic disease. *Br Med J* 1963;2:1107–1109.
15. Adamsons K Jr. Fetal surgery. *N Engl J Med* 1966;275:204–206.
16. Harrison MR, Filly RA, Parer JT, Faer MJ, Jacobson JB, de Lorimier AA. Management of the fetus with a urinary tract malformation. *J Am Med Assoc* 1981;246(6):635–639.
17. Harrison MR, Golbus MS, Filly RA. Management of the fetus with a correctable congenital defect. *J Am Med Assoc* 1981;246:774–777.

INDEX